Pediatric Oncology

Each volume of the series "Pediatric Oncology" covers the whole spectrum of the disease concerned, from research issues to clinical management, and is edited by internationally highly respected experts in a comprehensive and clearly structured way. The user-friendly layout allows quick reference to in-depth information. The series is designed for all health-care personnel interested in high-level education in pediatric oncology.

More information about this series at http://www.springer.com/series/5421

Timothy P. Cripe • Nicholas D. Yeager
Editors

Malignant Pediatric Bone Tumors - Treatment & Management

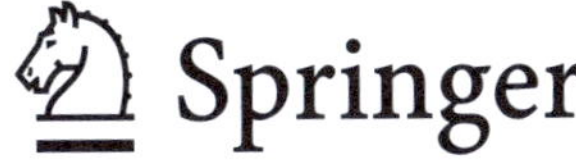

Springer

Editors
Timothy P. Cripe
Division of Pediatric Hematology/
Oncology/Blood and Marrow
Transplantation
Nationwide Children's Hospital
Columbus, OH
USA

Nicholas D. Yeager
Division of Pediatric Hematology/
Oncology/Blood and Marrow
Transplantation
Nationwide Children's Hospital
Columbus, OH
USA

ISSN 1613-5318   ISSN 2191-0812   (electronic)
Pediatric Oncology
ISBN 978-3-319-37187-0   ISBN 978-3-319-18099-1   (eBook)
DOI 10.1007/978-3-319-18099-1

Printed on acid-free paper

Springer International Publishing AG Switzerland is part of Springer Science+Business Media
(www.springer.com)

*TPC: For my wife, Linda, and children, Kevin, Jeff,
and Natalie. Without you all, nothing would have meaning.
For my patients, through whose journey we can better learn
to relieve the suffering of those patients who follow them.
NDY: For all the patients whose lives I have had the privilege
of being a small part of through the years, your spirit inspires
me every day. Also, for my friends and family who have
supported me and brought color to my life, thank you.
We thank Tami Davis and Kelly Bays for their outstanding
administrative assistance.*

Foreword

Malignant bone tumors in children, adolescents, and young adults are a vexing problem. Over the past century we have uncovered enormous information about these cancers, and have made substantial progress using multidisciplinary approaches to cure patients with localized disease. Yet we still lose a vast majority of patients whose cancer has spread beyond its initial confines to other organs. For both types of patients, regardless of the outcome, the journey is arduous. The patient must be surrounded by layers and layers of teams to accurately make the diagnosis, administer state-of-the-art therapies, provide psychosocial support, and, if all goes well, deal with long-term issues.

We assembled this book as both an evidence-based and experiential-based guide to the care of patients with malignant bone tumors. We asked a large team of experts, the majority of whom have worked together for many years and have thus collectively honed their skills, to give you, the reader, their wisdom and knowledge gleaned from both the medical and surgical literature and their vast clinical experiences. The chapters roughly follow the patient's journey chronologically from the development of symptoms to diagnosis to treatment to future horizons.

We hope this book provides a framework for current and future generations of health-care providers to enable their patients with malignant bone tumors to obtain the best possible medical, surgical, and psychological care.

Columbus, OH, USA　　　　　　　　　　　　Timothy P. Cripe, MD, PhD
Columbus, OH, USA　　　　　　　　　　　　　Nicholas D. Yeager, MD

Contents

1 Signs and Symptoms 1
Andrew A. Martin and Patrick J. Leavey

2 Diagnostic Studies of Pediatric Bone Tumors: Pathology and Imaging 9
O. Hans Iwenofu, Stephen M. Druhan, and Michael A. Arnold

3 Basic Principles of Biopsy 51
Thomas J. Scharschmidt and Joel L. Mayerson

4 The Evaluation of Lung Nodules in Pediatric Bone Tumors 57
Nicholas D. Yeager and Anthony N. Audino

5 Fertility Preservation and Reproductive Health in Pediatric Bone Tumor Patients 65
Stacy L. Whiteside

6 Chemotherapy Regimens for Patients with Newly Diagnosed Malignant Bone Tumors 83
Ryan D. Roberts, Mary Frances Wedekind, and Bhuvana A. Setty

7 Radiation Management 109
Ashley Sekhon, Karl Haglund, and Michael Guiou

8 Histological Response and Biological Markers 125
Kellie B. Haworth and Bhuvana A. Setty

9 Surgical Approach: Limb Salvage Versus Amputation 143
Vincent Y. Ng and Thomas J. Scharschmidt

10 Rehabilitation Following Orthopaedic Surgery in Children with Bone Tumors 155
Michelle A. Miller and Nathan Rosenberg

11 Patient Navigation of the Pediatric Bone Tumor Patient Across the Continuum of Care 171
Paula M. Sanborn

12   **Psychosocial Effects of Pediatric Bone Tumors
     and Recommendations for Supportive Care**   201
     Cynthia A. Gerhardt, Amii C. Steele,
     Amanda L. Thompson, and Tammi K. Young-Saleme

13   **Post-therapy Surveillance of Bone Tumors**   211
     Bhuvana A. Setty

14   **Recurrent Bone Tumors**   221
     Joanne Lagmay and Nicholas D. Yeager

15   **Novel Therapies on the Horizon**   265
     Timothy P. Cripe, Kellie B. Haworth,
     and Peter J. Houghton

16   **Survivorship**   293
     Stacy L. Whiteside and Anthony N. Audino

Contributors

Michael A. Arnold, MD, PhD Department of Pathology and Laboratory Medicine/Anatomic Pathology, Nationwide Children's Hospital, Columbus, OH, USA

Anthony N. Audino, MD Division of Hematology/Oncology/BMT, Nationwide Children's Hospital, Columbus, OH, USA

Timothy P. Cripe, MD, PhD Division of Hematology/Oncology/BMT, Nationwide Children's Hospital, Columbus, OH, USA

Stephen M. Druhan, MD Department of Radiology, Nationwide Children's Hospital, Columbus, OH, USA

Cynthia A. Gerhardt, PhD Center for Biobehavioral Health, The Research Institute at Nationwide Children's Hospital, Columbus, OH, USA

Michael W. Guiou, MD Department of Radiation Oncology, The Ohio State University Comprehensive Cancer Center, Columbus, OH, USA

Karl Haglund, MD, PhD Department of Radiation Oncology, The Ohio State University Comprehensive Cancer Center, Columbus, OH, USA

Kellie B. Haworth, MD Division of Hematology/Oncology/BMT, Nationwide Children's Hospital, Columbus, OH, USA

Peter J. Houghton, PhD Center for Childhood Cancer and Blood Diseases, The Research Institute at Nationwide Children's Hospital, Columbus, OH, USA

O. Hans Iwenofu, MD Division of Soft Tissue and Bone Pathology, Department of Pathology, The Ohio State University College of Medicine, Columbus, OH, USA

Joanne Lagmay, MD Division of Pediatric Hematology/Oncology, Shands Hospital for Children, University of Florida, Gainesville, FL, USA

Patrick J. Leavey, MD Department of Pediatric Hematology and Oncology, University of Texas Southwestern Medical Center, Dallas, TX, USA

Andrew A. Martin, MD Department of Pediatric Hematology and Oncology, University of Texas Southwestern Medical Center, Dallas, TX, USA

Joel L. Mayerson, MD Division of Musculoskeletal Oncology, Department of Orthopaedics, The Ohio State University, Columbus, OH, USA

Michelle A. Miller, MD Department of Physical Medicine, Nationwide Children's Hospital, Columbus, OH, USA

Vincent Y. Ng, MD Division of Musculoskeletal Oncology, Department of Orthopaedics, University of Maryland Medical Center, Baltimore, MD, USA

Ryan D. Roberts, MD, PhD Division of Hematology/Oncology/BMT, Nationwide Children's Hospital, Columbus, OH, USA

Nathan Rosenberg, MD Department of Physical Medicine, Nationwide Children's Hospital, Columbus, OH, USA

Paula Sanborn, BSN Division of Hematology/Oncology/BMT, Nationwide Children's Hospital, Columbus, OH, USA

Thomas J. Scharschmidt, MD Division of Musculoskeletal Oncology, Department of Orthopaedics, The Ohio State University, Columbus, OH, USA

Ashley Sekon, MD Department of Radiation Oncology, The Ohio State University Comprehensive Cancer Center, Columbus, OH, USA

Bhuvana A. Setty, MD Division of Hematology/Oncology/BMT, Nationwide Children's Hospital, Columbus, OH, USA

Amii C. Steele, PhD Division of Hematology/Oncology and Blood Marrow Transplant, Levine Children's Hospital, Charlotte, NC, USA

Amanda L. Thompson, PhD Center for Cancer and Blood Disorders, Children's National Medical Center, Washington, DC, USA

Mary Frances Wedekind, MD Department of Pediatrics, Nationwide Children's Hospital, Columbus, OH, USA

Stacy L. Whiteside, CPNP-AC Division of Hematology/Oncology/BMT, Nationwide Children's Hospital, Columbus, OH, USA

Nicholas D. Yeager, MD Division of Hematology/Oncology/BMT, Nationwide Children's Hospital, Columbus, OH, USA

Tammi K. Young-Saleme, PhD Division of Psychology/Neuropsychology, Nationwide Children's Hospital, Columbus, OH, USA

Signs and Symptoms

1

Andrew A. Martin and Patrick J. Leavey

Contents

1.1 **Introduction** 1

1.2 **Age** 2

1.3 **Sex and Ethnicity** 2

1.4 **Sites of Tumors** 3

1.5 **Signs and Symptoms** 4

1.6 **Diagnostic Evaluation** 5

1.7 **Predisposition Syndromes** 5

References................................ 6

Abstract

The majority of pediatric bone tumors are benign; however, malignant bone tumors account for a significant amount of morbidity and mortality among children and adolescents. Due to their often indolent presentation the diagnosis is often delayed. This chapter will highlight the signs and symptoms of malignant bone tumors including osteosarcoma, Ewing sarcoma, and chondrosarcoma. Malignant bone tumors vary by age, sex, ethnicity and tumor location. The typical presenting symptoms are similar for most malignant bone tumors with a few distinct variations between the subtypes. The initial diagnostic evaluation will be reviewed and subsequent chapters will go into more detail regarding the radiographic and pathologic diagnosis. There are a few syndromes with a known predisposition to malignant bone tumors that will be highlighted.

1.1 Introduction

Pediatric bone tumors, although rare, are the sixth most common neoplasm in children. Seven hundred individuals under 20 years of age are diagnosed with a primary bone malignancy each year in the United States, with an annual incidence rate of 8.7 per million children/adolescents (1999). The most common diagnosis in this age group is osteosarcoma, with approximately 400

A.A. Martin, MD (✉) • P.J. Leavey, MD
Department of Pediatric Hematology and Oncology, University of Texas Southwestern Medical Center, 5323 Harry Hines Boulevard, Dallas, TX 75390, USA
e-mail: Andrew.martin@utsouthwestern.edu; Patrick.leavey@utsouthwestern.edu

© Springer International Publishing Switzerland 2015

T.P. Cripe, N.D. Yeager (eds.), *Malignant Pediatric Bone Tumors - Treatment & Management*, Pediatric Oncology, DOI 10.1007/978-3-319-18099-1_1 patients identified each year, followed by Ewing sarcoma with around 200 (2006). International incidence rates are similar to those of the United States although osteosarcoma is less common in some Asian and Latin American populations, while Ewing sarcoma is less common in individuals of African descent and in Eastern Asia populations (Parkin et al. 1993). Chondrosarcoma is the third most frequent malignant bone tumor seen in patients under 20 years. The remainder of pediatric bone tumors is comprised of a population of rare histologically specified and unspecified malignancies. Despite their relative infrequency, malignant bone tumors convey a significant morbidity and mortality to this age group. It is estimated that there are 3,000 primary malignant bone tumors diagnosed each year in the United States and 1,500 deaths resulting from them (Siegel et al. 2014). The overall survival for patients with nonmetastatic osteosarcoma is upwards of 75 % but is only 10–30 % for patients with metastatic disease at presentation (Harris et al. 1998). The overall survival for patients with Ewing sarcoma is similar to that of osteosarcoma (Granowetter et al. 2009; Orr et al. 2012). Survival Epidemiology and End Results (SEER) data over several decades described only modest overall improvements in outcome from the 1970s to 1990s and a worse outcome for males compared to females (1999; 2006). One factor in this lack of improvement may be that diagnosis is often delayed, as it can be difficult to delineate the symptoms associated with malignant bone tumors from other more common ailments associated with this age group (Brasme et al. 2014; Goyal et al. 2004; Guerra et al. 2006).

1.2   Age

Malignant bone tumors, both Ewing sarcoma and osteosarcoma, increase in frequency with increasing age with a peak incidence at 15 years (1999; Meyers and Gorlick 1997; Sneppen and Hansen 1984). They represent less than 1 % of all malignancies in children under 4 years, and the incidence declines again after the adolescent peak (Stiller et al. 2006).

Osteosarcoma has a second age peak in older adulthood frequently related to Paget's disease (Ottaviani and Jaffe 2009; Mirabello et al. 2009). Within the pediatric age group, malignant bone cancer represents 5 % of all cancers in children 5–9 years, 11 % in children 10–14 years, and 8 % in children 15–19 years (1999). Although a similar increase incidence with age is seen for chondrosarcoma (Stiller et al. 2006), both chondrosarcoma and the other histologic specified and unspecified tumors remain rare throughout childhood (1999). The peak incidence for osteosarcoma is 10–19 years old with a second peak in the 1970s (Mirabello et al. 2009). Ewing sarcoma has a less profound peak incidence from 10 to 15 years old, and more than a quarter of cases occur in children under 10 years of age, and another quarter occur in adults greater than 20 years of age (Miller 1981; Glass and Fraumeni 1970). There is no older age peak associated with Ewing sarcoma (Figs. 1.1 and 1.2).

1.3   Sex and Ethnicity

There is a slight male predominance in malignant bone tumors overall, 1.19:1 (male to female) (1999), which also is true for each histologic subgroup: 1.27:1 for Ewing, 1.16:1 for osteosarcoma, and 1.5:1 for chondrosarcoma. These differences become even more pronounced in the adolescent age group (15–19 years old) with 2.03:1, 1.92:1, and 1.71:1 male to female predominance for Ewing, osteosarcoma, and chondrosarcoma, respectively (2006; Stiller et al. 2006).

A striking difference in incidence of Ewing sarcoma has been demonstrated between the white non-Hispanics and Hispanics groups and the African American/Black and Asian/Pacific Islander groups. Ewing sarcoma is extremely rare in groups of African and Southeast Asian descent; in fact, a SEER report demonstrated no cases of EWS in adolescents and young adults in these ethnic groups (2006). In osteosarcoma the ethnic predilection is reversed and slightly

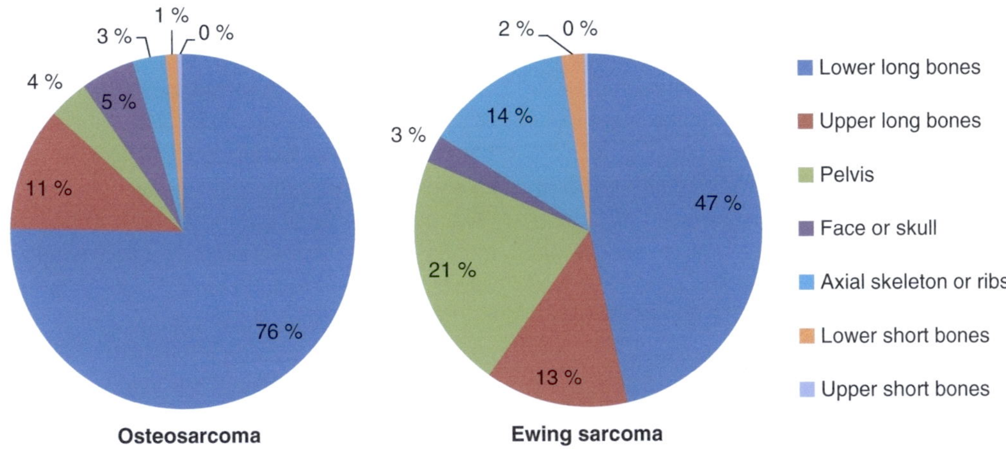

Fig. 1.1 Location of primary tumors in osteosarcoma and Ewing sarcoma (percentage)

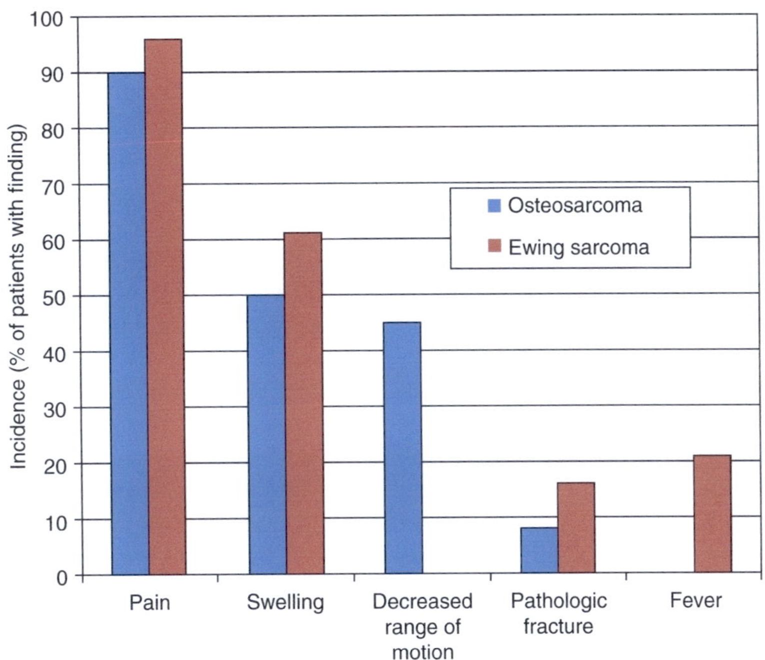

Fig. 1.2 Presenting symptoms in osteosarcoma and Ewing sarcoma (percentage)

more common in African American children, but the difference between the two is much smaller (1:1.33; white to black, respectively) (1999). Given the higher overall incidence of osteosarcoma than Ewing sarcoma, the total bone tumor ethnic ratio between white and black is 1.3:1 (1999).

1.4 Sites of Tumors

Osteosarcoma most commonly occurs in the long bones of the lower limb, while Ewing sarcoma and chondrosarcoma more commonly occur in the axial skeleton as well as long bones (1999; 2006). More specifically, osteosarcoma generally presents in the metaphyseal region of long bones, with the distal femur, proximal tibia, and proximal humerus being the most common sites in order of frequency. Ewing sarcoma is more likely to be seen in the diaphyseal regions of long bones and flat bones, with 40 % of Ewing tumors occurring in the axial skeleton (Arndt and Crist 1999). Non-skeletal presentations occur within the Ewing sarcoma family of tumors (ESFT) as well and generally demonstrate the same histologic findings as well as the characteristic EWS/FLI1 translocation. Askin tumors are ESFTs that involve the chest wall and clearly present a site-specific local control challenge (Shamberger et al. 2003). Ewing sarcoma also occurs in extraosseous sites, and while they were originally treated according to rhabdomyosarcoma chemotherapy regimens, patients with this subtype of the ESFT are now treated using Ewing sarcoma-specific regimens (Zagar et al. 2008; Raney et al. 1997). Such extraosseous tumors may occur in the soft tissue, retroperitoneum, skin, and solid organs such as the kidney (Orr et al. 2012; Zollner et al. 2013).

1.5 Signs and Symptoms

Pain and swelling are the primary presenting features for both osteosarcoma and Ewing sarcoma. Approximately 70 % of patients present with pain, and about 20 % have a concomitant palpable mass (Widhe and Widhe 2000). In a report from the University of Sao Paolo, investigators described that almost 90 % of patients had pain, but pain at rest was noted in less than 10 % of patients. A tumor mass was noted in 57 % of patients (Guerra et al. 2006). Night time pain, classically thought to be an indicator of malignancy, only occurs in 20 % of patients with bone sarcoma (Widhe and Widhe 2000), and preceding trauma, which can be diagnostically misleading, was reported in almost 50 % of patients with osteosarcoma. Patients with extraosseous Ewing sarcoma typically present features with pain and swelling in two-thirds of patients. Rare presentations in this group include shortness of breath, difficulty walking, urinary obstruction, or constipation (Orr et al. 2012). Constitutional symptoms including fever, weight loss, fatigue, and loss of appetite occurred in 31 % of patients with skeletal Ewing sarcoma and 20 % of patients with extraosseous Ewing sarcoma and are more frequent in patients with metastatic disease (Biswas et al. 2014). Patients with Ewing sarcoma of the paraspinal region may develop epidural invasion and present with signs of neurologic compromise from spinal cord or nerve root compression, including paralysis and bowel or bladder dysfunction. Such patients require emergent evaluation and laminectomy for neurological recovery. Patients with pelvic and chest wall tumors may not present with a palpable mass due to the fact that the growth of the tumor is likely internal or intracavity. Consequently patients with chest wall tumors may present with cardiorespiratory symptoms if there is significant lung compression and mediastinal shift. Both osteosarcoma and Ewing sarcoma can also metastasize to the lungs and skeletal bones, although metastatic lung nodules are rarely large enough at presentation to cause respiratory symptoms. Patients may also present with a pathological fracture at time of initial diagnosis. Plain radiographs were acquired on almost two-thirds of patients reported by Widhe et al. (Widhe and Widhe 2000), and many of these were done to exclude the trauma/fracture. Only 2 patients out of 100 with osteosarcoma were found to actually have a pathological fracture at diagnosis, and no patients out of the 47 with Ewing sarcoma were found to have a fracture. The typical differential diagnosis for patients who present as described above includes tendinitis, tumor, or trauma, and more uncommonly bursitis, Osgood-Schlatter disease, or Legg-Calve-Perthes disease, among many others (Widhe and Widhe 2000).

Patients with osteosarcoma have an average delay of 15 weeks from development of symptoms to diagnosis, while delays of up to 34 weeks have been reported for patients with Ewing sarcoma (Widhe and Widhe 2000; Sneppen and Hansen 1984; Goyal et al. 2004). The older age distribution for malignant bone tumors, the typical denial of symptoms in adolescence, and the frequent challenges in delineating a malignant lesion from a simple trauma, infection, or other inflammatory condition likely contribute to delays in the recognition of symptoms and diagnosis (Widhe and Widhe 2000; Goyal et al. 2004; Sneppen and Hansen 1984). Initial recommendations of simple rest and analgesics may also prolong time to diagnosis since temporary improvements in pain and tenderness are frequently seen with such measures and may reinforce the impression of benign etiology such as tendinitis (Widhe and Widhe 2000). Reassuringly, the data suggest that such delays do not result in adverse survival outcome for patients (Brasme et al. 2014; Martin et al. 2007).

Patients with recurrent skeletal lesions typically present with symptoms similar to those at presentation, suggesting that routine surveillance with bone scan for patients off therapy is unnecessary (Meyer et al. 2008; Powers et al. 2014).

1.6 Diagnostic Evaluation

Malignant bone tumors are rare, and there is a broad differential for bone pain especially in the pediatric and adolescent age group; therefore, the suspicion of such tumors by primary care physicians is low. Suspicion for malignancy at first medical visit has been noted for only 31 % of patients diagnosed with osteosarcoma and 19 % of patients with Ewing sarcoma (Widhe and Widhe 2000). Conventional imaging features with plain x-ray help differentiate benign bone lesions from malignant disease. Typical features of malignancy including cortical bone disruption, periosteal elevation, subperiosteal new bone formation, lytic and sclerotic changes in bone, soft tissue mass, and soft tissue ossification (classical sunburst appearance with malignant osteosarcoma), which is discussed in detail in Chap. 2 (Murphey et al. 1997). Widhe et al. reported that 67 % and 60 % of patients ultimately diagnosed with osteosarcoma and Ewing sarcoma, respectively, had x-ray imaging performed after their first primary care visit (Widhe and Widhe 2000). Unfortunately the false-negative rate, at this initial image, was 9 % for osteosarcoma and 43 % for Ewing sarcoma. Other imaging required for

the evaluation of a newly diagnosed patient with a primary bone malignancy includes MRI of the primary tumor to determine osseous, joint, and soft tissue tumor extent, along with other important characteristics for surgical planning such as neurovascular encroachment. Also required is a CT of the chest to evaluate for parenchymal metastatic lung disease and a technetium bone scan or CT-PET for distant skeletal and bone marrow disease (Meyer et al. 2008; Franzius et al. 2000). Radiological features typical for osteosarcoma (sunburst appearance, metaphyseal lesion) and Ewing sarcoma (onion skin appearance to periosteal elevation and diaphyseal lesion) can be considered in addition to clinical features such as age and ethnicity to predict tumor type. However, while sensitive, these features are not specific and a histological diagnosis is critical for a correct diagnosis and treatment planning. Laboratory evaluation of tumor markers such as alkaline phosphatase and LDH also provide some prognostic information (Bielack et al. 2002). Bone marrow aspirate and biopsy are still conventionally required to stage patients with Ewing sarcoma, but may soon be replaced with CT-PET which is very sensitive to presence of bone marrow disease (Hawkins et al. 2005; Newman et al. 2013).

1.7 Predisposition Syndromes

Rarely pediatric bone tumors (typically osteosarcoma) may be associated with predisposition syndromes such as Li-Fraumeni syndrome (p53 tumor suppressor germ line mutation), Rothmund-Thomson syndrome (RECQL4 gene mutation), radiation exposure, hereditary retinoblastoma (mutation in the Rb1 gene), osteochondroma, fibrous dysplasia, chronic osteomyelitis, Werner syndrome (loss of function mutation in WRN gene resulting in premature aging), and Bloom syndrome (BLM gene mutation encodes for RECQL3 helicase DNA repair enzyme) (Ottaviani and Jaffe 2009). Signs and symptoms of such predisposing conditions will likely be readily obvious to a careful cancer-focused patient history and careful physical examination.

Although surveillance guidelines are not well established for the aforementioned predisposition syndromes, a majority of institutions employ institution-specific screening guidelines (Teplick et al. 2011).

References

Arndt C, Crist WM (1999) Common musculoskeletal tumors of childhood and adolescence. N Engl J Med 341:342–352

Bielack SS, Kempf-Bielack B, Delling G et al (2002) Prognostic factors in high-grade osteosarcoma of the extremities or trunk: an analysis of 1,702 patients treated on neoadjuvant cooperative osteosarcoma study group protocols. J Clin Oncol 20:776–790

Biswas B, Shukla NK, Deo SV et al (2014) Evaluation of outcome and prognostic factors in extraosseous Ewing sarcoma. Pediatr Blood Cancer 61(11):1925–1931

Bleyer A, O'leary M, Barr R, Ries LAG (eds) (2006) Cancer epidemiology in older adolescents and young adults 15 to 29 years of age, Including SEER Incidence and Survival: 1975–2000, No. 06-5767 edn. National Institutes of Health, Bethesda

Brasme JF, Chalumeau M, Oberlin O et al (2014) Time to diagnosis of Ewing tumors in children and adolescents is not associated with metastasis or survival: a prospective multicenter study of 436 patients. J Clin Oncol 32:1935–1940

Franzius C, Sciuk J, Daldrup-Link HE et al (2000) FDG-PET for detection of osseous metastases from malignant primary bone tumours: comparison with bone scintigraphy. Eur J Nucl Med 27:1305–1311

Glass AG, Fraumeni JF Jr (1970) Epidemiology of bone cancer in children. J Natl Cancer Inst 44:187–199

Goyal S, Roscoe J, Ryder WD et al (2004) Symptom interval in young people with bone cancer. Eur J Cancer 40:2280–2286

Granowetter L, Womer R, Devidas M et al (2009) Dose-intensified compared with standard chemotherapy for non-metastatic Ewing sarcoma family of tumors: a Children's Oncology Group Study. J Clin Oncol 27:2536–2541

Guerra RB, Tostes MD, Da Costa Miranda L et al (2006) Comparative analysis between osteosarcoma and Ewing's sarcoma: evaluation of the time from onset of signs and symptoms until diagnosis. Clin (Sao Paulo) 61:99–106

Harris MB, Gieser P, Goorin AM et al (1998) Treatment of metastatic osteosarcoma at diagnosis: a Pediatric Oncology Group Study. J Clin Oncol 16:3641–3648

Hawkins DS, Schuetze SM, Butrynski JE et al (2005) [18F] Fluorodeoxyglucose positron emission tomography predicts outcome for Ewing sarcoma family of tumors. J Clin Oncol 23:8828–8834

Martin S, Ulrich C, Munsell M et al (2007) Delays in cancer diagnosis in underinsured young adults and older adolescents. Oncologist 12:816–824

Meyer JS, Nadel HR, Marina N et al (2008) Imaging guidelines for children with Ewing sarcoma and osteosarcoma: a report from the Children's Oncology Group Bone Tumor Committee. Pediatr Blood Cancer 51:163–170

Meyers PA, Gorlick R (1997) Osteosarcoma. Pediatr Clin N Am 44:973–989

Miller RW (1981) Contrasting epidemiology of childhood osteosarcoma, Ewing's tumor, and rhabdomyosarcoma. Natl Cancer Inst Monogr 56:9–15

Mirabello L, Troisi RJ, Savage SA (2009) Osteosarcoma incidence and survival rates from 1973 to 2004: data from the Surveillance, Epidemiology, and End Results Program. Cancer 115:1531–1543

Murphey MD, Robbin MR, Mcrae GA et al (1997) The many faces of osteosarcoma. Radiographics 17: 1205–1231

Newman EN, Jones RL, Hawkins DS (2013) An evaluation of [F-18]-fluorodeoxy-D-glucose positron emission tomography, bone scan, and bone marrow aspiration/biopsy as staging investigations in Ewing sarcoma. Pediatr Blood Cancer 60:1113–1117

Orr WS, Denbo JW, Billups CA et al (2012) Analysis of prognostic factors in extraosseous Ewing sarcoma family of tumors: review of St. Jude Children's Research Hospital experience. Ann Surg Oncol 19:3816–3822

Ottaviani G, Jaffe N (2009) The epidemiology of osteosarcoma. Cancer Treat Res 152:3–13

Parkin DM, Stiller CA, Nectoux J (1993) International variations in the incidence of childhood bone tumours. Int J Cancer 53:371–376

Powers JM, Cost C, Cederberg K et al (2014) Bone scintigraphy in osteosarcoma: a single institution experience. J Pediatr Hematol Oncol 36(8):e543–e545

Raney RB, Asmar L, Newton WA Jr et al (1997) Ewing's sarcoma of soft tissues in childhood: a report from the Intergroup Rhabdomyosarcoma Study, 1972 to 1991. J Clin Oncol 15:574–582

Ries LAG, Smith MA, Gurney JG, Linet M, Tamra T, Young JL, Bunin GR (eds). Cancer Incidence and Survival among Children and Adolescents: Inited states SEER Program 1975–1995, National cancer Institute, SEER Program, NIH Pub. No. 99–4649, Bethesda, MD, 1999

Shamberger RC, Laquaglia MP, Gebhardt MC et al (2003) Ewing sarcoma/primitive neuroectodermal tumor of the chest wall: impact of initial versus delayed resection on tumor margins, survival, and use of radiation therapy. Ann Surg 238:563–567; discussion 567–568

Siegel R, Ma J, Zou Z et al (2014) Cancer statistics. CA Cancer J Clin 64:9–29

Sneppen O, Hansen LM (1984) Presenting symptoms and treatment delay in osteosarcoma and Ewing's sarcoma. Acta Radiol Oncol 23:159–162

Stiller CA, Bielack SS, Jundt G et al (2006) Bone tumours in European children and adolescents, 1978–1997. Report from the automated childhood cancer information system project. Eur J Cancer 42:2124–2135

Teplick A, Kowalski M, Biegel JA et al (2011) Educational paper: screening in cancer predisposition syndromes: guidelines for the general pediatrician. Eur J Pediatr 170:285–294

Widhe B, Widhe T (2000) Initial symptoms and clinical features in osteosarcoma and Ewing sarcoma. J Bone Joint Surg Am 82:667–674

Zagar TM, Triche TJ, Kinsella TJ (2008) Extraosseous Ewing's sarcoma: 25 years later. J Clin Oncol 26: 4230–4232

Zollner S, Dirksen U, Jurgens H et al (2013) Renal Ewing tumors. Ann Oncol 24:2455–2461

Diagnostic Studies of Pediatric Bone Tumors: Pathology and Imaging

2

O. Hans Iwenofu, Stephen M. Druhan, and Michael A. Arnold

Contents

2.1 **Introduction**.   10
2.1.1 Basic Radiological Evaluation of Pediatric Bone Tumors.   10

2.2 **Epiphyseal Lesions**   11
2.2.1 Chondroblastoma   11
2.2.2 Langerhans Cell Histiocytosis   12
2.2.3 Osteomyelitis   12
2.2.4 Giant Cell Tumor   13

2.3 **Metaphyseal Lesions**.   17
2.3.1 Unicameral (Simple) Bone Cyst.   17
2.3.2 Aneurysmal Bone Cyst.   18
2.3.3 Telangiectatic Osteosarcoma   18
2.3.4 Conventional Osteosarcoma.   20
2.3.5 Metaphyseal Ewing Sarcoma Versus Small Cell Osteosarcoma   24

2.3.6 Ewing Sarcoma Versus Lymphoblastic Lymphoma   26
2.3.7 Langerhans Cell Histiocytosis Versus Chronic Osteomyelitis   27

2.4 **Diaphyseal Lesions**   32
2.4.1 Ewing Sarcoma Versus Osteomyelitis   32
2.4.2 Langerhans Cell Histiocytosis Versus Chronic Osteomyelitis   35
2.4.3 Periosteal Osteosarcoma.   38
2.4.4 Osteoid Osteoma and Osteoblastoma.   38
2.4.5 Nonossifying Fibroma   38
2.4.6 Fibrous Dysplasia.   39
2.4.7 Adamantinoma Versus Osteofibrous Dysplasia   42

References.   48

O.H. Iwenofu, MD
Division of Soft Tissue and Bone Pathology,
Department of Pathology, The Ohio State University
College of Medicine,
E418A Doan Hall 410 W. 10th Avenue, Columbus,
OH 43210, USA
e-mail: Hans.iwenofu@osumc.edu

S.M. Druhan, MD
Department of Radiology, Nationwide Children's
Hospital, 700 Children's Drive, Columbus,
OH 43205, USA
e-mail: Stephen.druhan@nationwidechildrens.org

M.A. Arnold, MD, PhD (✉)
Department of Pathology and Laboratory Medicine/
Anatomic Pathology, Nationwide Children's Hospital,
700 Children's Drive, Columbus, OH 43205, USA
e-mail: Michael.arnold@nationwidechildrens.org

Abstract

The unique pattern of distribution of bone tumors and the nature of their interaction with native bone creates distinct radiologic-pathologic correlates that are critical in the diagnostic evaluation of these lesions. The rarity of these lesions makes them especially daunting for the general pathologist and radiologist faced with the diagnostic evaluation of these entities. This chapter presents a richly illustrated synopsis of common pediatric bone lesions based on a rational integrated approach incorporating the gross anatomy of the lesions (via radiologic imaging) and pathologic analysis. This chapter presents entities and their mimics based on their anatomic location within the bone just as they

© Springer International Publishing Switzerland 2015
T.P. Cripe, N.D. Yeager (eds.), *Malignant Pediatric Bone Tumors - Treatment & Management*,
Pediatric Oncology, DOI 10.1007/978-3-319-18099-1_2

would present in "real life". This integrated approach, with emphasis on overlapping features of different entities, provides practical guidance for health care providers and trainees.

2.1 Introduction

Prompt and accurate diagnosis of bone tumors requires integrating clinical, radiographic, and pathologic data. The first clues encountered in this process are often the radiographic features of a lesion. The location along the bone (diaphyseal, metaphyseal, or epiphyseal), within the bone (surface, cortex, or medulla), and radiographic density can quickly narrow the differential diagnosis. The typical locations of common bone tumors are shown in Fig. 2.1. This chapter is organized to allow the reader to approach lesions by region of the involved bone, emphasizing the radiographic and pathologic features that distinguish key differential diagnoses at each location. Although the remainder of this book focuses on malignant lesions, it is important to know the differential diag-

nosis and various manifestations of benign lesions when confronted with radiographic findings.

2.1.1 Basic Radiological Evaluation of Pediatric Bone Tumors

The initial evaluation of any benign or malignant bone tumor usually begins with radiography. Aside from confirming the presence of a bone tumor, radiographs delineate features of the tumor to generate a differential diagnosis, guiding further imaging evaluation and management. The differential diagnosis of pediatric bone tumors can be significantly focused by the age of the patient in conjunction with the location of the lesion (Table 2.1) and radiographic characteristics that distinguish aggressive from nonaggressive lesions. Additionally, unifocal lesions versus a multifocal process can also help narrow the differential diagnosis (Table 2.2). Typically, benign lesions have a nonaggressive radiographic appearance, while malignant lesions will have a more aggressive radiographic appearance. There are certainly exceptions to this rule, including nontumoral processes such as osteomyelitis that can mimic an aggressive tumor. The radiographic appearance of an aggressive or nonaggressive tumor depends upon how the surrounding bone reacts to the underlying lesion. Nonaggressive lesions are usually slow growing and give the surrounding bone time to develop around the lesion, resulting in well-defined margins with a narrow zone of transition to surrounding intact bone. A slow-growing benign tumor can show expansion of the surrounding bone contour, without bony destruction, and without a soft tissue mass component. If a benign lesion does elicit surrounding periosteal reaction, the reaction will generally demonstrate a mature, well-formed, and less aggressive appearance.

Malignant bone tumors generally demonstrate aggressive radiographic features that reflect the fast-growing nature of the lesion, limiting the ability of the surrounding bone to react or "catch up" with the underlying aggressive process. These features include a wide zone of transition with poorly defined margins as well as frank bone destruction, outpacing the ability of the surrounding bone to remodel or develop a sclerotic margin. Such an appearance can reflect soft tissue mass extension

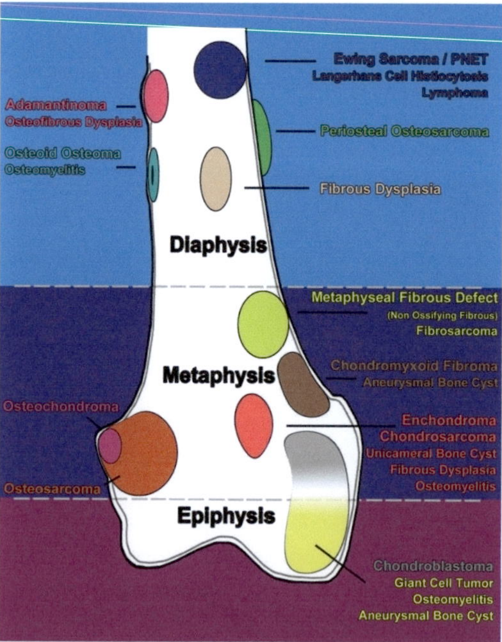

Fig. 2.1 Common locations of pediatric bone tumors. The location of a bone tumor is frequently the first information available to narrow the differential diagnosis of a bone lesion. This illustration demonstrates the common location of many pediatric bone tumors

Table 2.1 Pediatric bone tumors by their frequent locations in long bones

Epiphysis	Chondroblastoma
	Giant cell tumor (after physeal fusion)
	Langerhans cell histiocytosis (rare)
Metaphysis	Aneurysmal bone cyst
	Chondromyxoid fibroma
	Enchondroma
	Ewing sarcoma (more commonly metadiaphyseal or diaphyseal)
	Langerhans cell histiocytosis
	Leukemia
	Metastases
	Nonossifying fibroma/fibrous cortical defect
	Osteochondroma
	Osteoid osteoma
	Osteosarcoma
	Parosteal osteosarcoma
	Simple (unicameral) bone cyst
Diaphysis	Adamantinoma
	Ewing sarcoma
	Fibrous dysplasia
	Langerhans cell histiocytosis
	Nonossifying fibroma/fibrous cortical defect (in older patients)[a]
	Osteochondroma (in older patients)[a]
	Osteofibrous dysplasia
	Osteoid osteoma
	Periosteal osteosarcoma
	Simple (unicameral) bone cyst[a]

[a]These lesions begin in the metaphysis and with growth may "migrate" into the metadiaphysis and diaphysis

Table 2.2 Multifocal pediatric bone lesions

Brown tumors (hyperparathyroidism)
Cystic angiomatosis/lymphangiomatosis
Enchondroma (Ollier disease, Maffucci syndrome)
Fibrous dysplasia (McCune-Albright syndrome)
Infantile myofibromatosis
Langerhans cell histiocytosis
Leukemia
Metastases
Multifocal osteosarcoma
Nonossifying fibromas/fibrous cortical defects
Osteochondroma (osteochondromatosis)
Osteomyelitis/CRMO (chronic recurrent multifocal osteomyelitis)[a]

[a]While not a bone tumor, multifocal osteomyelitis and CRMO should be considered when multifocal bone lesions are encountered

from the bone as well as a permeative or moth-eaten appearance of bone destruction. Aggressive forms of periosteal reaction also indicate a fast-growing aggressive process. These patterns include "onionskin" or multilayered periosteal reaction composed of multiple concentric parallel layers of new bone adjacent to the cortex (Fig. 2.2a), as well as spiculated periosteal reaction which can appear either as a "sunburst" pattern of divergent ossified fibers radiating out from the periosteum (Fig. 2.2b) or a "hair-on-end" pattern with ossified fibers radiating perpendicular to the cortex (Fig. 2.2c). Additionally, aggressive periosteal reaction can appear as a "Codman triangle," which represents ossification of only the elevated periosteum at the margins of the aggressive process which then tapers down to the intact bone producing a triangular appearance (Fig. 2.2c).

2.2 Epiphyseal Lesions

The epiphysis generally has the least number of lesions associated with it, and this chapter will focus on chondroblastoma, Langerhans cell histiocytosis, osteomyelitis (usually subacute or chronic), and giant cell tumor (in skeletally mature patients after physeal fusion).

2.2.1 Chondroblastoma

Chondroblastomas appear as well-defined eccentric lucent lesions within the epiphyses of long bones. Additionally, they can occur in epiphyseal equivalents including apophyses and the patella (Turcotte et al. 1993). There are several radiographic characteristics which help distinguish chondroblastoma from other epiphyseal lucent lesions. On MRI, these lesions follow cartilage signal on all pulse sequences aside from occasional examples containing internal calcific matrix that demonstrates no signal. Additionally, painful lesions can demonstrate surrounding inflammatory response including bone marrow edema signal on MRI as well as bone marrow edema signal distant from the lesion (Figs. 2.3, 2.4, and 2.5). Biopsies show a benign cartilaginous neoplasm composed principally of sheets of mononuclear cells and osteoclast-type giant cells. The

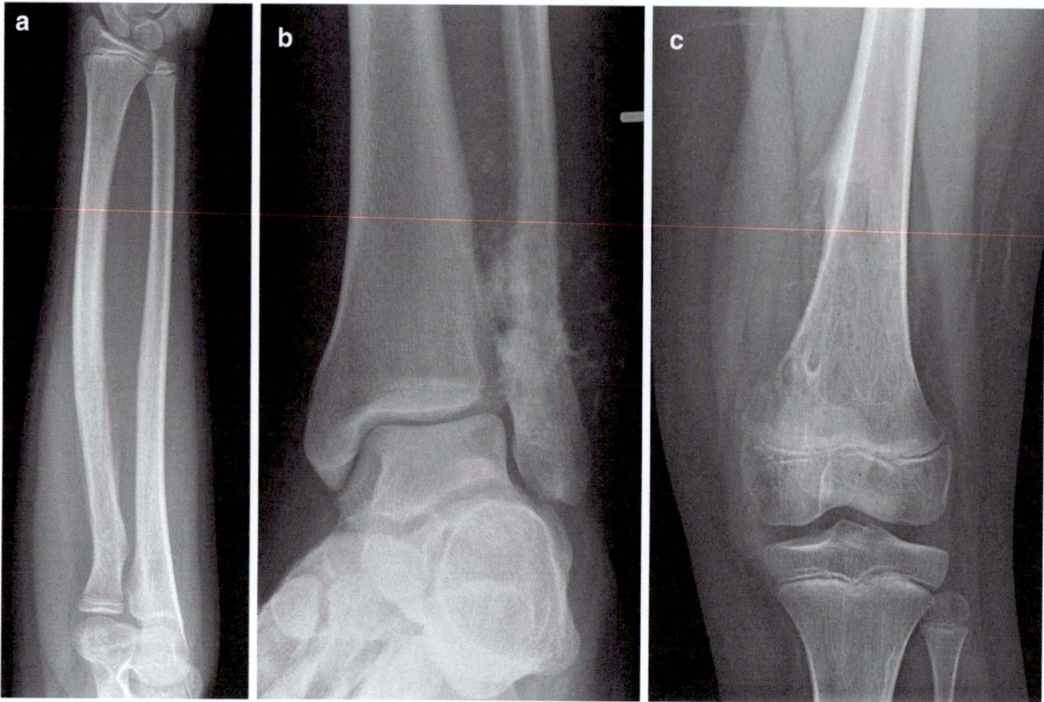

Fig. 2.2 Radiographic features of aggressive lesions. (**a**) This aggressive appearing lesion involving the proximal radial diaphysis demonstrates a permeative, "moth-eaten" appearance of the bone with aggressive periosteal reaction showing layers of "onionskin" appearing periosteal new bone formation as the soft tissue mass extends from the underlying bone. (**b**) This oblique frontal radiograph of the ankle demonstrates a lesion in the distal fibular metaphysis with a classic "sunburst" appearance of aggressive periosteal reaction. (**c**) An aggressive "moth-eaten" lytic-appearing lesion is seen within the metaphysis of the distal femur demonstrating bony destruction and a large soft tissue component with a "Codman triangle" at the superior margin of the soft tissue mass as well as "hair-on-end" aggressive periosteal reaction

mononuclear cells frequently contain nuclear grooves which imparts a "coffee bean" appearance to the cells (Fig. 2.6). The presence of cartilaginous matrix and chicken-wire calcifications helps to facilitate the diagnosis. Not uncommonly, secondary aneurysmal bone cyst can develop and sometimes dominate the overall radiologic and histologic appearance to the extent that the diagnosis of chondroblastoma could be obscured (Fig. 2.6c).

2.2.2 Langerhans Cell Histiocytosis

Langerhans cell histiocytosis (LCH) is included within the differential of epiphyseal lesions in the pediatric population as these lesions can occur in all locations in long bones and in many other bones including the mandible, pelvis, ribs, and spine (Fig. 2.7). Epiphyseal lesions generally appear well circumscribed and lytic in appearance, potentially resembling chondroblastoma. LCH is a spectrum of disease and can have any radiographic appearance; lesions can have both an aggressive and nonaggressive radiographic features. In biopsies, LCH is characterized by distinctive histiocytes that are reactive for CD1a, Langerin, and S-100. The characteristic cells of LCH are often accompanied by mixed inflammatory cells, typically including predominantly eosinophils (Fig. 2.8), and can show histologic similarities with osteomyelitis as discussed further in Sect. 2.3.

2.2.3 Osteomyelitis

In tubular bones, hematogenous osteomyelitis is usually localized to the metaphysis and may spread from the metaphysis through the growth

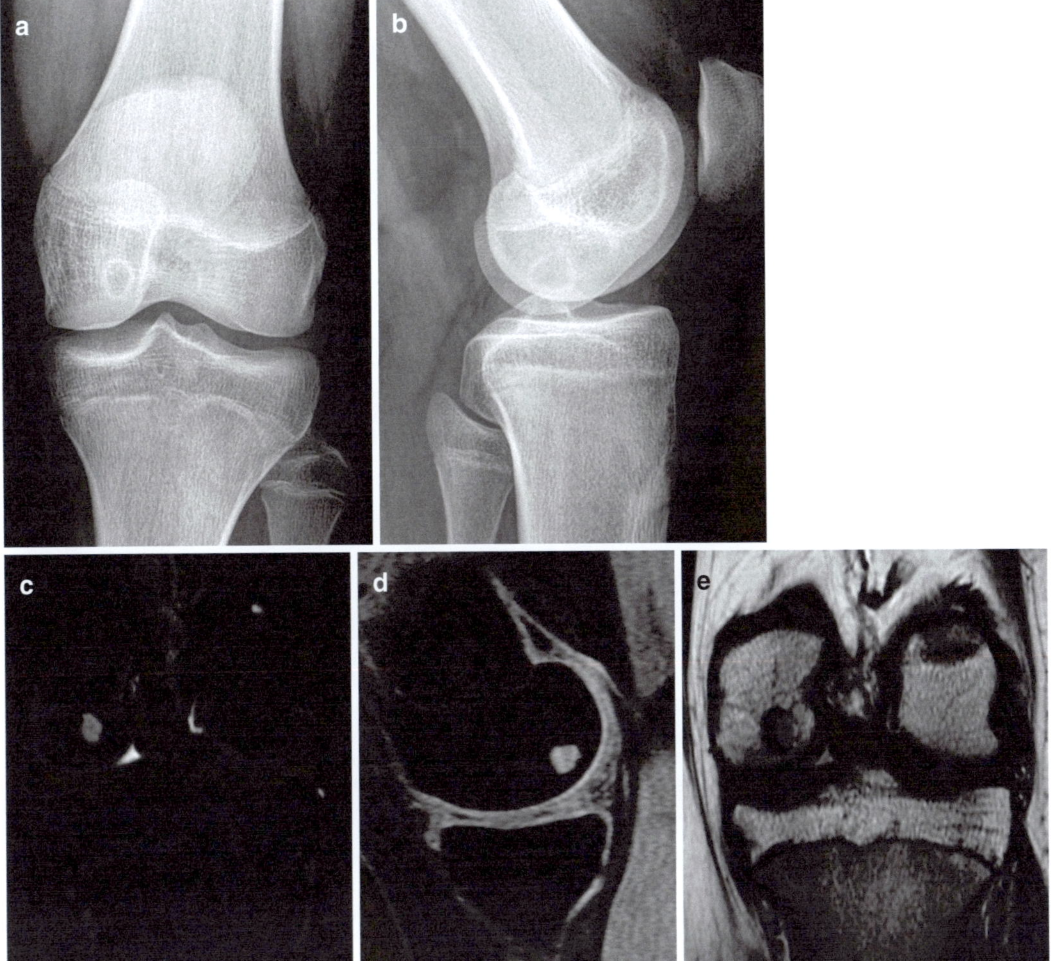

Fig. 2.3 Chondroblastoma of the distal femur. (**a, b**) Anterior-posterior (**a**) and lateral knee (**b**) radiographs demonstrate a lucent chondroblastoma with thin sclerotic borders within the medial condyle of the distal femoral epiphysis. (**c–e**) MRI sequences of the same patient (**a** coronal PD FS, **b** coronal T1, and **c** sagital 3C FSPGR FS) demonstrate a typical well-circumscribed lesion with surrounding low-signal consistent with the surrounding sclerosis. The lesion itself follows cartilage signal on all pulse sequences. Additionally in this painful lesion, bone marrow edema can be seen along the medial margin of the medial femoral condyle distant from the lesion itself, best appreciated on the coronal PD FS image (**a**)

plate to the epiphysis. In children a purely epiphyseal osteomyelitis is very rare; however, in infants younger than 15 months of age, epiphyseal osteomyelitis can occur more often given that metaphyseal vessels penetrate the growth plate and enter the epiphysis, allowing entry of causative organisms. The infection is usually subacute or chronic. An epiphyseal subacute or chronic osteomyelitis will generally appear lytic with sclerotic margin, overlapping with the appearance of other epiphyseal lesions. Metaphyseal osteomyelitis is discussed further in Sect. 2.3.

2.2.4   Giant Cell Tumor

Giant cell tumor (GCT) or osteo*clast*oma is an uncommon neoplasm that occurs most often in skeletally mature patients with only approximately 5 % occurring before skeletal maturity, mostly in

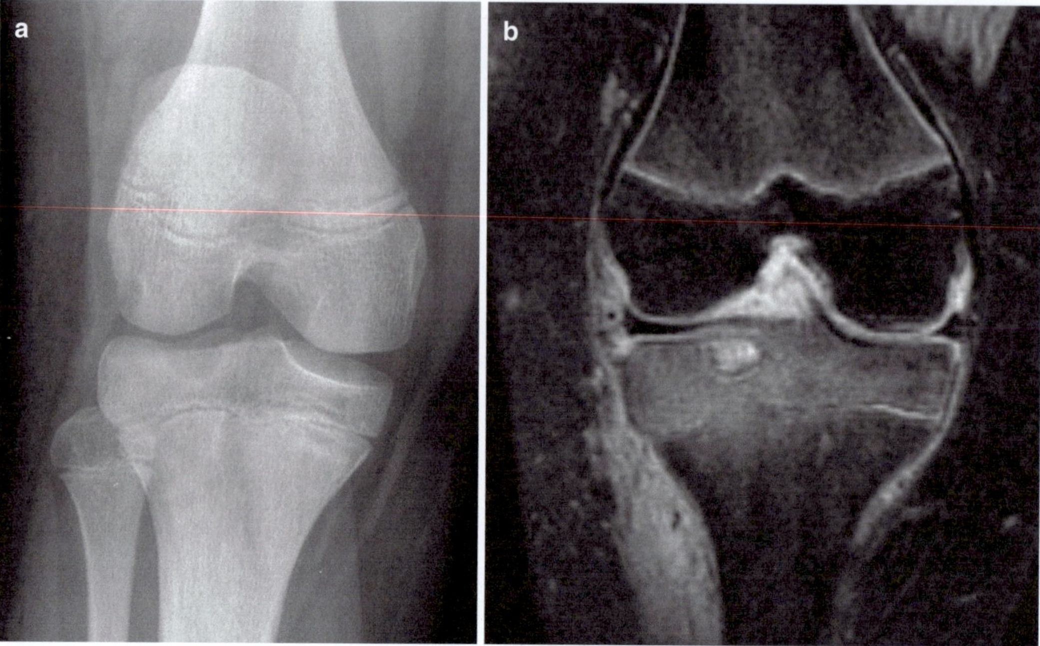

Fig. 2.4 Chondroblastoma of the proximal tibia. (**a**) An anterior-posterior radiograph demonstrates a well-defined lucent lesion with sclerotic borders within the lateral proximal tibial epiphysis, abutting the cortex. (**b**) MRI of the same patient (coronal PD FS) shows a well-circumscribed lesion within the lateral proximal tibial epiphysis with thin surrounding low-signal consistent with the surrounding sclerosis. The lesion itself follows cartilage signal. In this painful lesion, MRI demonstrates the significant surrounding inflammatory bone marrow edema signal as well as inflammation in the surrounding soft tissues

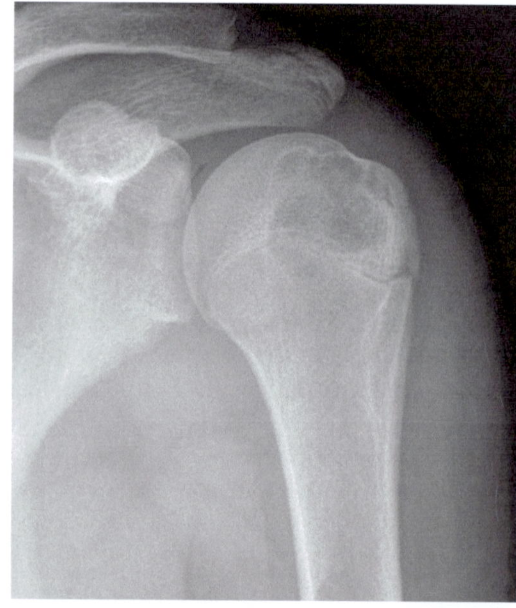

Fig. 2.5 Chondroblastoma of the proximal humerus. An anterior-posterior radiograph of the proximal humerus shows a well-defined lucent epiphyseal lesion with well-defined mildly lobulated borders showing thin rim of sclerosis within the proximal humeral epiphysis

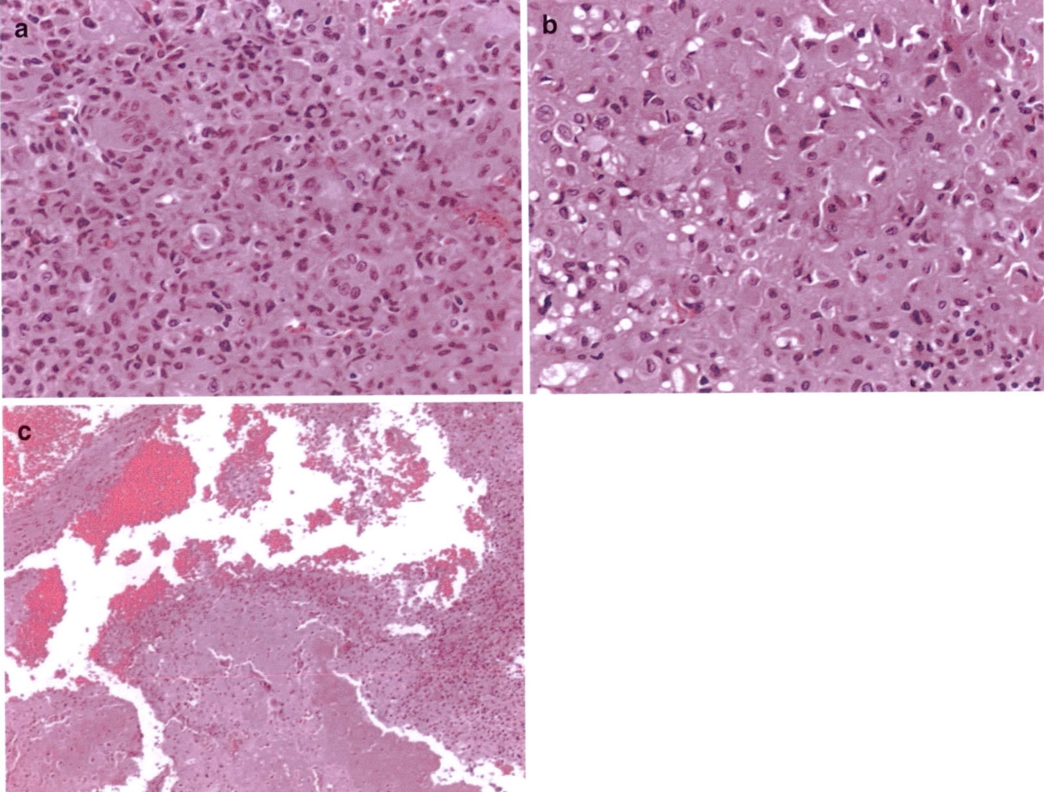

Fig. 2.6 Histologic features of chondroblastoma. (**a**) Chondroblastoma is composed of diffuse sheets of mononuclear cells admixed with osteoclast-type giant cells. (**b**) Prominent longitudinal grooves and "coffee bean" appearance of the cells are easily discernible, prototypic for this lesion. (**c**) Secondary aneurysmal bone cystlike changes in this chondroblastoma were extensive representing a histologic differential diagnosis of aneurysmal bone cyst

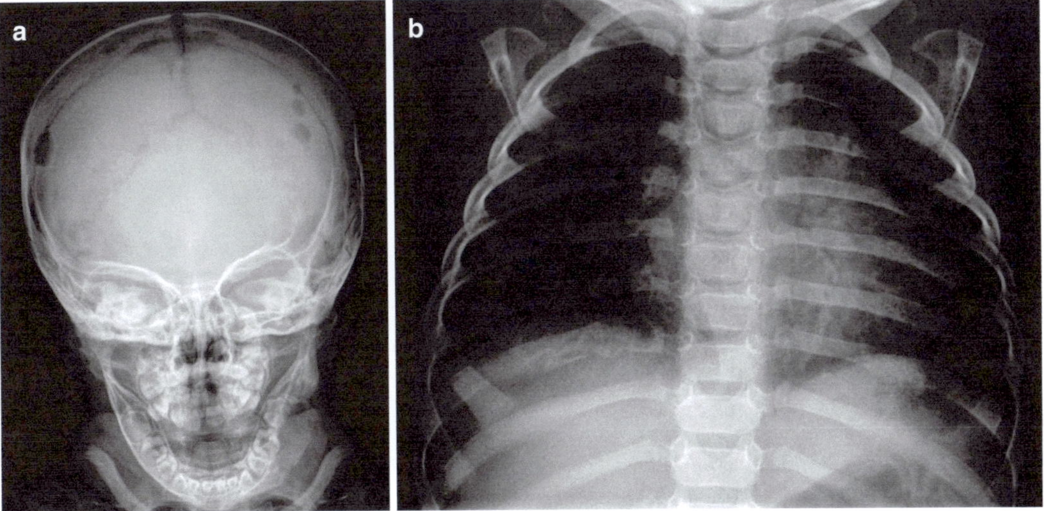

Fig. 2.7 Radiographic features of Langerhans cell histiocytosis. (**a**) Langerhans cell histiocytosis (LCH) involving the skull demonstrates multiple well-circumscribed lucent lesions with a "punched-out" appearance in this anterior-posterior view. Given multiple lesions, LCH is high in the differential diagnosis for this young child. (**b**) This anterior-posterior view of the chest demonstrates Langerhans cell histiocytosis of the rib, with an expansile lucency of the posterior right eighth rib

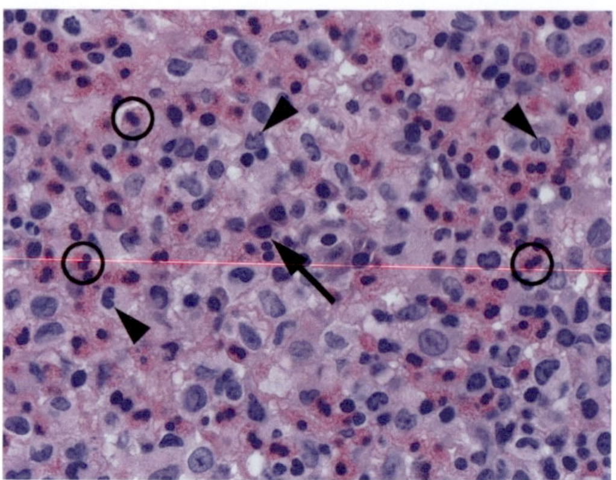

Fig. 2.8 Histologic features of Langerhans cell histiocytosis. The characteristic cells of Langerhans cell histiocytosis (LCH) have moderate eosinophilic to foamy cytoplasm and distinctive nuclei with folds, clefts, and grooves (*arrowheads*). LCH is typically accompanied by many eosinophils (*circles*); other inflammatory cells can be seen including plasma cells in this example (*arrow*). (H&E, 100× objective magnification)

the second decade of life. While it is a benign lesion, GCT tends to show locally aggressive behavior. In skeletally mature individuals, GCT is a well-circumscribed lucent lesion that is uniformly epiphyseal in location, usually abutting the articular surface, with variable extension into the metaphysis. In the rare case of GCT in a skeletally immature patient, GCT almost always appears metaphyseal in location and usually will abut the physis.

In histologic sections, GCT is characterized by multinucleated osteoclast-type giant cells (containing up to 50 nuclei) admixed with mononuclear cells (Fig. 2.9). While other giant cell-containing lesions enter the histologic differential diagnosis, the diagnosis of GCT is usually established by appropriate clinical and radiologic context in concert with the characteristic histologic features. This correlation is particularly important in GCT. The mononuclear cell population can show variable oval, round, or

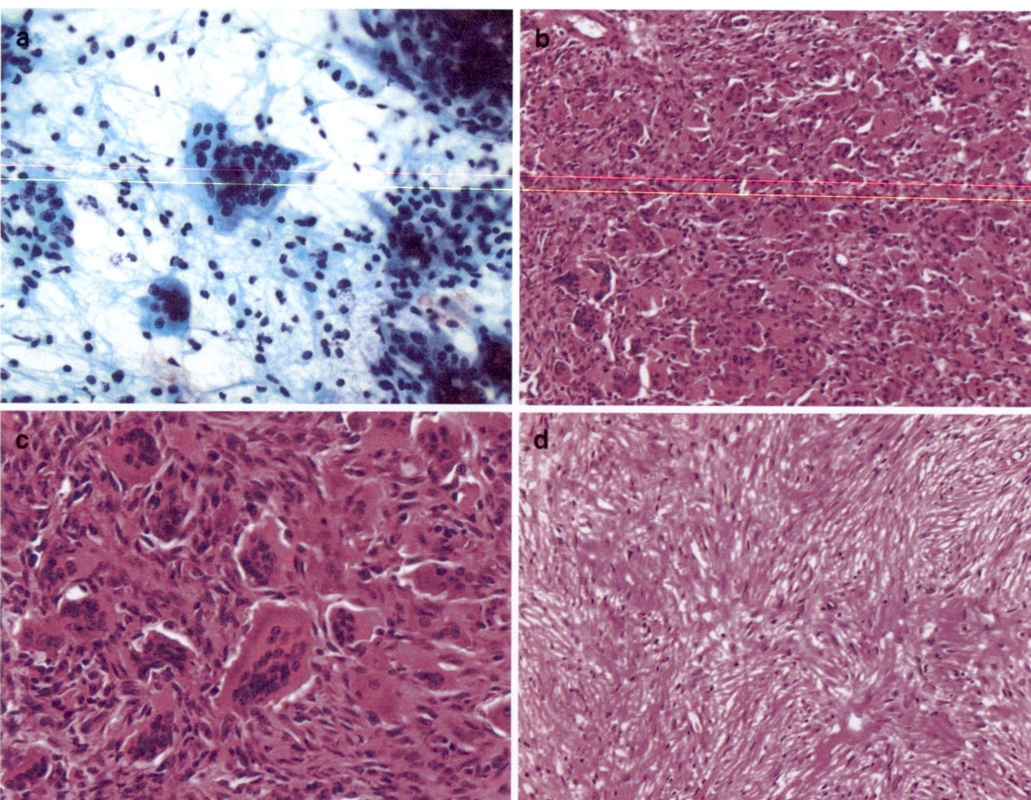

Fig. 2.9 Histologic features of giant cell tumor. (**a**) Papanicolaou stain of a fine-needle aspiration biopsy shows multinucleate osteoclast-type giant cells with admixed with mononuclear oval to spindle cells. (**b**) Histologic sections of giant cell tumor typically show numerous multinucleated osteoclast-type giant cells. (**c**) High-power view showing a multinucleated osteoclast-type giant cell containing 30–50 nuclei and adjacent mononuclear spindle cells. (**d**) A giant cell poor area within the same tumor shows a prominent spindle cell proliferation

spindled morphology. The proportion of the giant cells and mononuclear cells can be variable between and within lesions, and lesions with few giant cells can present diagnostic challenges, particularly in a limited biopsy specimen (Fig. 2.9d). Necrosis, mitosis, and tumor emboli in vessels can all be seen in GCT, but they do not correlate with malignant progression. Areas of reactive bone can be seen in these lesions particularly if there is an associated fracture. In a subset of cases, secondary aneurysmal bone cyst changes can occur simulating a solid variant of aneurysmal bone cyst. Immunohistochemistry is of very limited use in the histologic differential diagnosis of GCT due to the lack of a specific marker (de la Roza 2011; Dickson et al. 2008).

2.3   Metaphyseal Lesions

The differing lesions that may involve the metaphysis of long bones are many (see Table 2.1). This section will discuss simple or unicameral bone cyst (UBC), aneurysmal bone

cyst (ABC), osteosarcoma, Ewing sarcoma (more commonly metadiaphyseal or diaphyseal), LCH, and subacute/chronic osteomyelitis.

2.3.1   Unicameral (Simple) Bone Cyst

Unicameral or simple bone cysts (UBC) appear lucent on radiographs. They demonstrate well-defined borders with a sclerotic rim and may show mild expansion of the overlying thinned bony cortex. They usually occur centrally within the medullary space near the metaphysis and may "migrate away" from the metaphysis into the diaphysis during bone growth. Although they are called unicameral bone cysts, more mature cysts can demonstrate internal septations (Fig. 2.10). On contrast-enhanced imaging, these cysts do have a rim of vascular lining which does enhance while the internal fluid component does not. Additionally, given their internal fluid structure, a characteristic "fallen fragment sign" may be

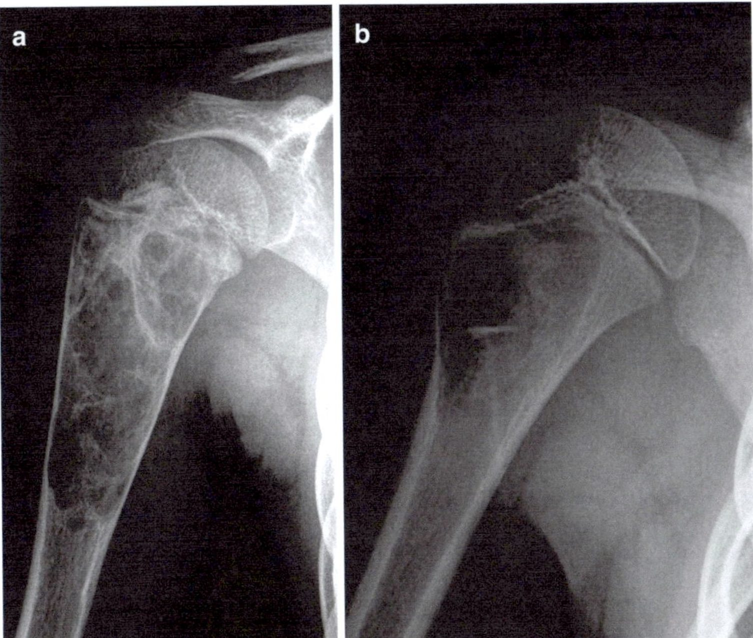

Fig. 2.10 Unicameral bone cysts of the proximal humerus. (**a**) Unicameral (simple) bone cyst is a benign lucent-appearing lesion often within the metaphysis with well-defined borders with no cortical destruction or periosteal reaction. This lesion demonstrates thin internal septations and mild expansion of the proximal humeral metaphysis. (**b**) The "fallen fragment sign" of unicameral bone cyst is the result of a pathologic fracture with cortical buckling and disruption extending through the well-defined lucent lesion. Bony fragment is seen layering dependently within the internal fluid of this unicameral bone cyst of the proximal humerus

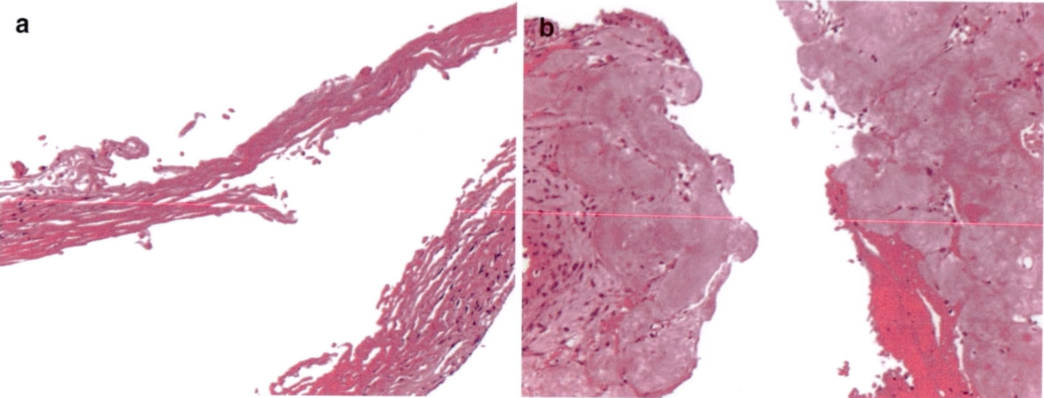

Fig. 2.11 Histologic features of unicameral bone cyst. Unicameral bone cyst is composed of cystic spaces with fibromembranous wall (**a**), with deposits of fibrin-like material in the cyst wall (**b**)

demonstrated through a pathologic fracture involving a UBC with the bone fragment layering dependently within the fluid (Fig. 2.10). Unicameral bone cysts are asymptomatic unless complicated by fracture; these lesions are the most common cause of pathologic fracture in children. UBC has a characteristic gross yellowish color and clear appearance. These lesions are often removed in piecemeal and consist of multiloculated cystic spaces devoid of true lining. The cyst wall is fibrous which may contain variable amounts of fibrin, multinucleate giant cells, and sometimes cementoid material (Fig. 2.11).

and the thin inner lining of the ABC will enhance, while the multiloculated fluid-containing spaces will not (Fig. 2.12d).

ABCs are grossly very hemorrhagic and sievelike, reminiscent of a sponge. Histologic section show multiloculated "cystic" spaces containing blood with no true lining with fibrous wall and variable amounts of osteoclastic-type giant cells, capillaries, spindle cells, and osteoid deposition that sometimes mineralize to form bone (Fig. 2.13). It is imperative to screen for secondary etiologies which may coexist in the same biopsy specimen.

2.3.2 Aneurysmal Bone Cyst

Aneurysmal bone cysts (ABCs) on radiographs appear lucent with sharp margins, showing a "soap-bubble" lesion with thin sclerotic borders (Fig. 2.12). The bony cortex may be very thinned to the point of nonvisualization; however, no bony destruction is seen, similar to unicameral bone cysts. ABCs are usually multiloculated and may demonstrate lacelike internal matrix. On MRI, the lesion will also demonstrate characteristic fluid-fluid levels due to layering degraded blood products, similar to UBC (Fig. 2.12c). On contrast-enhanced imaging, the internal septa

2.3.3 Telangiectatic Osteosarcoma

An important differential diagnosis is telangiectatic osteosarcoma, which shares similar histologic features to ABCs. Telangiectatic osteosarcoma is characterized by multiple blood-filled cysts and microscopically shows tumor cells arranged along delicate networks of sinusoidal vessels. These features can mimic aneurysmal bone cyst; however, the high-grade pleomorphic cells with anaplasia, coagulative necrosis, atypical mitotic figures, and osteoid matrix are often readily identified in telangiectatic osteosarcoma (Fletcher et al. 2013).

Fig. 2.12 Aneurismal bone cyst of the distal tibia. (**a**, **b**) Anterior-posterior (**a**) and lateral (**b**) radiographs of the distal tibia demonstrate an expansile lytic lesion eccentrically located and involving the posterior distal tibial metaphysis. This example has characteristic sharp geographic margins with thin rim of sclerosis and very faint lacelike internal matrix. No cortical break or destruction with no visible soft tissue component. (**c**, **d**) MRI sequences of the same patient (**c** axial T2WI with fat saturation, **d** sagittal post-gadolinium T1WI with fat saturation) demonstrate the sharp margins of the lesion, with a thin rim of decreased signal corresponding to sclerosis seen on radiographs. Multiple fluid-fluid levels within the cystic spaces, seen in panel **c**, represent layering of blood products and are characteristic, but not unique to aneurismal bone cysts. Typical thin enhancement of the margins and septa without a soft tissue component or cortical destruction are best seen in post-contrast T1-weighted images (panel **d**)

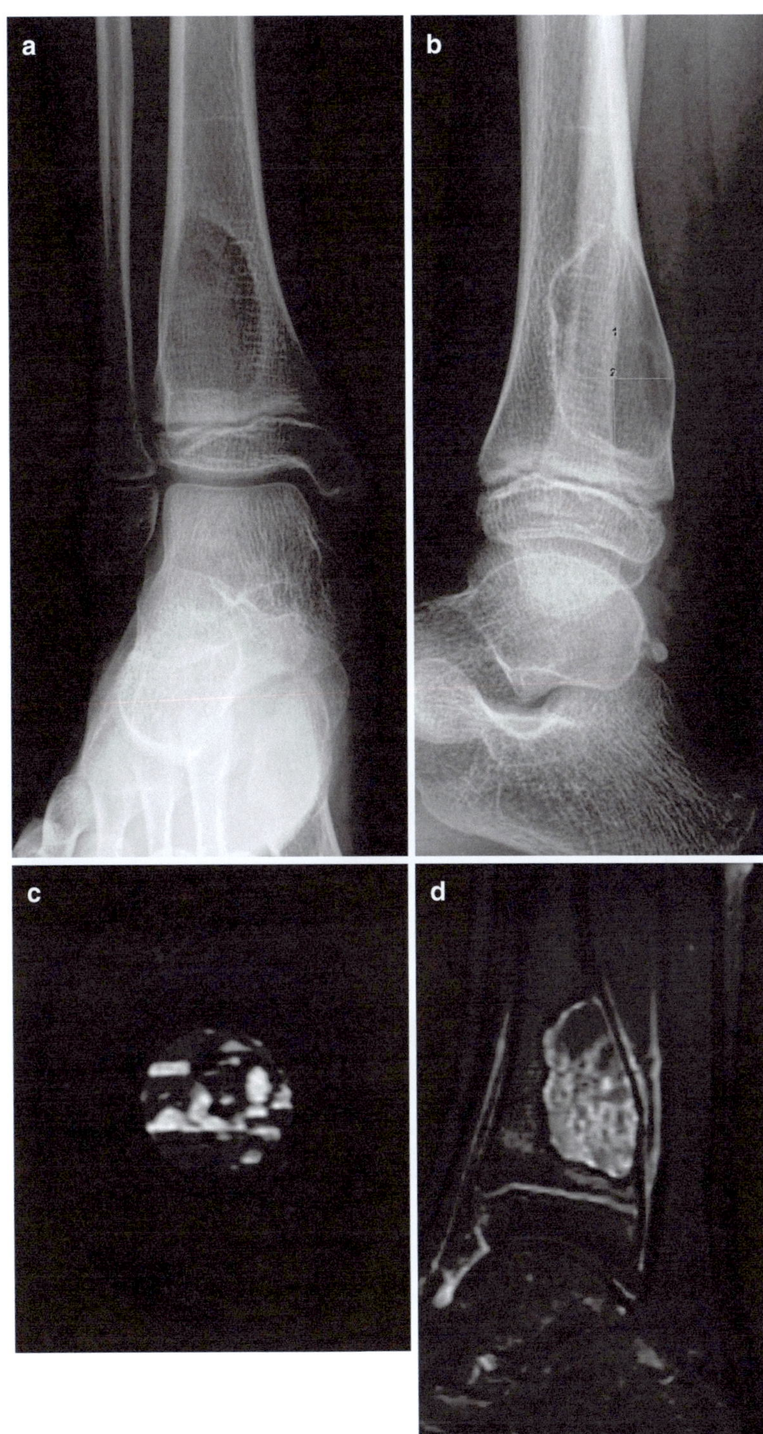

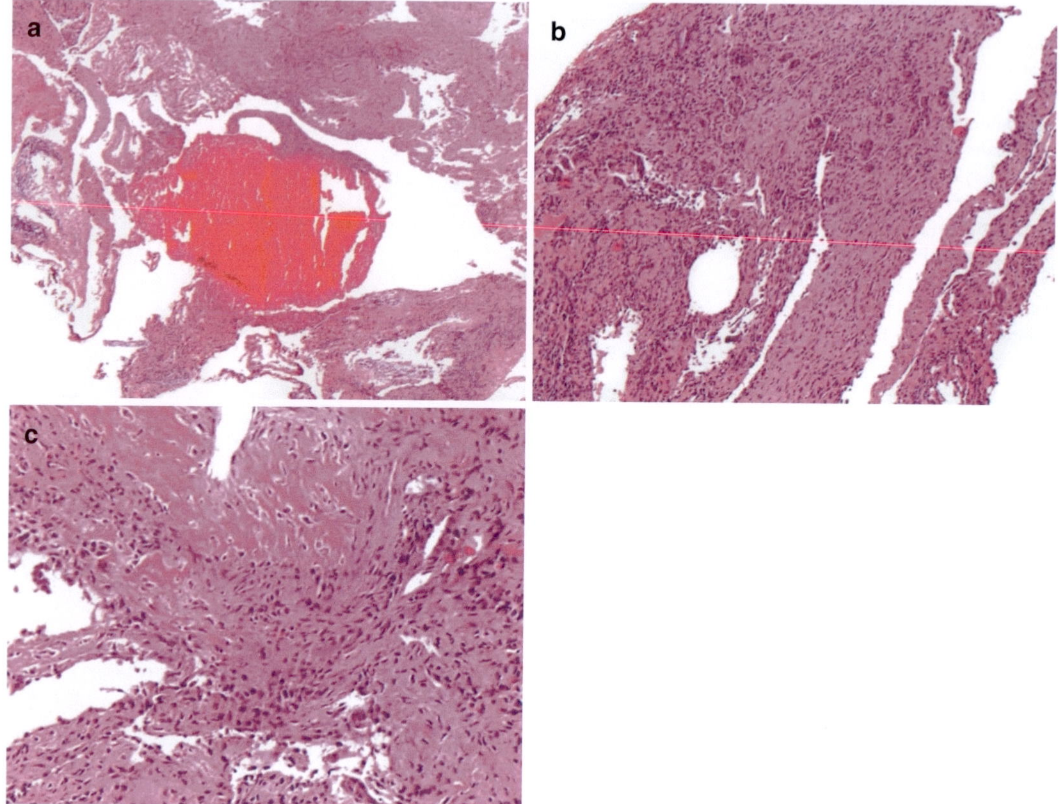

Fig. 2.13 Histologic features of aneurismal bone cyst. (**a**) Aneurysmal bone cyst contains blood-filled cystic spaces lined by fibrous septae. (**b**) Multinucleated giant cells are characteristically seen in the septae. Notably, cellular features of malignancy are absent. (**c**) Areas of osteoid deposition can be seen in aneurysmal bone cyst

Conversely, aneurysmal bone cyst can also show osteoid formation which can undergo mineralization, representing an important histologic differential diagnosis from osteosarcoma. In these instances, the absence of malignant cytologic features is an important histologic clue to the diagnosis of aneurysmal bone cyst.

2.3.4 Conventional Osteosarcoma

Conventional osteosarcoma can often be primarily diagnosed with radiography, with other imaging modalities typically reserved for staging and planning for surgical resection. Biopsy is performed for unequivocal confirmation of the diagnosis. In radiographs, osteosarcoma typically will appear as a large lesion with aggressive features showing a mixed lytic-sclerotic appearance, ill-defined margins, as well as bone destruction and a large soft tissue mass component. As a bone-forming tumor, conventional osteosarcoma classically has dense "cloud-like" matrix easily visible on radiographs (Fig. 2.14a, b). MRI can better delineate the soft tissue component and involvement of surrounding structures, useful for surgical planning (Fig. 2.14c). Additionally, osteosarcoma classically will demonstrate aggressive patterns of periosteal reaction including "sunburst" or "hair-on-end" pattern as well as "Codman triangles." The sunburst pattern develops when growth of the lesion outpaces the ability of the periosteum to lay down new bone, and the Sharpey's fibers stretch out in a divergent pattern from the bone (Fig. 2.14d), whereas "hair-on-end" periosteal reaction is oriented perpendicular to the bone. It is often seen with osteosarcoma but can also develop with other aggressive bony tumors such as Ewing sarcoma or osteoblastic metastases. The Codman triangles

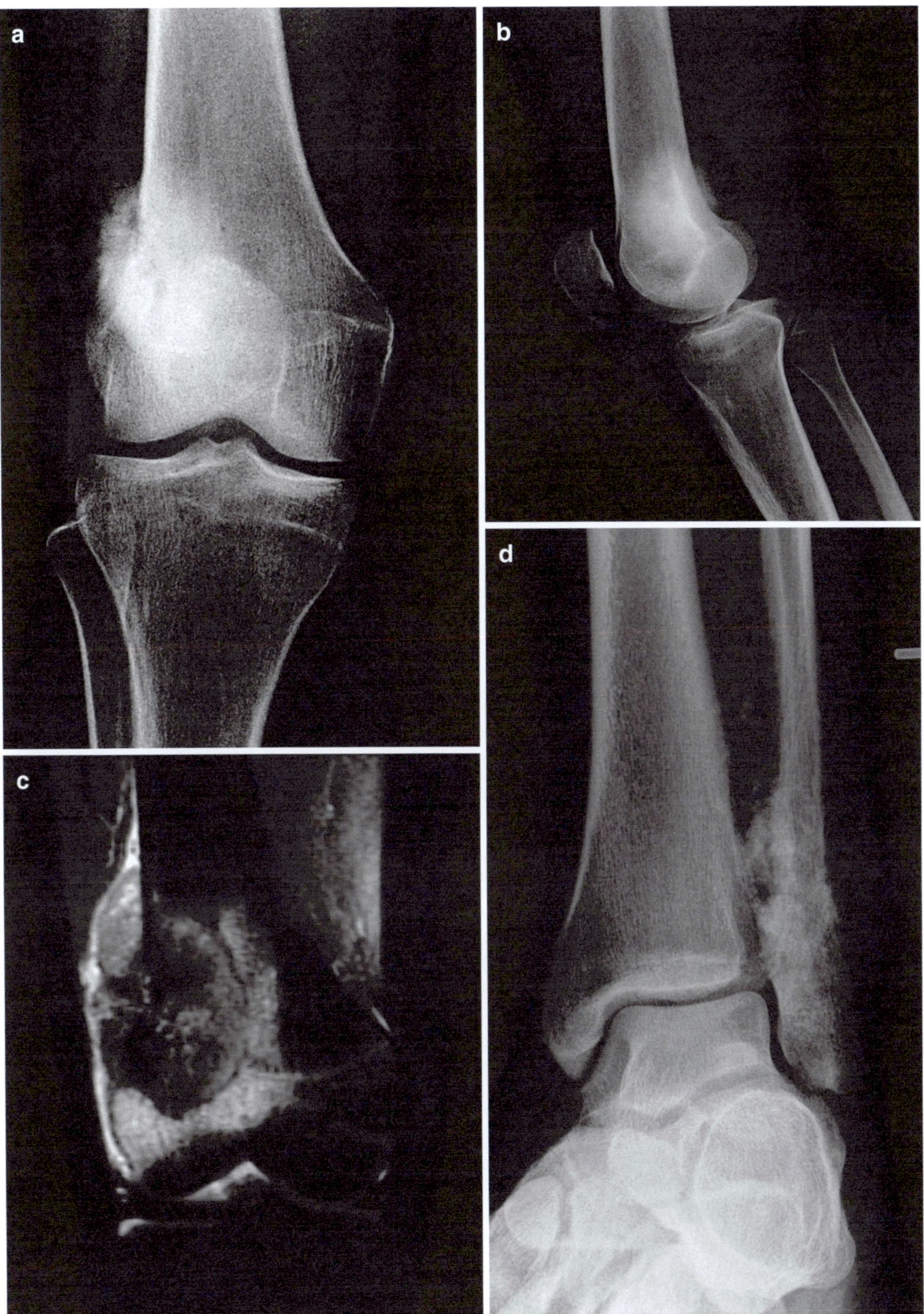

Fig. 2.14 Radiographic features of conventional osteosarcoma. Anterior-posterior (**a**) and lateral (**b**) radiographs of the knee demonstrate a large mass involving the distal femoral metaphysis with classic features of conventional osteosarcoma including dense "cloud-like" osseous matrix, cortical destruction with mass extension through the cortex. (**c**) Coronal T1 fat-saturated post-gadolinium imaging of the same patient better depicts the size of the soft tissue mass and extension of the osteosarcoma than radiography. Note the cortical destruction along the lateral aspect of the femur. (**d**) Oblique frontal radiograph of a conventional osteosarcoma involving the distal fibular metaphysis demonstrates a classic "sunburst" appearance of aggressive periosteal reaction

form on the edge of the periosteum in a fast-growing aggressive lesion or process. With aggressive lesions, the periosteum does not have time to completely ossify; thus, only the edge of the raised periosteum will ossify, producing the characteristic triangular appearance along the margins of the mass. While this is found often in osteosarcoma, this type of aggressive periosteal reaction can be found in many other aggressive lesions including Ewing sarcoma, osteomyelitis, metastatic disease, and other sarcomas. Osteosarcomas can occasionally appear purely lytic and exhibit little no periosteal reaction.

The histologic diagnosis of conventional osteosarcoma is established based on cells exhibiting malignant cytologic features associated with osteoid matrix material (Fletcher et al. 2013; Sanerkin 1980). Conventional osteosarcoma has a variety of histologic variants including osteoblastic, fibroblastic, chondroblastic, giant-cell rich, clear cell type, and epithelioid, yet none of these correlate with prognosis (Fig. 2.15) (Fletcher et al. 2013; Hauben et al. 2002). The malignant cells and associated osteoid permeate native bony trabeculae, often exhibiting anaplasia and atypical mitotic figures, and coagulative tumor necrosis involving the native bone trabeculae can be seen (Fig. 2.16). Osteoid matrix can be very focal or occasionally difficult to distinguish from other sclerosing sarcomas that produce thick collagen matrix. Generally, the role of immunohistochemistry in the diagnosis of osteosarcomas is limited and many pitfalls are known, including aberrant expression of markers such as cytokeratin that can mimic carcinoma (Okada et al. 2003). In cases where osteoid is scant or not easily discernible, immunohistochemical staining for SATB2 can be helpful to confirm bona fide osteoblastic differentiation (Fig. 2.17) (Conner and Hornick 2013). Recently, p16 expression has been shown to be predictive of tumor response to chemotherapy (Fig. 2.18) (Borys et al. 2012).

Osteoblastoma, especially aggressive forms, can show histologic features mimicking conventional osteosarcoma with plump epithelioid cells that can exhibit cytologic atypia. However, unlike osteosarcoma, osteoblastoma is typically a discrete lesion often in the diaphysis and does not invade surrounding native lamellar bone.

Parosteal osteosarcoma usually involves the metaphysis of long bones, most frequently the distal posterior aspect of the surface of the tibia. By definition, in the absence of dedifferentiation, parosteal osteosarcomas are low-grade malignant neoplasms composed of spindle cells with mild atypia which may manifest a cartilaginous cap thus mimicking an osteochondroma. However, parosteal osteosarcoma lacks the orderly arrangement typical of osteochondroma (Unni et al. 1976).

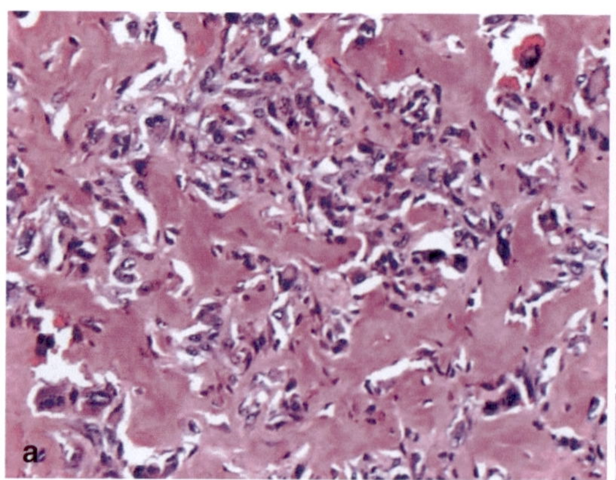
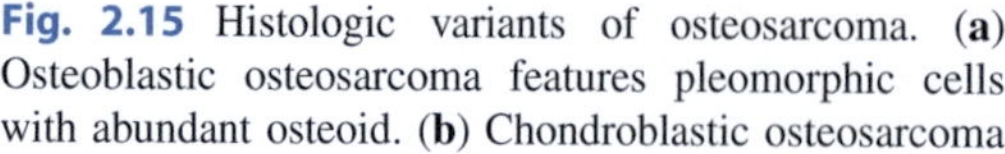
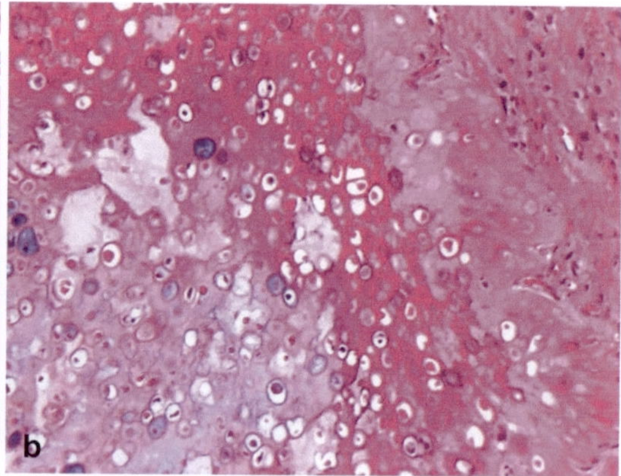

Fig. 2.15 Histologic variants of osteosarcoma. (**a**) Osteoblastic osteosarcoma features pleomorphic cells with abundant osteoid. (**b**) Chondroblastic osteosarcoma showing lobules of atypical chondrocytes merging imperceptibly with an area of osteoid deposition in the upper half of the image

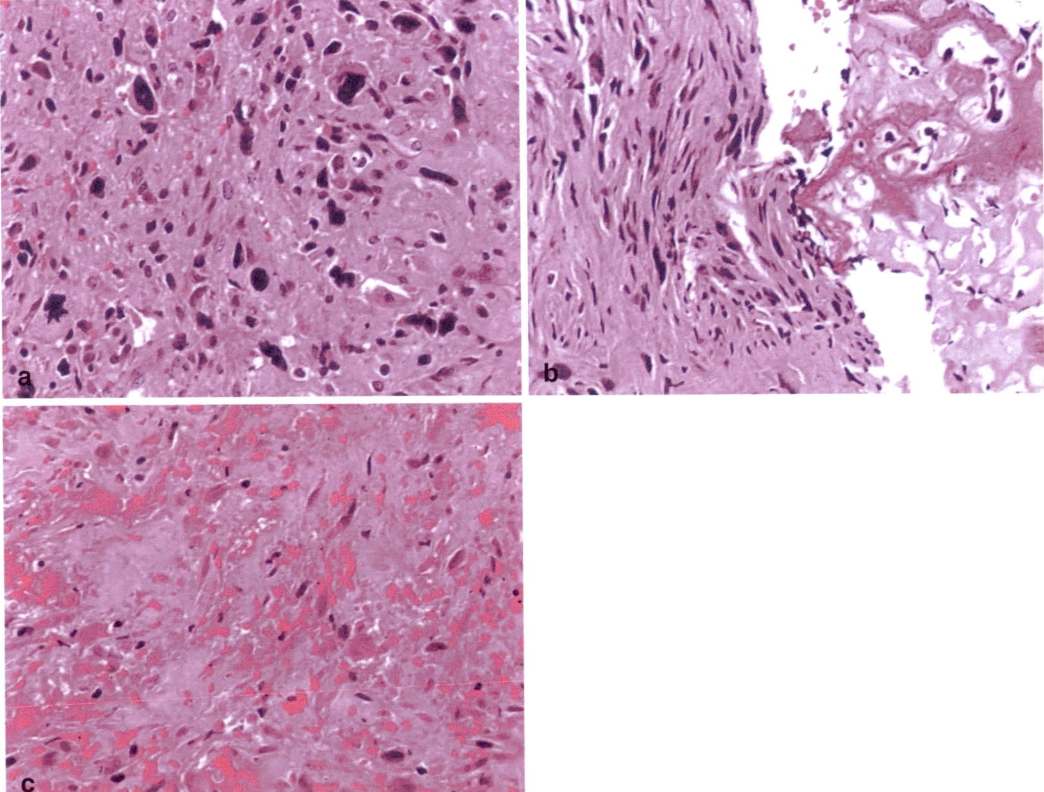

Fig. 2.16 Histologic features of conventional osteosarcoma. (**a, b**) Conventional osteosarcoma is a high-grade malignancy characterized by cells with nuclear hyperchromasia and pleomorphism (**a**) and lacy osteoid material adjacent to the malignant cells (**b** right half of the image). (**c**) Coagulative tumor necrosis is a frequent feature of conventional osteosarcoma

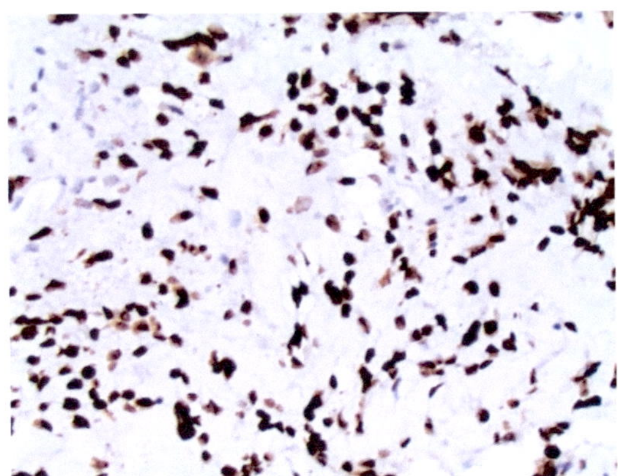

Fig. 2.17 SATB2 reactivity in osteosarcoma. (**a**) SATB2 is a marker of the osteoblast lineage and is typically diffusely reactive in conventional osteosarcoma

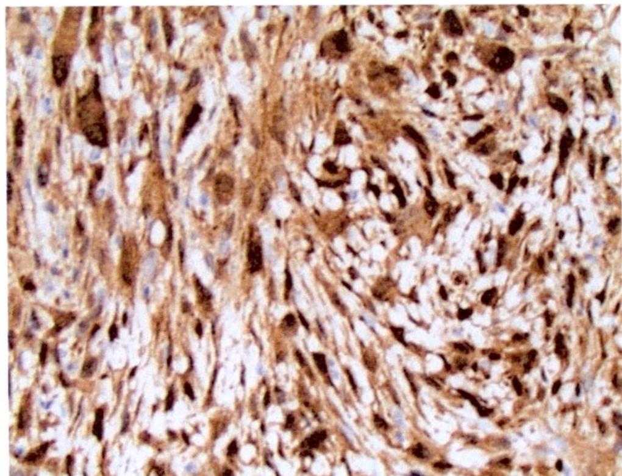

Fig. 2.18 P16 reactivity in osteosarcoma. Diffuse nuclear and cytoplasmic P16 expression may predict a favorable response to neoadjuvant chemotherapy

2.3.5 Metaphyseal Ewing Sarcoma Versus Small Cell Osteosarcoma

Small cell osteosarcoma is a poorly differentiated variant of osteosarcoma. Similar to conventional osteosarcoma, small cell osteosarcoma most often occurs in the metaphyseal region of long bones (Ayala et al. 1989; Green and Mills 2014; Nakajima et al. 1997) and can appear more lytic, lacking the typical "cloud-like" mineralization of the conventional osteosarcoma which contains more osteoid matrix (Fig. 2.19). Ewing sarcoma is more commonly diaphyseal and will be discussed further in Sect. 2.4. However, Ewing sarcoma can also present as a metaphyseal lesion with radiographic features that mimic osteosarcoma, including similar aggressive patterns of periosteal elevation such as Codman triangle (Fig. 2.20).

The poorly differentiated histologic appearance of small cell osteosarcoma can closely mimic Ewing sarcoma. Each of these lesions is composed of poorly differentiated cells with scant cytoplasm (Fig. 2.21). The presence of osteoid produced by tumor cells allows small cell

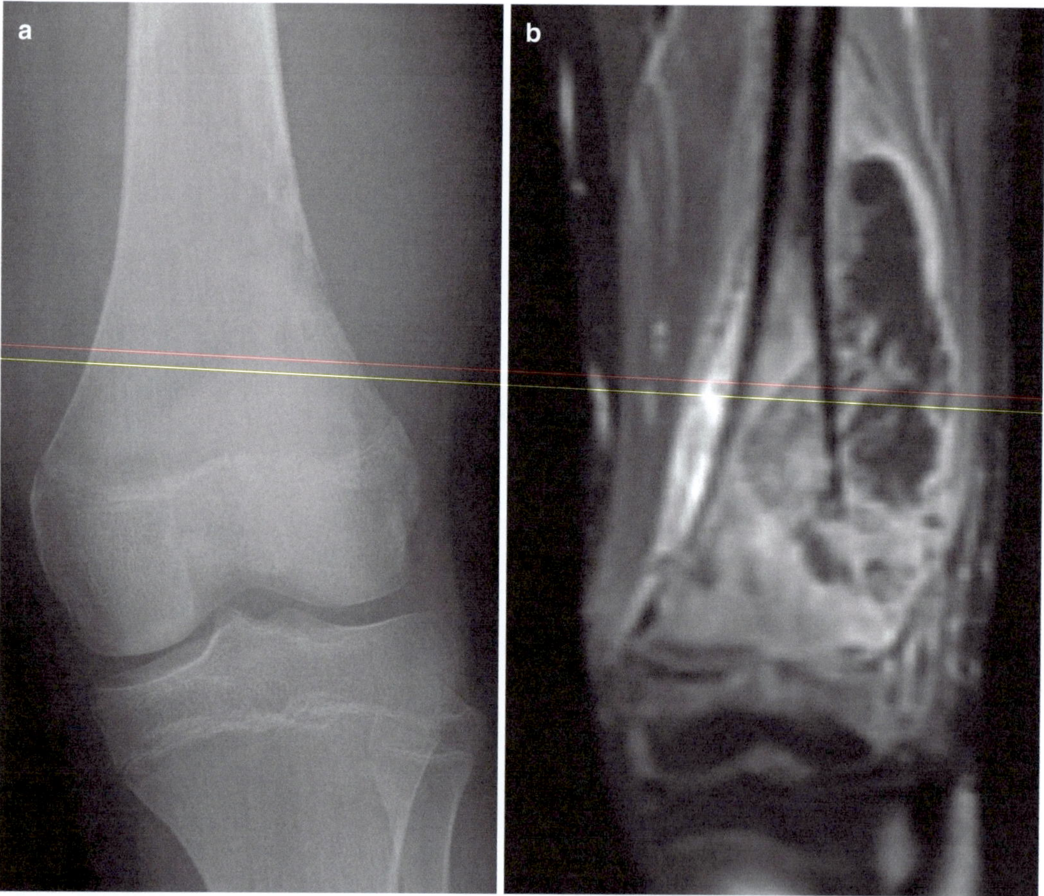

Fig. 2.19 Radiographic features of small cell osteosarcoma. (**a**) An anterior-posterior radiograph of the knee demonstrates an aggressive lesion with mixed lytic and sclerotic features and ill-defined margins. In this poorly differentiated osteosarcoma, the lack of osseous "cloud-like" mineralization typical of conventional osteosarcoma can overlap in appearance with an Ewing sarcoma involving the metaphysis. (**b**) MRI much better delineates the soft tissue component and intramedullary involvement than radiography of this poorly differentiated osteosarcoma. This coronal T1 post-contrast fat-saturated image of the distal femur shows a large aggressive destructive lesion. Note the necrotic component showing lack of central enhancement

osteosarcoma to be distinguished from Ewing sarcoma (Fig. 2.21a); however, osteoid is typically scant, corresponding with the radiographic lack of "cloud-like" mineralization classically associated with osteoid-rich conventional osteosarcoma. Immunohistochemical staining for markers such as FLI-1, more often reactive in Ewing sarcoma (Lee et al. 2011), or osteocalcin and Galectin-1 that are more often reactive in small cell osteosarcoma (Machado et al. 2013), can provide additional support for the diagnosis. CD99 immunohistochemical staining is variable and often cytoplasmic in small cell osteosarcoma

(Devaney et al. 1993; Machado et al. 2010). In contrast, Ewing sarcoma typically shows strong membranous CD99 reactivity (Fig. 2.22). However, membranous CD99 reactivity should not be regarded as diagnostic of Ewing sarcoma as CD99 reactivity is seen in many other tumor types, notably synovial sarcoma and lymphoblastic lymphoma. Definitive identification of Ewing sarcoma is possible based on the presence of specific chromosomal translocations, most often involving the *EWSR1* gene (Fletcher et al. 2013; Tsokos et al. 2012). Thus, florescent in situ hybridization (FISH) to detect *EWSR1*

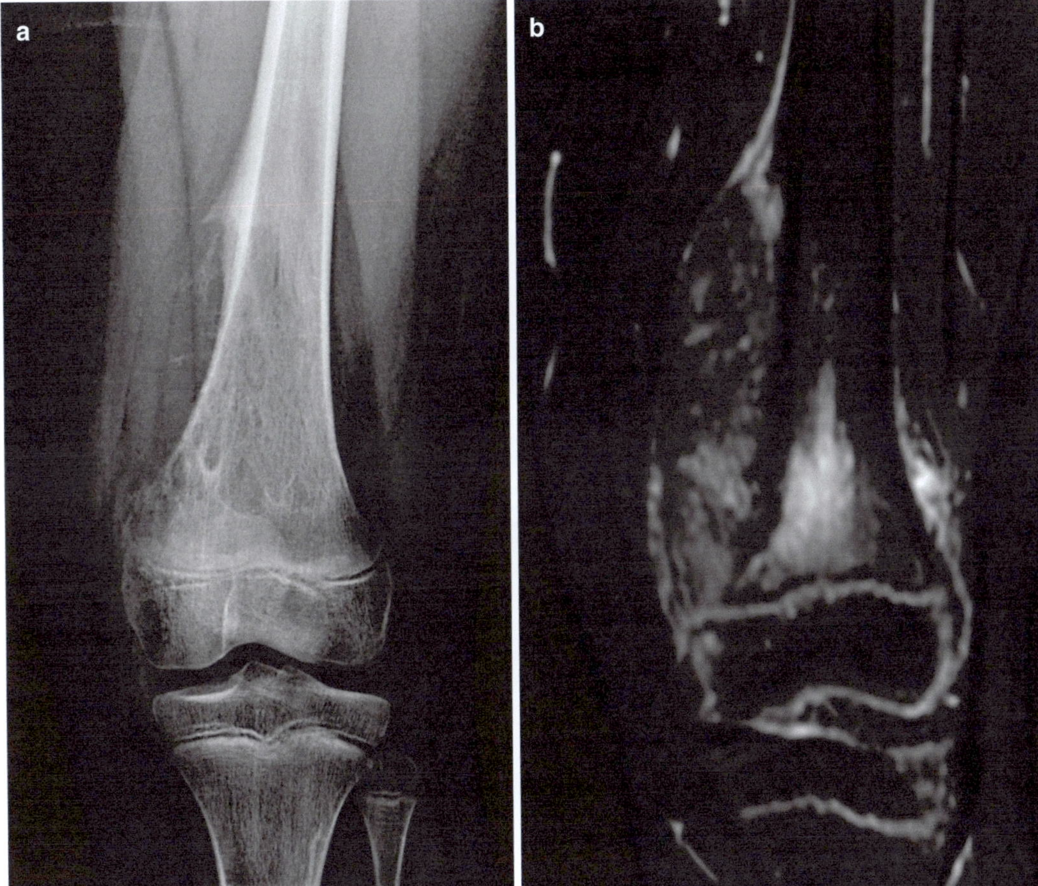

Fig. 2.20 Ewing sarcoma mimicking osteosarcoma. (**a**) An anterior-posterior radiograph of this Ewing sarcoma shows features that overlap with osteosarcoma. This aggressive "moth-eaten" lytic-appearing lesion within the metaphysis of the distal femur demonstrates bony destruction and a large soft tissue component with a "Codman triangle" at the superior margin of the soft tissue mass as well as "hair-on-end" aggressive periosteal reaction. (**b**) A coronal post-contrast T1 fat-saturated image of the same lesion demonstrates the large soft tissue component extending from the bone, bony destruction, as well as triangular-shaped enhancement at the superior margin of the tumor at the site of "Codman's triangle"

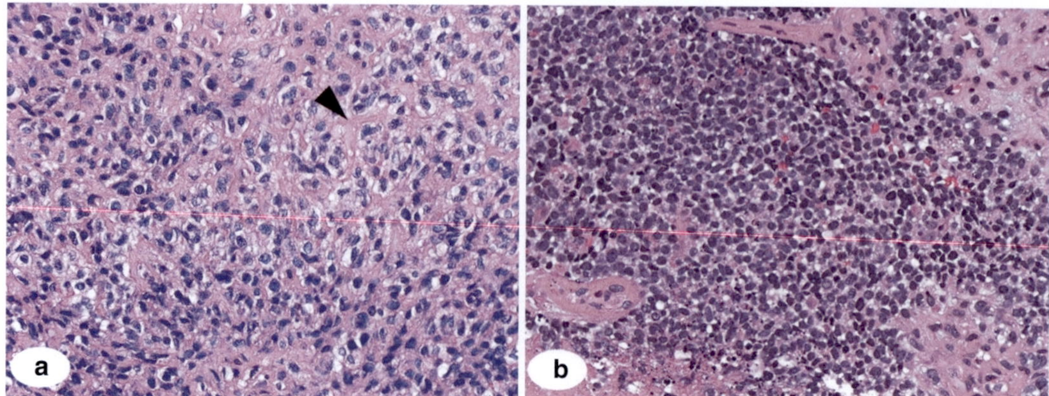

Fig. 2.21 Similar histologic appearances of small cell osteosarcoma and Ewing sarcoma. (**a**, **b**) Small cell osteosarcoma (**a**) and Ewing sarcoma (**b**) can each be composed of cells with similar monotonous round nuclei with scant cytoplasm. Small cell osteosarcoma can be distinguished from Ewing sarcoma by the presence of networks of lacy osteoid between the cells (**a** *arrowhead*)

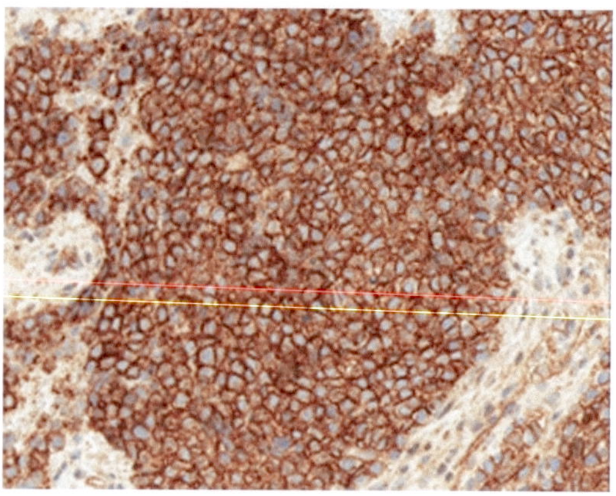

Fig. 2.22 Immunohistochemical staining for CD99 in Ewing sarcoma. CD99 reactivity in Ewing sarcoma typically demonstrates a strong, diffuse membranous pattern. This pattern is frequent in Ewing sarcoma; however, it is not specific to Ewing sarcoma

rearrangement and reverse-transcription-mediated polymerase chain reaction (RT-PCR) to detect the resulting fusion transcript are typically valuable in confirming the diagnosis of Ewing sarcoma. Exceptional cases of small cell osteosarcoma have been reported to show *EWSR1* rearrangements; however, the identified fusion gene partners in small cell osteosarcoma have not been reported in Ewing sarcoma (Debelenko et al. 2011; Dragoescu et al. 2013).

2.3.6 Ewing Sarcoma Versus Lymphoblastic Lymphoma

Ewing sarcoma and non-Hodgkin lymphomas involving the bone, such as lymphoblastic lymphoma, each show histologic features of monotonous infiltrates of round cells and each can grow in diffuse sheets. Patchy necrosis is often seen in Ewing sarcoma, typically sparing tumor cells adjacent to vessels, and dystrophic calcifications can be seen in areas of necrosis. The cells of Ewing sarcoma are cohesive, often showing indistinct cell borders and a small amount of foamy cytoplasm (Fig. 2.23). In contrast, lymphoblastic lymphomas are typically discohesive with artifactual separation between the cells and frequently display single-file infiltration or prominent crush artifacts (Fig. 2.24). The differences between Ewing sarcoma and lymphoma are often appreciable in aspirate smears or touch preparations. The cohesive nature of Ewing sarcoma produces three-dimensional clusters of cells (Fig. 2.25). Cells of most types of lymphomas tend to spread in a monolayer, and lymphoglandular bodies are often readily identifiable (Fig. 2.26).

Immunohistochemical staining to distinguish Ewing sarcoma from lymphoma can be accomplished with specific lymphoid markers. CD45 is typically diffuse in lymphomas, and specific

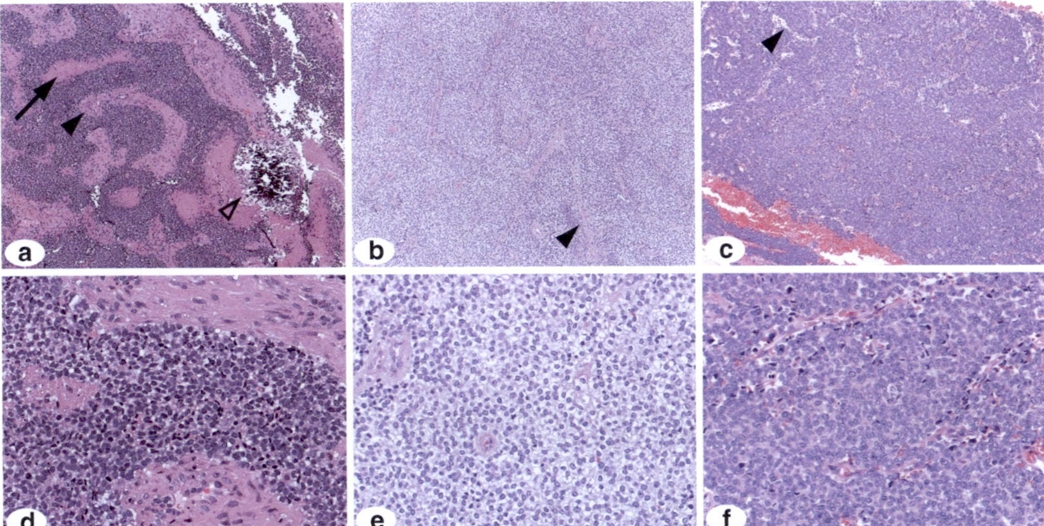

Fig. 2.23 Histologic features of Ewing sarcoma. Ewing sarcoma can display a spectrum of architectural and cytologic features. Ewing sarcoma most often grows in sheets with occasional calcifications (**a** *empty arrowhead*) and patchy areas of necrosis (**a** *arrow*). The vessels within the tumor can range from thick-walled vessels (**a** *arrowhead*) to thin-walled or delicate sinusoidal-like vessels (**b**, **c** *arrowheads*). Cells with round, monotonous nuclei and scant cytoplasm are characteristic of Ewing sarcoma. The cytoplasm contains variable amounts of glycogen, typically producing a foamy appearance with indistinct cell boarders (**d**); however, completely clear cytoplasm (**e**) or solidly eosinophilic (**f**) can also be seen

markers of B-cell lineage (CD19, CD20) or T-cell lineage (CD3) can confirm the lymphoid origin of the tumor. Ewing sarcoma is often characterized by reactivity for CD99; however, this represents a specific diagnostic pitfall in distinguishing Ewing sarcoma and lymphoblastic lymphomas; strong membranous CD99 reactivity is a frequent feature of lymphoblastic lymphomas (Riopel et al. 1994). Molecular testing, either RT-PCR or FISH for translocations specific to Ewing sarcoma, allows definitive identification of Ewing sarcoma.

2.3.7 Langerhans Cell Histiocytosis Versus Chronic Osteomyelitis

Langerhans cell histiocytosis (LCH) is a neoplasm seen primarily in children and young adults, typically presenting as a lytic bone lesion and often involving the skull (Fig. 2.27a) (Badalian-Very et al. 2013; Egeler and Nesbit 1995; Lieberman et al. 1996). However, LCH lesions can occur in all locations of long bones; rarely in the epiphysis and more commonly in the metaphysis or diaphysis. Many bones can be involved including the mandible, pelvis, ribs (Fig. 2.27b), and spine. LCH shows a spectrum of radiographic appearances, with lesions often having both aggressive and nonaggressive radiographic features. Metaphyseal lesions generally appear well circumscribed and lytic in appearance. The characteristic lesions of LCH are "punched-out" sharply circumscribed lytic cortical lesions with a sclerotic rim (Fig. 2.28). Biopsies of LCH will show abnormal histiocytes with distinctive cleaved and "bean-shaped" nuclei in a background of inflammation that frequently includes eosinophils (Fig. 2.29). The broad range of radiographic features of LCH can overlap with chronic osteomyelitis (Fig. 2.30). Similarly, the histologic features of these lesions significantly overlap. Biopsies of chronic osteomyelitis often contain eosinophils and reactive histiocytes (Fig. 2.31); however, the histiocytes of LCH are distinguished by their characteristic nuclear shape and reactivity for specific immunohistochemical markers:

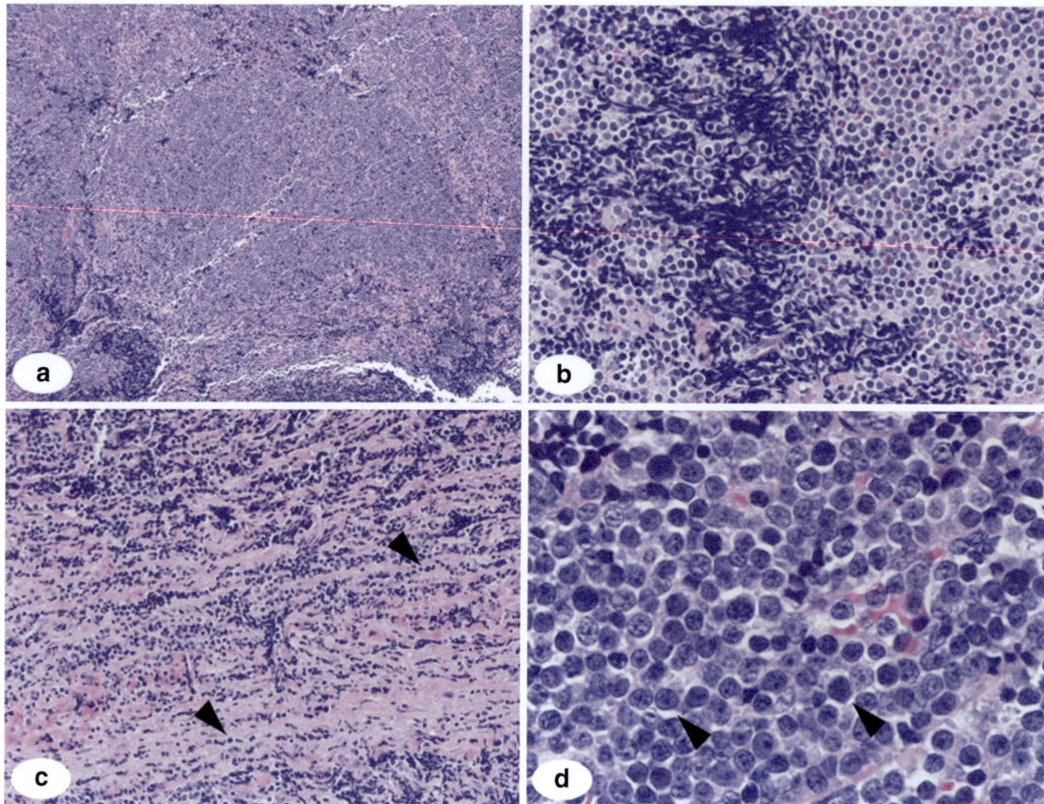

Fig. 2.24 Histologic features of lymphoblastic lymphoma. Lymphoblastic lymphoma grows in diffuse sheets with monotonous cells, similar to Ewing sarcoma (**a** H&E 10× objective magnification). Lymphoblasts are fragile, often resulting in crush artifacts (**b**). Single-file infiltration of surrounding tissues is also a common feature of lymphoma (**c** *arrowheads*). Lymphomas lack cell-cell junctions characteristic of many malignancies; thus, the discohesive nature of lymphomas results in visible artifactual spaces between the cells following formalin fixation and paraffin processing (**d** *arrowheads*)

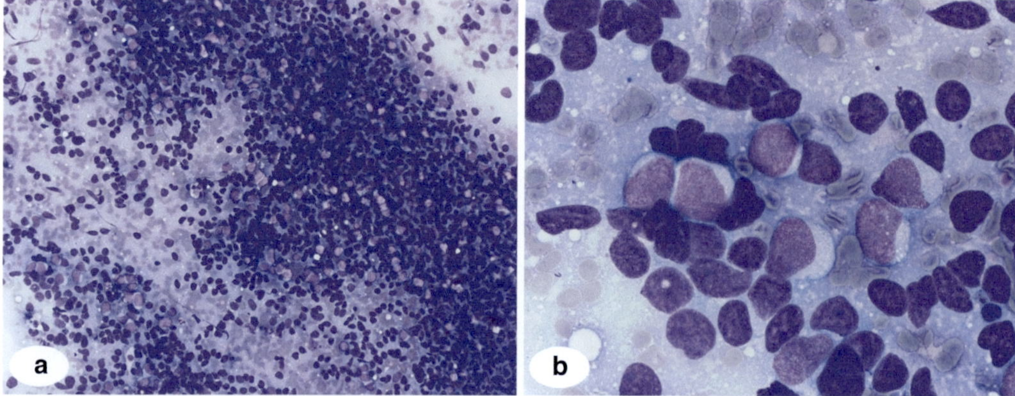

Fig. 2.25 Ewing sarcoma in aspirate smears and touch preparations. Smear and touch preparations of Ewing sarcoma typically contain cohesive clusters of cells in three-dimensional clusters (**a**). Individual tumor cells are often stripped of their cytoplasm, with occasional cells retaining their foamy cytoplasm (**b**)

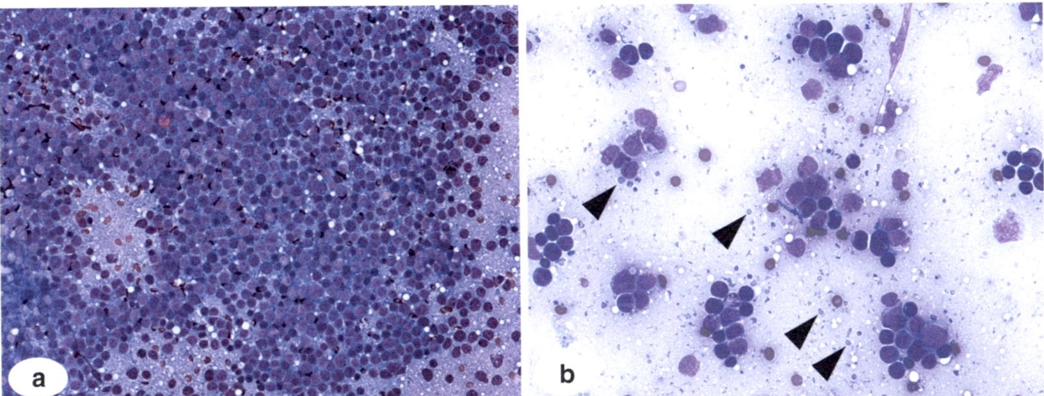

Fig. 2.26 Lymphoblastic lymphoma in aspirate smears and touch preparations. The discohesive nature of lymphoblastic lymphoma is easily appreciated in aspirate smear and touch preparations; lymphoblasts typically spread as monolayer of cells with scant cytoplasm (**a**). In areas of smears with fewer cells, the background is seen to contain broken fragments of cytoplasm, called lymphoglandular bodies, confirming the lymphoid origin of the neoplastic cells (**b** *arrowheads*)

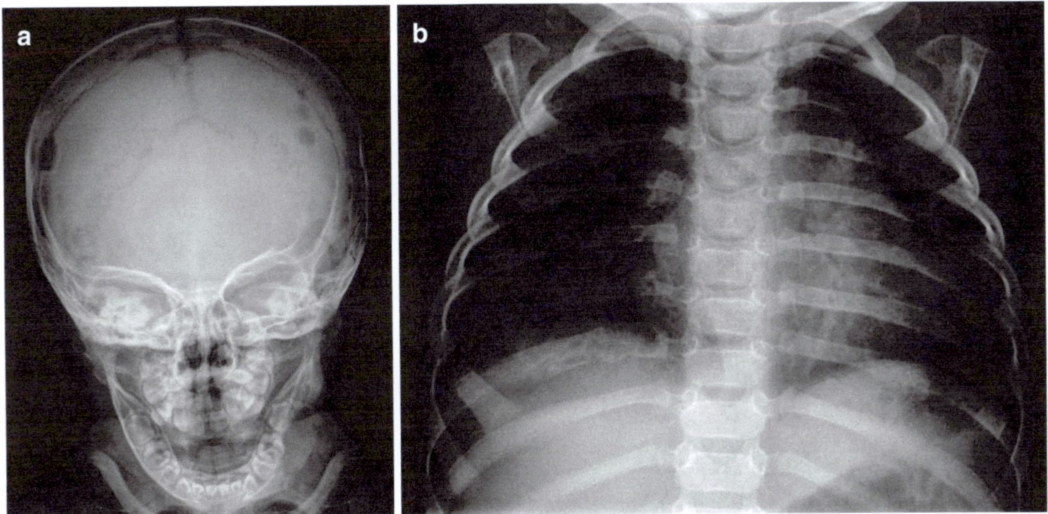

Fig. 2.27 Radiographic features of Langerhans cell histiocytosis. (**a**) Langerhans cell histiocytosis (LCH) involving the skull demonstrates multiple well-circumscribed lucent lesions with a "punched-out" appearance in this anterior-posterior view. Given multiple lesions, LCH is high in the differential diagnosis for this young child. (**b**) This anterior-posterior view of the chest demonstrates Langerhans cell histiocytosis of the rib, with an expansile lucency of the posterior right eighth rib

CD1a, S-100, and Langerin (Fig. 2.32) (Chikwava and Jaffe 2004; Geissmann et al. 2001; Nakajima et al. 1982). Microbiologic cultures of the bone lesion may identify the causative organism of chronic infection (Akinyoola et al. 2009; White et al. 1995).

Erdheim-Chester disease is a rare form of systemic histiocytosis that can involve the metaphysis in adults and is distinguished from LCH or osteomyelitis by the presence of xanthomatous histiocytes and multinucleated giant cells (Diamond et al. 2014).

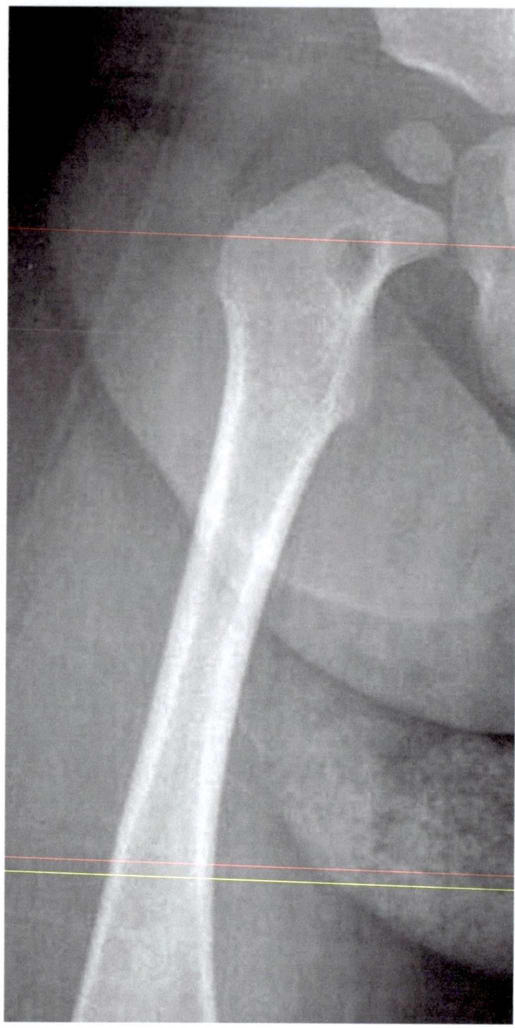

Fig. 2.28 Langerhans cell histiocytosis involving the femoral metaphysis. An anterior-posterior radiograph of the proximal femur demonstrates a well-circumscribed "punched-out" lytic lesion of LCH with sclerotic rim within the metaphysis

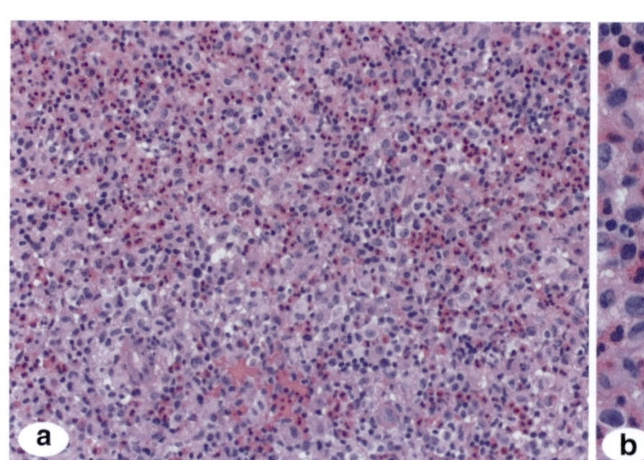

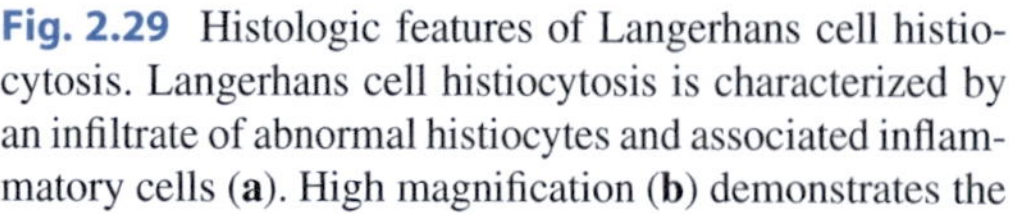

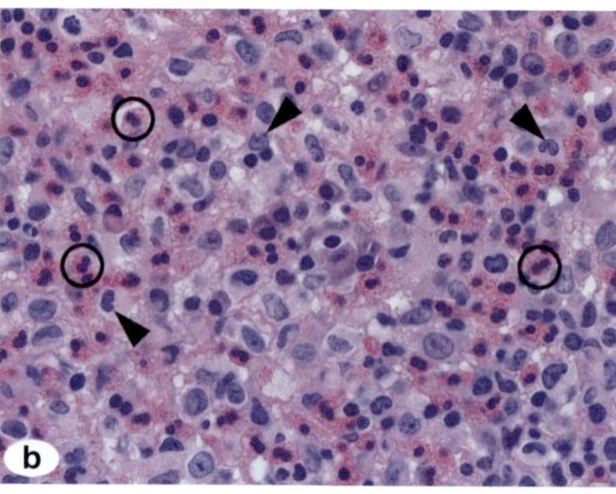

Fig. 2.29 Histologic features of Langerhans cell histiocytosis. Langerhans cell histiocytosis is characterized by an infiltrate of abnormal histiocytes and associated inflammatory cells (**a**). High magnification (**b**) demonstrates the irregular often "bean-shaped" contours of the abnormal histiocyte nuclei (*arrowheads*) and the many associated eosinophils (*circles*)

Fig. 2.30 Langerhans cell histiocytosis mimicking osteomyelitis. Anterior-posterior radiographs of this femur initially demonstrated a lytic lesion within the proximal femoral diaphysis with surrounding "onion-skin" periosteal reaction showing concentric layers (**a**). A follow-up radiograph (**b**) demonstrates progressive enlargement of destructive lytic lesion with ongoing periosteal reaction. Osteomyelitis can have a similar radiographic appearance

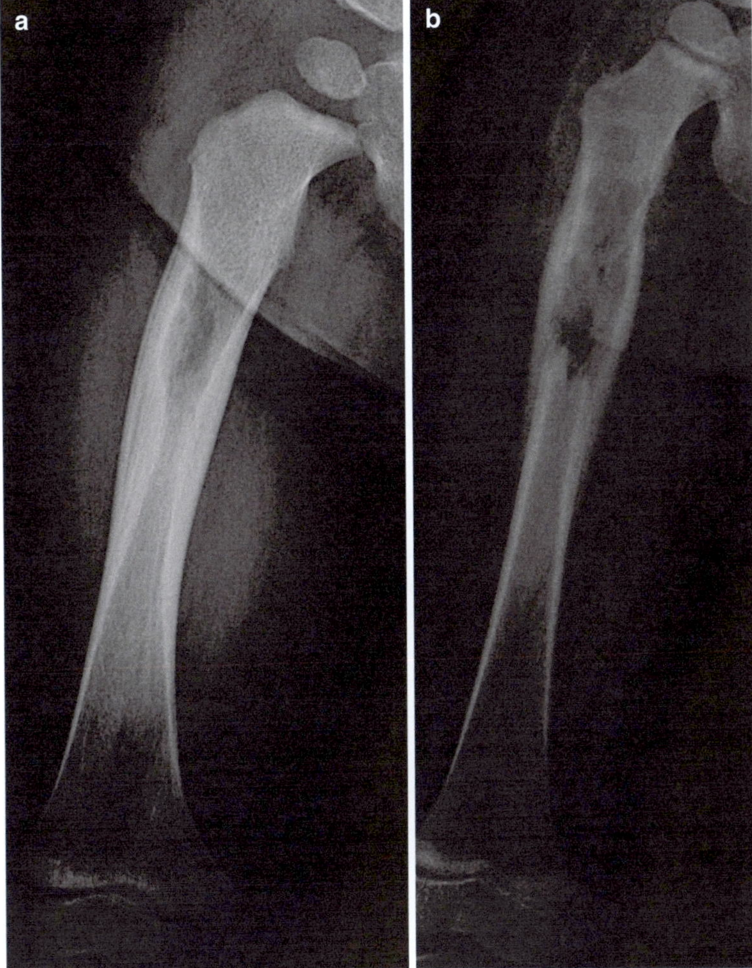

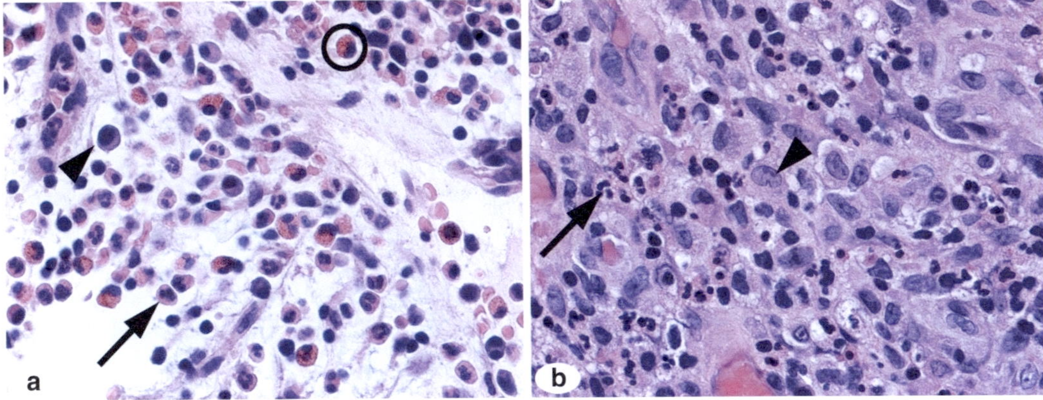

Fig. 2.31 Histologic features of chronic osteomyelitis. Chronic osteomyelitis can contain many inflammatory cell types in varying proportions. These examples show inflammation containing eosinophils (**a** *circle*), neutro-phils (**a**, **b** *arrows*), plasma cells (**a** *arrowhead*), and histiocytes (**b** *arrowhead*). Note that the reactive histiocytes seen in chronic osteomyelitis show predominantly rounded nuclear contours with occasional irregularity

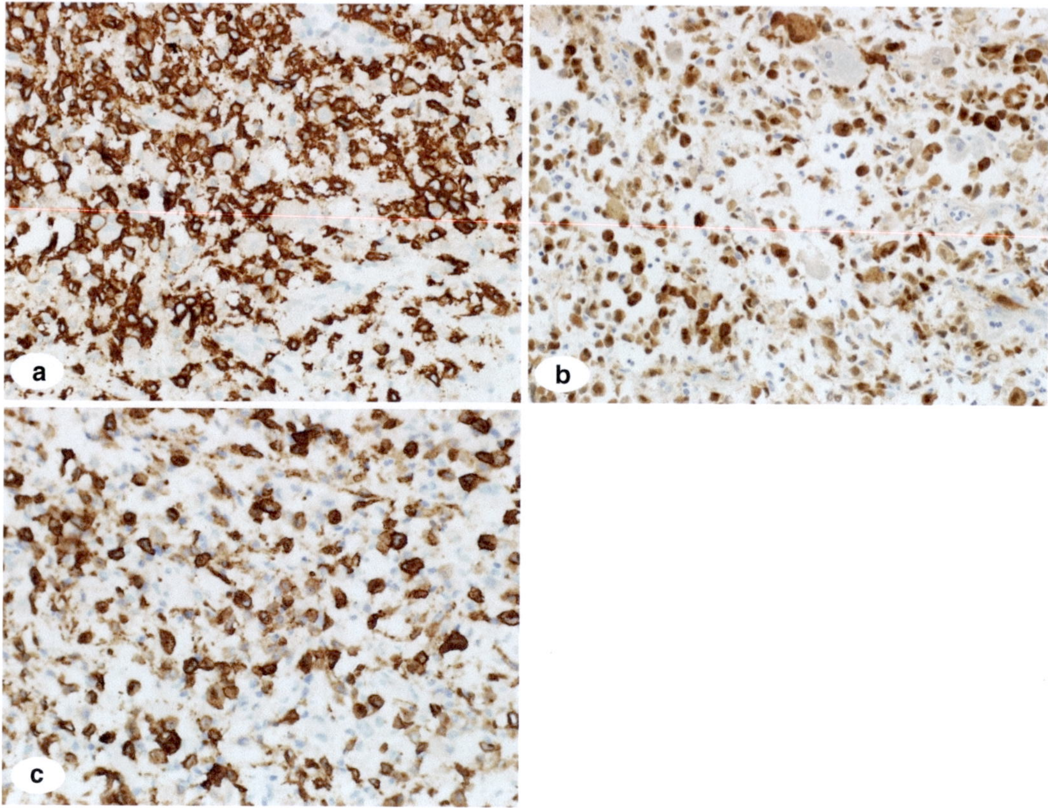

Fig. 2.32 Immunohistochemical features of Langerhans cell histiocytosis. The abnormal histiocytes of LCH are reactive for CD1a (**a**), S-100 (**b**), and Langerin (**c**)

2.4 Diaphyseal Lesions

A variety of benign and malignant lesions can involve the diaphysis in children. This section will discuss Ewing sarcoma, osteomyelitis, Langerhans cell histiocytosis, periosteal osteosarcoma, osteoid osteoma, osteoblastoma, nonossifying fibroma, and fibrous dysplasia.

2.4.1 Ewing Sarcoma Versus Osteomyelitis

Ewing sarcoma is a key differential diagnosis for lesions located in the diaphysis of long bones, as this is the most common location for Ewing sarcoma. Ewing sarcoma radiographically appears aggressive showing a lytic or mixed lytic and sclerotic lesion. Typical lesions show bone destruction and a permeative or "moth-eaten" appearance and often will show aggressive "onionskin" periosteal reaction of concentric layers, although can show other aggressive patterns of periosteal reaction as detailed in Sect. 2.3. On plain radiographs, the characteristics of Ewing sarcoma can overlap with osteomyelitis which can also demonstrate aggressive features (Fig. 2.33). However, additional imaging by MRI can demonstrate enhancing soft tissue extension without abscess, which would be less likely of an infectious process (Fig. 2.33c). In biopsies, Ewing sarcoma is readily distinguished from infection. Ewing sarcoma is composed of monotonous cells growing in sheets, in contrast to the variable lymphocytes, histiocytes, eosinophils, and neutrophils associated with osteomyelitis. Vessels within the Ewing sarcoma can range from delicate thin-walled capillaries to vessels

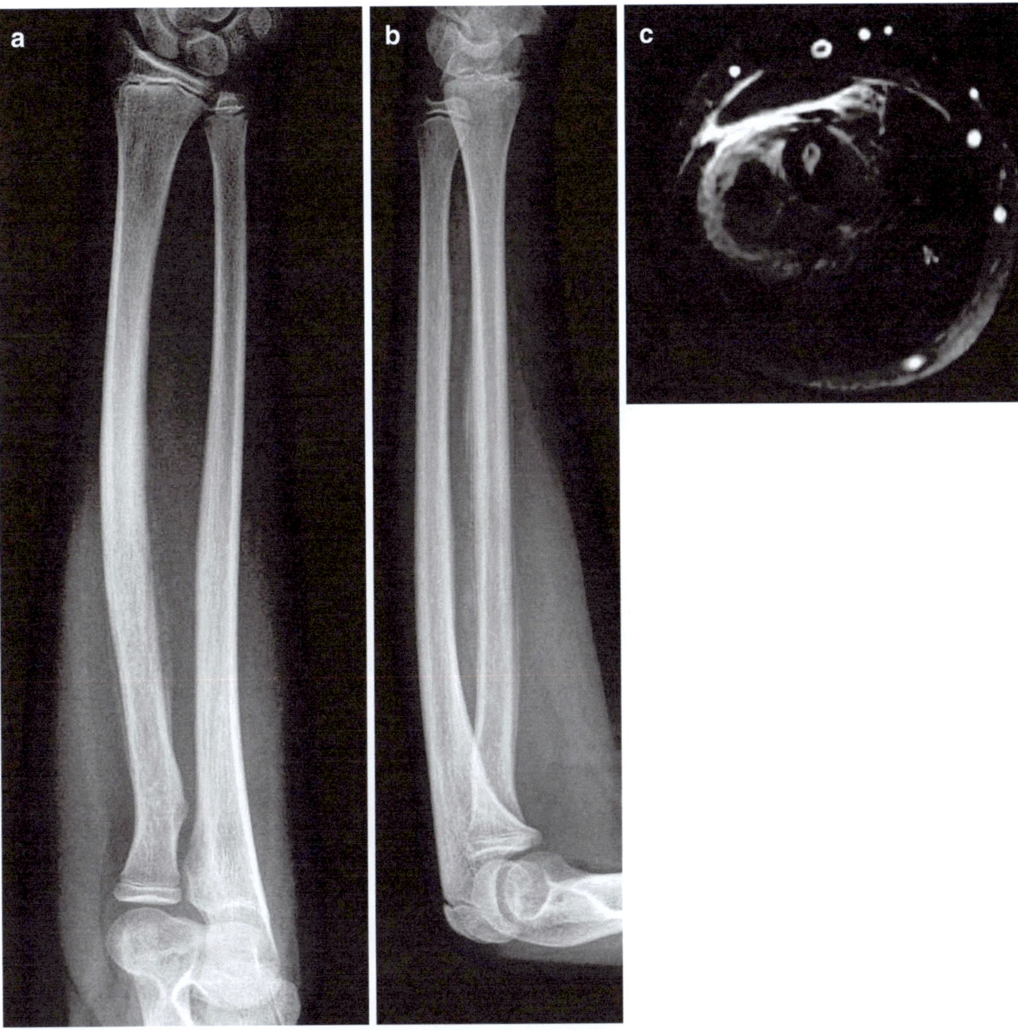

Fig. 2.33 Radiographic features of Ewing sarcoma involving the diaphysis. (**a, b**) Anterior-posterior and lateral radiographs of Ewing sarcoma of the radius show an aggressive appearing lesion involving the proximal diaphysis with a permeative, "moth-eaten" appearance of the lesion within the bone. Aggressive periosteal reaction is also present, featuring layers of "onionskin" appearing periosteal new bone formation as the soft tissue mass extends from the underlying bone. (**c**) An axial post-gadolinium T1 fat-saturated MRI image of the same patient demonstrates the large soft tissue component extending from the underlying diaphysis with cortical enhancement and bony destruction as well as surrounding peri-tumoral soft tissue enhancement

with a hypocellular fibrous sheath. Patchy necrosis is frequent in Ewing sarcoma, typically sparing tumor cells adjacent to vessels, and dystrophic calcifications can be seen in areas of necrosis. The tumor cells often show indistinct cell borders and a small amount of foamy cytoplasm (Figs. 2.34 and 2.35). Immunohistochemical staining for CD99 frequently demonstrates membranous staining (Fig. 2.36), and markers of neuroectodermal differentiation such as synaptophysin and neuron-specific enolase show varying degrees of reactivity (Tsokos et al. 2012). Of note, membranous CD99 reactivity is a typical feature of Ewing sarcoma, yet this pattern should not be regarded as diagnostic. Membranous CD99 reactivity is seen in many other tumor types, including synovial sarcoma and lymphomas.

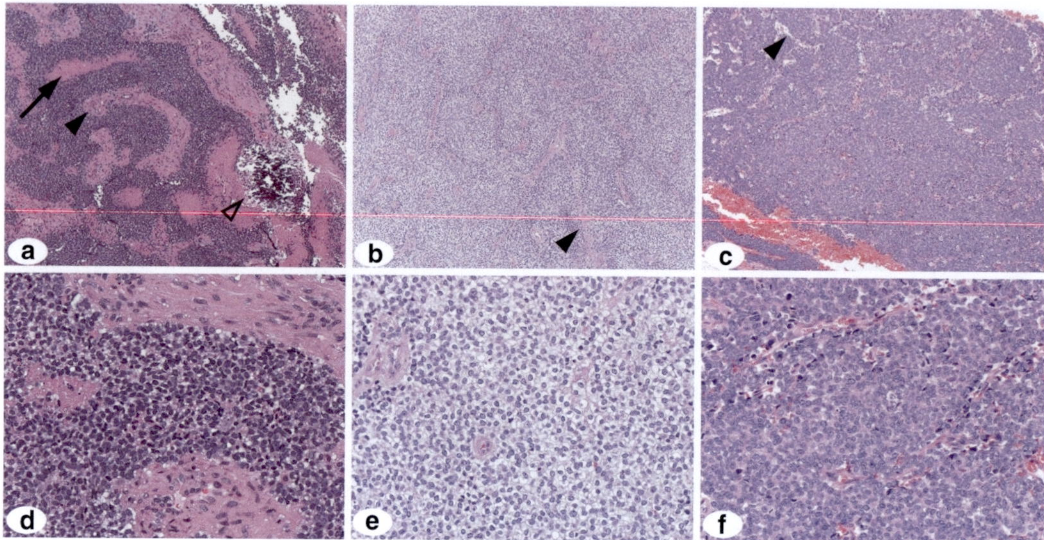

Fig. 2.34 Histologic features of Ewing sarcoma. Ewing sarcoma can display a spectrum of architectural and cytologic features. Ewing sarcoma most often grows in sheets, with occasional calcifications (**a** *empty arrow head*) and patchy areas of necrosis (**a** *arrow*). The vessels within the tumor can range from thick-walled vessels (**a** *arrowhead*) to thin-walled or delicate sinusoidal-like vessels (**b, c** *arrowheads*). Cells with round, monotonous nuclei and scant cytoplasm are characteristic of Ewing sarcoma. The cytoplasm contains variable amounts of glycogen, typically producing a foamy appearance with indistinct cell boarders (**d**); however, completely clear cytoplasm (**e**) or solidly eosinophilic (**f**) can also be seen

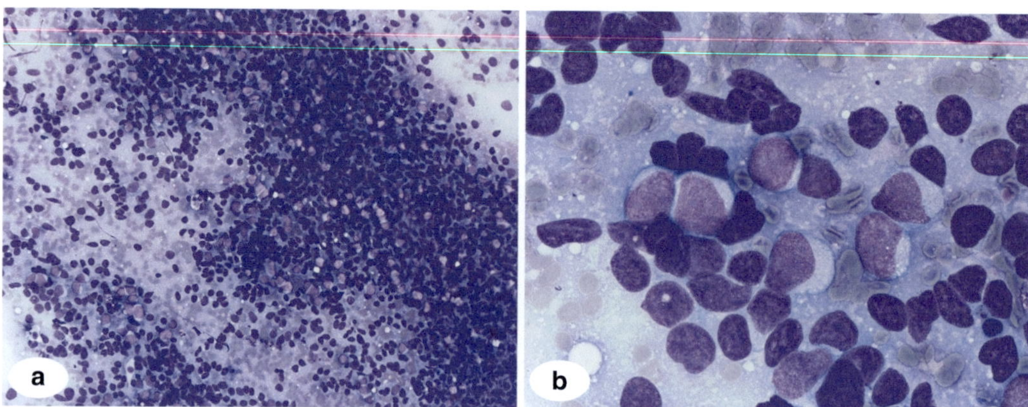

Fig. 2.35 Ewing sarcoma in aspirate smears and touch preparations. Smear and touch preparations of Ewing sarcoma typically contain cohesive clusters of cells in three-dimensional clusters (**a**). Individual tumor cells are often stripped of their cytoplasm, with occasional cells retaining their foamy cytoplasm (**b**)

Post-therapy Ewing sarcoma and osteosarcoma resection specimens require careful mapping to determine the percentage of viable tumor; several studies have identified necrosis in response to neoadjuvant therapy as predictor of patient outcome (Bacci et al. 2005; Daugaard et al. 1989; Delepine et al. 1997; Picci et al. 1997; Rosito et al. 1999). Margins should be inked, and bone margins removed prior to sawing the specimen into slabs. Orientation of the specimen should be noted and identified throughout handling to allow measurements from the gross tumor to the nearest margins and sampling of the margins for histologic sections. A central slab from the tumor should be mapped and submitted for microscopic examination to determine the percentage of viable tumor (Fig. 2.37).

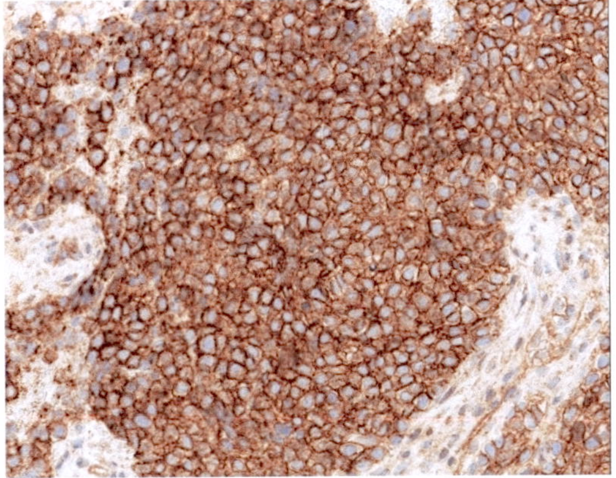

Fig. 2.36 Immunohistochemical staining for CD99 in Ewing sarcoma. CD99 reactivity in Ewing sarcoma typically demonstrates a strong, diffuse membranous pattern. This pattern is frequent in Ewing sarcoma; however, it is not specific to Ewing sarcoma

2.4.2   Langerhans Cell Histiocytosis Versus Chronic Osteomyelitis

Langerhans cell histiocytosis, as discussed in the previous section, can occur in many different bones and in all locations in long bones, most often within the metaphysis and diaphysis. Given that LCH can have a varied radiographic appearance from benign to aggressive, as can osteomyelitis, LCH and chronic infection involving the diaphyseal medullary bone can show overlapping radiographic features. Both may demonstrate an aggressive lytic lesion with surrounding periosteal reaction (Fig. 2.38). The histologic features can also show significant overlap, with mixed inflammatory cells including eosinophils and histiocytes (compare Figs. 2.39 and 2.40). The distinctive bean-shaped nuclei of LCH and reactivity for specific immunohistochemical markers such as CD1a, S-100, and Langerin can provide important clues to the correct diagnosis (Fig. 2.41) (Chikwava and Jaffe 2004; Geissmann et al. 2001; Nakajima et al. 1982). Microbiologic cultures of the bone lesion may identify the causative organism of a chronic infection (Akinyoola et al. 2009; White et al. 1995).

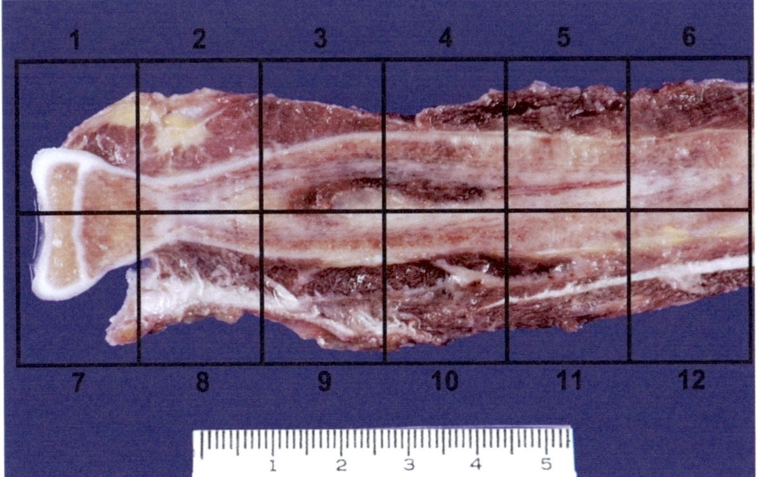

Fig. 2.37 Specimen mapping of Ewing sarcoma and osteosarcoma resection specimens. The percentage of tumor necrosis should be determined in resected sarcoma specimens following neoadjuvant chemotherapy. A central slab of the tumor should be mapped and submitted for histologic examination

Fig. 2.38 Langerhans cell histiocytosis mimicking osteomyelitis. Anterior-posterior radiographs of this femur initially demonstrated a lytic lesion within the proximal femoral diaphysis with surrounding "onionskin" periosteal reaction showing concentric layers (**a**). A follow-up radiograph (**b**) demonstrates progressive enlargement of destructive lytic lesion with ongoing periosteal reaction. Osteomyelitis can have a similar radiographic appearance

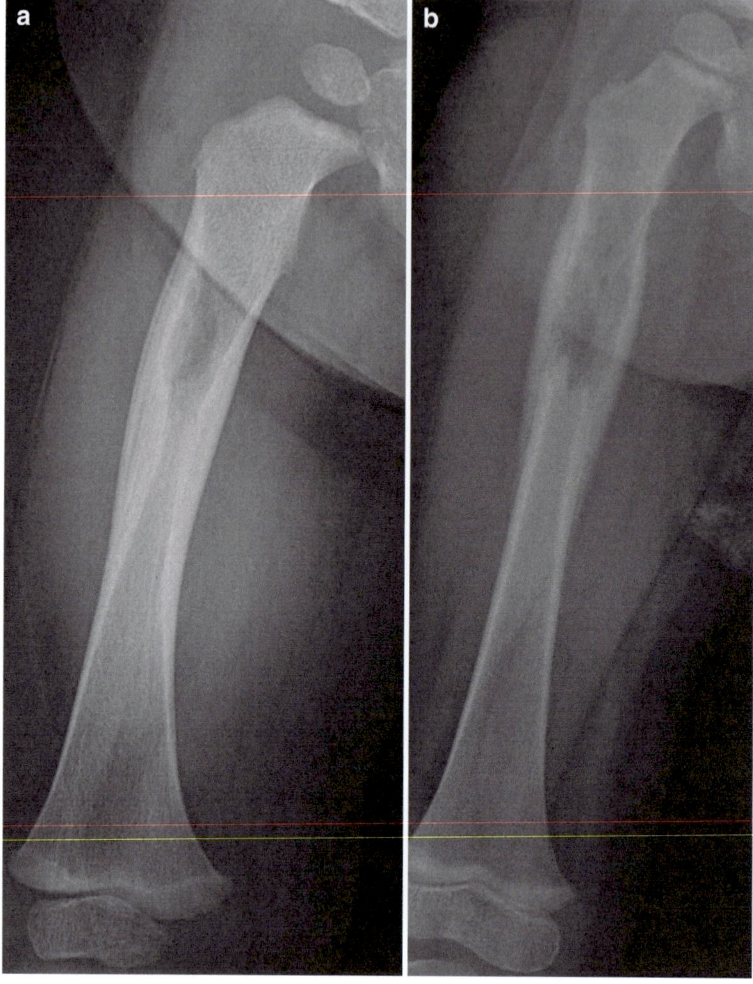

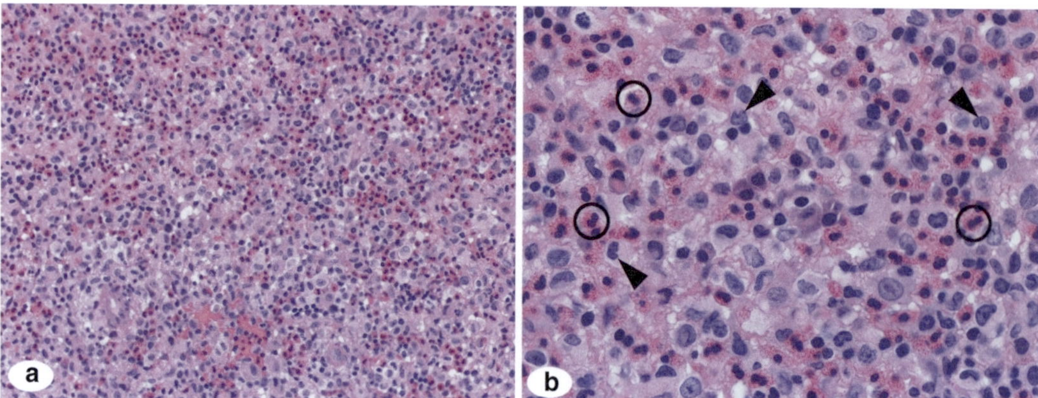

Fig. 2.39 Histologic features of Langerhans cell histiocytosis. Langerhans cell histiocytosis is characterized by an infiltrate of abnormal histiocytes and associated inflammatory cells (**a**). High magnification (**b**) demonstrates the irregular often "bean-shaped" contours of the abnormal histiocyte nuclei (*arrowheads*) and the many associated eosinophils (*circles*)

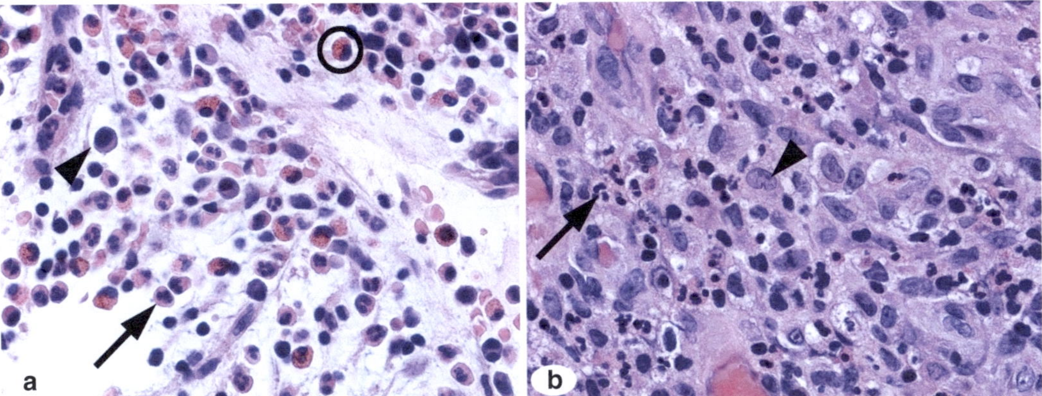

Fig. 2.40 Histologic features of chronic osteomyelitis. Chronic osteomyelitis can contain many inflammatory cell types in varying proportions. These examples show inflammation containing eosinophils (**a** *circle*), neutrophils (**a**, **b** *arrows*), plasma cells (**a** *arrowhead*), and histiocytes (**b** *arrowhead*). Note that the reactive histiocytes seen in chronic osteomyelitis show predominantly rounded nuclear contours with occasional irregularity

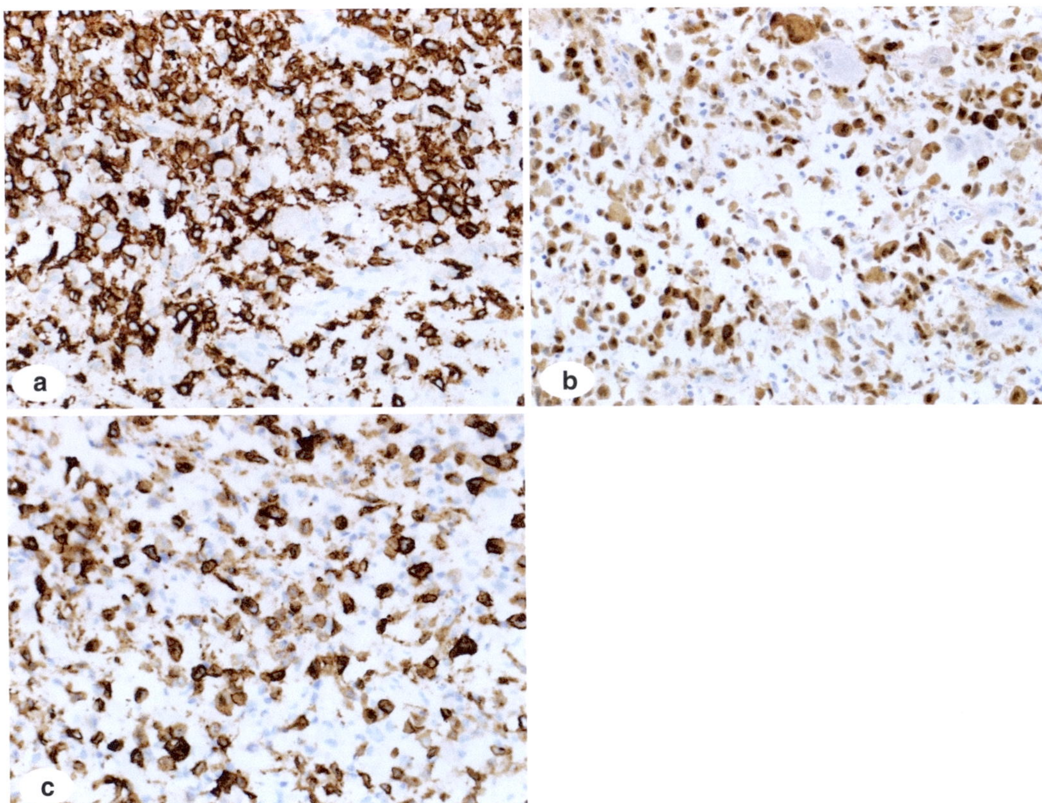

Fig. 2.41 Immunohistochemical features of Langerhans cell histiocytosis. The abnormal histiocytes of LCH are reactive for CD1a (**a** 40× objective magnification), S-100 (**b** 40× objective magnification) and Langerin (**c** 40× objective magnification)

2.4.3 Periosteal Osteosarcoma

Periosteal osteosarcoma has a predilection for the diaphyseal region of long bones unlike parosteal osteosarcoma, which commonly affects the metaphysis. Periosteal osteosarcoma predominantly affects the femur or tibia, and less often the humerus, radius, ulna, and pelvis (Fig. 2.42). Histologically, it is composed of lobules of cartilage exhibiting cytologic atypia with areas of osteoid matrix production and mineralization (Unni et al. 1976). The principal differential diagnosis includes periosteal chondrosarcoma or chondroma especially in core biopsy specimens. In these instances, integrating the radiologic characteristics of the lesion and the histology is critical to establishing the correct diagnosis.

2.4.4 Osteoid Osteoma and Osteoblastoma

Osteoid osteoma and osteoblastoma represent a spectrum of benign lesions distinguished by their size; osteoblastomas are currently classified as lesions 1.5 cm or larger, and smaller lesions are designated osteoid osteomas (Atesok et al. 2011). These lesions often present with nocturnal pain that is classically relieved by NSAIDs, due to inhibition of prostaglandin production (Byers 1968; Makley and Dunn 1982). Most lesions occur in the long bones of the lower extremities, though any bone can be affected (Byers 1968). The most common location of osteoid osteoma is the femur, and more often the femoral neck, with the tibia the next most common bone. They occur less frequently in the upper extremities, but when they do, they can affect the tubular bones of the hands. Less commonly they may affect the spine, where they often occur in the posterior vertebral arch. Imaging studies of these lesions can demonstrate highly characteristic features of a central nidus that is usually surrounded by dense sclerotic bone. The nidus may be entirely radiolucent or contain a central density within the radiolucent nidus. This finding is characteristic, and many lesions may be treated without a biopsy when findings correlate with clinical and physical exam findings. However,

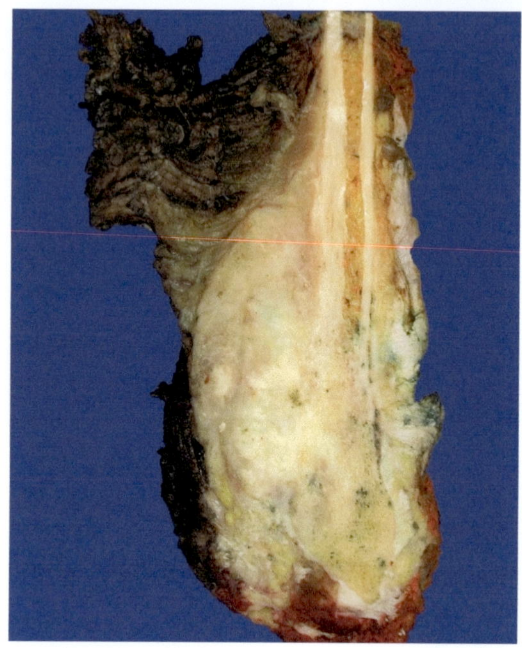

Fig. 2.42 Gross appearance of periosteal osteosarcoma. This periosteal osteosarcoma involving the metadiaphysis on the periosteal surface of the distal fibula shows a gray-tan cut surface

the characteristic central nidus can often be masked by the significant surrounding reactive sclerosis on radiography (Fig. 2.43), and cross-section CT imaging may be needed for diagnosis, which can often adequately demonstrate the characteristic findings (Fig. 2.43). Additionally, osteoid osteomas can demonstrate adjacent periosteal reaction and can mimic other lesions on radiography (Fig. 2.44). CT imaging often can demonstrate the characteristic findings (Fig. 2.44c). When biopsied, osteoid osteoma and osteoblastoma show similar histologic features. The central nidus is composed of vascular tissue with a network of osteoid (Green and Mills 2014), and the surrounding tissue contains woven bone and associated fibrous tissue (Fig. 2.45).

2.4.5 Nonossifying Fibroma

Nonossifying fibroma (NOF) is a benign fibrohistiocytic lesion with a sprinkling of osteoclast-type giant cells. The term metaphyseal fibrous

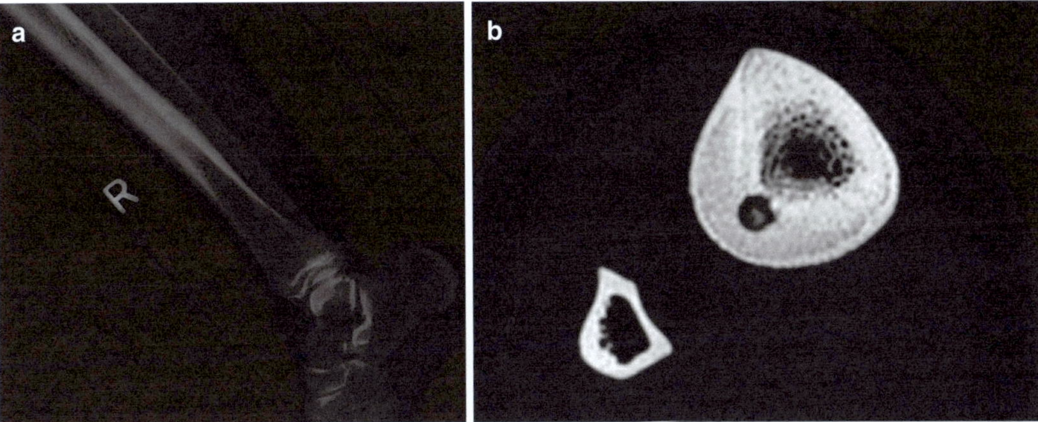

Fig. 2.43 Radiographic features of osteoid osteoma. (**a**) A lateral radiograph of the distal tibia and ankle demonstrates fusiform cortical thickening involving the posterior cortex of the distal tibial diaphysis with the suggestion of central radiolucency. These findings can overlap with stress fracture, and given clinical concern for osteoid oste- oma, CT was performed. (**b**) Axial CT image of the lower extremity centered at the tibial lesion demonstrates the cortical lesion within the tibial diaphysis demonstrates characteristic findings of an osteoid osteoma showing a radiolucent nidus with small central density surrounded by dense sclerotic bone

defect is used when the lesion is cortically based and NOF when there is medullary involvement. This lesion is histologically indistinguishable from benign fibrous histiocytoma which by defi- nition is typically diaphyseal in location (Fletcher et al. 2013). Histologically, it is composed of bland spindle cells in storiform arrays with asso- ciated osteoclast-type giant cells (Fig. 2.46). On occasion xanthomatous areas as well as hemosiderin-laden macrophages could be seen. This pattern could mimic fibrohistiocytic areas in a giant cell tumor and in fact may be histologi- cally indistinguishable.

2.4.6 Fibrous Dysplasia

Fibrous dysplasia is not a true neoplasm, although it can mimic a bone tumor or a bone cyst, espe- cially when it is unifocal and causes localized expansion of the bone. Any bone may be affected; however, most commonly it affects the craniofa- cial bones (often the skull base), rib, or long bones (most often the femur). Fibrous dysplasia is more often monostotic although it can be poly- ostotic, especially in the setting of McCune- Albright and Mazabraud syndromes (Fletcher et al. 2013; Ippolito et al. 2003). Lesions may be

metaphyseal, diaphyseal, or spanning both regions and will spare the epiphysis before phy- seal fusion. Radiographically, fibrous dysplasia in long bones causes expansion of the medullary cavity with endosteal scalloping, however, with- out bone destruction or periosteal reaction, bar- ring pathologic fracture. The lesions may demonstrate coarse trabeculation and a thin scle- rotic margin, forming a sclerotic "rind" about the lesion. Bowing of the affected bone may also occur. Within the lesion itself, fibrous dysplasia typically ranges from radiolucent to a "ground glass" appearance depending on the density of internal matrix (Fig. 2.47).

Fibrous dysplasia can result in a significant mass, yet with a distinct boundary from the sur- rounding native lamella bone (Fig. 2.48). Sharp circumscription is an important observation, as it helps to distinguish fibrous dysplasia from cen- tral low-grade osteogenic sarcoma which can have a "fibrous dysplasia-like" morphology and prominent gross and microscopic infiltration into surrounding normal bone. Histologically, fibrous dysplasia consists of a proliferation of irregular bone trabeculae and bland spindle cells without cellular atypia. The absence of osteoblastic rim- ming helps to distinguish it from another histo- logic mimic, osteofibrous dysplasia (Fig. 2.49).

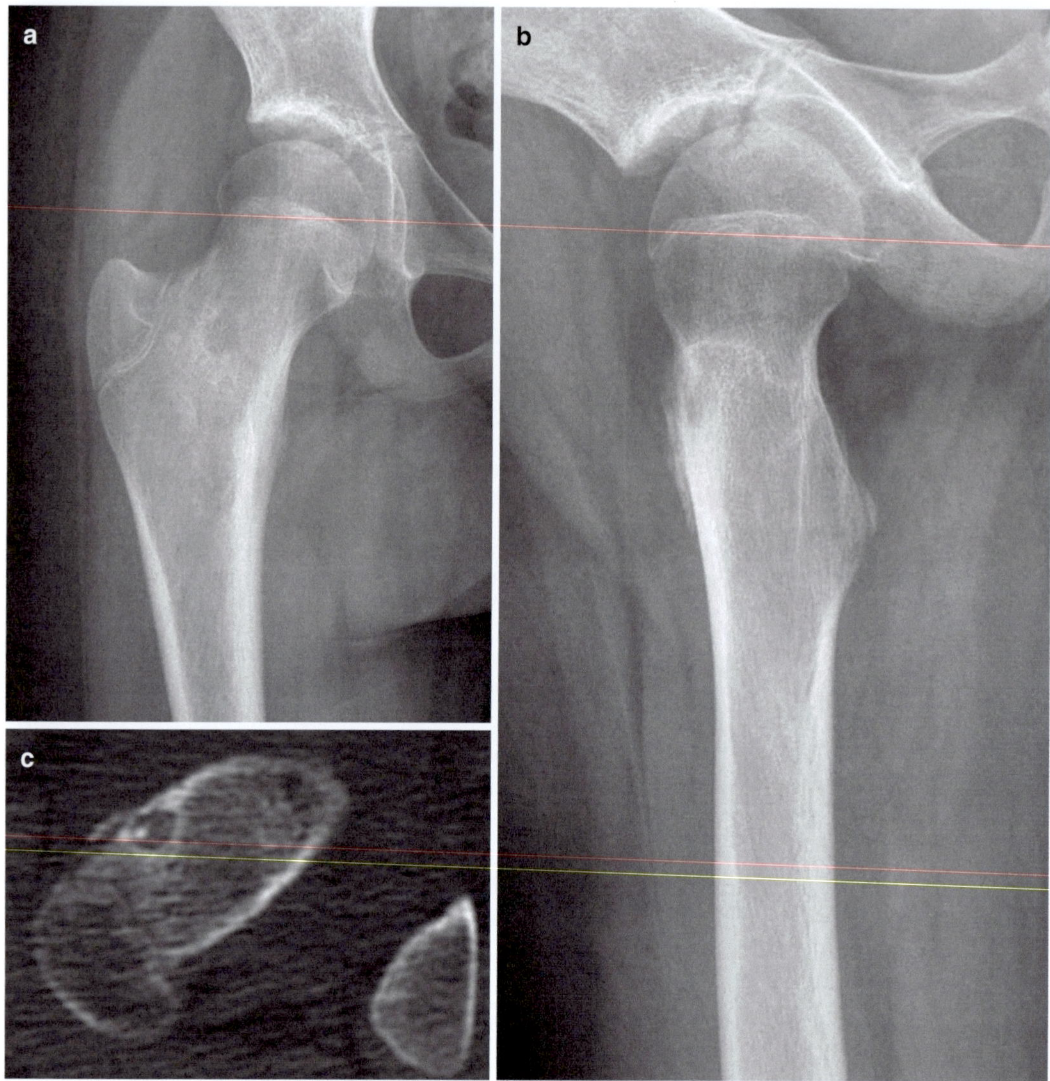

Fig. 2.44 Radiographic features of osteoid osteoma with periosteal reaction. (**a**, **b**) Anterior-posterior (**a**) and lateral (**b**) views of the proximal femur demonstrate a lucent lesion with surrounding sclerosis and adjacent periosteal reaction within the femoral neck. Other lesions, including LCH and infection, could have a similar appearance. (**c**) CT imaging of this same lesion demonstrates characteristic findings of osteoid osteoma. An axial CT image of the femoral neck centered at the lesion shows characteristic findings of an osteoid osteoma with a radiolucent nidus and small central density surrounded by sclerotic bone

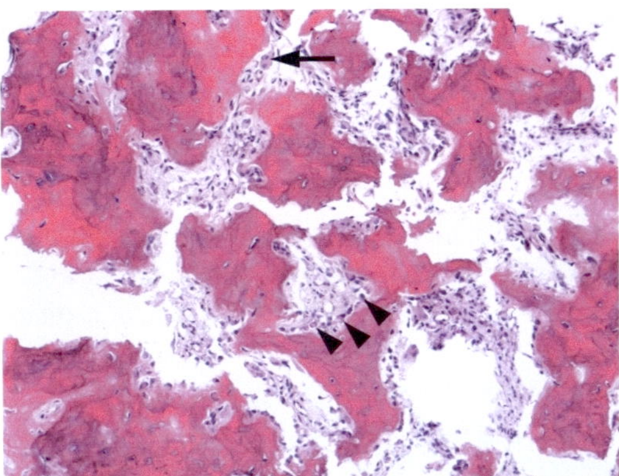

Fig. 2.45 Histologic features of osteoid osteoma and osteoblastoma. Osteoid osteoma and osteoblastoma show identical histologic features. The area surrounding the nidus represents the majority of the lesion and is composed of irregular woven bone with associated fibrovascular tissue. The woven bone is lined by osteoblasts (*arrowheads*) and occasional osteoclasts (*arrow*)

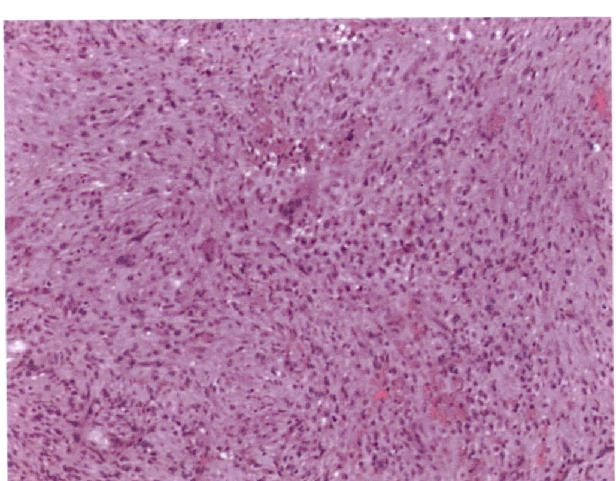

Fig. 2.46 Histologic features of nonossifying fibroma. Nonossifying fibroma is composed of bland spindle cells arranged in storiform arrays with occasional multinucleated cells present

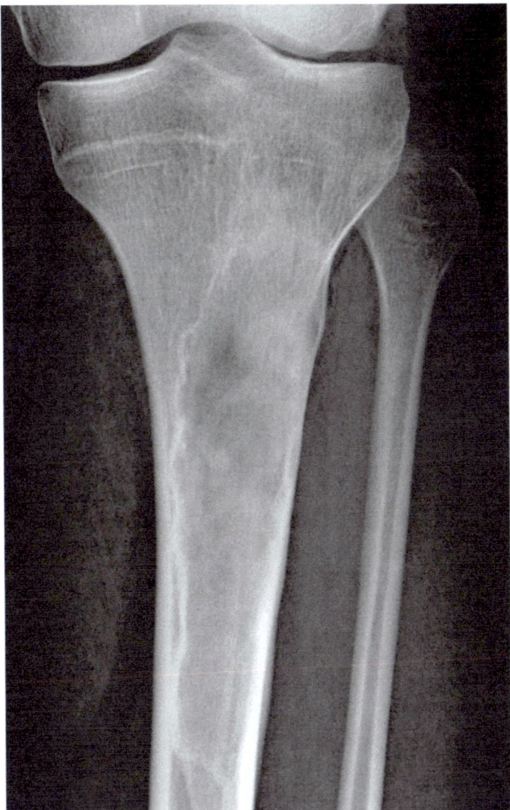

Fig. 2.47 Radiographic features of fibrous dysplasia. An anterior-posterior radiograph of the proximal tibia demonstrates a benign appearing slightly expansile lesion within the proximal tibia extending from the metaphysis into the diaphysis. The lesion demonstrates a "ground glass" appearance, with endosteal scalloping and a thin sclerotic border forming a "rind" about the lesion as well as mild lateral bowing of the diaphysis; all characteristic features of fibrous dysplasia

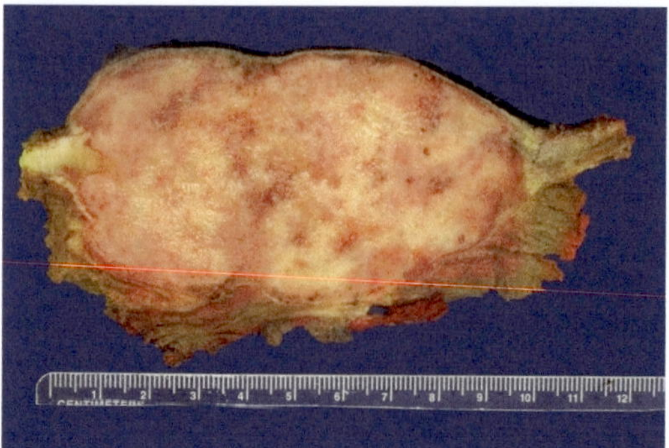

Fig. 2.48 Gross appearance of fibrous dysplasia. This example of fibrous dysplasia involving the rib shows an expansile mass with a gray-tan fibrous cut surface. Note the sharp circumscription from the surrounding bone

2.4.7 Adamantinoma Versus Osteofibrous Dysplasia

Adamantinoma is a rare malignancy with a predilection for the tibial diaphysis and less often the fibula. In radiographs, adamantinoma appears as an expansile mass with mixed lytic and sclerotic features (Fig. 2.50). Adamantinoma is a histologically distinct biphasic low-grade malignant tumor with two histologic types: classic adamantinoma and osteofibrous dysplasia-like (differentiated) adamantinoma (Fletcher et al. 2013). The classic type can exhibit four different phenotypes: (1) basaloid, (2) tubular, (3) spindle, and

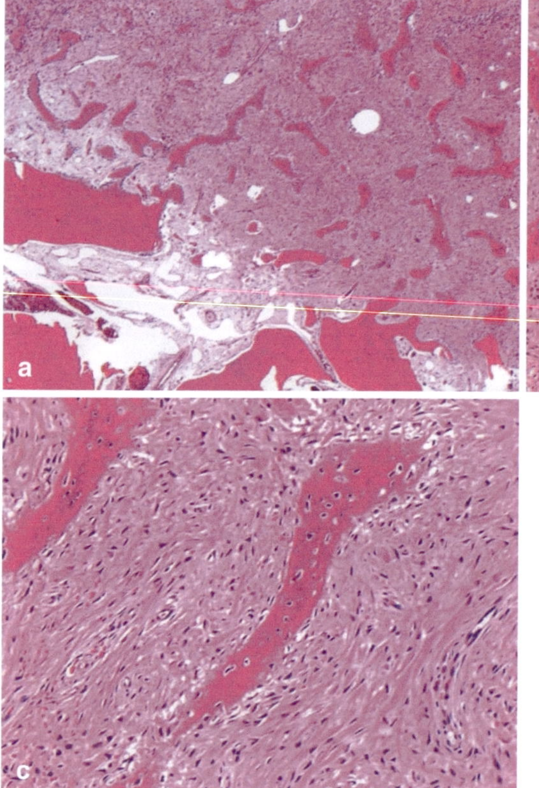

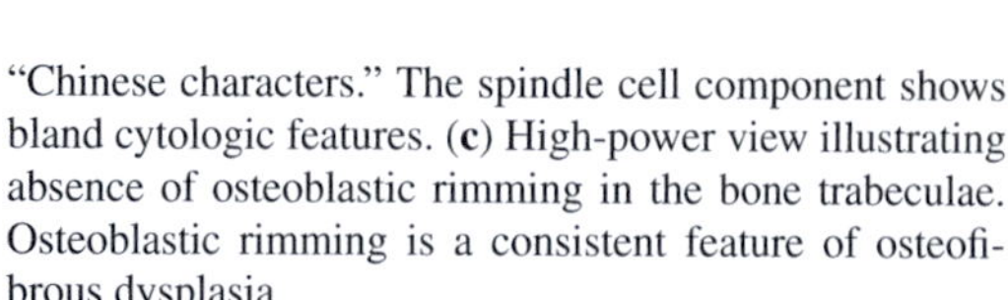

Fig. 2.49 Histologic features of fibrous dysplasia. (**a**) Low-power showing a proliferation of woven bone and spindle cells. The process is localized and does not invade surrounding larger native trabeculae in the lower left. (**b**) Irregular woven bone trabecular sometimes compared to "Chinese characters." The spindle cell component shows bland cytologic features. (**c**) High-power view illustrating absence of osteoblastic rimming in the bone trabeculae. Osteoblastic rimming is a consistent feature of osteofibrous dysplasia

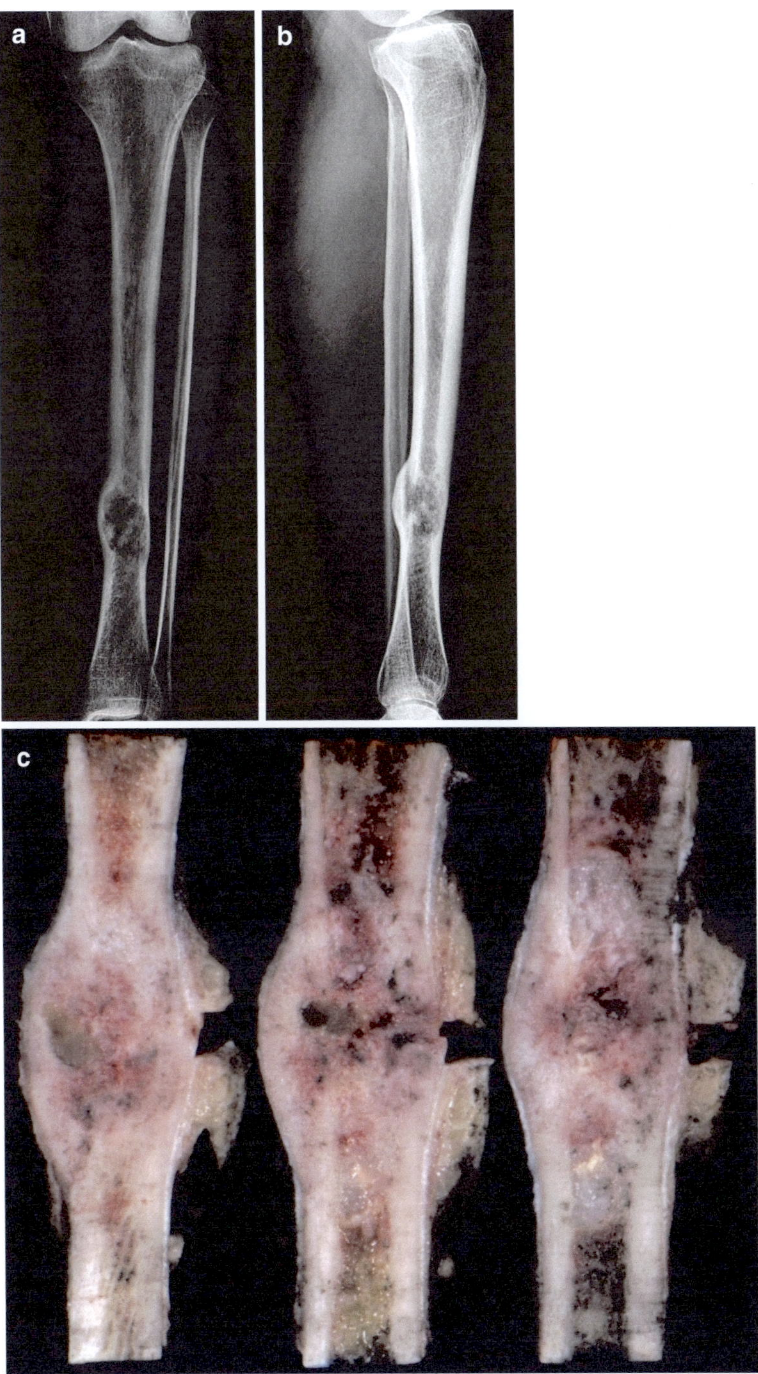

Fig. 2.50 Radiographic and gross features of adamantinoma. (**a**, **b**) This adamantinoma of the left tibia, seen in anterior-posterior (**a**) and lateral (**b**) radiographs, shows an expansile mixed lucent and sclerotic lesion involving the medullary cavity of the distal diaphysis of the left tibia. (**c**) Gross image showing a cut surface with variable solid gray-tan areas

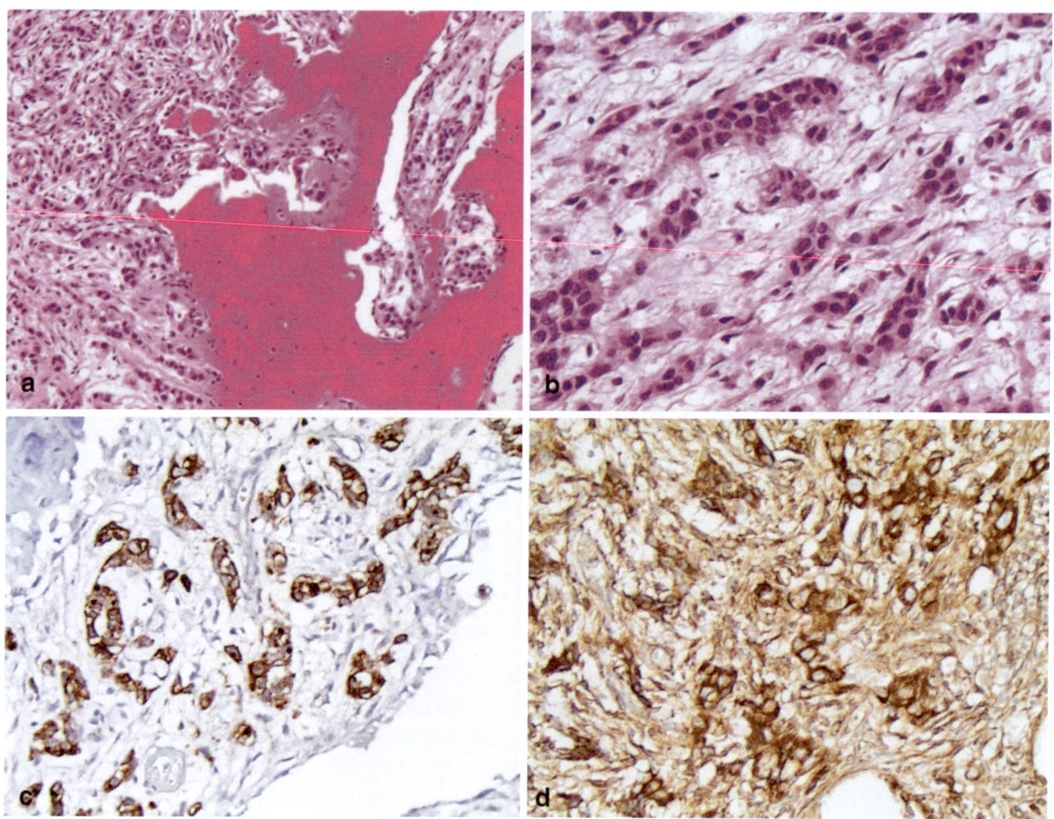

Fig. 2.51 Histologic features of adamantinoma. (**a, b**) Histologic sections showing malignant epithelial cells arrayed in a tubular pattern invading lamellar bone. (**c**) Cytokeratin AE1/AE3 staining shows diffuse cytokeratin reactivity limited to the epithelial cells. (**d**) Vimentin-staining highlights both the epithelial and mesenchymal components

(4) squamous. Usually, most tumors show variable combinations of different phenotypes (Fletcher et al. 2013). The basaloid pattern bears a striking resemblance to ameloblastoma of the jaw and consists of nests of epithelioid cells with peripheral palisading. The tubular phenotype consists of nests of epithelial cells forming tubular structures arrayed in a fibrotic stroma (Fig. 2.51). The spindle cell pattern can mimic a spindle cell sarcoma with cellular sweeping fascicles but typically lack the peripheral palisading seen in the basaloid pattern. The squamous pattern is often seen in the background of basaloid histomorphology with keratin pearls that can mimic squamous cell carcinoma.

Immunohistochemically, the epithelial cells express cytokeratin (particularly the basal type CK7, CK14, and CK19), vimentin, epithelial membrane antigen, p63, and podoplanin (D2-40) (Fig. 2.51) (Benassi et al. 1994; Czerniak et al. 1989; Dickson et al. 2011; Fletcher et al. 2013; Kashima et al. 2011; Sweet et al. 1992). Recurrent chromosomal abnormalities involving chromosomes 7, 8, 12, 19, and 21 have been described similar to osteofibrous dysplasia, suggesting possible histogenetic relationship (Bridge et al. 1994).

Osteofibrous dysplasia (OFD) is a rare lesion with a predilection for the tibia and fibula with significant radiographic overlap with adamantinoma. It occurs most commonly in the first two decades of life and on occasion at birth (Most et al. 2010). Clinically, patients present with swelling, anterior deformity, or pain especially if

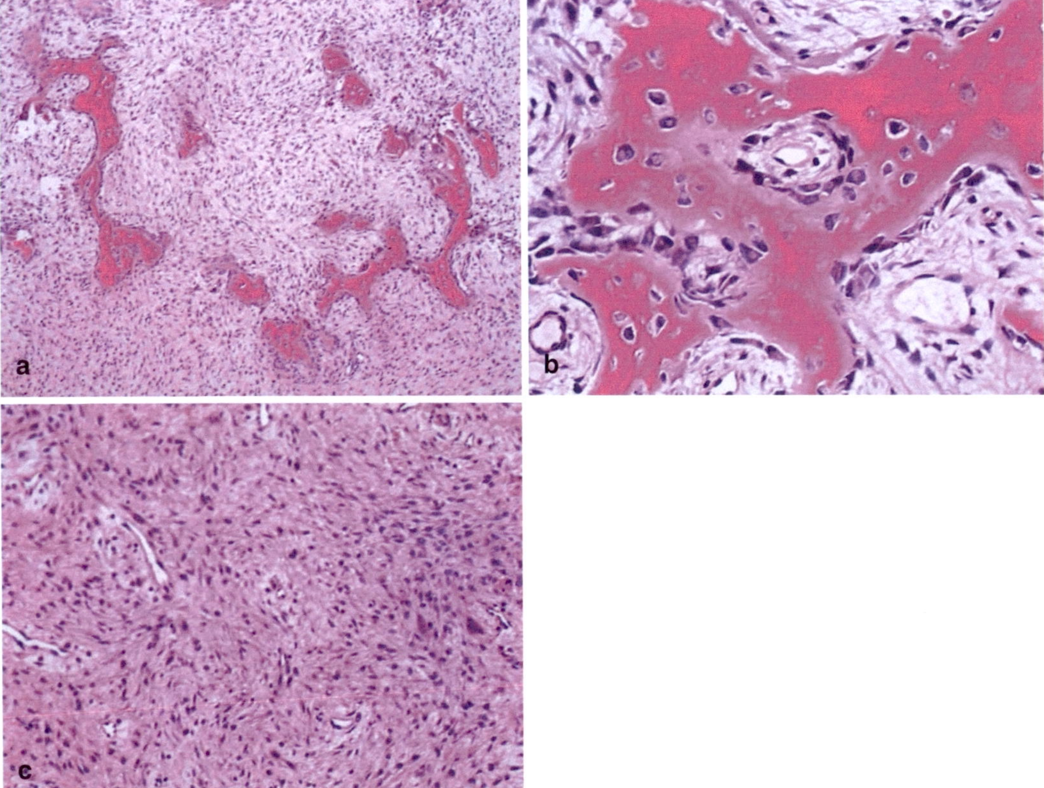

Fig. 2.52 Histologic features of osteofibrous dysplasia. (**a**) Osteofibrous dysplasia is characterized by bony trabeculae within a fibrous stroma. Epithelial nests are absent. (**b**) Bony trabeculae show prominent osteoblastic rimming, characteristic of osteofibrous dysplasia. (**c**) The fibrous component of osteofibrous dysplasia shows bland spindle cells in vague storiform arrays. No mitotic figures or cellular atypia are present

there is associated fracture. The radiologic appearance is usually nonaggressive and composed of multiloculated radiolucent expansion of the diaphyseal anterolateral cortex which may sometimes involve the medullary cavity but not soft tissue. The natural history of OFD is principally slow growth and eventual stabilization on attainment of skeletal maturity.

Grossly, OFD is a heterogeneous intracortical lesion composed of gritty white-yellow tissue. Histologic sections typical show bony trabeculae rimmed by osteoblasts with intervening fibrous tissue (Figs. 2.52 and 2.53). Osteoblastic rimming of bony trabeculae is a key feature that distinguishes OFD from fibrous dysplasia and location of the lesion combined with the presence of osteoblastic rimming facilitates prompt distinction of these lesions. By definition, discernible nests of epithelial cells are absent in OFD, distinguishing it from classic or differentiated adamantinoma. Immunohistochemical studies have demonstrated the presence of cytokeratin-positive cells in OFD (Benassi et al. 1994; Sweet et al. 1992) and cytogenetic studies have shown trisomies of chromosomes 7, 8, 9, and 12, suggesting that OFD may represent a clonal precursor of adamantinoma (Bridge et al. 1994) (Fig. 2.44).

The principal histologic differential diagnosis of OFD is osteofibrous dysplasia-like or differentiated adamantinoma. This can be especially challenging as both lesions share similar demographics, distribution, and radiographic and histologic features (Fig. 2.54). Osteofibrous

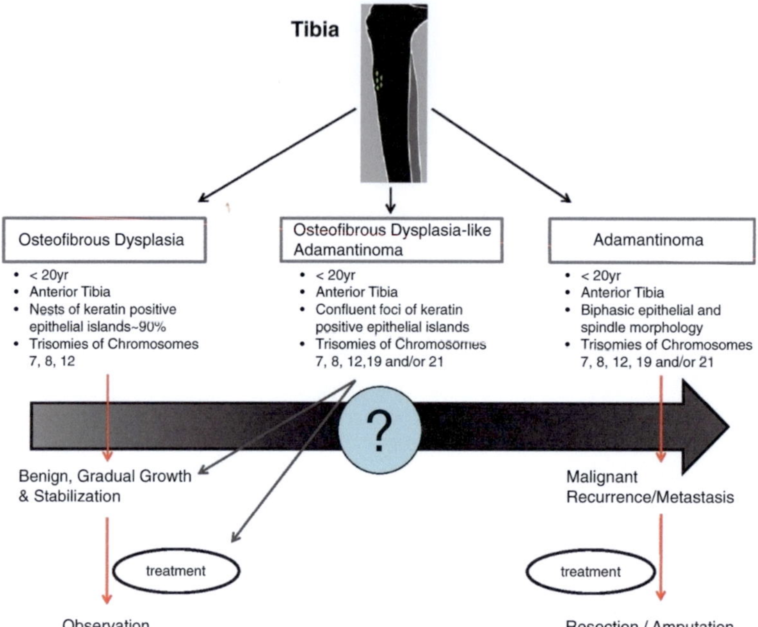

Fig. 2.53 A summary of the possible relationship between OFD, OFD-like adamantinoma and classic adamantinoma

dysplasia-like adamantinoma is a rare or poorly understood variant of adamantinoma that is characterized by OFD features with that nests of epithelial cells are seen present in a stroma similar to OFD (Fig. 2.55). Czerniak et al. believe this variant to represent a regressing form of classic adamantinoma (Czerniak et al. 1989). However, this variant is not known to metastasize. OFD-like adamantinoma closely mimics OFD, with the exception of nests of epithelial cells. By immunohistochemistry, confluent areas of cytokeratin-positive cells are easily demonstrated, much more extensively than the small nests of cytokeratin cells in OFD (Fig. 2.55).

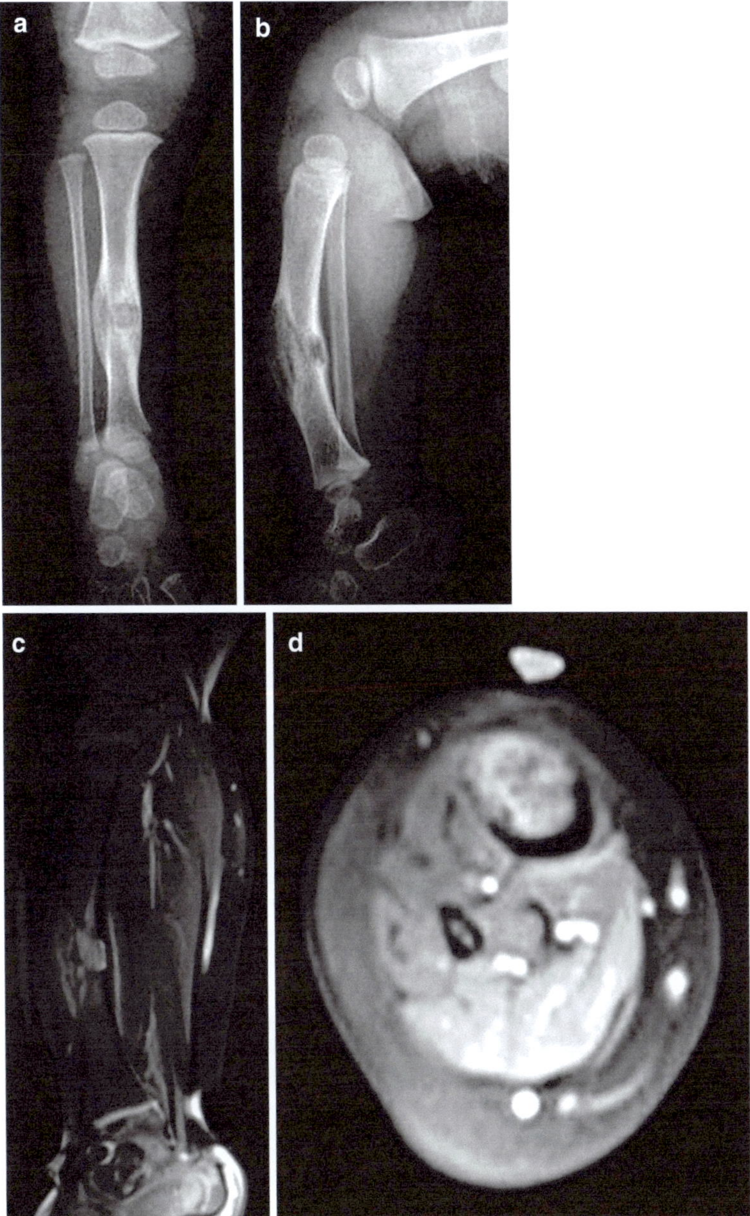

Fig. 2.54 Radiographic features of osteofibrous dysplasia-like adamantinoma. (**a**, **b**) Anterior-posterior (**a**) and lateral (**b**) and radiographs of the right tibia in this 13-month-old male show an expansile geographic v-shaped cortically based lesion in the diaphysis of the tibia with medullary involvement. (**c**, **d**) Post-contrast fat-saturated sagittal (**c**) and axial (**d**) views show a uniformly enhancing nonaggressive solid lesion centered in the cortex with medullary involvement

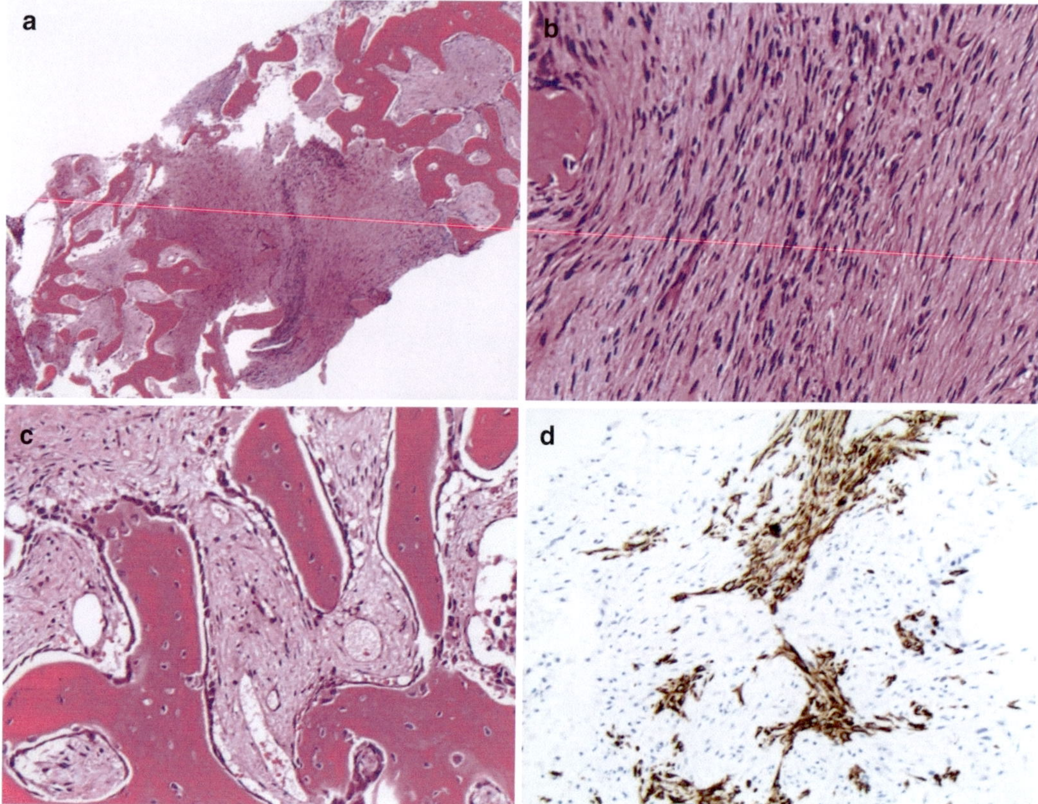

Fig. 2.55 Histologic features of osteofibrous dysplasia-like adamantinoma. (**a**) Histologic sections of osteofibrous dysplasia-like adamantinoma show a central cellular spindle cell proliferation with bony trabeculae. (**b**) Hyperchromasia of the spindle cells but without epithelial clusters are discernible on H&E sections. (**c**) Prominent osteoblastic rimming of the woven bone trabeculae. (**d**) Immunoperoxidase stain for cytokeratin AE1/AE3 shows confluent area of cytokeratin-positive cells

References

Akinyoola AL, Adegbehingbe OO, Aboderin AO (2009) Therapeutic decision in chronic osteomyelitis: sinus track culture versus intraoperative bone culture. Arch Orthop Trauma Surg 129(4):449–453. doi:10.1007/s00402-008-0621-y [Comparative Study]

Atesok KI, Alman BA, Schemitsch EH, Peyser A, Mankin H (2011) Osteoid osteoma and osteoblastoma. J Am Acad Orthop Surg 19(11):678–689 [Review]

Ayala AG, Ro JY, Raymond AK, Jaffe N, Chawla S, Carrasco H et al (1989) Small cell osteosarcoma. A clinicopathologic study of 27 cases. Cancer 64(10):2162–2173

Bacci G, Mercuri M, Longhi A, Ferrari S, Bertoni F, Versari M, Picci P (2005) Grade of chemotherapy-induced necrosis as a predictor of local and systemic control in 881 patients with non-metastatic osteosarcoma of the extremities treated with neoadjuvant chemotherapy in a single institution. Eur J Cancer 41(14):2079–2085. doi:10.1016/j.ejca.2005.03.036

Badalian-Very G, Vergilio JA, Fleming M, Rollins BJ (2013) Pathogenesis of Langerhans cell histiocytosis. Annu Rev Pathol 8:1–20. doi:10.1146/annurev-pathol-020712-163959 [Research Support, Non-U.S. Gov't Review]

Benassi MS, Campanacci L, Gamberi G, Ferrari C, Picci P, Sangiorgi L, Campanacci M (1994) Cytokeratin expression and distribution in adamantinoma of the long bones and osteofibrous dysplasia of tibia and fibula. An immunohistochemical study correlated to histogenesis. Histopathology 25(1):71–76

Borys D, Canter RJ, Hoch B, Martinez SR, Tamurian RM, Murphy B, Horvai A (2012) P16 expression predicts necrotic response among patients with osteosarcoma receiving neoadjuvant chemotherapy. Hum Pathol 43(11):1948–1954. doi:10.1016/j.humpath.2012.02.003 [Multicenter Study]

Bridge JA, Dembinski A, DeBoer J, Travis J, Neff JR (1994) Clonal chromosomal abnormalities in osteofibrous dysplasia. Implications for histopathogenesis and its relationship with adamantinoma. Cancer 73(6):1746–1752 [Case Reports Research Support, Non-U.S. Gov't]

Byers PD (1968) Solitary benign osteoblastic lesions of bone. Osteoid osteoma and benign osteoblastoma. Cancer 22(1):43–57

Chikwava K, Jaffe R (2004) Langerin (CD207) staining in normal pediatric tissues, reactive lymph nodes, and childhood histiocytic disorders. Pediatr Dev Pathol 7(6):607–614. doi:10.1007/s10024-004-3027-z [Comparative Study Research Support, Non-U.S. Gov't]

Conner JR, Hornick JL (2013) SATB2 is a novel marker of osteoblastic differentiation in bone and soft tissue tumours. Histopathology 63(1):36–49. doi:10.1111/his.12138

Czerniak B, Rojas-Corona RR, Dorfman HD (1989) Morphologic diversity of long bone adamantinoma. The concept of differentiated (regressing) adamantinoma and its relationship to osteofibrous dysplasia. Cancer 64(11):2319–2334

Daugaard S, Kamby C, Sunde LM, Myhre-Jensen O, Schiodt T (1989) Ewing's sarcoma. A retrospective study of histological and immunohistochemical factors and their relation to prognosis. Virchows Arch A Pathol Anat Histopathol 414(3):243–251

de la Roza G (2011) p63 expression in giant cell-containing lesions of bone and soft tissue. Arch Pathol Lab Med 135(6):776–779. doi:10.1043/2010-0291-OA.1

Debelenko LV, McGregor LM, Shivakumar BR, Dorfman HD, Raimondi SC (2011) A novel EWSR1-CREB3L1 fusion transcript in a case of small cell osteosarcoma. Genes Chromosomes Cancer 50(12):1054–1062. doi:10.1002/gcc.20923 [Case Reports Research Support, Non-U.S. Gov't]

Delepine N, Delepine G, Cornille H, Voisin MC, Brun B, Desbois JC (1997) Prognostic factors in patients with localized Ewing's sarcoma: the effect on survival of actual received drug dose intensity and of histologic response to induction therapy. J Chemother 9(5):352–363. doi:10.1179/joc.1997.9.5.352 [Clinical Trial]

Devaney K, Vinh TN, Sweet DE (1993) Small cell osteosarcoma of bone: an immunohistochemical study with differential diagnostic considerations. Hum Pathol 24(11):1211–1225

Diamond EL, Dagna L, Hyman DM, Cavalli G, Janku F, Estrada-Veras J, Haroche J (2014) Consensus guidelines for the diagnosis and clinical management of Erdheim-Chester disease. Blood 124(4):483–492. doi:10.1182/blood-2014-03-561381 [Review]

Dickson BC, Li SQ, Wunder JS, Ferguson PC, Eslami B, Werier JA, Kandel RA (2008) Giant cell tumor of bone express p63. Mod Pathol 21(4):369–375. doi:10.1038/modpathol.2008.29 [Research Support, Non-U.S. Gov't]

Dickson BC, Gortzak Y, Bell RS, Ferguson PC, Howarth DJ, Wunder JS, Kandel RA (2011) p63 expression in adamantinoma. Virchows Arch 459(1):109–113. doi:10.1007/s00428-011-1101-2

Dragoescu E, Jackson-Cook C, Domson G, Massey D, Foster WC (2013) Small cell osteosarcoma with Ewing sarcoma breakpoint region 1 gene rearrangement detected by interphase fluorescence in situ hybridization. Ann Diagn Pathol 17(4):377–382. doi:10.1016/j.anndiagpath.2012.08.004

Egeler RM, Nesbit ME (1995) Langerhans cell histiocytosis and other disorders of monocyte-histiocyte lineage. Crit Rev Oncol Hematol 18(1):9–35 [Review]

Fletcher CDM, World Health Organization., & International Agency for Research on Cancer (2013) WHO classification of tumours of soft tissue and bone, 4th edn. IARC Press, Lyon

Geissmann F, Lepelletier Y, Fraitag S, Valladeau J, Bodemer C, Debre M, Brousse N (2001) Differentiation of Langerhans cells in Langerhans cell histiocytosis. Blood 97(5):1241–1248 [Research Support, Non-U.S. Gov't]

Green JT, Mills AM (2014) Osteogenic tumors of bone. Semin Diagn Pathol 31(1):21–29. doi:10.1053/j.semdp.2014.01.001 [Review]

Hauben EI, Weeden S, Pringle J, Van Marck EA, Hogendoorn PC (2002) Does the histological subtype of high-grade central osteosarcoma influence the response to treatment with chemotherapy and does it affect overall survival? A study on 570 patients of two consecutive trials of the European Osteosarcoma Intergroup. Eur J Cancer 38(9):1218–1225 [Clinical Trial Randomized Controlled Trial]

Ippolito E, Bray EW, Corsi A, De Maio F, Exner UG, Robey PG, European Pediatric Orthopaedic, S (2003) Natural history and treatment of fibrous dysplasia of bone: a multicenter clinicopathologic study promoted by the European Pediatric Orthopaedic Society. J Pediatr Orthop B 12(3):155–177. doi:10.1097/01.bpb.0000064021.41829.94 [Multicenter Study Research Support, Non-U.S. Gov't]

Kashima TG, Dongre A, Flanagan AM, Hogendoorn PC, Taylor R, Athanasou NA (2011) Podoplanin expression in adamantinoma of long bones and osteofibrous dysplasia. Virchows Arch 459(1):41–46. doi:10.1007/s00428-011-1081-2 [Research Support, Non-U.S. Gov't]

Lee AF, Hayes MM, Lebrun D, Espinosa I, Nielsen GP, Rosenberg AE, Lee CH (2011) FLI-1 distinguishes Ewing sarcoma from small cell osteosarcoma and mesenchymal chondrosarcoma. Appl Immunohistochem Mol Morphol 19(3):233–238. doi:10.1097/PAI.0b013e3181fd6697

Lieberman PH, Jones CR, Steinman RM, Erlandson RA, Smith J, Gee T, Sperber M (1996) Langerhans cell (eosinophilic) granulomatosis. A clinicopathologic study encompassing 50 years. Am J Surg Pathol 20(5):519–552 [Research Support, U.S. Gov't, P.H.S.]

Machado I, Alberghini M, Giner F, Corrigan M, O'Sullivan M, Noguera R, Llombart-Bosch A (2010) Histopathological characterization of small cell osteosarcoma with immunohistochemistry and molecular genetic support. A study of 10 cases. Histopathology 57(1):162–167. doi:10.1111/j.1365-2559.2010.03589.x [Case Reports Letter Research Support, Non-U.S. Gov't]

Machado I, Lopez Guerrero JA, Navarro S, Mayordomo E, Scotlandi K, Picci P, Llombart-Bosch A (2013) Galectin-1 (GAL-1) expression is a useful tool to differentiate between small cell osteosarcoma and Ewing sarcoma. Virchows Arch 462(6):665–671. doi:10.1007/s00428-013-1423-3 [Research Support, Non-U.S. Gov't]

Makley JT, Dunn MJ (1982) Prostaglandin synthesis by osteoid osteoma. Lancet 2(8288):42 [Letter]

Most MJ, Sim FH, Inwards CY (2010) Osteofibrous dysplasia and adamantinoma. J Am Acad Orthop Surg 18(6):358–366 [Review]

Nakajima T, Watanabe S, Sato Y, Kameya T, Hirota T, Shimosato Y (1982) An immunoperoxidase study of S-100 protein distribution in normal and neoplastic tissues. Am J Surg Pathol 6(8):715–727 [Research Support, Non-U.S. Gov't]

Nakajima H, Sim FH, Bond JR, Unni KK (1997) Small cell osteosarcoma of bone. Review of 72 cases. Cancer 79(11):2095–2106

Okada K, Hasegawa T, Yokoyama R, Beppu Y, Itoi E (2003) Osteosarcoma with cytokeratin expression: a clinicopathological study of six cases with an emphasis on differential diagnosis from metastatic cancer. J Clin Pathol 56(10):742–746

Picci P, Bohling T, Bacci G, Ferrari S, Sangiorgi L, Mercuri M, Bertoni F (1997) Chemotherapy-induced tumor necrosis as a prognostic factor in localized Ewing's sarcoma of the extremities. J Clin Oncol 15(4):1553–1559 [Research Support, Non-U.S. Gov't]

Riopel M, Dickman PS, Link MP, Perlman EJ (1994) MIC2 analysis in pediatric lymphomas and leukemias. Hum Pathol 25(4):396–399

Rosito P, Mancini AF, Rondelli R, Abate ME, Pession A, Bedei L, Paolucci G (1999) Italian Cooperative Study for the treatment of children and young adults with localized Ewing sarcoma of bone: a preliminary report of 6 years of experience. Cancer 86(3):421–428 [Clinical Trial Multicenter Study Research Support, Non-U.S. Gov't]

Sanerkin NG (1980) Definitions of osteosarcoma, chondrosarcoma, and fibrosarcoma of bone. Cancer 46(1):178–185

Sweet DE, Vinh TN, Devaney K (1992) Cortical osteofibrous dysplasia of long bone and its relationship to adamantinoma. A clinicopathologic study of 30 cases. Am J Surg Pathol 16(3):282–290 [Comparative Study]

Tsokos M, Alaggio RD, Dehner LP, Dickman PS (2012) Ewing sarcoma/peripheral primitive neuroectodermal tumor and related tumors. Pediatr Dev Pathol 15(1 Suppl):108–126. doi:10.2350/11-08-1078-PB.1 [Review]

Turcotte RE, Kurt AM, Sim FH, Unni KK, McLeod RA (1993) Chondroblastoma. Hum Pathol 24(9):944–949

Unni KK, Dahlin DC, Beabout JW (1976) Periosteal osteogenic sarcoma. Cancer 37(5):2476–2485

White LM, Schweitzer ME, Deely DM, Gannon F (1995) Study of osteomyelitis: utility of combined histologic and microbiologic evaluation of percutaneous biopsy samples. Radiology 197(3):840–842. doi:10.1148/radiology.197.3.7480765

Basic Principles of Biopsy

3

Thomas J. Scharschmidt and Joel L. Mayerson

Contents

3.1   **Basic Principles**. 51

3.2   **Initial Workup** 52
3.2.1 Laboratory Studies. 52
3.2.2 Imaging Studies 53

3.3   **Types of Biopsy**. 53
3.3.1 Fine Needle Aspiration 53
3.3.2 Core Needle 54
3.3.3 Open Surgical Biopsy. 54

3.4   **Pitfalls/Complications** 55

Conclusion 56

References. 56

Abstract

Biopsy of a possible malignant bone sarcoma is the final most important planning procedure prior to the initiation of treatment. The overall goal of the biopsy is to obtain diagnostic tissue in the least invasive way possible. This will minimize possible complications. Very specific techniques must be followed in order to minimize these complications. Specialized training in performing a biopsy for a malignant bone tumor is of utmost performance to diminish risk of the biopsy and minimize the amount of tissue that must be resected with the definitive treatment procedure. When the physician follows standard algorithms in performing the biopsy, the risk of complications is decreased by 5-fold. This procedure is best performed in the setting of a multidisciplinary tertiary treatment center with involvement from a radiologist, pathologist, and subspecialty trained surgeon.

3.1 Basic Principles

The biopsy is the penultimate treatment planning procedure in the management of bone sarcomas. In accordance with its importance in the diagnostic process, it must be performed in a very precise way using definitive techniques. The overall goal of the biopsy is to obtain diagnostic tissue in the most minimal way possible to avoid contamination of additional tissue and not complicate eventual planned resection. A biopsy should be preceded

T.J. Scharschmidt, MD (✉) • J.L. Mayerson, MD
Division of Musculoskeletal Oncology, Department of Orthopaedics, The Ohio State University, 376 W. 10th Ave., Prior Hall, Suite 725, Columbus, Ohio 43210
e-mail: Thomas.scharschmidt@osumc.edu; Joel.mayerson@osumc.edu

© Springer International Publishing Switzerland 2015
T.P. Cripe, N.D. Yeager (eds.), *Malignant Pediatric Bone Tumors - Treatment & Management*, Pediatric Oncology, DOI 10.1007/978-3-319-18099-1_3

by a thorough clinical and radiographic evaluation (Errani et al. 2013). A multidisciplinary team including a radiologist, pathologist, and surgeon should consult as a team to develop an appropriate differential diagnosis prior to proceeding with the procedure. Several technical considerations must be followed without deviation in order to prevent possible unintended complications in the biopsy procedure. The biopsy incision must be performed in line with the definitive surgical resection incision and in a longitudinal rather than transverse direction. This approach allows for optimal postoperative reconstruction options and prevents unnecessary functional loss during tumor resection. In general, the biopsy tract should be considered contaminated with tumor cells and thus should be planned to be resected during the definitive procedure. At best a poorly placed biopsy incision can add morbidity by requiring additional resection of non-involved tissues and at worst can lead to an unnecessary amputation. Strict hemostasis must be maintained at all times during the biopsy as excess bleeding can contaminate normal tissues that will need to be resected to clear the additional tumor burden. Diagnostic tissue must also be obtained during the procedure, usually confirmed by performing a frozen section in conjunction with the pathologist. This caution prevents a potentially unnecessary second procedure if there is a problem such as a completely necrotic or non-diagnostic specimen. Multiple samples should be obtained as these malignancies can be heterogeneous in nature. Two studies performed by the Musculoskeletal Tumor Society, initially in 1982 and subsequently in 1996, demonstrated that the risk of complications from a biopsy performed by a non-tertiary sarcoma team is five times higher than having the biopsy performed at a tertiary referral center by an experienced sarcoma team (Mankin et al. 2006). The rate of major errors in this study was 13.5 %, the rate of complications was 15.9 %, and the rate of potentially avoidable amputation was 3 % (Mankin et al. 1996).

3.2 Initial Workup

The diagnosis of all potential masses is obtained through taking a comprehensive history, performing a thorough physical exam, obtaining appropriate cross-sectional imaging, and reviewing histologic material (when indicated). An accurate differential diagnosis can usually be formulated after the history and physical is performed. Jaffe wrote in his textbook on musculoskeletal tumors in 1958 that the biopsy should be regarded as the final diagnostic procedure and not a shortcut to the diagnosis. Appropriate imaging can help narrow the differential, and then, if tumor is still suspected, histologic analysis will usually confirm the diagnosis.

Pertinent questions include: how long has the mass been present? Stability over time favors a benign diagnosis, as sarcomas usually grow rapidly over a period of weeks to months (of course, there are exceptions to every rule). Is it painful? A constant, dull, unrelenting pain is common with bone sarcomas. Night pain that awakens the patient from sleep is also described (Guillon et al. 2011). Is there any history of trauma or prior history of cancer? Trauma may result in the development of myositis ossificans or a calcified hematoma. Also, occasionally trauma or injury may draw attention to a previously existing mass. Are there any concurrent systemic symptoms? Osteosarcomas rarely presented with additional or constitutional symptoms, but Ewing sarcomas may present with fevers, malaise, and other flu-like symptoms.

Once a complete history has been obtained, a physical exam is performed. Specific to the mass, important characteristics are: size, depth, consistency, and mobility. A fixed mass may suggest an underlying bony origin. The neurovascular exam of the affected extremity should be documented, as should the range of motion and function of the limb.

3.2.1 Laboratory Studies

There are no specific laboratory studies that are of significant benefit in the evaluation of potentially malignant bone sarcomas. Infectious processes can manifest with an elevated white blood cell count, erythrocyte sedimentation rate, and C-reactive protein. Lactate dehydrogenase levels can be elevated in small round blue cell tumors.

Alkaline phosphatase could be elevated and prognostic in osteosarcomas (Moore and Luu 2014). Calcium and phosphorus levels can be abnormal in tumoral calcinosis and uric acid levels can be elevated in gout. In general, these tests are non-specific and are of limited use in the evaluation of bone sarcomas.

The decision to proceed with imaging and/or biopsy is made after performing a history and physical exam. Reassuring findings that can lead to continued conservative observation include: absence of pain, stability of size, incidental finding, and masses that develop after trauma. Any mass in which the diagnosis is in question should be worked up further with imaging and/or biopsy.

3.2.2   Imaging Studies

The initial imaging study should consist of plain radiographs in two planes. Aggressive features (periosteal reaction, bone destruction, malignant osteoid formation) can usually be readily identified on radiographs (Fig. 3.1). After x-ray, magnetic resonance imaging (MRI) with gadolinium enhancement is the modality of choice for diagnostic evaluation. Proximity of neurovascular structures, extent of marrow involvement, parameters of soft tissue extension, and potential skip lesions can all be detected on MRI. Whole body bone scan or PET scan can be utilized to screen for distant metastases. Other uses for PET in the diagnosis and prognosis of these tumors are still being defined (Bastiaannet et al. 2004).

3.3   Types of Biopsy

After the initial workup is complete, the physician must decide whether to proceed with biopsy for tissue diagnosis. Only lesions that are definitively benign based on physical exam or imaging characteristics can avoid biopsy. All other lesions, or lesions in which the diagnosis is unclear should undergo tissue sampling. Adequate preoperative imaging is crucial to formulate proper differential and biopsy approach. The imaging should not be older than 4–6 weeks as malignant tumors can rapidly grow. Once the decision to proceed with biopsy has been made, there are

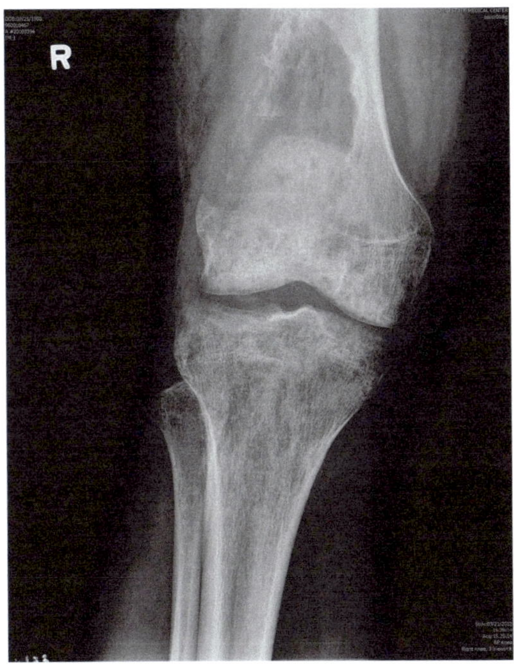

Fig. 3.1 Plain radiograph of the knee demonstrating an aggressive appearing lesion in the distal femur. Note the bone destruction, osteoid formation, and periosteal reaction

several potential methods that can be employed to obtain the tissue. Before the biopsy is performed, the definitive resection should be considered to allow proper placement of the biopsy tract. If the performing surgeon is not comfortable with the definitive surgical resection, then they should not perform the biopsy and should refer the patient to a specialized center (Springfield and Rosenberg 1996). The main consideration is to use the technique that will provide the highest diagnostic accuracy while minimizing complications. Choices of biopsy method include: fine needle aspiration (FNA), core needle biopsy, open incisional biopsy, and excisional biopsy.

3.3.1   Fine Needle Aspiration

Fine needle aspirations typically use 22- to 25-gauge needles and several passes are made into the periphery of the tumor. There are several distinct advantages of fine needle aspiration over other biopsy methods. It is less costly, can be performed in the office without anesthetic, and an

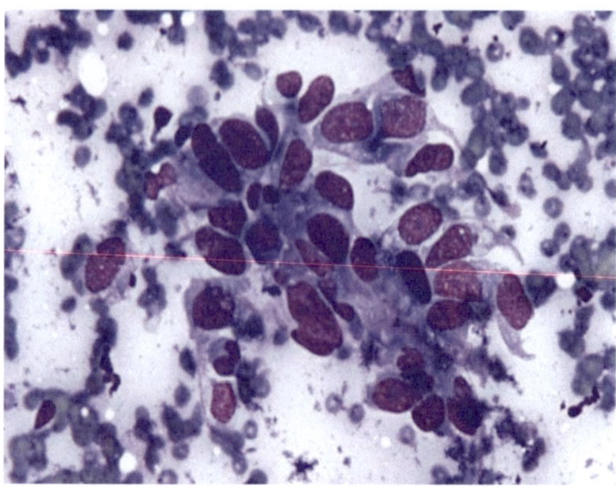

Fig. 3.2 Example of sample obtained from fine needle aspiration (FNA). The office-based biopsy yields a small sample of cells

immediate answer can be secured during the patient's office visit (Kaffenberger et al. 2010). Image guidance is not needed for FNA of palpable lesions that are safely away from vital underlying structures such as blood vessels but non-palpable lesions are better biopsied with image guidance. Either an ultrasound or a CT scanner can be used as the imaging modality of choice depending upon the expertise of the physician performing the biopsy. The main limitation of the fine needle aspiration is that it does not provide the evaluation of the tissue architecture (Fig. 3.2). A recently published study reported a diagnostic sensitivity and specificity of 89 % with fine needle aspiration (Ng et al. 2010). Other manuscripts have presented lower success rates with 79 % sensitivity and 72 % specificity (Kasraeian et al. 2010). These two studies demonstrate the most important rate-limiting step involved with the accuracy of FNA biopsy for musculoskeletal tumors, an expert cytopathologist. If there is no well-trained cytopathologist within the institution, utilization of fine needle aspiration biopsy is not a realistic option for diagnosis.

3.3.2   Core Needle

A second type of needle biopsy, called core needle biopsy, is slightly more invasive than a fine needle aspiration but can still be performed in the office without the need for surgical intervention (Adams et al. 2010). A 14-gauge needle is utilized. In this technique a local anesthetic is necessary. This additional needlestick minimally increases the risk of complication such as an allergic reaction. The costs of a core needle biopsy is slightly higher than FNA secondary to increased tissue handling needs that are required for its successful completion, but still much less than an open biopsy (Skrzynski et al. 1996). This biopsy technique can be performed either with or without image guidance depending upon the presence of a non-palpable or palpable mass. A recently published paper has also documented the sensitivity and specificity of this technique at 79 % and 82 % respectively (Kasraeian et al. 2010). Based on these success rates, a trained musculoskeletal pathologist, rather than a cytologist, is a minimum requirement and there is an additional cadre of pathologists that have been required to have the expertise to evaluate this type of specimen (Heslin et al. 1997).

3.3.3   Open Surgical Biopsy

Open biopsy is the gold standard technique as a study when diagnostic tissue for a bone lesion is required (Kasraeian et al. 2010). This procedure provides additional volume of the available specimen as well as a generally higher sensitivity and specificity with respect to diagnosis (Fig. 3.3). A representative sample is taken through the smallest possible longitudinal incision. It does have some downsides though; the risk of infection is higher, the cost is higher, and the risk of bleeding complications is increased. Additional bleeding within the wound bed can cause the possibility of further contamination by malignant cells. Any resultant hematoma should be considered contaminated and must be resected with the eventual definitive procedure. In addition, an open biopsy must be performed in an operating room using strict aseptic technique. The use of an operating room has additional costs as well. There are two types of open biopsy that can be performed. An excisional biopsy is performed by removing the entire tumor. An incisional biopsy

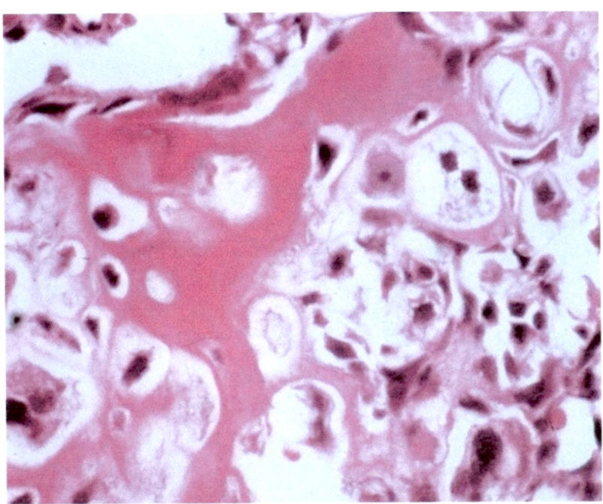

Fig. 3.3 Example of open biopsy demonstrating an osteosarcoma. Compared to an FNA, the open biopsy yields more tissues, and cellular architecture of the tumor can be analyzed

removes a portion of the tumor to obtain diagnosis, and is the most common biopsy used for the diagnosis of bone sarcomas. It can be combined with frozen section analysis to ensure that diagnostic tissue has been obtained. It is generally accepted that the extraosseous component of the tumor is representative of the diagnosis and is adequate. Sampling of the intraosseous portion requires violation of the bone cortex and may pre-dispose the patient to pathologic fracture. This should only be done if there is no extraosseous portion. If the intraosseous portion requires sampling, the smallest corticotomy needed to gain diagnosis should be used.

An excisional biopsy should only be considered as the correct initial procedure to obtain diagnostic tissue if all cross-sectional imaging studies demonstrate and are definitive for the presence of a benign lesion such as an osteochondroma. Specimen sent for culture must also occur whenever infection is in the clinical, radiographic, or histologic diagnostic differential diagnosis. If the diagnosis is in question at the time of planned resection, frozen section should again be used. When frozen section analysis does not allow for a definitive diagnosis to be made, the procedure should be stopped, the wound closed, and further surgical intervention to be planned after the pathologist has provided a final diagnosis. Exact hemostasis is an absolute requirement to prevent bleeding and wider contamination of the surrounding soft tissues by malignant cells. Proper biopsy procedure must be followed to prevent a wider resection and even possibly an unnecessary amputation.

3.4 Pitfalls/Complications

The main complications to be considered during biopsy include non-diagnostic tissue, hematoma, infection, and pathologic fracture. The rates of each of these are different based on the technique of biopsy employed.

Non-diagnostic samples can be avoided with the use of frozen section, which allows real-time evaluation of the sample to ensure viable tissue. The rate of non-diagnostic samples increases with the less invasive (FNA and core needle) types of biopsies (Mankin et al. 1996; Kasraeian et al. 2010). In addition, with any of the techniques, multiple passes in different directions should be obtained to minimize non-diagnostic procedures.

Hematomas can occur when strict hemostasis is not obtained at the time of the biopsy. For malignant tumors, any resultant hematoma must be considered contaminated with tumor cells and must be resected with the definitive surgery. This complication may lead to a larger surgery, more functional loss, and potentially amputation (Mankin et al. 2006).

The risk of infection also increases with the magnitude of the biopsy. The risk is minimal with FNA or core needle, but has been reported to be up to 10 % for open biopsy. This is an important consideration because an acquired infection will likely lead to a delay of chemotherapy.

Pathologic fracture is another complication that can lead to devastating outcomes and potentially amputation. This risk is minimized by utilizing the minimal invasive technique possible to obtain adequate tissue for diagnosis, and also taking the sample from the extraosseous mass. If a corticotomy is required for diagnosis, the smallest hole possible with rounded edges should be used to minimize fracture risk. Rounded ends provide more residual strength compared to squared corners (Clark et al. 1977).

Conclusion

The goal of the biopsy is to obtain diagnostic tissue while minimizing complications such as tissue contamination, delay of future treatment, and pathologic fracture. The appropriate biopsy technique in individualized for the patient based on the location and the size of the tumor. Choices include fine needle aspiration, core needle, and open surgical biopsy. Each is associated with risks and benefits, but in general, the minimal technique that will provide the highest diagnostic accuracy should be employed.

References

Adams SC, Potter BK, Pitcher DJ et al (2010) Office-based core needle biopsy of bone and soft tissue malignancies: an accurate alternative to open biopsy with infrequent complications. Clin Orthop Relat Res 468:2774–2780

Bastiaannet E, Groen H, Jager PL et al (2004) The value of FDG-PET in the detection, grading and response to therapy of soft tissue and bone sarcomas; a systematic review and meta-analysis. Cancer Treat Rev 30:83–101

Clark CR, Morgan C, Sonstegard DA et al (1977) The effect of biopsy-hole shape and size on bone strength. J Bone Joint Surg Am 59:213–217

Errani C, Traina F, Perna F et al (2013) Current concepts in the biopsy of musculoskeletal tumors. Sci World J 2013:538152

Guillon MA, Mary PM, Brugiere L et al (2011) Clinical characteristics and prognosis of osteosarcoma in young children: a retrospective series of 15 cases. BMC Cancer 11:407

Heslin MJ, Lewis JJ, Woodruff JM et al (1997) Core needle biopsy for diagnosis of extremity soft tissue sarcoma. Ann Surg Oncol 4:425–431

Kaffenberger BH, Wakely PE Jr, Mayerson JL (2010) Local recurrence rate of fine-needle aspiration biopsy in primary high-grade sarcomas. J Surg Oncol 101:618–621

Kasraeian S, Allison DC, Ahlmann ER et al (2010) A comparison of fine-needle aspiration, core biopsy, and surgical biopsy in the diagnosis of extremity soft tissue masses. Clin Orthop Relat Res 468: 2992–3002

Mankin HJ, Mankin CJ, Simon MA (1996) The hazards of the biopsy, revisited. Members of the musculoskeletal tumor society. J Bone Joint Surg Am 78: 656–663

Mankin HJ, Lange TA, Spanier SS (2006) THE CLASSIC: The hazards of biopsy in patients with malignant primary bone and soft-tissue tumors. The Journal of Bone and Joint Surgery, 1982;64:1121-1127. Clin Orthop Relat Res 450:4–10

Moore DD, Luu HH (2014) Osteosarcoma. Cancer Treat Res 162:65–92

Ng VY, Thomas K, Crist M et al (2010) Fine needle aspiration for clinical triage of extremity soft tissue masses. Clin Orthop Relat Res 468:1120–1128

Skrzynski MC, Biermann JS, Montag A et al (1996) Diagnostic accuracy and charge-savings of outpatient core needle biopsy compared with open biopsy of musculoskeletal tumors. J Bone Joint Surg Am 78:644–649

Springfield DS, Rosenberg A (1996) Biopsy: complicated and risky. J Bone Joint Surg Am 78:639–643

The Evaluation of Lung Nodules in Pediatric Bone Tumors

4

Nicholas D. Yeager and Anthony N. Audino

Contents

4.1　**Introduction** 57

4.2　**Methods of Imaging the Lungs in Pediatric Bone Tumor Patients** 58
4.2.1　Computed Tomography 58
4.2.2　FDG-PET 59

4.3　**Management of Lung Nodules** 59
4.3.1　Management of Lung Nodules in Osteosarcoma Patients 59
4.3.2　Management of Lung Nodules in Ewing Sarcoma Patients 60

4.4　**Indications for Biopsy** 61

References............................. 61

Abstract

One of the most important prognostic variables for patients with primary bone malignancy is the presence or absence of metastatic disease at presentation. About 20 % of patients with osteosarcoma, and 25 % of patients with Ewing's sarcoma will have metastases at presentation, and the lung is the most common site of distant involvement for both diseases. The sensitivity of modern imaging techniques has allowed the identification of tiny lung nodules in cancer patients, including many which may not be malignant at all and may actually represent scarring from prior infection or small lymph nodes. Because the impact of pulmonary involvement on prognosis and management in primary bone sarcoma patients is profound, it is important to characterize the lesions as completely as possible when they are identified. In this section, the imaging characteristics, identification strategies, effects on management, and indications for biopsy of lung nodules in patients with bone malignancy are reviewed.

4.1　Introduction

Patients with primary bone malignancy who present with metastatic disease continue to have very poor outcomes regardless of what systemic chemotherapeutic or local control strategies are utilized. Approximately 20 % of patients with

N.D. Yeager, MD (✉) • A.N. Audino, MD
Division of Hematology/Oncology/BMT,
Nationwide Children's Hospital,
700 Children's Drive, Columbus, OH 43205, USA
e-mail: Nicholas.yeager@nationwidechildrens.org;
Anthony.audino@nationwidechildrens.org

© Springer International Publishing Switzerland 2015
T.P. Cripe, N.D. Yeager (eds.), *Malignant Pediatric Bone Tumors - Treatment & Management*,
Pediatric Oncology, DOI 10.1007/978-3-319-18099-1_4

osteosarcoma (OS) and 25 % of Ewing's sarcoma (EWS) patients present with metastatic disease, and the most common site of involvement for both is the lungs (Meyers and Gorlick 1997; Grier 1997; Volker et al. 2007). Not only does the presence of lung disease have a profound impact on prognosis, it also heavily influences the therapeutic approach to these patients, with both immediate and long term implications for the affected individuals. With advancements in imaging technology, an important part of planning treatment for bone tumor patients is the interpretation of pulmonary nodules identified during the initial evaluation. In this chapter, methods of pulmonary imaging are reviewed, as well as the clinical impact of lung disease on patients with OS and EWS.

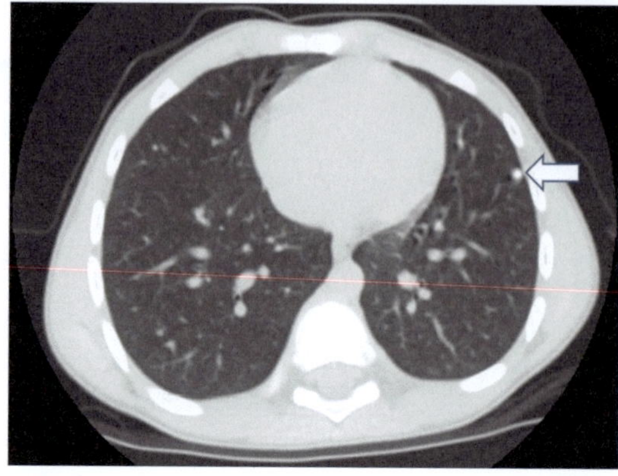

Fig. 4.1 A single, calcified metastatic osteosarcoma nodule in the left lung (identified with *arrow*)

4.2 Methods of Imaging the Lungs in Pediatric Bone Tumor Patients

4.2.1 Computed Tomography

Computed tomography (CT) is generally utilized as the primary method of evaluating for pulmonary involvement. CT has been shown to be more reliable in the identification of lung nodules than chest x-ray, and modern multi-detector high-resolution techniques have demonstrated adequate sensitivity and specificity in the identification of pulmonary lesions (Cohen et al. 1982; Franzius et al. 2001). Pulmonary imaging with this modality is generally performed without contrast, unless known or suspected lesions are adjacent to the mediastinal vessels, and it is important that imaging be obtained before a sedated procedure is performed to avoid false positive results from atelectasis. Malignant lung nodules are typically well demarcated, ovoid or round lesions most often seen at the periphery (Fig. 4.1) (Herold et al. 1996). CT imaging is not perfect however, and several limitations in its use have been identified. The cost and radiation exposure of CT are considerably higher than that of plain chest radiographs, particularly when multiple studies are obtained over time. Also, it has long been held that CT underestimates the number of metastatic lesions in the lung identified at

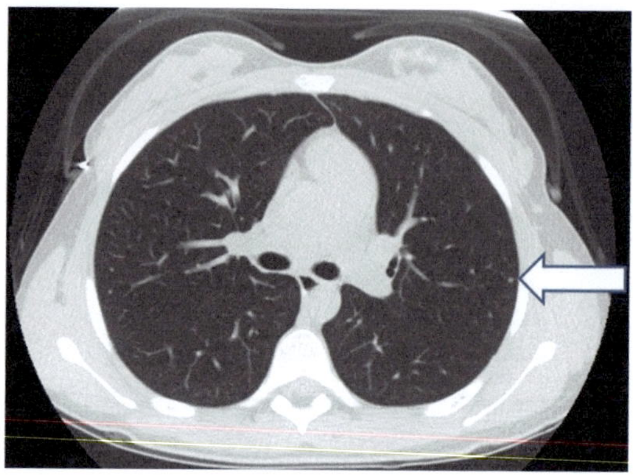

Fig. 4.2 A single, biopsy-proven benign left lung nodule (identified with *arrow*)

thoracotomy for patients with osteosarcoma, and a recent analysis confirmed that this continues to be the case despite more precise imaging protocols (Parsons et al. 2004; Cerfolio et al. 2009; Ellis et al. 2011). Conversely, the significance of small nodules identified on CT can be unclear, particularly in older adolescents, young adults, and those living in areas with endemic fungal infections. In fact, for patients with osteosarcoma, up to 24 % of previously identified nodules may be benign at the time of definitive resection, especially small nodules (<5 mm) along the fissures which tend to be lymph nodes rather than tumor (Fig. 4.2) (Bacci et al. 2008). Factors associated with an increased likelihood of representing true malignancy include nodule size ≥5 mm, more than three total nodules, bilateral involvement, peripheral location, and the presence of

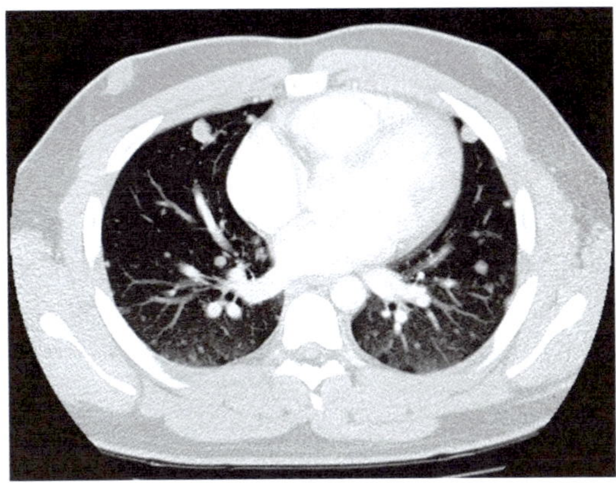

Fig. 4.3 Multiple metastatic Ewing nodules

calcifications for patients with osteosarcoma (Fig. 4.3) (Absalon et al. 2008; Brader et al. 2011; Murrell et al. 2011).

4.2.2 FDG-PET

^{18}F-fluorodeoxyglucose positron emission tomography (FDG-PET) is increasingly being used as a staging tool for patients with cancer, including malignant bone tumors. Unfortunately, while traditional FDG-PET is very useful in the evaluation of chemotherapeutic response and is an excellent screening tool for lymph node and bone metastases, its utility in the evaluation of lung nodules is limited. A standardized uptake value (SUV) of 2.5 has been used as a cut off to distinguish benign from malignant lesions (Cistaro et al. 2012). Multiple studies have demonstrated the sensitivity of FDG-PET in the identification of malignant lung nodules to be inferior to that of CT, especially for smaller lesions (Franzius et al. 2001; Volker et al. 2007; Fortes et al. 2008). It is particularly unreliable for nodules less than 8–10 mm in size, with reported sensitivity rates as low as 25–29.6 % (Absalon et al. 2008; Brader et al. 2011). The addition of computed tomography to FDG-PET (FDG-PET/CT) has allowed improved accuracy in the evaluation of lung nodules with this modality. Sensitivity and specificity rates of 90.3 % and 87.5 %, respectively, have been reported with PET/CT, but unfortunately, this modality still demonstrates limitations in the evaluation of tiny nodules less than 6 mm in size (Cistaro et al. 2012).

4.3 Management of Lung Nodules

4.3.1 Management of Lung Nodules in Osteosarcoma Patients

As previously noted, about 20 % of patients will present with identifiable metastatic disease at diagnosis, with pulmonary disease being present in over 80 % of these cases (Kempf-Bielack et al. 2005). Without systemic therapy, more than 80 % of patients will develop lung recurrence regardless of local surgery (Link et al. 1986). Unfortunately, patients with metastatic disease have a dismal outcome overall, with long term survival rates of less than 20 % (Mialou et al. 2005). Several factors have been identified that influence outcomes in OS patients with lung disease, including the total number of nodules, unilateral or bilateral involvement, and the ability to achieve a complete surgical resection. Presenting with more than three to five pulmonary nodules has consistently been identified in several studies as being associated with inferior survival (Buddingh et al. 2010; Chen et al. 2008; Bacci et al. 2008; Daw et al. 2006). For those with three or fewer nodules, 5 year overall survival rates of 40 % or greater have been described in some analyses, as compared to less than 15 % for those with higher numbers of nodules. Likewise, bilateral involvement has been shown to confer a worse prognosis for OS patients, with 5 year disease-free survival rates of less than 10 % having been reported for those with bilateral lung metastases at presentation (Bacci et al. 2008). It has also been reported that patients who present with centrally located nodules (defined as lesions adjacent to a first degree bronchus or blood vessel) have an inferior prognosis compared to those with peripheral lesions (Letourneau et al. 2011b).

The therapeutic intervention that has been shown to have the most significant impact on survival for patients with pulmonary metastases is the ability to achieve a surgical complete remission. While chemotherapy is necessary for any attempt at cure for patients with OS, without resection of all lung disease long-term disease survival is nearly impossible (Bacci et al. 2008; Buddingh et al. 2010; Kager et al. 2003). The accepted surgical approach to lung nodule resection is via thoracotomy, which allows for direct palpation of lung tissue to identify lesions not identified on pre-operative imaging. Despite advancements in imaging technology, studies continue to demonstrate that CT often underestimates the number of nodules found when thoracotomy is performed (Kayton et al. 2006; Cerfolio et al. 2009). Thus, while thorascopic approaches to nodule resection may have less morbidity, the importance of complete surgical resection of all metastatic disease continues to support thoracotomy as the standard for the management of OS patients (Castagnetti et al. 2004). Thoracoscopy may have a role when the diagnosis of metastatic disease is in question and the nodules are large enough to be amenable to this approach. The role of bilateral thoracotomy in the management of patients who present with unilateral disease continues to be an area of debate. Data on the optimal management of patients with unilateral disease at presentation is lacking, but a report published by Su et al. supported the performance of a contralateral thoracotomy for patients who recurred with unilateral disease less than 2 years from diagnosis. In this study, seven of nine (78 %) of patients with recurrence <2 years from diagnosis went on to develop contralateral disease, while only one of five (20 %) of patients who developed unilateral disease more than 2 years from diagnosis went on to develop contralateral recurrence. A survey of surgeons and oncologists performed by the Connective Tissue Oncology Society revealed that thoracotomy of the unaffected side has not been routine practice of most surgeons and oncologists, and at least one subsequent retrospective analysis showed no advantage to contralateral surgery (Su et al. 2004; Vo 2014). Further prospective studies are necessary to develop firm recommendations on this topic, though such trials are unlikely to be undertaken due to the invasive nature of the intervention.

4.3.2 Management of Lung Nodules in Ewing Sarcoma Patients

Approximately 25 % of patients with EWS present with metastatic disease at diagnosis and similar to OS patients, hematogenous spread into the lungs is the most common site of distant disease. Despite improvements in survival with intensification of systemic chemotherapy for localized disease, outcomes remain poor for patients with metastatic EWS, with event-free survival consistently shown to be about 20 % (Pinkerton et al. 2001; Miser et al. 2004). Patients with metastatic disease exclusive to the lungs, however, have demonstrated better outcomes with disease-free survival of 30–40 % when treated with standard therapy (Pinkerton et al. 2001; Miser et al. 2004). Further, intensification of systemic therapy for patients with primary lung metastasis, utilizing high dose chemotherapy/ stem cell rescue has been advocated by some, but the results of prospective studies have been mixed, and at this time, this approach should be considered investigational (Meyers et al. 2001; Drabko et al. 2012; Oberlin et al. 2006).

Local therapy is an important component of any treatment strategy aimed at prolonging survival in patients with metastatic EWS (Thorpe et al. 2012). While there have been no prospective studies designed to elucidate the optimal approach to local therapy, both surgery and radiation therapy can be considered, and may have a role in the management of pulmonary metastases. Several retrospective analyses have suggested benefit to the use of whole lung radiotherapy at doses of 12–18 Gy, and it has become standard practice in most centers (Paulussen et al. 1998a, b; Paulino et al. 2013; Spunt et al. 2001). The risk of radiation pneumonitis at these doses is relatively low, and severe pulmonary complications are seen in less than 10 % of those treated (Bolling et al. 2008). Unfortunately, the risk of toxicity does increase with subsequent surgical procedures or further radiation boosts to previously treated lung tissue (Bolling et al. 2008). The role of surgical resection is less clear in EWS patients with lung disease compared to OS patients. Two small retrospective analyses have suggested a survival benefit to surgical resection of EWS lung nodules (Lanza et al. 1987; Letourneau et al. 2011a). In an analysis performed by Letourneau et al. there was a suggestion that surgical resection of pulmonary nodules was associated with increased survival compared to patients treated with radiation, either alone or in conjunction with surgery (Letourneau et al. 2011a). The patient numbers in this analysis were quite small however, and the retrospective nature of the study prevents strong conclusions from being made. Further study is necessary to determine the optimal approach to local therapy for these patients.

4.4   Indications for Biopsy

Because pulmonary metastatic disease has such a significant impact on the prognosis and management of patients with bone cancer, attempts should be made to determine the etiology of lung nodules when possible. In many cases, the presence of lung disease is clear: large nodules greater than 5 mm in size involving both lungs, calcified in patients with OS, or nodules large enough to be positive on PET, likely need no further work-up at diagnosis to plan treatment. In cases where the diagnosis may be in question, the nodules will generally be amenable to video assisted thorascopic surgery (VATS) or CT guided biopsy. These techniques can establish a tissue diagnosis with minimal healing time, allowing for a more rapid initiation of chemotherapy. For small nodules, VATS following the preoperative placement of microcoils or guidewires via CT guidance can be an effective way to biopsy lesions smaller than 5 mm in size (Fig. 4.4) (Heran et al. 2011; Murrell et al. 2011). Alternatively, lesions smaller than 5 mm in size can be observed following treatment with chemotherapy. Should the nodules increase in size with treatment, biopsy should be performed. In patients with osteosarcoma, complete resolution of nodules with chemotherapy occurs less than 10 % of the time (Bacci et al. 2008). Most nodules will remain stable, and

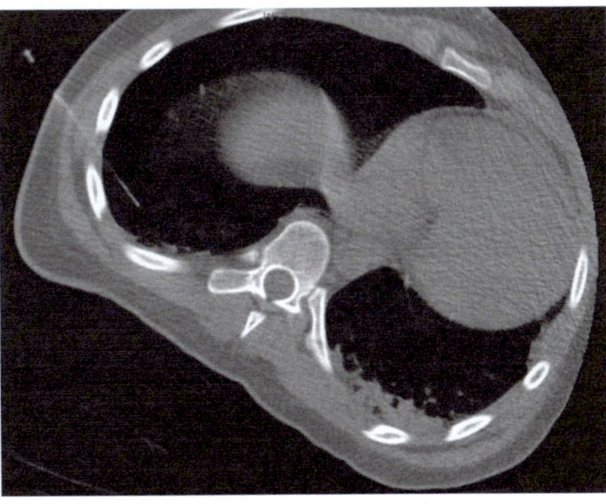

Fig. 4.4 CT guided localization of a tiny osteosarcoma lung nodule

potentially become more calcified. Resolution of pulmonary disease is much more likely for patients with Ewing's sarcoma with resolution following induction chemotherapy seen in almost 50 % of patients (Luksch et al. 2012). A lack of complete resolution in this cohort was associated with a much worse prognosis. While a good response to chemotherapy in patients with EWS supports a diagnosis of metastatic disease, it may be difficult to completely exclude the possibility of other etiologies, such as infection or atelectasis, with resolution. Because most of these patients will likely receive whole lung irradiation which carries potential for morbidities, it is important to try to characterize the lesions at diagnosis if at all possible.

References

Absalon MJ, Mccarville MB, Liu T, Santana VM, Daw NC, Navid F (2008) Pulmonary nodules discovered during the initial evaluation of pediatric patients with bone and soft-tissue sarcoma. Pediatr Blood Cancer 50:1147–1153

Bacci G, Rocca M, Salone M, Balladelli A, Ferrari S, Palmerini E, Forni C, Briccoli A (2008) High grade osteosarcoma of the extremities with lung metastases at presentation: treatment with neoadjuvant chemotherapy and simultaneous resection of primary and metastatic lesions. J Surg Oncol 98:415–420

Bolling T, Schuck A, Paulussen M, Dirksen U, Ranft A, Konemann S, Dunst J, Willich N, Jurgens H (2008) Whole lung irradiation in patients with exclusively pulmonary metastases of Ewing tumors. Toxicity analysis and treatment results of the EICESS-92 trial. Strahlenther Onkol 184:193–197

Brader P, Abramson SJ, Price AP, Ishill NM, Zabor EC, Moskowitz CS, LA Quaglia MP, Ginsberg MS (2011) Do characteristics of pulmonary nodules on computed tomography in children with known osteosarcoma help distinguish whether the nodules are malignant or benign? J Pediatr Surg 46:729–735

Buddingh EP, Anninga JK, Versteegh MI, Taminiau AH, Egeler RM, VAN Rijswijk CS, Hogendoorn PC, Lankester AC, Gelderblom H (2010) Prognostic factors in pulmonary metastasized high-grade osteosarcoma. Pediatr Blood Cancer 54:216–221

Castagnetti M, Delarue A, Gentet JC (2004) Optimizing the surgical management of lung nodules in children with osteosarcoma: thoracoscopy for biopsies, thoracotomy for resections. Surg Endosc 18: 1668–1671

Cerfolio RJ, McCarty T, Bryant AS (2009) Non-imaged pulmonary nodules discovered during thoracotomy for metastasectomy by lung palpation. Eur J Cardiothorac Surg 35:786–791; discussion 791

Chen F, Miyahara R, Bando T, Okubo K, Watanabe K, Nakayama T, Toguchida J, Date H (2008) Prognostic factors of pulmonary metastasectomy for osteosarcomas of the extremities. Eur J Cardiothorac Surg 34:1235–1239

Cistaro A, Lopci E, Gastaldo L, Fania P, Brach Del Prever A, Fagioli F (2012) The role of 18F-FDG PET/CT in the metabolic characterization of lung nodules in pediatric patients with bone sarcoma. Pediatr Blood Cancer 59:1206–1210

Cohen M, Grosfeld J, Baehner R, Weetman R (1982) Lung CT for detection of metastases: solid tissue neoplasms in children. AJR Am J Roentgenol 139:895–898

Daw NC, Billups CA, Rodriguez-Galindo C, Mccarville MB, Rao BN, Cain AM, Jenkins JJ, Neel MD, Meyer WH (2006) Metastatic osteosarcoma. Cancer 106:403–412

Drabko K, Raciborska A, Bilska K, Styczynski J, Ussowicz M, Choma M, Wojcik B, Zaucha-Prazmo A, Gorczynska E, Skoczen S, Wozniak W, Chybicka A, Wysocki M, Gozdzik J, Kowalczyk J (2012) Consolidation of first-line therapy with busulphan and melphalan, and autologous stem cell rescue in children with Ewing's sarcoma. Bone Marrow Transplant 47:1530–1534

Ellis MC, Hessman CJ, Weerasinghe R, Schipper PH, Vetto JT (2011) Comparison of pulmonary nodule detection rates between preoperative CT imaging and intraoperative lung palpation. Am J Surg 201:619–622

Fortes DL, Allen MS, Lowe VJ, Shen KR, Wigle DA, Cassivi SD, Nichols FC, Deschamps C (2008) The sensitivity of 18F-fluorodeoxyglucose positron emission tomography in the evaluation of metastatic pulmonary nodules. Eur J Cardiothorac Surg 34:1223–1227

Franzius C, Daldrup-Link HE, Sciuk J, Rummeny EJ, Bielack S, Jurgens H, Schober O (2001) FDG-PET for detection of pulmonary metastases from malignant primary bone tumors: comparison with spiral CT. Ann Oncol 12:479–486

Grier HE (1997) The Ewing family of tumors. Ewing's sarcoma and primitive neuroectodermal tumors. Pediatr Clin North Am 44:991–1004

Heran MK, Sangha BS, Mayo JR, Blair G, Skarsgard ED (2011) Lung nodules in children: video-assisted thoracoscopic surgical resection after computed tomography-guided localization using a microcoil. J Pediatr Surg 46:1292–1297

Herold CJ, Bankier AA, Fleischmann D (1996) Lung metastases. Eur Radiol 6:596–606

Kager L, Zoubek A, Potschger U, Kastner U, Flege S, Kempf-Bielack B, Branscheid D, Kotz R, Salzer-Kuntschik M, Winkelmann W, Jundt G, Kabisch H, Reichardt P, Jurgens H, Gadner H, Bielack SS (2003) Primary metastatic osteosarcoma: presentation and outcome of patients treated on neoadjuvant Cooperative Osteosarcoma Study Group protocols. J Clin Oncol 21:2011–2018

Kayton ML, Huvos AG, Casher J, Abramson SJ, Rosen NS, Wexler LH, Meyers P, Laquaglia MP (2006) Computed tomographic scan of the chest underestimates the number of metastatic lesions in osteosarcoma. J Pediatr Surg 41:200–206; discussion 200–206

Kempf-Bielack B, Bielack SS, Jurgens H, Branscheid D, Berdel WE, Exner GU, Gobel U, Helmke K, Jundt G, Kabisch H, Kevric M, Klingebiel T, Kotz R, Maas R, Schwarz R, Semik M, Treuner J, Zoubek A, Winkler K (2005) Osteosarcoma relapse after combined modality therapy: an analysis of unselected patients in the Cooperative Osteosarcoma Study Group (COSS). J Clin Oncol 23:559–568

Lanza LA, Miser JS, Pass HI, Roth JA (1987) The role of resection in the treatment of pulmonary metastases from Ewing's sarcoma. J Thorac Cardiovasc Surg 94:181–187

Letourneau PA, Shackett B, Xiao L, Trent J, Tsao KJ, Lally K, Hayes-Jordan A (2011a) Resection of pulmonary metastases in pediatric patients with Ewing sarcoma improves survival. J Pediatr Surg 46:332–335

Letourneau PA, Xiao L, Harting MT, Lally KP, Cox CS Jr, Andrassy RJ, Hayes-Jordan AA (2011b) Location of pulmonary metastasis in pediatric osteosarcoma is predictive of outcome. J Pediatr Surg 46:1333–1337

Link MP, Goorin AM, Miser AW, Green AA, Pratt CB, Belasco JB, Pritchard J, Malpas JS, Baker AR, Kirkpatrick JA et al (1986) The effect of adjuvant chemotherapy on relapse-free survival in patients with osteosarcoma of the extremity. N Engl J Med 314:1600–1606

Luksch R, Tienghi A, Hall KS, Fagioli F, Picci P, Barbieri E, Gandola L, Eriksson M, Ruggieri P, Daolio P, Lindholm P, Prete A, Bisogno G, Tamburini A, Grignani G, Abate ME, Podda M, Smeland S, Ferrari S (2012) Primary metastatic Ewing's family tumors: results of the Italian Sarcoma Group and Scandinavian Sarcoma Group ISG/SSG IV Study including myeloablative chemotherapy and total-lung irradiation. Ann Oncol 23:2970–2976

Meyers PA, Gorlick R (1997) Osteosarcoma. Pediatr Clin North Am 44:973–989

Meyers PA, Krailo MD, Ladanyi M, Chan KW, Sailer SL, Dickman PS, Baker DL, Davis JH, Gerbing RB, Grovas A, Herzog CE, Lindsley KL, Liu-Mares W, Nachman JB, Sieger L, Wadman J, Gorlick RG (2001) High-dose melphalan, etoposide, total-body irradiation, and autologous stem-cell reconstitution as consolidation therapy for high-risk Ewing's sarcoma does not improve prognosis. J Clin Oncol 19:2812–2820

Mialou V, Philip T, Kalifa C, Perol D, Gentet JC, Marec-Berard P, Pacquement H, Chastagner P, Defaschelles AS, Hartmann O (2005) Metastatic osteosarcoma at diagnosis: prognostic factors and long-term outcome–the French pediatric experience. Cancer 104:1100–1109

Miser JS, Krailo MD, Tarbell NJ, Link MP, Fryer CJ, Pritchard DJ, Gebhardt MC, Dickman PS, Perlman EJ, Meyers PA, Donaldson SS, Moore S, Rausen AR, Vietti TJ, Grier HE (2004) Treatment of metastatic Ewing's sarcoma or primitive neuroectodermal tumor of bone: evaluation of combination ifosfamide and etoposide – a Children's Cancer Group and Pediatric Oncology Group study. J Clin Oncol 22:2873–2876

Murrell Z, Dickie B, Dasgupta R (2011) Lung nodules in pediatric oncology patients: a prediction rule for when to biopsy. J Pediatr Surg 46:833–837

Oberlin O, Rey A, Desfachelles AS, Philip T, Plantaz D, Schmitt C, Plouvier E, Lejars O, Rubie H, Terrier P, Michon J, Société Française des Cancers de l'Enfant (2006) Impact of high-dose busulfan plus melphalan as consolidation in metastatic Ewing tumors: a study by the Societe Francaise des Cancers de l'Enfant. J Clin Oncol 24:3997–4002

Parsons AM, Detterbeck FC, Parker LA (2004) Accuracy of helical CT in the detection of pulmonary metastases: is intraoperative palpation still necessary? Ann Thorac Surg 78:1910–1916; discussion 1916–1918

Paulino AC, Mai WY, Teh BS (2013) Radiotherapy in metastatic ewing sarcoma. Am J Clin Oncol 36:283–286

Paulussen M, Ahrens S, Burdach S, Craft A, Dockhorn-Dworniczak B, Dunst J, Frohlich B, Winkelmann W, Zoubek A, Jurgens H (1998a) Primary metastatic (stage IV) Ewing tumor: survival analysis of 171 patients from the EICESS studies. European Intergroup Cooperative Ewing Sarcoma Studies. Ann Oncol 9:275–281

Paulussen M, Ahrens S, Craft AW, Dunst J, Frohlich B, Jabar S, Rube C, Winkelmann W, Wissing S, Zoubek A, Jurgens H (1998b) Ewing's tumors with primary lung metastases: survival analysis of 114 (European Intergroup) Cooperative Ewing's Sarcoma Studies patients. J Clin Oncol 16:3044–3052

Pinkerton CR, Bataillard A, Guillo S, Oberlin O, Fervers B, Philip T (2001) Treatment strategies for metastatic Ewing's sarcoma. Eur J Cancer 37:1338–1344

Spunt SL, Mccarville MB, Kun LE, Poquette CA, Cain AM, Brandao L, Pappo AS (2001) Selective use of whole-lung irradiation for patients with Ewing sarcoma family tumors and pulmonary metastases at the time of diagnosis. J Pediatr Hematol Oncol 23: 93–98

Su WT, Chewning J, Abramson S, Rosen N, Gholizadeh M, Healey J, Meyers P, La Quaglia MP (2004) Surgical management and outcome of osteosarcoma patients with unilateral pulmonary metastases. J Pediatr Surg 39:418–423; discussion 418–423

Thorpe SW, Weiss KR, Goodman MA, Heyl AE, Mcgough RL (2012) Should aggressive surgical local control be attempted in all patients with metastatic or pelvic Ewing's sarcoma? Sarcoma 2012:953602

Vo A (2014) Pediatric osteosarcoma lung metastasis: variations in clinical management [abstract]. Proceedings of the 105th annual meeting of the American Association for Cancer Research 74:Abstract nr 4045

Volker T, Denecke T, Steffen I, Misch D, Schonberger S, Plotkin M, Ruf J, Furth C, Stover B, Hautzel H, Henze G, Amthauer H (2007) Positron emission tomography for staging of pediatric sarcoma patients: results of a prospective multicenter trial. J Clin Oncol 25: 5435–5441

Fertility Preservation and Reproductive Health in Pediatric Bone Tumor Patients

5

Stacy L. Whiteside

Contents

5.1   Introduction   65

5.2   Male Fertility   66
5.2.1 Effects of Chemotherapy and Radiation
       on Male Fertility.   66

5.3   Female Fertility.   67
5.3.1 Effects of Chemotherapy and Radiation on
       Female Fertility   68

5.4   Pediatric Bone Tumor Experience   68
5.4.1 Childhood Cancer Survivor
       Study (CCSS).   68
5.4.2 Ewing Sarcoma   69
5.4.3 Osteosarcoma.   69

5.5   Clinical Guidelines.   70

5.6   Risk Identification   71

5.7   Pretreatment Options for Males   71

5.8   Pretreatment Options for Females   73

5.9   Post-treatment Family Planning
      Options   76

5.10 Contraception.   79

5.11 Challenges and Barriers to Providing
      Fertility Preservation Options.   79
5.11.1 Lack of Information   79
5.11.2 Ethical Considerations   79

Conclusion   80

References.   80

Abstract

The majority of children, adolescents, and young adults with pediatric bone tumors will become long-term survivors. However, many treatment modalities utilized in the modern era of chemotherapy put their future fertility in significant jeopardy. Chemotherapy that includes alkylating agents, radiation to the pelvis or CNS, and aggressive surgeries are commonly used in an attempt to cure childhood bone tumors. Survivors of cancer place a high priority on fertility and report high levels of psychological distress associated with fertility loss. Options are available to preserve fertility prior to chemotherapy when possible, but multiple barriers exist which reduce the likelihood of fertility preservation utilization.

5.1   Introduction

In the current era of multi-modal therapies for malignant bone tumors in children, adolescents, and young adults, 5-year survival rates are approaching 70 % for patients with non-metastatic

S.L. Whiteside, CPNP-AC
Division of Hematology/Oncology/BMT,
Nationwide Children's Hospital,
700 Children's Drive, Columbus, OH 43205, USA
e-mail: Stacy.whiteside@nationwidechildrens.org

© Springer International Publishing Switzerland 2015
T.P. Cripe, N.D. Yeager (eds.), *Malignant Pediatric Bone Tumors - Treatment & Management*,
Pediatric Oncology, DOI 10.1007/978-3-319-18099-1_5

disease (Edge 2014). Chemotherapy that includes alkylating agents, radiation to the pelvis or CNS, and aggressive surgeries are commonly used in an attempt to cure childhood bone tumors. These treatments can have many adverse effects on the reproductive and endocrine systems including altered pubertal development, impaired hormonal regulation, and impaired fertility and sexual functioning, significantly reducing quality of life (Metzger et al. 2013). Long-term effects of therapy should be considered and discussed with patients and families at diagnosis, before and during therapy, and during follow-up to enable patients to take advantage of emerging technologies to protect their future fertility or make informed decisions regarding their treatment options. Adolescent and young adults with cancer consistently rank information about fertility preservation as very important and among the top issues they face (Gupta et al. 2013). However, these conversations can be challenging for providers, parents and patients. Organizations including the American Society of Clinical Oncology (ASCO), the American Society for Reproductive Medicine (ASRM), and the American Academy of Pediatrics (AAP) have developed guidelines to assist clinicians in implementing these discussions early into the diagnosis and treatment process. It is critical that providers have access to the wealth of available tools and information available in a timely and efficient manner.

5.2   Male Fertility

Male fertility requires the intact functioning of the testes, hypothalamic-pituitary-gonadal (HPG) axis, and genitourinary organs. Spermatogenesis, the process of maturation of spermatozoa from immature spermatogonial germ cells, occurs in the seminiferous tubules of the testes with support of the Sertoli cells. This process is dependent on high levels of intratesticular testosterone, which promotes sperm production and development of secondary sex characteristics. Testosterone is produced by the interstitial Leydig cells that surround the epithelium. At the start of puberty, the hypothalamus produces gonadotropin-releasing hormone (GnRH) which causes the anterior pituitary to release follicle stimulating hormone (FSH) and luteinizing hormone (LH). FSH primarily influences the function of the Sertoli cells, while LH drives the Leydig cells. With the onset of this hormonal activity, the formerly dormant germ cells begin the lifelong process of self-renewal and differentiation into spermatogonia (Jahnukainen et al. 2011). The complete process of maturation takes approximately 74 days. Once initiated, germ cells in the mature testes constantly renew and differentiate into sperm, assuring that there are germ cells at different developmental stages in the mature testes at all times after puberty. In contrast, in the prepubertal testes turnover is limited to early germ cells, making them highly sensitive to cytotoxic therapy (Knopman et al. 2010). Spermatozoa are stored in the epididymis until ejaculation.

5.2.1   Effects of Chemotherapy and Radiation on Male Fertility

Impact on male fertility can be secondary to impaired spermatogenesis from gonadotoxic chemotherapy, gonadotropin deficiency from CNS-directed therapy, or functional abnormalities of the genitourinary organs related to spinal/pelvic surgery or radiation. A primary risk factor for reduced fertility is alkylating agent associated gonadal toxicity. The magnitude of this risk is determined by the specific alkylating agent and the cumulative dosing. Although there is individual variation in risk of gonadotoxicity after exposure to alkylating agents, the cumulative dosing likely to produce azoospermia has been established for most agents. Cumulative doses of cyclophosphamide greater than $5–7.5$ g/m^2 are associated with abnormal semen parameters, and azoospermia is consistently observed after total cyclophosphamide dose greater than 19 g/m^2, ifosfamide greater than 60 g/m^2, procarbazine greater than 4 g/m^2, busulfan greater than 600 mg/m^2, melphalan greater than 140 mg/m^2, and cisplatin greater than 600 mg/m^2 (Kenney et al. 2001, 2012; Williams et al. 2008; Aubier et al. 1989; Meistrich et al. 1992). Alkylating agents used in combination have an additive effect on gonadotoxicity. Post-treatment azoospermia may be permanent, but recovery of normal spermatogenesis years after treatment is possible. Early studies based upon histologic assessment of testicular tissue implied that the immature testis was relatively resistant to chemotherapy (Ginsberg 2011). However, recent studies have demonstrated that the prepubertal testes and the pubertal testes are highly vulnerable to cytotoxic agents given for cancer therapy (Hobbie et al. 2005; Howell and Shalet 1998).

Radiation, similar to chemotherapy, interferes with rapidly dividing cells, making the germ cells of spermatogenesis a target. The effects of radiation are dictated by dosage, age, and radiation field. The testicular germinal epithelium is especially sensitive to radiation. Spermatogenesis can be impaired by direct testicular irradiation, including total body irradiation, or by scatter from treatment fields in the pelvis, bladder, inguinal/femoral, or abdominal/flank (Kenney et al. 2012). Impaired spermatogenesis is observed after testicular doses as low as 100 cGy, and recovery is unlikely after doses exceeding 4–6 Gy (Gracia and Woodruff 2012; Kenney et al. 2012; Lee and Shin 2013). Gonadotropin deficiency, secondary to disruption of the HPG axis or cranial radiation doses greater than 30 Gy is also associated with reduced fertility.

Lastly, pelvic surgeries with potential to impact erectile function have significant ramifications on options for future fertility. Retroperitoneal lymph node dissection, cystectomy, pelvic exenteration, or any similar deep pelvic surgery may result in damage to the vas deferens, ejaculatory duct, or seminal vesicles which collectively comprise the excurrent ductal system of the testis (Gracia and Woodruff 2012). These procedures may also result in cavernous nerve injury with erectile dysfunction, autonomic nerve damage with ejaculatory dysfunction, and physical interruption or obstruction of the sperm delivery pathway (Gracia and Woodruff 2012). Improvements in surgical technique, including nerve sparing modifications and retroperitoneal resections have helped to decrease the risk of erectile dysfunction and ejaculatory dysfunction (See Table 5.1).

5.3   Female Fertility

Female fertility requires a functioning HPG axis, ovaries, and a uterus. Reproductive potential however, is mainly limited by available oocytes.

Table 5.1 Gonadotoxic chemotherapy agents used in pediatric bone tumors

High risk
Cyclophosphamide
Ifosfamide
Melphalan
Busulfan
Intermediate risk
Cisplatin with low cumulative dose
Carboplatin with low cumulative dose
Adriamycin
Low risk
Actinomycin D
Vincristine
Methotrexate

The process of oogenesis begins before birth with a peak in oocyte number at 20 weeks gestation (6–7 million), followed by progressive atresia and a quantitative oocyte drop to 1–2 million at birth, followed by 300,000 at menarche (Gracia and Woodruff 2012; Knopman et al. 2010). In normal menstruating women, ovarian function depends on pituitary gonadotropin production. Secretion of gonadotropin-releasing hormone (GnRH) from the hypothalamus stimulates the release of follicle stimulating hormone (FSH) and luteinizing hormone (LH) from the pituitary. With each cycle, multiple follicles are selected to enter the growing pool and begin to mature, but only one will become the dominant follicle selected for ovulation, while the remaining follicles undergo atresia (Gracia and Woodruff 2012; Knopman et al. 2010). The dominant follicle produces estradiol, which triggers an LH surge and results in the mature oocyte being released into the fallopian tube where fertilization occurs. Follicle development and atresia is a continuous process occurring throughout the reproductive lifespan. When a healthy woman reaches her mid to late 30s, a threshold number of follicles are reached at which reproductive potential drops significantly, follicular depletion accelerates, and the remaining oocytes are of overall poorer quality. Finally, with continued decline of ovarian reserve, a second threshold occurs when a woman is in her late 40s or early 50s, the start of menopause, when it is no longer possible to have biologic children (Gracia and Woodruff 2012).

5.3.1 Effects of Chemotherapy and Radiation on Female Fertility

Chemotherapy and radiation therapy destroy ovarian follicles, and predispose treated females to premature ovarian failure. The negative effect of chemotherapy on female fertility is dependent on the age of the patient at the time of treatment, the specific chemotherapeutic agent(s) used, and the cumulative dosing (Gracia and Woodruff 2012; Trudgen and Ayensu-Coker 2014). Similar to males, alkylating agents are the most gonadotoxic to female fertility. In contrast to males, significantly higher doses of alkylators are required to cause infertility in females. However, gonadotoxicity in females is more age dependent than males. Specifically, older age has a greater negative impact, as there is an overall smaller follicular pool during cancer therapy (Ginsberg 2011). The natural depletion of the number of follicles present in an individual female's ovaries can be accelerated by cancer treatment. If the degree of depletion is near complete, then the result is acute ovarian failure defined by early menopause with consequent infertility that occurs during or shortly after treatment (Gracia and Woodruff 2012). If the degree of depletion is more moderate, then the individual is at risk for premature menopause, where females remain fertile following cancer therapy but have an overall shortened reproductive life span.

Radiation to the ovaries, either through direct pelvic radiation, abdominal or spine radiation, or scatter radiation, in doses as low as 1–2 Gy in girls and 4–6 Gy in adult females can have permanent negative effects on the ovaries by causing depletion of follicles (Gracia and Woodruff 2012). Irradiation may also impact fertility by causing damage to the uterine musculature and vascular structures, thereby limiting the ability of the survivor to carry a pregnancy to term. High dose cranial irradiation in the dose range of 35–40 Gy or greater, can cause hypogonadism through effects on the hypothalamus and pituitary. This exposure results in dysregulation of hormonal pathways responsible for menstruation and fertility.

Table 5.2 Gonadotoxic radiation dosage used in pediatric bone tumors

High risk
Total body irradiation for bone marrow transplant/ stem cell transplant
Pelvic or whole abdominal radiation dose ≥6 Gy in adult women
Pelvic or whole abdominal radiation dose ≥10 Gy in postpubertal girls
Pelvic or whole abdominal radiation dose ≥15 Gy in prepubertal girls
Intermediate risk
Testicular radiation dose I–6 Gy from scattered pelvic or abdominal radiation
Pelvic or whole abdominal radiation dose 5–10 Gy in postpubertal girls
Pelvic or whole abdominal radiation dose 10–15 Gy in prepubertal girls
Craniospinal radiotherapy dose ≥25 Gy

Finally, the surgical resection of reproductive organs has obvious implications for infertility when hysterectomies or oophorectomies become necessary (See Table 5.2).

5.4 Pediatric Bone Tumor Experience

Most patients with aggressive pediatric bone tumors will receive a treatment regimen that includes high doses of chemotherapy with alkylating agents and other chemotherapeutic drugs that can impair fertility, aggressive surgical resection, and sometimes radiation therapy. Reproductive outcomes in childhood cancer survivors have not been studied extensively with large cohorts of patients, and most information comes from small single-institutional studies.

5.4.1 Childhood Cancer Survivor Study (CCSS)

The primary exception from small studies is the Childhood Cancer Survivor Study (CCSS) which reported on multiple outcomes for cancer survivors including late mortality, subsequent malignant neoplasms, chronic health conditions, fertility, and health status using matched sibling controls (Ginsberg et al. 2010b). Childhood cancer survivors from the CCSS were half as likely as their matched control siblings to sire a pregnancy with an overall reported rate of premature ovarian failure of 6 % (Chemaitilly et al. 2006; Larsen et al. 2003; Longhi et al. 2000, 2003). High risk exposures identified in the study included radiation greater than 7.5 Gy to the testes and high doses of alkylating agents including cyclophosphamide dose greater than 7.5 g/m (Green et al. 2010). In fact, when controlled for these factors, survivors were equally likely as their matched control siblings to sire a pregnancy (Green et al. 2010).

5.4.2 Ewing Sarcoma

Three hundred forty-one survivors of Ewing sarcoma (EWS) were separately analyzed within this cohort for their fertility status. Infertility was common among both male and female EWS survivors. Female survivors were 35 % less likely to report a pregnancy than siblings of childhood cancer survivors, even after excluding women who were surgically sterile (Ginsberg et al. 2010b). Similarly, male EWS survivors were 62 % less likely to report siring a child than male siblings (Ginsberg et al. 2010b). Contemporary therapy for EWS includes high dose cyclophosphamide and ifosfamide, so we can anticipate that the rate of infertility will not be much different for patients treated today. Another 58 patient analysis of sarcoma patients including 22 with EWS reviewed semen analyses before, during, and after treatment with chemotherapy with multi-agent chemotherapy including cyclophosphamide (Meistrich et al. 1992). While pretreatment levels were similar to the control subjects, azoospermia occurred within 4 months of treatment (Meistrich et al. 1992). The cumulative dose of cyclophosphamide was the most significant determinant of recovery to normospermic levels; approximately 70 % of those who had received doses less than 7.5 g/m^2 recovered, but only 10 % recovered when doses exceeded 7.5 g/m^2 (Meistrich et al. 1992). In a retrospective

study of 17 male sarcoma survivors treated with high dose cyclophosphamide within a multi-agent chemotherapy regimen, a total dose of cyclophosphamide of 7.5 g/m^2 was also associated with a decreased risk of an abnormal sperm count with an incidence of azoospermia of 58.8 % (Kenney et al. 2001). This analyses also demonstrated that exposure prior to the onset of puberty did not appear to protect males from subsequent gonadal damage. All of the patients exposed to 25 g/m^2 of cyclophosphamide or higher were azoospermic irrespective of their pubertal status at the time of treatment (Kenney et al. 2001).

5.4.3 Osteosarcoma

In patients with osteosarcoma, exposure to Ifosfamide has also been analyzed in several case series. Kenney et al. reviewed six patients with non-metastatic osteosarcoma who were treated with multi-agent chemotherapy (Kenney et al. 2001). They reported their results as consistent with previously reported studies that used semen analysis as their measure of spermatogenesis, demonstrating 52–89 % of survivors with abnormal sperm counts after treatment with Ifosfamide 24–45 g/m^2 (Kenney et al. 2001). The United Kingdom Children's Cancer Study Group (UKCCSG) reviewed gonadal function of patients who were treated for Ewing or soft tissue sarcoma with regimens containing ifosfamide as the only potential gonadotoxic agent (Williams et al. 2008). Male patients who received high dose Ifosfamide (greater than 60 g/m^2) showed 73 % to be subfertile and 27 % azoospermic (Williams et al. 2008). Hormone profiles were consistent with germ cell failure, 31 % had increased FSH, while Leydig cell function remained preserved (Williams et al. 2008). The female cohort for the study had different treatment regimens including ifosfamide (Longhi et al. 2003). Unfortunately, very few patients were willing to undergo semen analysis and/or hormone testing, so the study was only able to conclude that Ifosfamide seems to be a major cause of infertility in male osteosarcoma patients with a dose-dependent relationship between higher doses of ifosfamide with higher probability of becoming sterile (Longhi et al. 2003). They also noted that Cisplatin causes azoospermia or oligospermia with a gradual recovery of spermatogenesis in 50 % of patients after 2 years and 80 % after 5 years following cumulative dose of 600 mg/m^2 (Longhi et al. 2003). In contrast, the Rizzoli Institute also reviewed the reproductive function of female survivors of localized osteosarcoma. Twenty-four of their 92 patients were prepubertal at the time of chemotherapy and underwent menarche at a mean age of 13 (range 11–16), consistent with the mean age of menarche of the normal population in Italy (Longhi et al. 2000). Of the postpubertal patients, 69 % experienced amenorrhea during chemotherapy, 66/68 patients resumed menstrual activity by the end of chemotherapy, whereas the 2 patients age 39 and 43 at the start of treatment had permanent amenorrhea (Longhi et al. 2000). Of the 92 patients, only 2 patients reported a willingness to conceive without achieving a pregnancy and 20 others had successful pregnancies with healthy offspring (Longhi et al. 2000). A Finnish study demonstrated similar findings in a small cohort of female osteosarcoma survivors with all patients having amenorrhea at the completion of chemotherapy, but 90 % had some returned menses within 3–12 months of follow-up (Wikstrom et al. 2003). The three patients who had irregular menses cycles upon resumption of menstruation represented the highest cumulative dose of Ifosfamide (54.5 g/m^2, 63.5 g/m^2, and 60.4 g/m^2) (Wikstrom et al. 2003). Importantly, resumption of menses does not directly correlate to fertility and pregnancy, and thus is a limitation of this small study.

5.5 Clinical Guidelines

Several organizations have published guidelines for fertility preservation in cancer patients. The ethics committee of the American Society for Reproductive Medicine produced the first guideline on fertility preservation and reproduction in 2005. It addressed the roles of cancer specialists and fertility specialists in the counseling and referral of cancer patients including safety and efficacy of options, special considerations for minor patients, and ethical considerations in the disposition of stored gametes, embryos, and gonadal tissue (Robertson et al. 2005). The American Society of Clinical Oncology (ASCO) followed with their guideline for practicing oncologists in 2006, which was updated in 2013 (http://www.asco.org/guidelines/fertility). The American Academy of Pediatrics published a guideline in 2008 (Fallat and Hutter 2008) that is currently being revised for publication, reviewing the technical aspects of fertility preservation in pediatric and adolescent patients as well as the ethical considerations. Specifically, the AAP recommendations are as follows:

Evaluation of candidacy for fertility preservation should involve a team of specialists, including a pediatric oncologist and/or radiation oncologist, a fertility specialist, an ethicist, and a mental health professional.

1. Cryopreservation of sperm should be offered whenever possible to male patients or families of male adolescents.
2. Current fertility-preservation options for female children and adolescents should be considered experimental and are offered only in selected institutions in the setting of a research protocol.
3. In considering actions to preserve a child's fertility, parents should consider a child's assent, the details of the procedure involved, and whether such procedures are of proven utility or experimental in nature. In some cases, after such consideration, acting to preserve a child's fertility may be appropriate.
4. Instructions concerning disposition of stored gametes, embryos, or gonadal tissue in the event of the patient's death,

unavailability, or other contingency should be legally outlined and understood by all parties, including the patient if possible.

5. Concerns about the welfare of a resultant offspring with respect to future cancer risk should not be a cause for denying reproductive assistance to a patient.

5.6 Risk Identification

Once the definitive cancer diagnosis is made, fertility risk identification may proceed as the proposed treatment plan unfolds. As previously discussed, fertility risk factors include age, chemotherapeutic agents used, radiation dose, and possible surgical interventions. Oncologists have many risk assessment tools at their disposal. The NCCN guidelines for Adolescent and Young Adult Oncology recommend the risks to fertility be discussed prior to the initiation of chemotherapy and a referral for fertility preservation occur within 24 h for who choose to pursue it (Coccia et al. 2014). It also refers providers to the on-line risk assessment tool at www.livestrong.org/we-can-help/fertility-services.

Based on these recommendations, Fig. 5.1 shows an overview of the stratification of fertility considerations based on planned anti-cancer therapy and Fig. 5.2 is an algorithm for screening new oncology patients for fertility counseling and referrals.

5.7 Pretreatment Options for Males

Cryopreservation of ejaculated semen is the recommended fertility preservation method for adult males and pubertal boys. Mature spermatozoa can be found at Tanner III stage with a testis volume above 5 ml, although 20 % of males at Tanner stage II or above with testicular volumes greater than 10–12 ml have achieved spermiation, with the ability to provide sperm for cryopreservation (Gracia and Woodruff 2012). Cryopreservation of two to three samples collected following a period of abstinence of 48 h between samples is recommended prior to starting treatment to ensure optimal DNA integrity and sperm quality (Gracia and Woodruff 2012; Rodriguez-Wallberg and Oktay 2014; Leonard et al. 2004).

In cases of ejaculation failure, sperm may be extracted via *testicular sperm extraction (TESE)*, a surgical procedure where sperm is extracted via an open incision through the scrotum and one or multiple biopsies of testicular tissue are obtained

Cancer surgery	Fertility-sparing surgery preserving gonads. Preservation of the uterus in females. Use of cryopreservation may be considered prior to surgery if the risk of gonadal damage is high
Radiation therapy to pelvic organs and gonads	Shielding aimed at reducing damage of reproductive organs and surgical ovarian transposition Use of cryopreservation may be considered prior to radiotherapy
Cytotoxic treatment with high risk of gonadal damage	Use of cryopreservation methods such as sperm banking for males, freezing of embryos and oocytes for females and gonadal tissue freezing

Fig. 5.1 Fertility preservation options to consider based on treatment

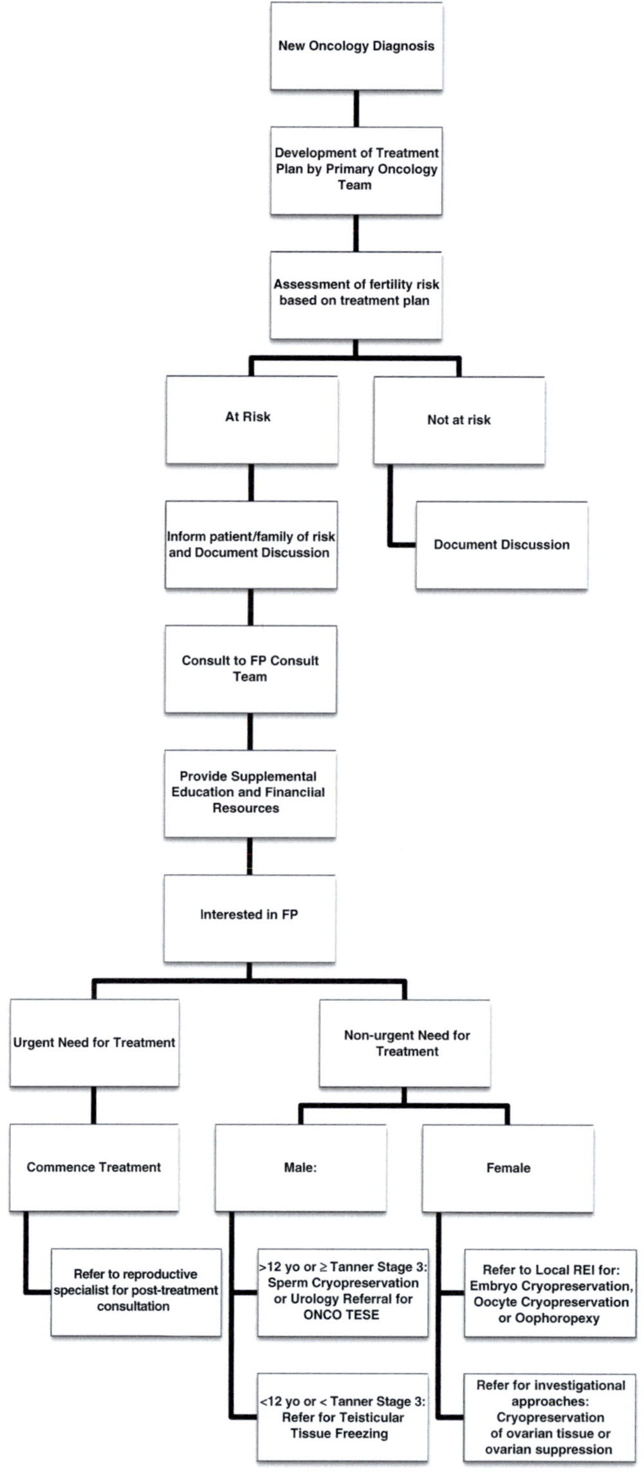

Fig. 5.2 Work-flow algorithm for fertility preservation during cancer therapy

and sperm can be harvested and placed in media for analysis and cryopreservation (Quinn and Vadaparampil 2012; Schrader et al. 2003). Patients with neurologic compromise can undergo *vibrostimulatory ejaculation* if the sacral reflex is intact. In the absence of an intact spinal pathway, *electroejaculation* can be performed, although this requires anesthesia if the patient does not have a complete spinal cord injury (Gracia and Woodruff 2012). In electroejaculation, a rectal probe is used to transmit electrical stimulation to the short postsynaptic sympathetic fibers in the walls of the ejaculatory organs leading to ejaculation (Berookhim and Mulhall 2014).

Collecting sperm prior to cancer therapy has a unique set of challenges. Patients are facing cancer or other serious medical issues. The context in which patients are asked to provide specimens is fraught with stress. They are often feeling ill, emotionally overwhelmed, are in pain, and are possibly under the influence of narcotics or other medications. They may be hospitalized and have limited privacy for masturbation. Patients may be unable to perform under severe time constraints and pressure, particularly adolescent boys, and there may be religious or personal objections to masturbation that are difficult to overcome (Ogle et al. 2008). Every attempt should be made to facilitate the collection of ejaculated sperm. Patients should be provided private and relaxing physical conditions whenever possible. It is important to avoid discussing the details of sample collection with adolescents in the presence of their families. Separate discussions with the adolescent patient and family members help avoid introducing unnecessary embarrassment that might present yet another barrier to successful collection. Sexually stimulating audiovisual materials, such as magazines or videos, should be provided to the patient if appropriate.

Testicular tissue cryopreservation is the only available option in prepubertal patients who have not yet initiated spermatogenesis. Investigators are examining cryopreservation of testicular tissue through either cell suspension or whole tissue as a possible option for fertility preservation (Gracia and Woodruff 2012). The tissue can be obtained via testicular biopsy. Although prepubertal germ cells do not contain mature spermatozoa, they do demonstrate the presence of spermatogonial diploid stem cells, which maintain the capacity to differentiate into mature cells given the appropriate microenvironment. Investigators from the Children's Hospital of Philadelphia published reports of prepubertal boys who underwent testicular biopsy with tissue cryopreservation (Ginsberg et al. 2010a). Despite this and other similar experimental protocols reporting preservation of prepubertal tissue, no study to date has demonstrated a technique to transform this immature, cryopreserved tissue into functional gametes either in vivo or in vitro (Ginsberg et al. 2010a). Furthermore, hypothetical risks associated with tissue preservation exist. Given the underlying malignancy in patients undergoing testicular tissue extraction, there is concern regarding the potential for reseeding the cancer when cryopreserved tissue is reintroduced into the native host. Thus, testicular tissue cryopreservation is performed strictly under an experimental, IRB-approved protocol, as no clinically proven means to use such tissue for reproductive purposes exists at this time (Gracia and Woodruff 2012) (See Table 5.3).

5.8 Pretreatment Options for Females

Embryo cryopreservation is the most established fertility preservation method for females. The ovaries are stimulated with FSH injections and LH for approximately a week and a half (Quinn and Vadaparampil 2012). Ultrasounds and blood tests are used throughout this time to monitor development of ovarian follicles. When the follicles are appropriately sized, an injection of human chorionic gonadotropin (hCG) triggers ovulation and the eggs are aspirated transvaginally from the follicles just prior to ovulation (Quinn and Vadaparampil 2012). Oocytes are then fertilized by either intracytoplasmic sperm

Table 5.3 Fertility preservation options for males

	Definition	Pubertal status	Time requirement	Success rates	Cost	Timing	Special considerations
Sperm banking (masturbation)	Sperm is obtained through masturbation, then frozen	After puberty	Outpatient procedure	Generally high The most established technique for men	Approx. $1,500 for 3 samples; storage fees average $300–$500/year	Before treatment	Deposits can be made every 24–48 h. May consider TESE or electroejaculation if male unable to ejaculate
Radiation shielding of gonads	Use of shielding to reduce the dose of radiation delivered to the testes	Before and after puberty	In conjunction with radiation treatments	Possible with select radiation fields and anatomy	Generally included in the cost of radiation treatments	During treatment	Expertise required; does not protect against effects of chemotherapy
Testicular tissue freezing	Tissue obtained through biopsy and frozen for future use	Before and after puberty	Outpatient procedure	No available human success rates	$500–$2,500 for surgery; $300–$1,000 for freezing; $300–$500/year for storage	Before treatment	May be only option for prepubescent boys. Experimental use with IRB approved protocol
Testicular sperm extraction (TESE)	Use of biopsy to obtain individual sperm from testicular tissue	Tanner stage II	Outpatient procedure	30–70 % in postpubescent patients	$4,000–$16,000 (in additional to costs for IVF)	Before or after treatment	Center should be able to freeze sperm found at the time of biopsy
Donor sperm	Sperm donated by a man for artificial insemination or IVF	After puberty	Readily available for purchase	50–80 %	$200–$500 per vial (in addition to costs for IUI or IVF)	After treatment	Can choose donor based on wide range of characteristics
Adoption	Process that creates a legal parent-child relationship	After puberty	Varies depending on the type of adoption	N/A	$2,500–$35,000	After treatment	Medical history often a factor

injection or in vitro fertilization and cryopreserved for later use. Typically embryo cryopreservation takes approximately 2–6 weeks to accomplish, dependent on the phase of the patient's menstrual cycle at presentation to a reproductive specialist. Embryo cryopreservation carries high out of pocket costs, requires a male partner or sperm donor, and can cause delays in initiation of cancer treatment.

Oocyte cryopreservation can be utilized if there is no male partner or sperm donor. The oocytes are harvested as described in embryo cryopreservation, with or without hormonal stimulation. While initial pregnancy rates were not as high as with embryo cryopreservation, oocyte freezing techniques continue to improve prompting the ASRM to no longer consider oocyte cryopreservation to be an experimental procedure (Pfeifer 2013).

Oophoropexy is a surgical procedure done to spare ovarian function in patients who undergo pelvic radiation (Williams et al. 1999). The laparoscopic procedure moves the ovaries out of potential radiation fields to minimize exposure and damage during radiation treatment. Reduction of radiation exposure has been reported to be decreased by approximately 50–90 % (Gracia and Woodruff 2012).

Ovarian tissue cryopreservation provides a viable alternative option for patients who wish to preserve their fertility but expedite their cancer therapy, or for prepubertal girls who have no other options to preserve their future fertility (Gracia and Woodruff 2012). This process involves harvesting ovarian cortex tissue which contains thousands of follicles containing immature eggs. The tissue can be removed laparoscopically as an outpatient surgery and either reimplanted into the pelvis (orthotopic transplantation,) in subcutaneous tissue or muscle (heteroscopic transplantation) (Gracia and Woodruff 2012; Pfeifer et al. 2013, 2014; Quinn and Vadaparampil 2009; West et al. 2009), or follicles can be matured in vitro and fertilized years after cancer therapy is complete. This method of fertility preservation is investiga-

tional, and only offered through clinical trials at limited institutions under IRB supervision. An important consideration of this technology is the potential of reintroducing malignant cells of harvested ovarian tissue. Metastatic Ewing sarcoma has been reported in the ovary (Sullivan et al. 2012). One of the largest series of cryopreserved ovarian tissue in the world at Copenhagen University Hospital reviewed 16 surviving sarcoma patients tissue to evaluate the risk of residual cancer cells in the ovarian cortex intended for transplantation. Tissue of nine patients with Ewing sarcoma, one patient with chondrosarcoma, and four patients with osteosarcoma was examined by light microscopy, RT-PCR for presence of EWS-FLI1, and finally xenotransplantation with no evidence of malignant contamination (Smitz 2004). They concluded that it is safe to transplant ovarian tissue from patients who previously suffered from a sarcoma, but recommended evaluation of a sample of tissue for malignant cell contamination prior to transplantation (Smitz 2004). Another series of eight patients evaluated cryopreserved ovarian samples from Ewing sarcoma patients with histology examination and RT-PCR for EWS-FLI1. Histology did not reveal any malignant cells; however, one sample did show a positive result for the EWS-FLIi transcript (Abir et al. 2010). The authors concluded that because EWS is highly metastatic, ovarian tissue should be carefully examined both by histological and molecular techniques before ovarian transplantation (Abir et al. 2010). There have been two transplantations of ovarian tissue to patients recovered from EWS and no relapses have been observed due to the replacement of the ovarian tissue (Anderson et al. 2008). One patient was transplanted two years after completing treatment, resulting in 3 live births and no relapse for greater than seven years (Anderson et al. 2008). The other patient was diagnosed with EWS at age 9 and had one ovary cryopreserved. It was transplanted 4.5 years after it was cryopreserved to induce pubertal development by endogenous hormone secretion (Ernst et al. 2013). She successfully underwent pubertal development and menstruation 1 year after transplantation (Ernst et al. 2013).

Ovarian suppression is theorized to protect the ovaries by suppressing the pituitary-ovarian axis simulating prepubertal hormonal milieu, reducing recruitment of follicles and thereby creating a quiescent ovarian state, making them less susceptible to the damage of chemotherapeutic agents (Blumenfeld et al. 2008, 2014; Falcone et al. 2004; Gracia and Woodruff 2012). To date, 20 studies have reported on nearly 2,000 patients treated with gonadotropin releasing hormone analogues (GnRH-a) in parallel to chemotherapy including 5 prospective randomized controlled trials (RCTs) and 15 non-randomized controlled trials reporting a significant decrease in premature ovarian failure rates in survivors of various cancers (Blumenfeld et al. 2014; Ibrahim et al. 2008). However, nine studies including six randomized controlled trials did not support the effectiveness of GnRH-a treatment (Blumenfeld et al. 2014; Ibrahim et al. 2008). Seven meta-analysis have concluded that GnRH-a use may be beneficial and decrease the risk of premature ovarian failure, including the most recent Cochrane analysis which concluded that GnRH-a was effective in protection of menstruation and ovulation after chemotherapy (Blumenfeld et al. 2014). The authors concluded that the use of GnRH-a should be considered for women of reproductive age receiving chemotherapy, stating they were effective in protecting the ovaries from chemotherapy and should be given before or during treatment, although no significant difference in pregnancy rates was seen (Ibrahim et al. 2008). Unfortunately at this time, no studies have been able to consistently demonstrate improvement in pregnancy rates. Until data can demonstrate a significant improvement in pregnancy outcomes for women receiving GnRH-a is produced, GnRH-a cotreatment with chemotherapy as an exclusive means to preserve fertility should be recommended with caution (Gracia and Woodruff 2012) (See Table 5.4).

5.9 Post-treatment Family Planning Options

While the majority of survivors of pediatric bone tumors will retain their fertility, a significant proportion of survivors will suffer from infertility or subfertility making traditional conception difficult or impossible.

Sperm recipientcy is the most frequently used and successful method of family building available for males (Quinn and Vadaparampil 2012). This technique involves using donor sperm to inseminate the female partner of a male cancer survivor. Mancini et al. found that young adult cancer survivors who did not preserve sperm reported a lower physical and mental quality of life, and furthermore, patients who were not informed that sperm cryopreservation was an option prior to cancer treatment universally report being dissatisfied with their medical treatment.

Oocyte recipientcy is the process involving the use of a donated ova which can be fertilized either with a female cancer survivor's partner's sperm or donor sperm, then transferred into the survivor's uterus to carry the pregnancy. Should the survivor no longer have a uterus, a gestational surrogate can receive the embryos and carry the pregnancy to term.

Surrogacy is a viable option for intended parents who are either unable to carry a baby to term or conceive without assistance. Traditional surrogates use their own eggs and sperm donated either by the intended father or a sperm donor. A gestational surrogate, often called a gestational carrier, does not use her own ova and achieves a pregnancy through in vitro fertilization. The gametes may be provided by both of the intended parents, an egg donor and the intended father, donated eggs and donated sperm, donor sperm and the intended mother's oocytes, or donated embryos (Quinn and Vadaparampil 2012).

Finally, cancer survivors may elect to use *adoption*. Adoption can be a difficult process for a prospective parent with a cancer history, and some agencies require survivors to be cancer free for a

Table 5.4 Fertility preservation options for females

	Definition	Pubertal status	Time requirement	Success rates	Cost	Timing	Special considerations
Embryo freezing	Harvesting eggs, in vitro fertilization of embryos for later implantation	After puberty	Approx. 2 weeks Outpatient surgical procedure	Approx. 40 % per transfer; varies by age and carrier Thousands of babies born	Approx. $12,000/ cycle; storage fees and pregnancy costs additional	Before or after treatment	Need partner of donor sperm
Egg freezing	Harvesting and freezing of unfertilized eggs	After puberty	Approx. 2 weeks Outpatient surgical procedure	Approx. 21.6 % per embryo transfer	Approx. $12,000/ cycle; storage fees and pregnancy costs additional	Before or after treatment	May be attractive to single women or those opposed to embryo creation
Ovarian tissue freezing	Freezing of ovarian tissue and reimplantation after cancer treatment; possible in vitro maturation of oocytes	Before or after puberty	Outpatient surgical procedure	At least 38 live births reported as of October 2014	$12,000 for procedure; storage fees and reimplantation costs additional	Before or after treatment	Not suitable if high risk of ovarian metastases Only preservation option for prepubescent girls; experimental use with IRB approved protocols
Radiation shielding of gonads	Use of shielding to reduce scatter radiation to the reproductive organs	Before or after puberty	In conjunction with radiation treatment	Only possible with selected radiation fields and anatomy	Generally included in cost of radiation	During treatment	Expertise required Does not protect against effects of chemotherapy
Ovarian transposition	Surgical repositioning of ovaries away from the radiation field	Before or after puberty	Outpatient procedure	Approx. 50 % due to altered blood flow and scattered radiation	Unknown; may be covered by insurance	Before treatment	Expertise required
Ovarian suppression	Gonadotropin releasing hormone (GnRH) analogues or antagonists used to suppress ovaries	After puberty	In conjunction with chemotherapy	Unknown; conflicting results reported Larger randomized trials in progress	$500/month	During treatment	Does not protect from radiation effects; experimental

(continued)

Table 5.4 (continued)

	Definition	Pubertal status	Time requirement	Success rates	Cost	Timing	Special considerations
Donor embryos	Embryos donated by a couple	After puberty	Varies; is done in conjunction with IVF	Unknown; higher than that of frozen embryo IVF transfers	$5,000–$7,000 (in addition to costs for IVF)	After treatment	Donor embryo available through IVF clinics or private agencies
Donor eggs	Eggs donated by a woman	After puberty	Varies; is done in conjunction with IVF	40–50 %	$5,000–$15,000 (in addition to costs for IVF)	After treatment	Patient can choose donor based on various characteristics
Gestational surrogacy	Woman carries a pregnancy for another woman or couple	After puberty	Varies; time is required to find surrogate and implant embryo	Similar to IVF- approx. 30 %	$10,000–$100,000	After treatment	Legal status varies by state
Adoption	Process that creates a legal parent--child relationship	After puberty	Varies depending on type of adoption	N/A	$2,500–$35,000	After treatment	Medical history often a factor

minimum of 5 years before attempting to adopt. However, organizations such as Northwestern's Oncofertility Consortium have developed a list of "cancer friendly" agencies that are more flexible and willing to work with cancer survivors. Infertile cancer survivors can experience significant depression and anxiety similar to the general infertile population, thus appropriate mental health referrals and counseling should be encouraged.

5.10 Contraception

Except in rare cases, adolescents and young adults with cancer have the same sexual, marital, and romantic aspirations as their healthy peers. Thus, they share the same information needs as their peers regarding effective contraception, avoiding unwanted pregnancies, and sexually transmitted infections (STIs). Many cytotoxic drugs, as well as radiotherapy, are teratogenic and mutagenic and conception during chemotherapy may result in abortion of the embryo or gross congenital abnormalities of the fetus, emphasizing the need for effective contraception in sexually active young

people undergoing treatment for cancer (Murphy et al. 2013). Available contraceptive methods are summarized in Table 5.5.

5.11 Challenges and Barriers to Providing Fertility Preservation Options

5.11.1 Lack of Information

Despite the evidence that fertility loss in survivors of cancer is related to psychological distress and impaired quality of life, many cancer patients and their families still do not receive adequate information or referral to a reproductive specialist for fertility preservation (Rodriguez-Wallberg and Oktay 2014). While it has been acknowledged that information may be lost given the overwhelming nature of the diagnosis, studies of health care providers have also suggested that risks of infertility are not routinely and universally discussed. Among pediatric oncology providers, only 35 % reported consulting with reproductive specialists. Reasons for not discussing risks for infertility include lack of time, lack of information regarding level of gonadotoxicity of different regimens, cost, lack of referral network, and general discomfort of provider in discussing the topic (Levine 2011; Nahata et al. 2012; Quinn et al. 2009a, b; Rodriguez-Wallberg and Oktay 2014). Providers also cited patient factors impacting their discussions including language or cultural barriers, belief that fertility preservation is too anxiety-provoking or stressful, poor patient prognosis, concern for cost for family, and concern about age of patient (Kelvin et al. 2012).

5.11.2 Ethical Considerations

Multiple ethical issues surround fertility preservation techniques, particularly for pediatric and adolescent patients who have not yet reached the age of 18. These patients present the additional concern for the child's ability to contribute to the complex decisions related to fertility preservation and future disposition of reproductive materials. Young chil-

Table 5.5 Options for contraception

	Examples
Abstinence	n/a
Behavioral method	No method
	Withdrawal
	Periodic abstinence
Oral contraception	Oral combined pill (OCP)
	Progestin-only pill (POP)
	Emergency contraception ("Morning after pill")
	Oral progestogens
Injectable contraceptives	Depo-provera
Implant contraceptives	Norplant, jadelle, implanon
Intra-uterine devices (IUDs)	Copper IUD
	Levonorgestrel
Barrier methods	Female
	Diaphragm
	Cervical cap
	Vaginal sponge
	Female condoms
	Vaginal spermicides
	Male
	Male condoms

dren obviously are unable to contribute to the decision making process and available options are experimental and should be discussed with caution and under IRB approval with parents or guardians. Older children may have a much more active role in the informed consent process and careful consideration should be made to include them in the process depending on their developmental level. These conversations can be awkward and embarrassing to teens and young adults, and should occur without parents present whenever possible using clear and simple language.

Oncologists' reluctance to discuss fertility issues with patients with a poor prognosis has been reported in multiple studies with the general consensus being that fertility preservation is not important at a time when a patient is fighting for survival (Saito et al. 2005). Providers may worry that discussing fertility preservation will give patients a false hope about their prognosis. At the same time, pursuing fertility preservation may be a source of hope and happiness for patients during difficult times.

Lastly, and perhaps one of the most difficult areas of fertility preservation, is the question of posthumous assisted reproduction (PAR). This refers to the utilization of cryopreserved reproductive materials to conceive a child with the use of assisted reproductive technologies after the death of the patient. The ASRM guidelines state that "Precise instructions should be given about the disposition of stored gametes, embryos, or gonadal tissue in the event of the patient's death, unavailability, or other contingency" (Robertson 2005). Under the law, gametes and embryos are classified as a type of property, and people whose genetic material the gametes or embryos contain are the default owners of this property. As property, gametes and embryos can be bequeathed to others upon their death. Given this legal understanding, disputes over reproductive material may have to be resolved in court if a bioethics consultant or others cannot first help resolve the matter (Gracia and Woodruff 2012). Unfortunately, it is not possible to predict the outcome of these cases because there is no set precedent in this matter and individual judges have ruled quite differently in similar cases. With regard to minors, the repro-

ductive material is technically the property of the child, and parents should not be allowed to use or discard their child's reproductive material before the child turns 18. If a minor child passes away, the child's reproductive material should be immediately destroyed or donated to science.

Clinicians who care for cancer patients should understand and anticipate questions regarding the ethical issues surrounding fertility preservation, working closely with bioethicists and legal counsel to address their patients' concerns about fertility preservation options.

Conclusion

The majority of children, adolescents, and young adults with pediatric bone tumors will become long-term survivors. Survivors of cancer place a high priority on fertility and report high levels of psychological distress associated with fertility loss (Murphy et al. 2013). Options are available to preserve fertility among those at risk of infertility secondary to cancer treatment, but several barriers exist which reduce the likelihood of fertility preservation utilization. Health care providers should be prepared to discuss the negative impact of cancer therapy on reproductive health with their patients and families in the same way other risks of cancer treatment are discussed. The possibility of using fertility preservation methods should be presented to all patients, and appropriate referrals provided. Interdisciplinary collaboration between oncologists, reproductive endocrinologists, urologists, and gynecologists, development of local clinical guidelines, and availability of educational materials and activities should be encouraged to ensure that patient needs are being met.

References

Abir R, et al (2010) Occasional involvement of the ovary in Ewing sarcoma. Hum Reprod 25(7):1708–1712

Anderson CY et al (2008) Two successful pregnancies following autotransplantation of frozen/thawed ovarian tissue. Hum Reprod 23(10):2266–2272

Aubier F, Flamant F, Brauner R et al (1989) Male gonadal function after chemotherapy for solid tumors in childhood. J Clin Oncol 7:304–309

Berookhim BM, Mulhall JP (2014) Outcomes of operative sperm retrieval strategies for fertility preservation among males scheduled to undergo cancer treatment. Fertil Steril 101:805–811

Blumenfeld Z, Avivi I, Eckman A et al (2008) Gonadotropin-releasing hormone agonist decreases chemotherapy-induced gonadotoxicity and premature ovarian failure in young female patients with Hodgkin lymphoma. Fertil Steril 89:166–173

Blumenfeld Z, Katz G, Evron A (2014) 'An ounce of prevention is worth a pound of cure': the case for and against GnRH-agonist for fertility preservation. Ann Oncol 25:1719–1728

Chemaitilly W, Mertens AC, Mitby P et al (2006) Acute ovarian failure in the childhood cancer survivor study. J Clin Endocrinol Metab 91:1723–1728

Coccia PF, Pappo AS, Altman J et al (2014) Adolescent and young adult oncology, version 2.2014. J Natl Compr Canc Netw 12:21–32, quiz 32

Edge SB (2014) The NCCN guidelines program and opportunities for quality improvement. J Natl Compr Canc Netw 12(Suppl 1):S1–S4

Ernst E et al (2013) Case Report: stimulation of puberty in a girl with chemo and radiation therapy induced ovarian failure by transplantation of a small part of her frozen/thawed ovarian tissue. Eur J Cancer 49(4):911–914

Falcone T, Attaran M, Bedaiwy MA et al (2004) Ovarian function preservation in the cancer patient. Fertil Steril 81:243–257

Fallat ME, Hutter J (2008) Preservation of fertility in pediatric and adolescent patients with cancer. Pediatrics 121:e1461–e1469

Ginsberg JP (2011) Educational paper: the effect of cancer therapy on fertility, the assessment of fertility and fertility preservation options for pediatric patients. Eur J Pediatr 170:703–708

Ginsberg JP, Carlson CA, Lin K et al (2010a) An experimental protocol for fertility preservation in prepubertal boys recently diagnosed with cancer: a report of acceptability and safety. Hum Reprod 25:37–41

Ginsberg JP, Goodman P, Leisenring W et al (2010b) Long-term survivors of childhood Ewing sarcoma: report from the childhood cancer survivor study. J Natl Cancer Inst 102:1272–1283

Gracia C, Woodruff TK (2012) Oncofertility medical practice: clinical issues and implementation. Springer, New York

Green DM, Kawashima T, Stovall M et al (2010) Fertility of male survivors of childhood cancer: a report from the Childhood Cancer Survivor Study. J Clin Oncol 28:332–339

Gupta AA, Edelstein K, Albert-Green A et al (2013) Assessing information and service needs of young adults with cancer at a single institution: the importance of information on cancer diagnosis, fertility preservation, diet, and exercise. Support Care Cancer 21:2477–2484

Hobbie WL, Ginsberg JP, Ogle SK et al (2005) Fertility in males treated for Hodgkins disease with COPP/ABV hybrid. Pediatr Blood Cancer 44:193–196

Howell S, Shalet S (1998) Gonadal damage from chemotherapy and radiotherapy. Endocrinol Metab Clin N Am 27:927–943

Ibrahim SF, Osman K, Das S et al (2008) A study of the antioxidant effect of alpha lipoic acids on sperm quality. Clinics (Sao Paulo) 63:545–550

Jahnukainen K, Ehmcke J, Hou M et al (2011) Testicular function and fertility preservation in male cancer patients. Best Pract Res Clin Endocrinol Metab 25:287–302

Kelvin JF, Kroon L, Ogle SK (2012) Fertility preservation for patients with cancer. Clin J Oncol Nurs 16:205–210

Kenney LB, Laufer MR, Grant FD et al (2001) High risk of infertility and long term gonadal damage in males treated with high dose cyclophosphamide for sarcoma during childhood. Cancer 91:613–621

Kenney LB, Cohen LE, Shnorhavorian M et al (2012) Male reproductive health after childhood, adolescent, and young adult cancers: a report from the Children's Oncology Group. J Clin Oncol 30:3408–3416

Knopman JM, Papadopoulos EB, Grifo JA et al (2010) Surviving childhood and reproductive-age malignancy: effects on fertility and future parenthood. Lancet Oncol 11:490–498

Larsen EC, Muller J, Schmiegelow K et al (2003) Reduced ovarian function in long-term survivors of radiation- and chemotherapy-treated childhood cancer. J Clin Endocrinol Metab 88:5307–5314

Lee SH, Shin CH (2013) Reduced male fertility in childhood cancer survivors. Ann Pediatr Endocrinol Metab 18:168–172

Leonard M, Hammelef K, Smith GD (2004) Fertility considerations, counseling, and semen cryopreservation for males prior to the initiation of cancer therapy. Clin J Oncol Nurs 8:127–131, 145

Levine J (2011) Fertility preservation in children and adolescents with cancer. Minerva Pediatr 63:49–59

Longhi A, Porcu E, Petracchi S et al (2000) Reproductive functions in female patients treated with adjuvant and neoadjuvant chemotherapy for localized osteosarcoma of the extremity. Cancer 89:1961–1965

Longhi A, Macchiagodena M, Vitali G et al (2003) Fertility in male patients treated with neoadjuvant chemotherapy for osteosarcoma. J Pediatr Hematol Oncol 25:292–296

Meistrich ML, Wilson G, Brown BW et al (1992) Impact of cyclophosphamide on long-term reduction in sperm count in men treated with combination chemotherapy for Ewing and soft tissue sarcomas. Cancer 70:2703–2712

Metzger ML, Meacham LR, Patterson B et al (2013) Female reproductive health after childhood, adolescent, and young adult cancers: guidelines for the assessment and management of female reproductive complications. J Clin Oncol 31:1239–1247

Murphy D et al (2013) Why Healthcare Providers Should Focus on the Fertility of AYA Cancer Survivors: It's Not Too Late! Front Oncol 3:248

Nahata L, Cohen LE, Yu RN (2012) Barriers to fertility preservation in male adolescents with cancer: it's time for a multidisciplinary approach that includes urologists. Urology 79:1206–1209

Ogle SK, Hobbie WL, Carlson CA et al (2008) Sperm banking for adolescents with cancer. J Pediatr Oncol Nurs 25:97–101

Pfeifer S, Goldberg J, Mcclure R, Lobo R, Thomas M, Widra E, Licht M, Collins J, Cedars M, Racowsky C, Vernon M, Davis O, Gracia C, Catherino W, Thornton K, Rebar R, La Barbera A (2013) Mature oocyte cryopreservation: a guideline. Fertil Steril 99:37–43

Pfeifer S, Goldberg J, Lobo R, Pisarska M, Thomas M, Widra E, Sandlow J, Licht M, Rosen M, Vernon M, Catherino W, Davis O, Dumesic D, Gracia C, Odem R, Thornton K, Reindollar R, Rebar R, La Barbera A (2014) Ovarian tissue cryopreservation: a committee opinion. Fertil Steril 101:1237–1243

Quinn GP, Vadaparampil ST (2009) Fertility preservation and adolescent/young adult cancer patients: physician communication challenges. J Adolesc Health 44:394–400

Quinn GP, Vadaparampil ST (2012) Reproductive health and cancer in adolescents and young adults. Springer, Dordrecht

Quinn GP, Vadaparampil ST, King L et al (2009a) Impact of physicians' personal discomfort and patient prognosis on discussion of fertility preservation with young cancer patients. Patient Educ Couns 77:338–343

Quinn GP, Vadaparampil ST, Lee JH et al (2009b) Physician referral for fertility preservation in oncology patients: a national study of practice behaviors. J Clin Oncol 27:5952–5957

Robertson JA, Bonnicksen AL, Amato P, Brzyski RG, Damewood MD, Greenfield D, Keye WR, Marshall LA, Mastroianni L, Morales AJ, Rebar RW, Steinbock B, Tipton S, Wolf SM (2005) Fertility preservation and reproduction in cancer patients. Fertil Steril 83:1622–1628

Rodriguez-Wallberg KA, Oktay K (2014) Fertility preservation during cancer treatment: clinical guidelines. Cancer Manag Res 6:105–117

Saito K et al (2005) Sperm cryopreservation before cancer chemotherapy helps in the emotional battle against cancer. Cancer 104(3):521–524

Schrader M, Muller M, Sofikitis N et al (2003) "Oncotese": testicular sperm extraction in azoospermic cancer patients before chemotherapy-new guidelines? Urology 61:421–425

Smitz J (2004) Oocyte developmental competence after heterotopic transplantation of cryopreserved ovarian tissue. Lancet 363:832–833

Sullivan HC et al (2012) Unusual presentation of metastatic Ewing sarcoma to the ovary in a 13 year old: A case report and review. Fetal Pediatr Pathol 31(3):159–163

Trudgen K, Ayensu-Coker L (2014) Fertility preservation and reproductive health in the pediatric, adolescent, and young adult female cancer patient. Curr Opin Obstet Gynecol 26:372–380

West ER, Zelinski MB, Kondapalli LA et al (2009) Preserving female fertility following cancer treatment: current options and future possibilities. Pediatr Blood Cancer 53:289–295

Wikstrom AM, Hovi L, Dunkel L et al (2003) Restoration of ovarian function after chemotherapy for osteosarcoma. Arch Dis Child 88:428–431

Williams RS, Littell RD, Mendenhall NP (1999) Laparoscopic oophoropexy and ovarian function in the treatment of Hodgkin disease. Cancer 86:2138–2142

Williams D, Crofton PM, Levitt G (2008) Does ifosfamide affect gonadal function? Pediatr Blood Cancer 50:347–351

Chemotherapy Regimens for Patients with Newly Diagnosed Malignant Bone Tumors

6

Ryan D. Roberts, Mary Frances Wedekind, and Bhuvana A. Setty

Contents

6.1 **Introduction** 83

6.2 **Chemotherapy for Ewing's Sarcoma** 85
6.2.1 Ewing and PNET 85
6.2.2 Identification of Active Agents 85
6.2.3 Collaborative Groups 86
6.2.4 Multi-agent Chemotherapy 87
6.2.5 Current Standard of Care 89
6.2.6 Ongoing and Upcoming Trials 90

6.3 **Chemotherapy for Osteosarcoma** 91
6.3.1 Identification of Active Agents 91
6.3.2 Collaborative Groups 93
6.3.3 Multi-agent Chemotherapy 94
6.3.4 Approaches to Systemic Therapy 94
6.3.5 Current Standard of Care 100
6.3.6 Ongoing and Upcoming Trials 101

6.4 **Treatment of Metastatic Disease** 101

Conclusions 102

References 103

R.D. Roberts, MD, PhD (✉) • B.A. Setty, MD
Division of Hematology/Oncology/BMT,
Nationwide Children's Hospital,
700 Children's Drive, Columbus, OH 43205, USA
e-mail: Ryan.roberts@nationwidechildrens.org;
Bhuvana.setty@nationwidechildrens.org

M.F. Wedekind, MD
Department of Pediatrics,
Nationwide Children's Hospital,
700 Children's Drive, Columbus, OH 43205, USA
e-mail: Mary.wedekind@nationwidechildrens.org

Abstract

The advent of chemotherapy brought dramatic improvements to the care of patients stricken with malignant bone tumors. Early experimentation with cytotoxic medications identified a number of agents with activity in both Ewing's sarcoma and osteosarcoma. Survival rates in patients treated with these new agents improved five- to six-fold over the course of less than a decade. Therapies identified during the early years of chemotherapy continue to form the backbone upon which most modern regimens are built. Efforts to further improve outcomes have proved difficult. Modest, incremental gains have come only through experimentation involving large populations of patients made possible through the emergence of international cooperative groups. Advances in supportive care have facilitated the gradual intensification of treatment regimens both in terms of dose intensity and interval compression. Patients with refractory or metastatic disease continue to fare poorly. New approaches to the treatment of these patients are desperately needed.

6.1 Introduction

Throughout most of the twentieth century, the treatment of patients with malignant bone tumors was primarily the realm of surgeons and, during and early part of the twenty-first century, that of

© Springer International Publishing Switzerland 2015
T.P. Cripe, N.D. Yeager (eds.), *Malignant Pediatric Bone Tumors - Treatment & Management*,
Pediatric Oncology, DOI 10.1007/978-3-319-18099-1_6

radiation oncologists. Patients stricken with ossifying sarcomas, originially described by Ewing as "diffuse endotheliomas of bone" (Ewing 1924) either underwent resection (usually by amputation) or received primary radiation therapy. Nearly all patients succumbed to their disease, and survival was discussed in terms of months. Those whose lesions were treated with radical surgery or radiation therapy alone almost always developed widespread metastatic disease. Isolated lesions could be treated with radiation, which often alleviated symptoms and occasionally prolonged survival, but rarely achieved cure.

Under these circumstances, patients diagnosed with Ewing's sarcoma experienced long-term survival rates of about 10 % (Jenkin 1966). As this tumor was determined to be radiosensitive, many patients were treated with aggressive radiation therapy, but most still did not survive beyond 2 years. Improvements in radiation techniques pushed survival curves upward of 20 % (Phillips and Higinbotham 1967), but struggled to make more definitive improvements. Despite these advances, most patients' disease eventually progressed and led to metastatic disease, which continued to be universally fatal.

Patients diagnosed with osteosarcoma also fared poorly. Their tumors were treated surgically as they proved to be less radiosensitive. Patients undergoing radical surgical procedures such as amputation experienced survival rates of 11–17 % for patients without identifiable pulmonary metastasis (Weinfeld and Dudley 1962; Dahlin and Coventry 1967; Marcove et al. 1970; Link et al. 1986). Patients who developed metastasis, whether prior to diagnosis or several months after amputation, essentially all died from their disease.

To practitioners caring for patients with malignant bone tumors, the need for systemic treatment of these diseases was apparent. Advances in surgical techniques and radiation technology provided stepwise improvements in the control of primary tumors and even of some types of metastasis. These advances did not, however, lead to remarkable improvements in outcome. Most patients still went on to develop metastatic disease despite the ever-more aggressive treatments. The strong tendency for these tumors to recur at distant metastatic sites suggested that dissemination occurred prior to resection and hinted at the potential value of systemic therapies, provided that medications having significant activity against these tumors could be discovered.

The early successes of chemotherapy as treatment for leukemia, for lymphoma, and then for some solid tumors fueled the hope that these discoveries might prove useful for patients with malignant bone tumors. The poor outcomes seen with many of the early attempts to treat osteosarcoma and Ewing's sarcoma with systemic chemotherapy led many to conclude that these tumors were not sensitive to these drugs. Further experimentation led to the identification of active agents and the subsequent development of combination regimens that has revolutionized the care of patients with malignant bone tumors. Modern chemotherapy has markedly improved outcomes in these patients. Chemotherapy has become an integral and essential part of the modern multimodal approach, which combines the most effective elements of systemic therapy with advanced methods for local control through surgery and radiation. Chemotherapy has improved survival and has been valuable in facilitating local control, preventing the emergence of disseminated disease, and providing ever-expanding options for the palliative care of patients by slowing tumor progression and reducing gross tumor burden.

Despite the significantly better outcomes afforded by modern chemotherapy, there still remain many opportunities for improvement. While event-free survival rates for patients with localized disease now exceed 70 % in some studies (Lewis et al. 2007; Meyers et al. 2008; Womer et al. 2012), metastatic disease has proven to be poorly responsive to current systemic therapies. Short-term survival for patients with metastatic disease remains 40 % at best (Goorin et al. 2002), with 5-year overall survival of around 20 % (Grier et al. 2003; Casey et al. 2009; Aljubran et al. 2009). The biological underpinnings of metastatic spread have become a very active field of research, and many current experimental therapy approaches are focusing on preventing the emergence of metastasis (Khanna et al. 2014).

This chapter summarizes the clinical trials and other developments from which the concepts that drive current approaches to chemotherapy for malignant bone tumors have been derived. It outlines the treatments that form our current standard of care and discusses some of the questions raised by the results of recent trials as well as those being asked by current and ongoing studies.

6.2 Chemotherapy for Ewing's Sarcoma

6.2.1 Ewing and PNET

Originally thought to represent independent entities, Ewing's sarcoma and primitive neuroectodermal tumor (PNET) of the bone are now understood to represent a single entity. Evidence for this singularity comes from the fact that both have similar responses to treatment (Miser et al. 1987a, b), similar histologic appearance with essentially identical expression of oncogene markers (McKeon et al. 1988; Ambros et al. 1991), and identical chromosomal translocations which are thought to drive their biology (Turc-Carel et al. 1983; Whang-Peng et al. 1984). They have been treated identically for many years, and no distinction is made between the two in this chapter.

6.2.2 Identification of Active Agents

Cyclophosphamide This is a nitrogen mustard and alkylating agent and was one of the first agents shown to have efficacy in patients with Ewing's sarcoma. A number of reports throughout the early 1960s described responses to cyclophosphamide (Pinkel 1962; Sutow and Sullivan 1962; Jenkin 1966). Most of these reports noted a slowing in the progression of metastatic disease in patients receiving the drug. Several authors of these early studies argued that its effects might be more significant if used earlier in the disease at times of lower tumor burden.

Vincristine Several studies performed in the 1960s showed efficacy of vincristine, a vinca alkaloid and mitotic spindle inhibitor, in patients with Ewing's sarcoma. This included some responses in patients who had disease that was resistant or refractory to other treatment regimens (James and George 1964; Sutow 1968). While the magnitude of the antitumor effect seen with vincristine monotherapy is relatively small, its modest side effect profile and mechanism of action that generates synergy with many other chemotherapeutic agents made it popular in many multi-agent protocols. One of the first such protocols used a treatment regimen that employed indefinite cycles of vincristine and cyclophosphamide in an adjuvant fashion after treatment with radiation (Hustu et al. 1968). The first five patients demonstrated a very positive outcome with a disease-free survival (DFS) of 12–38 months.

Doxorubicin The development of anthracyclines, DNA intercalating agents which inhibit topoisomerase II function, in the late 1960s and early 1970s prompted multiple studies of their effects in Ewing's sarcoma. Studies with both doxorubicin (Oldham and Pomeroy 1972; Evans et al. 1974) and daunorubicin (Evans et al. 1974) showed efficacy of anthracyclines in Ewing's sarcoma. While early trials were hampered by increased incidence of cardiac disease, many of those untoward effects are now avoided by limiting cumulative doses. The intensification of doxorubicin dosing has proved to be of immense importance in the treatment of this disease. A meta-analysis of patients with Ewing's sarcoma treated with chemotherapy throughout the 1970s and 1980s (Smith et al. 1991) identified doxorubicin as the most important agent in these treatments.

Ifosfamide (and etoposide) Ifosfamide is another nitrogen mustard derivative and DNA alkylating agent. It was initially utilized primarily as a replacement for cyclophosphamide in attempts to intensify therapy in standard regimens for high-risk patients (Deméocq et al. 1989; Jürgens et al. 1989). It has become an agent routinely utilized in the care of patients with Ewing's sarcoma. Ifosfamide is commonly used in combination with etoposide, a topoisomerase inhibitor, which has little efficacy as a monotherapy, but has shown to have synergistic efficacy when used in conjunction with ifosfamide (Miser et al. 1987b). Subsequent evidence for the specific activity of ifosfamide and etoposide (IE) in Ewing's sarcoma came with window studies performed in patients with newly diagnosed disease (Meyer et al. 1992). While some smaller historical control studies have produced results that argue to the contrary (Oberlin et al. 1992; Bacci et al. 1998), large well-controlled studies have established the utility of IE in the treatment of Ewing's sarcoma (discussed below).

6.2.3 Collaborative Groups

Ewing's sarcoma remains a relatively rare disease. The need to increase the number of patients enrolled in clinical trials and to increase the rate at which trials can accrue has served as the impetus for the formation of multiple collaborative groups, which bring together multiple institutions, often across multiple nations, to facilitate advancements in the treatment of Ewing's sarcoma. These groups have included the Intergroup Ewing's Sarcoma Study (IESS) group, a conglomeration of North American clinical trials groups, the Cooperative Ewing's Sarcoma Study (CESS) group, combined efforts of a number of central European countries, the Scandinavian Study Group (SSG), and others.

A summary of the collaborative group studies undertaken to date is outlined in Table 6.1. Important findings from those studies and the ways

Table 6.1 Ewing's sarcoma trials discussed in the text

Study	Years	No. of patients	Regimen	Findings
IESS-I (Nesbit et al. 1981, 1990)	1973–1978	342	VAC vs. VACD vs. VAC + Pulm XRT	Patients receiving DOX experienced best outcomes Patients receiving DOX developed fewer metastases than those receiving XRT Pelvic lesions have worse prognosis
IESS-II (Burgert et al. 1990)	1978–1982	214	VACD (DOX high-dose intermittent vs. moderate-dose continuous)	Improved disease control and survival with more aggressive chemotherapy Early intensity improves outcomes Increased cardiovascular toxicity with high-dose DOX
ET-1 (Craft et al. 1997)	1978–1986	142	VACD (± surgery)	Intensified neoadjuvant regimen improved resection of pelvic masses Extremely poor outcomes for metastatic disease Surgical outcomes better than radiation alone?
CESS 81 (Jürgens et al. 1988)	1981–1985	93	VACD	Decreased metastasis with early initiation of therapy Increased local recurrence without complete resection despite radiation
CESS-86 (Paulussen et al. 2001)	1986–1991	301	Standard risk: VACD High risk: VAD/IFOS	High-risk patients experienced same 10-year OS (52 % vs. 51 %) Histologic response prognostic of outcome
ET-2 (Craft et al. 1998)	1987–1993	243	VCR + DOX + IFOS + DACT	CPM to IFOS and increased DOX improved outcomes
REN2 (Bacci et al. 1998)	1988–1991	82	VACD/IE	No benefit with adding IE relative to outcomes in REN1
INT-0091 (Grier et al. 2003)	1988–1992	518	VACD vs. VACD/IE	IE improved outcomes in nonmetastatic disease No benefit to IE in metastatic disease
INT-0154 (Granowetter et al. 2009)	1995–1998	478	VDC + IE (standard dose vs. increased dose)	Increased dose therapy did not improve outcome
AEWS-0031 (Womer et al. 2012)	2001–2005	587	VDC + IE ± G-CSF (standard vs. interval compressed)	Interval compression improved outcome without increasing toxicity

DACT dactinomycin, *DOX* doxorubicin, *G-CSF* (granulocyte colony-stimulating factor), *IE* ifosfamide + etoposide, *IFOS* ifosfamide, *VAC* vincristine + dactinomycin + cyclophosphamide, *VAD* vincristine + dactinomycin + doxorubicin, *VACD* vincristine + dactinomycin + cyclophosphamide + doxorubicin, *VCR* vincristine in which they have educated our current standard of care are discussed in the sections that follow.

6.2.4 Multi-agent Chemotherapy

With the identification throughout the late 1960s and early 1970s of multiple agents having activity against Ewing's sarcoma, a number of small case series reported increasingly noteworthy successes utilizing multi-agent and multimodal therapies. A number of investigators reported responses, including durable remissions, in patients treated with VAC (vincristine, dactinomycin, cyclophosphamide) (Jaffe et al. 1976) and VACD (VAC plus doxorubicin) (Rosen et al. 1974). The report from Memorial Sloan Kettering was particularly impressive, describing 12 children treated with VACD, all of whom remained alive without disease for 10–37 months. Their report included three patients who initially presented with metastatic disease who also responded to therapy. These initial reports clearly opened the field for investigation into the appropriate and optimal application of adjuvant multi-agent and multimodal therapy. These studies also identified the management of toxicity as a primary obstacle to the widespread use of multi-agent chemotherapy, with high rates of congestive heart failure, infections complicating therapy, profound nausea and vomiting, as well as other side effects. Much of the research activity in subsequent years focused on managing these toxicities to make regimens more tolerable without sacrificing efficacy.

Establishment of the VACD backbone In 1973, a collaborative effort between pediatric cancer groups was formed called the Intergroup Ewing's Sarcoma Study. From 1973 to 1978, they performed their first clinical trial, which compared VAC to VACD and to VAC with prophylactic pulmonary radiotherapy (Nesbit et al. 1981). Analysis at 2.5 years found significant advantages to treatment with doxorubicin or pulmonary radiotherapy when compared to VAC alone (Nesbit et al. 1981). Repeat analysis after 6 years of follow-up further confirmed the benefits of adding doxorubicin to VAC therapy. In that analysis, patients receiving VACD experienced overall survival (OS) rates of 65 %, compared with only 28 % with VAC alone (Nesbit et al. 1990). While there was some survival advantage seen with the addition of pulmonary radiotherapy (OS of 53 %), the gains were much greater with doxorubicin, and the number of patients developing metastatic disease was much higher without it. Local recurrence rates remained unacceptably high—approximately 15 % across all groups. Subgroup analysis found that patients with pelvic disease fared much worse than patients with axial disease. At 5 years, OS was 34 % for pelvic disease versus 57 % in non-pelvic disease (Nesbit et al. 1990). This study, now known as IESS-1, firmly established the importance of doxorubicin in the treatment of patients with Ewing's sarcoma. These results helped to confirm on a larger scale similar results reported by others (Rosen et al. 1978).

Building on the success of IESS-1, the intergroup subsequently set out to compare two competing regimens, one using intermittent high-dose therapy and another using continuous moderate-dose therapy. This second study, IESS-2, was performed between 1978 and 1982. Given the huge improvements in outcome seen in patients receiving doxorubicin, patients randomized to the high-dose therapy arm received a regimen similar to that used in IESS-1, only with increased doses of doxorubicin and cyclophosphamide. Five-year follow-up showed even greater gains in survival for patients receiving the intensified dose, with overall survival rates of 77 %, compared to 63 % in the moderate-dose therapy group (Burgert et al. 1990). Patients receiving the higher doses also experienced better disease control, with only 21 % of patients developing metastasis compared to 30 % of those in the moderate-dose therapy group. It was notable that increasing doses did not result in increased toxicities, with comparable adverse effects seen in both groups.

Trials conducted by multiple other cooperative groups confirmed the value of dose-intensive doxorubicin. Limiting their study to that of patients with localized bony disease, the group from St. Jude reported excellent results by adding doxorubicin both neoadjuvantly and adjuvantly in their ES-79 trial. Patients receiving doxorubicin had improved metastatic control, tumor regression, and overall survival. The five-year overall survival for these patients approached 80 % (Hayes et al. 1989). Results were similar in the collaborative POG 8346 study, where doxorubicin was administered in both the neoadjuvant and adjuvant settings. Response rate was found to be 88 % after neoadjuvant therapy (Donaldson et al. 1998). The 5-year OS of this group, which included those with pelvic and metastatic disease, was 55 %. Patients with localized disease had 5-year OS of 65 %.

The cooperative European group's CESS-81 study likewise showed a 70 % response rate with 3-year DFS of responders at 79 % using a VACD-based regimen (Jürgens et al. 1988). Post hoc analysis performed in this study suggested that early intensification reduced rates of metastasis. Results from this study emphasized the need to improve local control. The establishment of centralized radiation planning mid-study reduced local recurrence rates of approximately 50 % early in the study to less than 25 % over the entire 6-year observation period (Jürgens et al. 1988). The ET-1 study, organized by investigators in the United Kingdom, again confirmed the need for intense early chemotherapy with VACD (Craft et al. 1997). This study further emphasized the need for aggressive local control, which is discussed in Chap. 9. The investigators made a point to emphasize the incredibly poor outcomes of patients with metastatic disease. While 45 of the 120 patients with localized disease were alive at 10 years, only 2 of the 20 patients presenting with metastatic disease survived 10 years beyond diagnosis, despite this aggressive chemotherapy regimen.

Management of pelvic disease Given the poor outcomes noted in previous studies for patients with pelvic and sacral Ewing, the IESS-II study sought to improve outcomes in patients with pelvic disease. In this study, all patients with pelvic disease received intensified therapy with intermittent dosing using VACD. The need for appropriate local control was emphasized, and all patients with unresectable disease or with positive margins received intensive radiation with 55 Gy to the tumor bed with generous margins (Evans et al. 1991). Reported separately from the rest of the IESS-II trial, patients with pelvic disease receiving treatment under this intensified regimen experienced 5-year remission-free survival rates of 55 %, a dramatic improvement over the 23 % seen in the first IESS trial. These modifications in therapy, with intensification of chemotherapy and an emphasis on effective local control, pushed the 5-year OS in patients with pelvic disease very near than seen in patients with localized disease of the extremity. One should note, however, that multiple patients in this treatment cohort experienced late relapses at 6 years and later—a phenomenon particularly common to pelvic disease and a problem that continues to this day and that should be considered in the early reporting of trial results.

Addition of ifosfamide and etoposide Seeking to capitalize on promising early reports of the activity of ifosfamide in Ewing's sarcoma (discussed above), the two American groups (CCG and POG) conducted a collaborative study to investigate whether the addition of IE to standard therapy would improve outcome (Grier et al. 2003). INT-0091 demonstrated a survival benefit for patients with localized disease receiving courses of alternating VACD and IE. The addition of IE in this study increased the 5-year event-free survival (EFS) from 54 to 69 % in patients with localized disease. There was no benefit seen for patients with metastatic disease, with both the control and experimental groups experiencing a 22 % 5-year survival.

The group from the United Kingdom took a slightly different approach to the integration of ifosfamide in their ET-2 trial. Rather than alternating courses of VACD with IE, patients enrolled in ET-2 received cycles of ifosfamide, vincristine, and doxorubicin (IVAD) throughout both the neoadjuvant and adjuvant phases of therapy. In the last several cycles, dactinomycin replaced doxorubicin in order to limit cumulative doses of doxorubicin. The five-year OS improved from 44 % in ET-1 to 62 % in ET-2 (Craft et al. 1998). Importantly, the benefits of ifosfamide-based therapy also extended to patients who presented with metastatic disease. Five-year survival for this group increased from 9 to 23 %. Patients receiving ifosfamide in this study also experienced decreased incidence of local relapse. It is likely that this large benefit was more of a function of the markedly poor survival seen in the small number of patients with metastatic disease enrolled in ET-1 than it was a superiority of the IVAD regimen, as the two studies reported essentially identical results in patients with metastatic disease.

Dose intensification Analyses performed in the early 1990s suggested that outcomes in patients with Ewing's sarcoma depended largely on the dose intensity of chemotherapy, especially with regard to doxorubicin (Smith et al. 1991). From 1995 to 1998, the INT-0154 study sought to determine whether increasing the doses of medications in the already-established VDC + IE backbone could improve outcomes in patients with localized disease (Granowetter et al. 2009). Unfortunately, there were no benefits seen with intensification of therapy by this method, despite the increased numbers of toxicities observed. The five-year EFS was 70 % for the intensified regimen vs. 72 % for the standard regimen.

Interval compression An alternate means of dose intensification was born with the development during the 1990s of marrow-stimulating agents such as filgrastim, which proved effective in accelerating marrow recovery. Using these medications, chemotherapy could be given more often. It was hypothesized that more frequent administration of cytotoxic agents would allow less time for recovery and expansion of chemotherapy-resistant clones within tumors. Preliminary studies testing this theory (Womer et al. 2000) suggested that "interval compression" facilitated by the routine use of colony-stimulating factors and less stringent count recovery criteria for the initiation of subsequent cycles could improve both EFS (73 %) and OS (85 %). Investigators designed the AEWS0031 study to determine the value of interval compression in a large-scale randomized setting. Patients enrolled in the study received the same chemotherapy dosage of VDC + IE either in traditional 3-week cycles or every 2 weeks by accelerating count recovery after chemotherapy with filgrastim (Womer et al. 2012). Interval compression improved both EFS and OS in patients with localized disease (from 65 to 73 % and 77 to 83 %, respectively). Importantly, interval compression did not increase toxicity. This regimen of interval compression with VDC + IE forms the backbone of current standard therapy regimens in North America and elsewhere.

6.2.5 Current Standard of Care

The treatment of patients with newly diagnosed Ewing's sarcoma continues to build on a backbone of vincristine, doxorubicin, and cyclophosphamide. INT 0091 and ET-2 established a role for ifosfamide and etoposide as well. AEWS0031 demonstrated the value of interval compression. The most recent standard regimen, built on the successful evolution of these studies, is illustrated in Fig. 6.1. Treatment under this protocol consists of alternating cycles of VDC and IE, which repeat for a total of 14 cycles of therapy. Recovery is supported by the administration of G-CSF (granulocyte-colony stimulating factor) at the conclusion of each cycle. Subsequent cycles begin 14 days after the beginning of the last cycle or as soon as the patient demonstrates adequate hematologic recovery (defined by platelets greater than 75,000/μL and absolute neutrophil count (ANC) greater than 750/μL). Local control with surgery and/or radiation therapy is recommended after the sixth cycle of chemotherapy. If necessary, radiation can begin during cycle 7. Doxorubicin is omitted from the last two cycles of VDC to reduce cumulative anthracycline exposure.

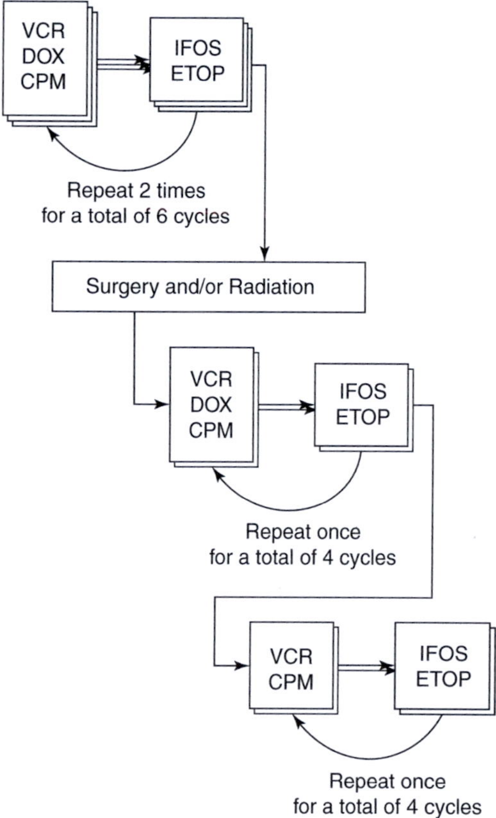

Fig. 6.1 Schematic overview of treatment recommendations for Ewing's sarcoma. Based on the experimental arm used in AEWS0031, this interval compressed regimen is currently considered the standard of care in North America and elsewhere. See text for dosing details

Standard dosing for these agents is as follows:

- VCR: vincristine 2 mg/m² (max 2 mg), day 1
- DOX: doxorubicin 37.5 mg/m²/day, days 1 and 2
- CPM: cyclophosphamide 1,200 mg/m², day 1 with MESNA for uroprotection
- IFOS: ifosfamide 1,800 mg/m²/day, days 1–5 with MESNA for uroprotection
- ETOP: etoposide 100 mg/m²/day IV infusion over 1–2 h, days 1–5
- G-CSF: filgrastim 5 mcg/kg/day SQ, max 300 mcg, beginning 24–36 h after the last dose of chemotherapy, continued for at least 7 days or until the ANC is at least 750, or pegfilgrastim 100 mcg/kg SQ, max 6 mg, once 24–36 h after the last dose of chemotherapy

The failure of multiple attempts to improve outcomes by increasing doses of these agents above those used in typical modern regimens suggests that conventional doses of these agents probably lie somewhere near the ceiling of their therapeutic windows.

6.2.6 Ongoing and Upcoming Trials

A number of European centers favor induction using vincristine, ifosfamide, doxorubicin, and etoposide (VIDE, as used in the Euro-E.W.I.N.G. 99 study); this is considered to be an acceptable alternative standard of care. Euro-E.W.I.N.G 99 was designed to determine the safety and efficacy of this intensified induction regimen utilizing VIDE. It was also designed to compare the efficacy of consolidation using vincristine/dactinomycin/ifosfamide (VAI) with that of mega therapy consolidation using busulfan/melphalan in patients with isolated pulmonary metastases or poor responses to induction chemotherapy and to compare the tolerability and efficacy of consolidation therapy with VAI with that of consolidation with VAC in good responders. Investigators noted a lower-than-expected rate of poor response to induction therapy early in the study, which threatened accrual to the intermediate-risk arm. The study was opened to members of the Children's Oncology Group under AEWS0331 in 2004 and was recently closed to accrual. Initial reports from this study have shown that the VIDE induction regimen can be given safely (Juergens et al. 2006) and that the prognostic value of different EWS fusion types may be questionable (Le Deley et al. 2010).

The successor to AEWS0031, AEWS1031, began recruiting in late 2010. This study aims to test the effects of incorporating topotecan, an inhibitor of topoisomerase, into the VDC + IE backbone, essentially alternating topotecan and doxorubicin in each subsequent cycle. The rationale for this study comes from activity observed for combined cyclophosphamide/topotecan regimens in patients with refractory/relapsed Ewing's sarcoma (Hunold et al. 2004; Saylors et al. 2001) and from animal studies demonstrating more-than-additive activity when topotecan is combined with vincristine (Thompson et al. 1999).

The study will continue to utilize interval compression supported by routine utilization of growth factor with less stringent count recovery requirements. Recruitment is ongoing. Results will not be known for several years to come.

6.3 Chemotherapy for Osteosarcoma

Prior to the advent of chemotherapy, only a small fraction of patients survived encounters with osteosarcoma. With the introduction of adjuvant chemotherapy in the 1960s and early 1970s, combined modality treatments improved the outlook. In little more than a decade, survival surged to over 60 %. Since the 1980s, however, improvements on these outcomes have proved elusive (Allison et al. 2012) despite myriad large-scale efforts testing promising therapies. Multiple agents that appeared promising in preclinical and early clinical studies proved disappointing in phase III trials. Efforts to intensify treatments have bought little change in survival, while efforts to reduce intensity and spare patients from many of the most harmful side effects had very negative impacts on outcomes. The search for more cures has been plagued by controversies concerning the very value of adjuvant chemotherapy and by study results that have proved difficult to interpret. There is a clear need for new therapies that can prevent and treat metastatic disease as current therapies remain ineffective in the treatment of disseminated osteosarcoma. Following is an overview summarizing approaches to the systemic treatment of osteosarcoma, including the early history of systemic therapy and identification of active agents, the approaches to therapy that have been tested in cooperative group trials, current standards of care, and emerging concepts that are being addressed in ongoing clinical trials.

6.3.1 Identification of Active Agents

Cyclophosphamide Having observed the responses of patients with leukemia and various solid tumors, physicians started using cyclophosphamide to treat osteosarcoma during the early 1960s (Pinkel 1962; Finklestein et al. 1969; Sutow et al. 1971). While these early studies reported responses to cyclophosphamide in some patients, only about 15 % of patients showed objective responses. Treatment with higher doses or for longer periods of time was limited by a number of toxicities, especially hemorrhagic cystitis and persistent emesis. These limitations to use were eventually overcome with improvements in supportive care and preventive treatments, especially the advent of effective antiemetics (Cunningham et al. 1987) and of agents which can prevent urotoxicity (Scheef et al. 1979). Throughout the development of combination therapies, cyclophosphamide remained a staple of medical therapy, though it has since been largely abandoned, as its use has not enhanced outcomes beyond those obtained with current standard therapies.

Dactinomycin In some of the first studies using animal models of osteogenic sarcoma, the RNA polymerase inhibitor dactinomycin showed significant activity against the Ridgway osteogenic sarcoma model (Schwartz et al. 1966, 1968). While concern over treatment-related toxicities prevented early adoption of dactinomycin for treating patients with osteosarcoma, some human studies were performed using the agent as a radiosensitizer that did show activity (Cupps et al. 1969). Interest in dactinomycin was renewed after VAC (vincristine, dactinomycin, and cyclophosphamide) showed efficacy in patients with rhabdomyosarcoma. Early studies utilizing VAC plus radiation therapy for patients with metastatic pulmonary disease achieved durable remissions in small numbers of patients (Sutow et al. 1975).

Methotrexate Building on reports of the efficacy of antifolates in children with non-Hodgkin's lymphoma and in adults with lung carcinomas, oncologists from the Children's Hospital Boston group assessed the effects of high-dose methotrexate in patients with osteosarcoma. Their case series, published in 1973, showed the responses of ten patients with osteosarcoma (mostly metastatic) to an escalating dose regimen of high-dose methotrexate with citrovorum rescue (Jaffe et al.

1973). Nine of ten patients showed some response, including two patients who showed complete regression of lung metastases without radiation. By 1975, Rosen et al. showed improvement of 3-year EFS to 52 % by using high-dose methotrexate (HDMTX) with doxorubicin and cyclophosphamide, which together formed one of the first multi-agent protocols, deemed the T4 protocol (Delépine et al. 1990). Subsequent trials demonstrated a clear relationship to dose and response, which has driven multiple efforts to maximize methotrexate exposure (Winkler et al. 1984; Saeter et al. 1991). Methotrexate remains an integral component of standard therapy regimens to this day.

Doxorubicin came of age during the early 1970s. Investigators from the Acute Leukemia Group assessed the efficacy of this agent in patients with osteosarcoma and showed that single-agent doxorubicin coupled with amputation increased disease-free survival to 45 % after 32 months (Cortes et al. 1974). Multiple subsequent studies showed marked efficacy of doxorubicin, including augmentation of response when added to other effective agents (Bacci et al. 1993; Smeland et al. 2003). The importance of doxorubicin for treating osteosarcoma was clarified by the COSS-82 study (Winkler et al. 1988). This study aimed to determine whether patients could be spared to highly toxic chemotherapy by withholding neoadjuvant doxorubicin (and cisplatin), supposing that poor histologic responders could be salvaged by introducing these agents to their adjuvant regimens. Results showed that patients who did not receive neoadjuvant doxorubicin fared poorly. The subsequent addition of doxorubicin to regimens of those who had poor histologic responses could not salvage their outcomes. This highlighted the importance of early dose intensity of doxorubicin in the treatment of osteosarcoma.

A meta-analysis performed on published studies in the late 1980s suggested that of all the agents employed in the treatment of osteosarcoma to date, doxorubicin had the greatest effect on outcome (Smith et al. 1991). The analysis also suggested that the dose intensity (amount of drug per unit time) had greater effect than total dose. Attempts were made early in the use of doxorubicin to push the dose of doxorubicin higher, though these efforts caused unacceptably high rates of cardiotoxicity (Von Hoff 1979). Analysis suggested that cumulative doses less than 240 mg/m^2 were generally safe, but that rates of cardiotoxicity increased markedly with higher doses (Von Hoff 1979; Lipshultz et al. 1995). Data also suggested that decreasing the rate of administration could reduce the risk for developing cardiomyopathies (Lipshultz et al. 1995), but this has not played out in pediatric studies (Lipshultz et al. 2012). Doxorubicin continues to prove itself a very important drug in the treatment of osteosarcoma, with many believing it to be the most important single agent in modern regimens (Eselgrim et al. 2006).

The primary dose-limiting toxicity of doxorubicin has always been the development of cardiac failure and chemotherapy-related cardiotoxicity. Dexrazoxane has been developed as a cardioprotective agent. When given prior to chemotherapy, it can significantly reduce the rates of cardiotoxicity (Kalam and Marwick 2013) without reducing the therapeutic efficacy of doxorubicin. The use of dexrazoxane is recommended in patients receiving cumulative doses of anthracyclines that present a significant risk for substantial cardiac damage (van Dalen et al. 2005). Dexrazoxane continues to be increasingly utilized in protocols recommending higher doses of doxorubicin, which has become a routine (Anderson 2005; Mulrooney et al. 2009).

Cisplatin A platinum-based DNA cross-linking agent, it was introduced in the late 1970s and quickly found favor with those treating osteosarcoma. In 1978, Ochs et al. reported responses in six of eight patients with disease recurrence after treatment with HDMTX and doxorubicin (Ochs et al. 1978). Several other studies have confirmed response rates in relapsed disease of approximately 40 % (Baum et al. 1979; Winkler et al. 1983). Ettinger et al. treated 12 newly diagnosed patients with cisplatin and doxorubicin in a neoadjuvant fashion and observed durable responses in most patients, with no evidence of disease in

10 out of 12 patients at a median follow-up of 23 months (Ettinger et al. 1981). In the COSS-82 study, the combination of doxorubicin/cisplatin was found to be far superior to BCD (bleomycin, cyclophosphamide, dactinomycin) (Winkler et al. 1988). While tolerated doses can be limited by nephrotoxicity and ototoxicity, cisplatin remains a primary agent for the treatment of osteosarcoma, a primary component of the MAP (methotrexate, adriamycin [doxorubicin], platinum [cisplatin]) backbone used in most modern regimens.

Ifosfamide (and etoposide) Ifosfamide, another nitrogen mustard derivative, has been used as an alkylating agent in chemotherapy protocols since the early 1980s. A report by Marti et al. in 1985 sparked interest in ifosfamide as treatment for osteosarcoma. They reported clinical responses in one-third of patients with recurrent osteosarcoma (Marti et al. 1985). The COSS-86 study incorporated ifosfamide into the neoadjuvant treatment regimen and showed an improvement in histologic tumor response when added to the MAP backbone (Winkler et al. 1990). Investigators found evidence for synergy between ifosfamide and etoposide in recurrent sarcomas (Miser et al. 1987b), and data from the Rizzoli IOR-II study suggested that the combination may have improved outcomes for poor responders (Bacci et al. 1993). Based on these data, the Scandinavian group replaced the upfront regimen (MAP) with ifosfamide and etoposide (IE) alone as the salvage regimen for poor responders in the SSG-VIII study (Smeland et al. 2003). Unfortunately, their results showed that patients receiving IE alone as salvage therapy fared much worse than patients who continued to receive MAP. The INT-0133 study set out to definitively determine whether there was any benefit to augmenting the MAP backbone by adding ifosfamide. The results of that study were difficult to interpret (Meyers et al. 2005) due to an interaction in the statistical analysis of the factorial study design. In the most recent follow-up data (Meyers et al. 2008), however, it appears that the addition of ifosfamide by itself to the backbone regimen did not improve outcomes. Given these

unclear results, many have continued to use ifosfamide or IE in the treatment of patients with osteosarcoma, though the data to support this has not been robust. The EURAMOS-1 study was designed to directly answer this question by comparing MAP-IE to MAP alone in a large cohort of poor histologic responders (Marina et al. 2014). The results of that study suggest that augmentation of standard MAP therapy with IE provides no clear survival benefit for patients with poor histologic response (see Chap. 8), while it definitively carries a cost of increased toxicity. Whether or not this more intensive regimen would be beneficial for patients with a good histologic response (i.e., those proved to be the most chemoresponsive) has not been tested.

Some suggest that ifosfamide may be more effective for osteosarcoma when given in doses much higher (15–18 mg/m^2) than those typically used in most protocols (12 mg/m^2). Whether high-dose ifosfamide truly provides additional benefit, and whether those benefits are warranted given the significant additional renal and hematologic toxicity, remains controversial. Trials directly comparing the efficacy of high-dose ifosfamide to standard-dose ifosfamide have produced conflicting results (Berrak et al. 2005; Ferrari et al. 2005; Kudawara et al. 2013). Some have expressed that the marked toxicities observed with these therapies do not justify even the best results noted in the previous studies. Regardless, many patients with recurrent, refractory, and metastatic disease have been treated with high-dose ifosfamide and etoposide, and this is generally considered an appropriate treatment.

6.3.2 Collaborative Groups

While osteosarcoma is the most common primary malignant tumor of the bone, it remains a relatively rare disease when compared to other malignancies and disease entities. The need to increase patient numbers in order to expedite and enhance the study of treatments for osteosarcoma was apparent early, and multiple collaborative groups formed across the United States and

Europe. These have included the German-Austrian-Swiss study group, which has produced the COSS trials; the Scandinavian group, which has produced the SSG trials; the Italian group from the Rizzoli Institute; the European Osteosarcoma Intergroup (EOI) headquartered in Great Britain; and the North American groups, now consolidated under the Children's Oncology Group, among others. More recent trials have been conducted under the umbrella of EURAMOS, which has organized all of these groups into one large international collaborative group for conducting clinical trials in patients with osteosarcoma.

A summary of the collaborative group studies undertaken to date is outlined in Table 6.2. Important findings from those studies and the ways in which they have influenced our current standard of care are given in the sections that follow.

6.3.3 Multi-agent Chemotherapy

BCD (bleomycin, cyclophosphamide, dactinomycin) During the early days of chemotherapy, BCD formed the backbone of many different chemotherapy regimens. Investigators at Memorial Sloan Kettering showed overall response rates of 62 % in a group of patients containing both patients with treatment failure and newly diagnosed patients (Mosende et al. 1977). The COSS-80 study compared the BCD with cisplatin and found the two regimens to have very similar efficacy (Winkler et al. 1984). Given the increased toxicities associated with the platinum-based compound, authors reporting the results of that study favored the ongoing use of BCD over cisplatin. These results, however, conflicted with prior studies. In COSS-82, investigators replaced neoadjuvant doxycycline and cisplatin with BCD in an effort to reduce treatment-related toxicities. Patients receiving the experimental BCD regimen fared much worse than those receiving the more toxic agents (27 % vs. 59 %). Clear differences in those receiving the BCD-containing salvage regimen further confirmed the inferiority of

BCD to other available therapies (Winkler et al. 1988). Since the publication of that study, BCD has largely been abandoned in the treatment of patients with osteosarcoma.

MAP (methotrexate, adriamycin [doxorubicin], platinum [cisplatin]) As illustrated above, high-dose methotrexate, doxorubicin, and cisplatin remain the three drugs with greatest efficacy in the treatment of patients with osteosarcoma. Variations on regimens combining these three agents have formed the backbone of chemotherapy protocols for osteosarcoma since the early 1980s (Link et al. 1986; Winkler et al. 1990) and continue to do so in modern practice.

6.3.4 Approaches to Systemic Therapy

Adjuvant therapy Improvements in patient outcomes during the 1960s and early 1970s were heralded as great achievements. Over the course of a little more than a decade, survival in patients with osteosarcoma had improved from 15 % to nearly 60 %. While most oncologists attributed these gains to the adjuvant use of chemotherapy, investigators from the Mayo Clinic reported studies in the early 1980s which caused many to question both the value of adjuvant chemotherapy and the validity of historical control studies. In their study, patients who underwent surgical resection alone experienced the same 42 % survival rate as patients who underwent 1 year of treatment with high-dose methotrexate (Edmonson et al. 1984). A subsequent meta-analysis of outcomes for patients treated surgically at their institution prompted investigators to conclude that there had been a "natural improvement" in the outcomes of patients with osteosarcoma, independent of systemic chemotherapy (Taylor et al. 1978, 1985). They suggested that improved diagnostic and surgical techniques developed over the previous decades were the primary drivers of the improved outcomes.

Significant controversy ensued, and the matter was not ultimately resolved until the publication of the multi-institutional osteosarcoma study (MIOS) in 1986 (Link et al. 1986). This carefully controlled study demonstrated clear benefit to patients treated with adjuvant chemotherapy, with 66 % of patients receiving the BCD + HDMTX regimen alive without disease at 2 years vs. 17 % EFS in those who did not receive this regimen. This study also made use of both a prospectively randomized control group and a historical control group. The results validated the use of historical controls in these types of studies, and a myriad of subsequent findings have affirmed the value of adjuvant chemotherapy.

Neoadjuvant therapy In the early 1980s, the group from Memorial Sloan Kettering introduced the concept of neoadjuvant chemotherapy through the T5–T7 protocols (Winkler et al. 1988). With the development of the new limb salvage surgeries, the time period between diagnosis and surgery was often prolonged in order to permit the manufacture of prostheses. To bridge that gap between diagnosis and definitive surgical resection, patients were started on chemotherapy. Further justification for pursuing neoadjuvant chemotherapy came from observations regarding patterns of metastasis: more than 80 % of patients presenting with localized disease who were treated with amputation alone developed metastases, suggesting that most patients had microscopic metastases within their lungs at diagnosis. Rosen's group argued that early administration of chemotherapy would be more effective in treating micrometastases and that waiting until after surgery to provide adjuvant chemotherapy would only permit those metastases to develop further and acquire resistance. Moreover, by administering chemotherapy in a neoadjuvant setting, one could assess the chemoresponsiveness of a patient's tumor by quantifying tumor necrosis at the time of resection. The prognostic value of neoadjuvant chemotherapy was subsequently borne out in multiple clinical trials (Bielack et al. 2002; Kager et al. 2003; Bacci et al. 2005).

An additional benefit of neoadjuvant chemotherapy with assessment of histologic response was to accelerate the development of chemotherapy protocols (Rosen 1985). By using percent necrosis at the time of resection as a surrogate for efficacy of the various regimens, the observation period required for assessing differences between regimens was dramatically shortened. This advance allowed new studies to benefit from the results of previous studies almost immediately.

As experience grew, there arose reasons to question the overall value of relying on histologic assessment of response to neoadjuvant chemotherapy as a lone surrogate for response to treatment. While it has been clear that the determination of histologic response to treatment has clear prognostic value, two problems emerged. First, no new agents have been found which can effectively salvage poor responders. Attempts to intensify adjuvant therapy for poor responders have generally yielded poor results (Picci et al. 1985; Saeter et al. 1991; Goorin et al. 2003; Bacci et al. 2005; Marina et al. 2014). This concept is discussed further in the following section. Secondly, efforts designed to increase tumor necrosis in the primary tumor, while effective at increasing necrosis, have not translated into concordant improvements in outcome. Perhaps this phenomenon has been most evident in studies investigating intra-arterial chemotherapy (Winkler et al. 1990; Meyers et al. 1998; Ferrari et al. 2005).

The utilization of neoadjuvant chemotherapy does provide additional benefits, which will likely fuel its continued use in the treatment of malignant bone tumors. Preoperative shrinkage and consolidation of the primary tumor often facilitates resection and limb salvage procedures. Starting patients with chemotherapy often avoids delays that can occur while waiting for surgical procedures to be scheduled and gives surgeons time to plan and prepare for a successful limb-sparing procedure.

Salvage chemotherapy Given the ability to evaluate response to therapy in a proactive fashion, some have proposed an approach which aims to limit toxicity by giving all patients a less intensive neoadjuvant regimen. Patients who show good response than complete therapy on the less intensive regimen, and patients who show poor response can then be salvaged using more

Table 6.2 Osteosarcoma trials discussed in the text

Study	Years	No. of patients	Regimen	Findings

T10 (Rosen et al. 1982)	1978–1982	57	Neo: HDMTX + DOX + BCD
			Adj:
			  GR: HDMTX + DOX + BCD
			  PR: DOX + CDDP + BCD
				Suggested value to "salvage" therapy, showing equivalent responses in PRs switched from HDMTX to CDDP CDDP more effective than HDMTX? 93 % DFS at a median of 20 months from start of chemo

COSS-80 (Winkler et al. 1983)	1979–1982	192	Neo: MTX + DOX + VCR + XRT Adj: MTX + DOX + VCR + BCD	No adverse outcomes from delaying definitive surgery No change in natural history of disease Definitive benefit of adjuvant chemotherapy

COSS-82 (Winkler et al. 1988)	1982–1984	141	Neo: HDMTX + BCD vs. MAP
			Adj:
			  GR: HDMTX + BCD or MAP
			  PR: DOX + CDDP or CDDP + IFOS + BCD
				BCD worse than DOX + CDDP
				Delayed administration of DOX led to poor outcomes
				Could not salvage poor responders by adding back DOX + CDDP
				Confirmed prognostic value of histologic necrosis

SSG-II (Saeter et al. 1991)	1982–1989	107	Neo: HDMTX
			Adj:
			  GR: HDMTX + DOX + BCD
			  PR: HDMTX + DOX + CDDP + BCD
				Single-agent MTX not effective as neoadjuvant therapy
				Confirmed dose-response for serum MTX and tumor necrosis
				Salvage chemotherapy was not effective

CCG 782 (Provisor et al. 1997)	1983–1986	268	Neo: HDMTX + BCD
			Adj:
			  GR: HDMTX + DOX + BCD
			  PR: DOX + CDDP + BCD
				Unable to confirm same outcomes as published for T10 protocol
				Validated histological response as prognostic tool
				Unable to salvage PR with CDDP

EOI-1 (Bramwell et al. 1992)	1983–1986	198	DOX + CDDP vs. MAP	No improvement in outcome with addition of HDMTX Similar outcomes using simplified regimen

IOR/OS-1 (Bacci et al. 1990)	1983–1986	127	Neo: MTX (HD vs. MD) + IA CDDP
			Adj:
			  GR: MTX + CDDP
			  FR: MTX + DOX + CDDP
			  PR: DOX + BCD
				Improved outcomes with HDMTX relative to standard dose
				Very poor outcomes in PR salvaged with DOX + BCD

MIOS (Link et al. 1986)	1986	36	DOX + CDDP + BCD	Improved outcomes with adjuvant multi-agent chemotherapy
COSS-86 (Winkler et al. 1990; Fuchs et al. 1998)	1986–1988	171	LR: MAP HR: MAP (IV vs. IA CDDP) + IFOS	Improved outcomes in patients receiving IFOS Increased histologic response with addition of IFOS No improved histologic response or survival benefit with IA CDDP

Study	Years	No. of patients	Regimen	Findings
IOR/OS-2 (Bacci et al. 1993)	1986–1989	164	Neo: MAP (IA CDDP) Adj: GR: MAP PR: MAP + IE	PR salvaged with MAP + IE had outcomes similar to GR Increased heart failure with DOX doses >390 mg/m^2
EOI-2 (Souhami et al. 1997)	1986–1991	391	DOX + CDDP vs. Neo: HDMTX + DOX + VCR Adj: HDMTX + DOX + CDDP + BCD	Equivalent outcomes with 2-drug regimen and T10 protocol Improved tolerability and decreased cost of simplified regimen
T12 (Meyers et al. 1998)	1986–1993	73	Neo: HDMTX + BCD ± DOX + CDDP Adj: MAP + BCD	Intensified neoadjuvant regimen produced modest increase in histologic response but no improvement in EFS
POG 8651 (Goorin et al. 2003)	1986–1993	100	MAP + BCD Surgery week 0 vs. week 10	Delaying definitive surgical resection did not affect outcome
SSG-VIII (Smeland et al. 2003)	1990–1997	113	Neo: HDMTX + DOX + CDDP Adj: GR: HDMTX + DOX + CDDP PR: IE	Improved outcomes when DOX and CDDP added to neoadjuvant therapy No improvement in outcome for PR by switching to IE response did not increase survival
IOR/OS-3 (Ferrari et al. 1999)	1993–1995	95	Neo: MAP (IA vs. IV CDDP) Adj: GR: MAP PR: MAP + IFOS	Decreased cardiotoxicity with cumulative doses of DOX <390 mg/m^2 PR effectively salvaged with IFOS IA CDDP improved histologic response, but not outcome
INT 0133 (Meyers et al. 2005, 2008; Chou et al. 2009)	1993–1997	662	MAP ± IFOS ± MTP-PE	No improvement in outcome with IFOS Increased overall survival with MTP-PE
EOI-3 (Lewis et al. 2007)	1993–2002	497	DOX + CDDP (3 weeks) vs. DOX + CDDP + G-CSF (2 weeks)	Interval compression improved histological response but not survival
ISG/SSG-1 (Ferrari et al. 2005)	1997–2000	182	MAP + HDIFOS	No improvement in survival with HDIFOS Major renal and hematologic toxicities with HDIFOS
EURAMOS-1 (Bielack et al. 2013; Marina et al. 2014)	2005–2011	1,335	Neo: MAP Adj: GR: MAP ± IFN PR: MAP ± IE	No improvement in RFS for GR receiving IFN No improvement in outcomes for PR receiving IE Increased toxicities with MAP + IE

Adj adjuvant therapy, *BCD* bleomycin + cyclophosphamide + dactinomycin, *CDDP* cisplatin, *DOX* doxorubicin, *G-CSF* granulocyte colony-stimulating factor, *GR* good responders, *IA* intra-arterial, *IE* ifosfamide + etoposide, *IFN* interferon alpha, *IFOS* ifosfamide, *IV* intravenous, *MAP* high-dose methotrexate + doxorubicin + cisplatin, *MTP-PE* muramyl tripeptide liposomal, *Neo* neoadjuvant therapy, *PR* poor responders intensive therapies. Interest in such an approach was piqued when Rosen et al. reported the results of the T10 trial. In this trial, patients showing poor response to neoadjuvant HDMTX, doxorubicin, and BCD were switched to cisplatin- and doxorubicin-based adjuvant therapy. Results showed very similar outcomes for patients receiving the salvage regimen compared to the group showing good response to neoadjuvant therapy (Rosen et al. 1982).

The COSS-82 study sought to build on the salvage concept by reducing the intensity of neoadjuvant therapy under the hypothesis that poor responders could be salvaged with an intensified regimen (Winkler et al. 1988). All patients on the experimental arm of this study received neoadjuvant HDMTX and BCD only. Patients who had poor histologic response transitioned to adjuvant therapy with cisplatin and doxorubicin. The results of that study showed that patients in the experimental groups experienced outcomes that were markedly inferior both to the control groups and to the historical controls, regardless of whether patients showed good histologic response or received salvage adjuvant therapy.

Similar results were shown in the Scandinavian SSG-II trial (Saeter et al. 1991). This study took a similar approach, de-intensifying the neoadjuvant regimen by using HDMTX alone. Efforts to transition poor responders to postoperative doxorubicin and cisplatin did not adequately salvage this group. SSG-II clearly showed the inadequacy of neoadjuvant chemotherapy with HDMTX monotherapy. The subsequent SSG-VIII trial sought to capitalize on this by intensifying neoadjuvant therapy to a regimen containing HDMTX, doxorubicin, and cisplatin (Smeland et al. 2003). That trial also investigated whether transitioning to alternative adjuvant therapy could improve outcomes in poor responders. Patients who had poor response were changed from cisplatin and doxorubicin to ifosfamide and etoposide. These patients did worse than those who stayed on initial therapy, despite the poor histologic response. This result contrasts with those seen in the IOR-II trial at the Rizzoli Institute, where poor responders were given a regimen that augmented doxorubicin and cisplatin therapy with the addition of ifosfamide and etoposide (Bacci et al. 1993). In that trial, poor responders who received augmented therapy experienced outcomes very similar to good responders. A subsequent study suggested that ifosfamide alone might salvage outcomes for poor responders (Ferrari et al. 1999). A clearer picture of the real benefits provided by intensification of adjuvant therapy has come with the completion of the EURAMOS-1 trial. This trial was designed to directly compare poor responders who received intensified chemotherapy with ifosfamide and etoposide with those who continued the MAP-based backbone therapy. The eagerly awaited results of this large cooperative trial have been released (Marina et al. 2014) and show that while intensification of therapy with ifosfamide and etoposide increases the toxicities and second malignancies that patients experience, it does not improve disease-free outcomes.

Intra-arterial chemotherapy Given the clear prognostic value of histologic response after neoadjuvant chemotherapy, some have predicted that therapies targeting increased necrosis might improve outcomes. One therapeutic strategy for increasing necrosis of the primary tumor is intra-arterial administration of chemotherapy. Several studies have used this approach to increase the local concentration of antineoplastics and thus improve histologic response. Multiple studies testing the validity of this approach have shown that while intra-arterial chemotherapy can improve histologic responses to neoadjuvant therapy, this improvement in histologic response is not associated with a similar improvement in survival (Winkler et al. 1990; Meyers et al. 1998; Ferrari et al. 2005). Intra-arterial chemotherapy is, however, associated with increased cost, increased patient discomfort, and increased complication rates. Such approaches to augmentation of therapy have largely been abandoned.

Dose intensification Much of the development of chemotherapy regimens for osteosarcoma has focused on the intensification of therapy. Advances have focused on intensification both through the increase of total cumulative doses and through the compression of interval timing. As discussed in each of the individual sections above, clear dose-response relationships exist for most of the active agents in osteosarcoma: doxorubicin, alkylating agents, methotrexate, and cisplatin. Intensification of these regimens often pits increases in efficacy against increases in toxicity, both of which accompany dose augmentation. Details relevant to intensification of each of these individual agents are discussed in their corresponding sections under Sect. 6.3.1. Some efforts to intensify systemic neoadjuvant chemotherapy have generated improvements in histologic response, though these have not always translated into bona fide improvements in clinical outcomes.

Simplified regimens Some groups, most notably the EOI, have advocated treatments which attempt to simplify chemotherapy regimens, reducing toxicities and side effects while maintaining outcomes. The first study conducted by their group, EOI-1, showed that patients receiving a short (six-cycle) regimen of doxorubicin and cisplatin fared better than those receiving a combined regimen with four cycles of cisplatin/doxorubicin alternating with four cycles of HDMTX (Bramwell et al. 1992). When outcomes seen for patients receiving the shortened regimen appeared to be comparable to many of the more prolonged regimens utilized at that time, EOI pushed forward with a study comparing the two-drug regimen to the then-standard-of-care T10 protocol, which utilized doxorubicin, cisplatin, HDMTX, and BCD. The results of that study showed essentially identical outcomes for the two groups (Souhami et al. 1997). Since that time, overall outcomes have improved and now have survival rates superior to those obtained with these simplified regimens. With the exception of EOI-3 (which examined the effects of interval compression of the simplified regimen using filgrastim) (Lewis et al. 2007), no subsequent studies of substantial size and quality have revisited the concept of the simplified regimen. The results shown through this series of investigations do raise some interesting questions. For example, while methotrexate clearly has single-agent activity in

osteosarcoma, EOI-1 would suggest that it may not provide additional benefit beyond that seen with doxorubicin and cisplatin alone. Answers to these questions will depend on the design of future trials that address them.

Immunotherapy Clinicians and scientists have long hypothesized a role for the immune system in the control of osteosarcoma. Some trials have incorporated agents such as inhaled GM-CSF and interferon (IFN)α. Among the most intriguing results obtained with immunotherapy have been the reports of IFNα-only adjuvant therapy given to patients at the Karolinska Institute. They reported 39 patients who were treated postoperatively with interferon alone yet enjoyed 10-year event-free survival rates of 43 % (Müller et al. 2005). EURAMOS-1 attempted to capitalize on these observations by treating a cohort of good responders with maintenance interferon therapy after completion of adjuvant MAP. A preliminary report of that study suggested that MAP plus interferon is not superior to MAP alone, with event-free survival of 77 and 74 % (Bielack et al. 2013). These results may have been handicapped by poor adherence to therapy; nearly one of every four patients randomized to receive interferon never started it, and nearly half of those who did discontinued it prior to completion of the study.

The most widely studied immunomodulatory agent in osteosarcoma has been mifamurtide (L-MTP-PE), which contains a synthetic analog of bacterial cell wall components encapsulated in liposomes for delivery directly to macrophages. In preclinical studies, L-MTP-PE causes histologic changes that induce peripheral fibrosis surrounding the tumor, inflammatory cell infiltration, and neovascularization (Bielack et al. 2004). The INT-0133 study initially set out to determine whether L-MTP-PE (with or without the addition of ifosfamide) would enhance survival outcomes when added to a backbone of MAP therapy. Unfortunately, the results from the INT-0133 study initially showed a statistical interaction in the 2×2 study design between ifosfamide and L-MTP-PE (Meyers et al. 2005), making the study underpowered as the design relied on the independence of each arm in the analysis.

Conclusions were therefore difficult to draw from the results. A subsequent statistical analysis undertaken after more follow-up data were collected suggested that there was, in fact, benefit derived from L-MTP-PE, but not from ifosfamide (Meyers et al. 2008). There was a statistically significant improvement in overall survival (78 % versus 70 %) and event-free survival in those receiving MTP-PE independent of the chemo regimen. A similar pattern was seen in patients with metastatic disease, with 5-year survival in patients receiving L-MTP-PE of 45 % compared to 26 % in patients not receiving L-MTP-PE (Chou et al. 2009). Given the number of patients enrolled, however, these differences did not reach statistical significance. With the initial confusion surrounding the results of INT-0133 and with current difficulty obtaining L-MTP-PE, whether it will ever be incorporated into mainstream therapy—and what exactly the benefits of incorporation might be—remains unclear.

Further discussion of immunotherapies can be found in Chap. 15.

6.3.5 Current Standard of Care

The treatment of patients with newly diagnosed osteosarcoma builds on a backbone of recurring cycles of doxorubicin, cisplatin, and high-dose methotrexate. There is now rather definitive evidence from the EURAMOS-1 trial suggesting that the addition of ifosfamide and etoposide provides no additional benefit to patients with localized disease who are poor responders to neoadjuvant chemotherapy. The standard that has emerged from the results of these studies is illustrated in Fig. 6.2. Treatment with this regimen consists of recurring cycles of doxorubicin and cisplatin followed 3 weeks later by two courses of high-dose methotrexate with leucovorin rescue. This course is repeated until the patient has completed six cycles (18 courses of chemotherapy). Surgical resection is undertaken after the second cycle when possible. Given the cumulative exposures resulting from these protocols, many recommend cardioprotection with dexrazoxane prior to doxorubicin infusions.

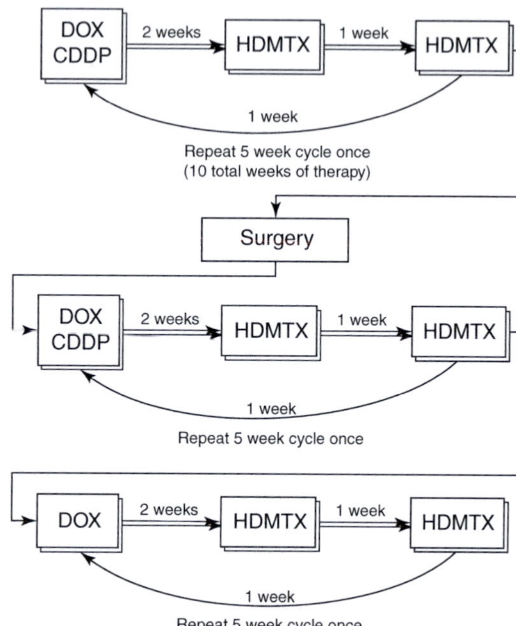

Fig. 6.2 Schematic overview of treatment recommendations for osteosarcoma. Based on the protocols used in the recent EURAMOS-1 study, this regimen formed the standard of care treatment arm for both groups. In the absence of conclusive evidence supporting further intensification of therapy in poor responders, this regimen should be considered standard of care for all patients with localized disease

Standard dosing for these agents is as follows:

- DOX: doxorubicin 37.5 mg/m²/day, days 1 and 2 of week 1 of each cycle. Dexrazoxane may be given immediately prior to each doxorubicin infusion for cardioprotection.
- CDDP: cisplatin 60 mg/m²/day, days 1 and 2 of week 1 of each cycle.
- HDMTX: methotrexate 12 g/m²/dose, day 1 of weeks 4 and 5 of each cycle. Leucovorin rescue should be started 24 h after the start of each MTX infusion and continued until MTX serum levels clear.

As with Ewing's sarcoma, the failure of multiple trials aimed at intensifying these therapies either by increasing doses of the above agents or by the addition of other cytotoxic agents has led many to conclude that the dose levels used in these modern protocols probably lie very near the ceiling of the therapeutic window.

6.3.6 Ongoing and Upcoming Trials

As illustrated above, treatment of osteosarcoma has greatly improved since the turn of the nineteenth century. The research efforts of countless scientists and clinical investigators have proved the value of a multidisciplinary approach combining the best of systemic chemotherapy and surgical resection have to offer. Frustratingly, outcomes for patients with osteosarcoma have stagnated over the last 40 years, despite multiple efforts to improve therapy (Allison et al. 2012). Future advances are likely to come from improved understanding of the biology of this disease and from novel approaches to treatment.

6.4 Treatment of Metastatic Disease

While improvements for patients with localized disease have been slow and incremental, they have been real. Unfortunately, there have been no real improvements in patients with disseminated disease. Whether patients present with metastatic disease or develop metastasis after initial therapy, prognosis remains incredibly poor with 2-year survival generally less than 20 % (Allison et al. 2012). The failure of multiple efforts to improve outcomes by intensification of therapy suggests that our current standard of care regimens likely maximize the effects that can be seen with modern cytotoxic agents. Much research rightfully continues to focus on improving outcomes for this group of patients. Real advances are likely to come only with novel and innovative new therapies that build on an improved understanding of the biology that drives metastatic disease.

Metastatic Ewing's sarcoma While aggressive treatment with cytotoxic agents has significantly improved the outcomes for patients with localized Ewing's sarcoma, there have been few improvements for patients with metastatic disease. Two-year EFS for patients with metastatic Ewing's sarcoma remains $\leq$20 %. Multiple trials have sought to improve outcomes through intensification of therapy. The most dramatic of these concepts has been that of "mega therapy," where dose-limiting hematopoietic toxicities are overcome by stem cell rescue, facilitating further dose escalation with conventional agents. These trials operated under the hypothesis that dose escalation would enhance tumor cell destruction and provide a corresponding increase in survival. One particular early study showed benefit to mega therapy (Burdach et al. 1993), though others have had difficulty replicating these results. It is probable that the decision to limit treatment to high-risk patients who were able to achieve remission, as well as the exceptionally poor outcomes in the control group (zero percent survival), skewed these results. From 1996 to 1998, CCG-7951 compared the regimen utilized in the INT-0091 study (VDC + IE, discussed in Sect. 6.2.4) with high-dose chemotherapy followed by autologous stem cell transplant in patients with high risk for Ewing's sarcoma. Good responders were given mega therapy consisting of TBI followed by melphalan and etoposide with autologous stem cell rescue (Meyers et al. 2001). When comparing all patients, the 2-year EFS of 20 % in patients receiving mega therapy was no different from those who did not. When comparison was limited only to patients who achieved stem cell transplant, the 2-year EFS was only slightly better at 25 %.

The Memorial Sloan Kettering P6 protocol used a similar VDC + IE induction protocol. Patients achieving good tumor response then received either TBI/melphalan or thiotepa/carboplatin followed by autologous stem cell transplant. They concluded that neither regimen maintained remission (Kushner and Meyers 2001), with 2-year EFS of 10 % and 3-year EFS at only 5 %. An extensive review published with the report of this study summarized the results of multiple smaller studies and concluded that none of these approaches to mega therapy provided much benefit. In the US collaborative group, neither prolonged induction, shorter induction, nor end intensification with TBI/melphalan/etoposide has improved EFS. From the NCI, short-term induction with TBI followed by end intensification did not improve outcomes. The cooperative group from the United Kingdom conducted a study using prolonged treatment with modest dosing with ifosfamide replacing cyclophosphamide but failed to demonstrate an improvement in EFS. In studies done by the German and European cooperative groups, adding etoposide to prolonged treatment also did not improve outcomes. There was a report from the group at St. Jude which showed improved outcomes using prolonged semicontinuous therapy at modest doses, achieving 3-year EFS of 54 %. Unfortunately, studies from France, the United States, and Chile were unable to replicate these results. The EBMTR has shown some improvement in outcomes using a hyper-myeloablative protocol containing busulfan, though no clear overall advantage could be found as long-term complications skewed the results (Burdach et al. 2000).

Others have shown some benefit with irinotecan and temozolomide (Wagner et al. 2004; Wagner and McAllister 2007; Casey et al. 2009). While survival was not significantly improved with irinotecan/temozolomide, some studies have noted symptomatic improvement in as many as 50 % of patients (Wagner and McAllister 2007). Many consider this regimen to be useful in palliation.

Metastatic osteosarcoma The prognosis of patients with metastasis in osteosarcoma remains very poor, with survival ranging from 20 to 40 % (Boye et al. 2014). Despite many efforts to improve outcomes for this group of patients, none have provided real advances that improve survival. Notable efforts to improve outcomes for patients with metastatic osteosarcoma include those using higher doses of MTX and ifosfamide (Bacci 2003) and adding trastuzumab (human epidermal growth factor receptor 2 antibody) to high-dose chemotherapy (Ebb et al. 2012). A Children's Oncology Group study published in 2002 showed a 2-year OS of 59 % for patients with newly diagnosed

metastatic osteosarcoma who received high-dose ifosfamide and etoposide (Goorin et al. 2002). This finding represented a marked improvement over the 30 % response rate seen previously with standard-dose ifosfamide alone (Harris et al. 1995) and the 33 % response rate seen for patients with recurrent disease treated with ifosfamide and etoposide (Miser et al. 1987b), but has not been reproduced. The degree to which these numbers resulted from treating untreated disease versus recurrent disease or from the combination of ifosfamide and etoposide versus the higher doses of ifosfamide has been a topic of debate. ISG/SSG-II showed that high-dose chemotherapy with stem cell rescue did not improve survival, despite causing significantly higher toxicities (Boye et al. 2014). Thus, despite this regimen being feasible, it showed no benefit in survival.

As with Ewing's sarcoma, there is a deep need for an improved understanding of the mechanisms of metastasis, including the mechanisms which render metastatic disease relatively resistant to therapy. Significant advances in the treatment of metastatic osteosarcoma are likely to come only with novel therapies born of an increased understanding of the biology of metastatic osteosarcoma.

Conclusions

The utilization of chemotherapy in the treatment of malignant bone tumors has profoundly improved the prognosis of patients affected with Ewing's sarcoma and osteosarcoma. Prior to chemotherapy, only one in every ten patients affected with these tumors would survive their disease. Now, seven in ten patients or more will live beyond their disease. The formation of cooperative groups has facilitated the study of therapeutic regimens, dramatically increasing the number of participants in clinical trials and shortening the time period over which iterative advancements can be made.

While survival for patients with malignant bone tumors improved dramatically with the advent of chemotherapy, subsequent gains have proved much more difficult to achieve.

Multiple efforts to intensify chemotherapy regimens for patients with newer or more potent cytotoxic agents, increased doses of established medications, and augmentation of therapy with alternative strategies have proved to be of modest benefit in the best cases. More frequently, they have only added toxicity. These results suggest that current regimens likely maximize the benefits that are possible using cytotoxic agents. Further gains will likely only be realized with the development of novel therapies that exploit a more intimate understanding of the biologic pathways that drive these diseases.

There is a particular need for therapies that can affect better outcomes in patients with metastatic disease. Increased research into the mechanisms that drive metastasis and resistance (which may go hand in hand biologically, not just clinically) will be paramount in the search for drugs and targets that more effectively treat metastatic and recurrent disease. Some have proposed that we should rethink our approach to evaluating therapeutic agents in the preclinical setting in order to identify drugs which might interfere in the metastatic process or in the microenvironmental interactions that seem to endow tumor cells with resistance to chemotherapy (Khanna et al. 2014). However, as advancements are pursued, there is clearly room to improve systemic therapies for patients with malignant tumors of the bone.

References

Aljubran AH, Griffin A, Pintilie M, Blackstein M (2009) Osteosarcoma in adolescents and adults: survival analysis with and without lung metastases. Ann Oncol 20:1136–1141. doi:10.1093/annonc/mdn731

Allison DC, Carney SC, Ahlmann ER et al (2012) A meta-analysis of osteosarcoma outcomes in the modern medical era. Sarcoma 2012:704872. doi:10.1155/2012/704872

Ambros IM, Ambros PF, Strehl S et al (1991) MIC2 is a specific marker for Ewing's sarcoma and peripheral primitive neuroectodermal tumors. Evidence for a common histogenesis of Ewing's sarcoma and peripheral primitive neuroectodermal tumors from MIC2 expression and specific chromosome aberration. Cancer 67:1886–1893

Anderson B (2005) Dexrazoxane for the prevention of cardiomyopathy in anthracycline treated pediatric cancer patients. Pediatr Blood Cancer 44:584–588

Bacci G (2003) Neoadjuvant chemotherapy for osteosarcoma of the extremities with metastases at presentation: recent experience at the Rizzoli Institute in 57 patients treated with cisplatin, doxorubicin, and a high dose of methotrexate and ifosfamide. Ann Oncol 14:1126–1134

Bacci G, Picci P, Ruggieri P et al (1990) Primary chemotherapy and delayed surgery (neoadjuvant chemotherapy) for osteosarcoma of the extremities. The Istituto Rizzoli Experience in 127 patients treated preoperatively with intravenous methotrexate (high versus moderate doses) and intraarterial cisplatin. Cancer 65:2539–2553

Bacci G, Picci P, Ferrari S et al (1993) Primary chemotherapy and delayed surgery for nonmetastatic osteosarcoma of the extremities. Results in 164 patients preoperatively treated with high doses of methotrexate followed by cisplatin and doxorubicin. Cancer 72:3227–3238

Bacci G, Picci P, Ferrari S et al (1998) Neoadjuvant chemotherapy for Ewing's sarcoma of bone: no benefit observed after adding ifosfamide and etoposide to vincristine, actinomycin, cyclophosphamide, and doxorubicin in the maintenance phase – results of two sequential studies. Cancer 82:1174–1183

Bacci G, Mercuri M, Longhi A et al (2005) Grade of chemotherapy-induced necrosis as a predictor of local and systemic control in 881 patients with nonmetastatic osteosarcoma of the extremities treated with neoadjuvant chemotherapy in a single institution. Eur J Cancer 41:2079–2085

Baum ES, Gaynon P, Greenberg L et al (1979) Phase II study of cis-dichlorodiammineplatinum(II) in childhood osteosarcoma: Children's Cancer Study Group Report. Cancer Treat Rep 63:1621–1627

Berrak SG, Pearson M, Berberoğlu S et al (2005) High-dose ifosfamide in relapsed pediatric osteosarcoma: therapeutic effects and renal toxicity. Pediatr Blood Cancer 44:215–219

Bielack SS, Kempf-Bielack B, Delling G et al (2002) Prognostic factors in high-grade osteosarcoma of the extremities or trunk: an analysis of 1,702 patients treated on neoadjuvant cooperative osteosarcoma study group protocols. J Clin Oncol 20:776–790

Bielack SS, Machatschek J-N, Flege S, Jürgens H (2004) Delaying surgery with chemotherapy for osteosarcoma of the extremities. Expert Opin Pharmacother 5:1243–1256. doi:10.1517/14656566.5.6.1243

Bielack S, Smeland S, Whelan J, Marina N (2013) MAP plus maintenance pegylated interferon alpha-2b (MAP-IFN) versus MAP alone in patients (pts) with resectable high-grade osteosarcoma and good. ASCO Proc

Boye K, Del Prever AB, Eriksson M et al (2014) High-dose chemotherapy with stem cell rescue in the primary treatment of metastatic and pelvic osteosarcoma:

final results of the ISG/SSG II study. Pediatr Blood Cancer 61:840–845

Bramwell VH, Burgers M, Sneath R et al (1992) A comparison of two short intensive adjuvant chemotherapy regimens in operable osteosarcoma of limbs in children and young adults: the first study of the European Osteosarcoma Intergroup. J Clin Oncol 10:1579–1591

Burdach S, Jürgens H, Peters C et al (1993) Myeloablative radiochemotherapy and hematopoietic stem-cell rescue in poor-prognosis Ewing's sarcoma. J Clin Oncol 11:1482–1488

Burdach S, Van Kaick B, Laws HIJ et al (2000) Allogeneic and autologous stem-cell transplantation in advanced Ewing tumors. An update after long-term follow-up from two centers of the European Intergroup study EICESS. Stem-Cell Transplant Programs at Düsseldorf University Medical Center, Germany and. Ann Oncol 11:1451–1462

Burgert BEO, Nesbit ME, Garnsey LA et al (1990) Multimodal therapy for the management of nonpelvic, localized Ewing's sarcoma of bone: intergroup study IESS-II. J Clin Oncol 8:1514–1524

Casey DA, Wexler LH, Merchant MS et al (2009) Irinotecan and temozolomide for Ewing sarcoma: the Memorial Sloan-Kettering experience. Pediatr Blood Cancer 53:1029–1034. doi:10.1002/pbc.22206

Chou AJ, Kleinerman ES, Krailo MD et al (2009) Addition of muramyl tripeptide to chemotherapy for patients with newly diagnosed metastatic osteosarcoma: a report from the Children's Oncology Group. Cancer 115:5339–5348. doi:10.1002/cncr.24566

Cortes EP, Holland JF, Wang JJ et al (1974) Amputation and adriamycin in primary osteosarcoma. N Engl J Med 291:998–1000. doi:10.1056/NEJM197411072911903

Craft A, Cotterill S, Bullimore J, Pearson D (1997) Long-term results from the first UKCCSG Ewing's tumour study (ET-1). Eur J Cancer 33:1061–1069. doi:10.1016/S0959-8049(97)00043-9

Craft A, Cotterill S, Malcolm A (1998) Ifosfamide-containing chemotherapy in Ewing's sarcoma: the Second United Kingdom Children's Cancer Study Group and the Medical Research Council Ewing's Tumor Study. Clin Oncol 16:3628–3633

Cunningham D, Hawthorn J, Pople A et al (1987) Prevention of emesis in patients receiving cytotoxic drugs by GR38032F, a selective 5-HT3 receptor antagonist. Lancet 1:1461–1463

Cupps RE, Ahmann DL, Soule EH (1969) Treatment of pulmonary metastatic disease with radiation therapy and adjuvant actinomycin D. Preliminary observations. Cancer 24:719–723. doi:10.1002/1097-0142(196910)24:4<719::AID-CNCR2820240409>3.0.CO;2-A

Dahlin DC, Coventry MB (1967) Osteogenic sarcoma: a study of six hundred cases. J Bone Joint Surg 49:101–110

Delépine N, Delépine G, Desbois J et al (1990) Osteogenic osteosarcoma: a model of curable disease by multidisciplinary approach of treatment. Biomed Pharmacother 44:243–248. doi:10.1016/0753-3322(90)90148-3

Deméocq F, Oberlin O, Benz-Lemoine E et al (1989) Initial chemotherapy including ifosfamide in the management of Ewing's sarcoma: preliminary results. A protocol of the French Pediatric Oncology Society (SFOP). Cancer Chemother Pharmacol 24(Suppl 1):S45–S47

Donaldson SS, Torrey M, Link MP et al (1998) A multidisciplinary study investigating radiotherapy in Ewing's sarcoma: end results of POG #8346. Int J Radiat Oncol 42:125–135. doi:10.1016/S0360-3016(98)00191-6

Ebb D, Meyers P, Grier H et al (2012) Phase II trial of trastuzumab in combination with cytotoxic chemotherapy for treatment of metastatic osteosarcoma with human epidermal growth factor receptor 2 overexpression: a report from the children's oncology group. J Clin Oncol 30:2545–2551

Edmonson J, Green S, Ivins J et al (1984) A controlled pilot study of high-dose methotrexate as postsurgical adjuvant treatment for primary osteosarcoma. J Clin Oncol 2:152–156

Eselgrim M, Grunert H, Kühne T et al (2006) Dose intensity of chemotherapy for osteosarcoma and outcome in the Cooperative Osteosarcoma Study Group (COSS) trials. Pediatr Blood Cancer 47:42–50. doi:10.1002/pbc.20608

Ettinger LJ, Douglass HO, Higby DJ et al (1981) Adjuvant adriamycin and cis-diamminedichloroplatinum (cis-platinum) in primary osteosarcoma. Cancer 47:248–254

Evans AE, Baehner RL, Chard RL et al (1974) Comparison of daunorubicin (NSC-83142) with adriamycin (NSC-123127) in the treatment of late-stage childhood solid tumors. Cancer Chemother Rep 58:671–676

Evans RG, Nesbit ME, Gehan EA et al (1991) Multimodal therapy for the management of localized Ewing's sarcoma of pelvic and sacral bones: a report from the second intergroup study. J Clin Oncol 9:1173–1180

Ewing J (1924) Further report of endothelial myeloma of bone. Proc NY Pathol Soc 24:93–100

Ferrari S, Mercuri M, Picci P et al (1999) Nonmetastatic osteosarcoma of the extremity: results of a neoadjuvant chemotherapy protocol (IOR/OS-3) with high-dose methotrexate, intraarterial or intravenous cisplatin, doxorubicin, and salvage chemotherapy based on histologic tumor response. Tumori 85:458–464

Ferrari S, Smeland S, Mercuri M et al (2005) Neoadjuvant chemotherapy with high-dose Ifosfamide, high-dose methotrexate, cisplatin, and doxorubicin for patients with localized osteosarcoma of the extremity: a joint study by the Italian and Scandinavian Sarcoma Groups. J Clin Oncol 23:8845–8852. doi:10.1200/JCO.2004.00.5785

Finklestein JZ, Hittle RE, Hammond GD (1969) Evaluation of a high dose cyclophosphamide regimen in childhood tumors. Cancer 23:1239–1242

Fuchs N, Bielack SS, Epler D et al (1998) Long-term results of the co-operative German-Austrian-Swiss osteosarcoma study group's protocol COSS-86 of intensive multidrug chemotherapy and surgery for osteosarcoma of the limbs. Ann Oncol 9:893–899

Goorin AM, Harris MB, Bernstein M et al (2002) Phase II/III trial of etoposide and high-dose ifosfamide in newly diagnosed metastatic osteosarcoma: a pediatric oncology group trial. J Clin Oncol 20:426–433. doi:10.1200/JCO.20.2.426

Goorin AM, Schwartzentruber DJ, Devidas M et al (2003) Presurgical chemotherapy compared with immediate surgery and adjuvant chemotherapy for nonmetastatic osteosarcoma: Pediatric Oncology Group Study POG-8651. J Clin Oncol 21:1574–1580

Granowetter L, Womer R, Devidas M et al (2009) Dose-intensified compared with standard chemotherapy for nonmetastatic Ewing sarcoma family of tumors: a Children's Oncology Group Study. J Clin Oncol 27:2536–2541. doi:10.1200/JCO.2008.19.1478

Grier HE, Krailo MD, Tarbell NJ et al (2003) Addition of ifosfamide and etoposide to standard chemotherapy for Ewing's sarcoma and primitive neuroectodermal tumor of bone. N Engl J Med 348:694–701. doi:10.1056/NEJMoa020890

Harris MB, Cantor AB, Goorin AM et al (1995) Treatment of osteosarcoma with ifosfamide: comparison of response in pediatric patients with recurrent disease versus patients previously untreated: a Pediatric Oncology Group study. Med Pediatr Oncol 24:87–92

Hayes FA, Thompson EI, Meyer WH et al (1989) Therapy for localized Ewing's sarcoma of bone. J Clin Oncol 7:208–213

Hunold A, Ahrens S, Boldering N (2004) Topotecan and cyclophosphamide for Ewing tumour relapse. SIOP Abstr. p O.025:333

Hustu HO, Holton C, James D, Pinkel D (1968) Treatment of Ewing's sarcoma with concurrent radiotherapy and chemotherapy. J Pediatr 73:249–251

Jaffe N, Farber S, Traggis D et al (1973) Favorable response of metastatic osteogenic sarcoma to pulse high-dose methotrexate with citrovorum rescue and radiation therapy. Cancer 31:1367–1373. doi:10.1002/1097-0142(197306)31:6<1367::AID-CNCR2820310611>3.0.CO;2-6

Jaffe N, Paed D, Traggis D et al (1976) Improved outlook for Ewing's sarcoma with combination chemotherapy (vincristine, actinomycin D and cyclophosphamide) and radiation therapy. Cancer 38:1925–1930

James D, George P (1964) Vincristine in children with malignant solid tumors. J Pediatr 64:534–541

Jenkin RDT (1966) Ewing's sarcoma a study of treatment methods. Clin Radiol 17:97–106. doi:10.1016/S0009-9260(66)80064-8

Juergens C, Weston C, Lewis I et al (2006) Safety assessment of intensive induction with vincristine, ifosfamide, doxorubicin, and etoposide (VIDE) in the treatment of Ewing tumors in the EURO-E.W.I.N.G. 99 clinical trial. 22–29. doi: 10.1002/pbc

Jürgens H, Exner U, Gadner H et al (1988) Multidisciplinary treatment of primary Ewing's sarcoma of bone. A 6-year experience of a European Cooperative Trial. Cancer 61:23–32

Jürgens H, Exner U, Kühl J et al (1989) High-dose ifosfamide with mesna uroprotection in Ewing's sarcoma. Cancer Chemother Pharmacol 24(Suppl 1):S40–S44

Kager L, Zoubek A, Pötschger U et al (2003) Primary metastatic osteosarcoma: presentation and outcome of patients treated on neoadjuvant Cooperative Osteosarcoma Study Group protocols. J Clin Oncol 21:2011–2018

Kalam K, Marwick TH (2013) Role of cardioprotective therapy for prevention of cardiotoxicity with chemotherapy: a systematic review and meta-analysis. Eur J Cancer 49:2900–2909

Khanna C, Fan TM, Gorlick R et al (2014) Towards a drug development path that targets metastatic progression in osteosarcoma. Clin Cancer Res. doi:10.1158/1078-0432.CCR-13-2574

Kudawara I, Aoki Y, Ueda T et al (2013) Neoadjuvant and adjuvant chemotherapy with high-dose ifosfamide, doxorubicin, cisplatin and high-dose methotrexate in non-metastatic osteosarcoma of the extremities: a phase II trial in Japan. J Chemother 25:41–48. doi:1 0.1179/1973947812Y.0000000055

Kushner BH, Meyers PA (2001) How effective is dose-intensive/myeloablative therapy against Ewing's sarcoma/primitive neuroectodermal tumor metastatic to bone or bone marrow? The Memorial Sloan-Kettering experience and a literature review. J Clin Oncol 19:870–880

Le Deley M-C, Delattre O, Schaefer K-L et al (2010) Impact of EWS-ETS fusion type on disease progression in Ewing's sarcoma/peripheral primitive neuroectodermal tumor: prospective results from the cooperative Euro-E.W.I.N.G. 99 trial. J Clin Oncol 28:1982–1988. doi:10.1200/JCO.2009.23.3585

Lewis IJ, Nooij MA, Whelan J et al (2007) Improvement in histologic response but not survival in osteosarcoma patients treated with intensified chemotherapy: a randomized phase III trial of the European Osteosarcoma Intergroup. J Natl Cancer Inst 99:112–128. doi:10.1093/jnci/djk015

Link MP, Goorin AM, Miser AW et al (1986) The effect of adjuvant chemotherapy on relapse-free survival in patients with osteosarcoma of the extremity. N Engl J Med 314:1600–1606. doi:10.1056/NEJM198606193142502

Lipshultz SE, Lipsitz SR, Mone SM et al (1995) Female sex and drug dose as risk factors for late cardiotoxic effects of doxorubicin therapy for childhood cancer. N Engl J Med 332:1738–1743. doi:10.1056/NEJM199506293322602

Lipshultz SE, Miller TL, Lipsitz SR et al (2012) Continuous versus bolus infusion of doxorubicin in children with ALL: long-term cardiac outcomes. Pediatrics 130:1003–1011. doi:10.1542/peds.2012-0727

Marcove RC, Mike V, Hajek JV et al (1970) Osteogenic sarcoma under the age of twenty-one. A review of one hundred and forty-five operative cases. J Bone Joint Surg 52:411–423

Marina N, Smeland S, Bielack SS, et al. (2014) MAPIE vs MAP as postoperative chemotherapy in patients with a poor response to preoperative chemotherapy for newly-diagnosed osteosarcoma: results from EURAMOS-1. Connect. Tissue Oncol Soc. Berlin, Germany, p 96

Marti C, Kroner T, Remagen W et al (1985) High-dose ifosfamide in advanced osteosarcoma. Cancer Treat Rep 69:115–117

McKeon C, Thiele CJ, Ross RA et al (1988) Indistinguishable patterns of protooncogene expression in two distinct but closely related tumors: Ewing's sarcoma and neuroepithelioma. Cancer Res 48: 4307–4311

Meyer WH, Kun L, Marina N et al (1992) Ifosfamide plus etoposide in newly diagnosed Ewing's sarcoma of bone. J Clin Oncol 10:1737–1742

Meyers PA, Gorlick R, Heller G et al (1998) Intensification of preoperative chemotherapy for osteogenic sarcoma: results of the Memorial Sloan-Kettering (T12) protocol. J Clin Oncol 16:2452–2458

Meyers PA, Krailo MD, Ladanyi M et al (2001) High-dose melphalan, etoposide, total-body irradiation, and autologous stem-cell reconstitution as consolidation therapy for high-risk Ewing's sarcoma does not improve. J Clin Oncol 19:2812–2820

Meyers PA, Schwartz CL, Krailo M et al (2005) Osteosarcoma: a randomized, prospective trial of the addition of ifosfamide and/or muramyl tripeptide to cisplatin, doxorubicin, and high-dose methotrexate. J Clin Oncol 23:2004–2011. doi:10.1200/JCO.2005.06.031

Meyers PA, Schwartz CL, Krailo MD et al (2008) Osteosarcoma: the addition of muramyl tripeptide to chemotherapy improves overall survival–a report from the Children's Oncology Group. J Clin Oncol 26:633–638. doi:10.1200/JCO.2008.14.0095

Miser J, Kinsella T, Triche T et al (1987a) Treatment of peripheral neuroepithelioma in children and young adults. J Clin Oncol 5:1752–1758

Miser JS, Kinsella TJ, Triche TJ et al (1987b) Ifosfamide with mesna uroprotection and etoposide: an effective regimen in the treatment of recurrent sarcomas and other tumors of children and young adults. J Clin Oncol 5:1191–1198

Mosende C, Gutierrez M, Caparros B, Rosen G (1977) Combination chemotherapy with bleomycin, cyclophosphamide and dactinomycin for the treatment of osteogenic sarcoma. Cancer 40:2779–2786. doi:10.1002/1097-0142(197712)40:6<2779::AID-CNCR2820400604>3.0.CO;2-E

Müller CR, Smeland S, Bauer HCF et al (2005) Interferon-alpha as the only adjuvant treatment in high-grade osteosarcoma: long term results of the Karolinska Hospital series. Acta Oncol 44:475–480

Mulrooney DA, Yeazel MW, Kawashima T et al (2009) Cardiac outcomes in a cohort of adult survivors of childhood and adolescent cancer: retrospective analysis of the Childhood Cancer Survivor Study cohort. BMJ 339:b4606

Nesbit ME, Perez CA, Tefft M et al (1981) Multimodal therapy for the management of primary, nonmetastatic Ewing's sarcoma of bone: an Intergroup Study. Natl Cancer Inst Monogr 56:255–262

Nesbit MEJ, Gehan E, Burgert EOJ et al (1990) Multimodal therapy for the management of primary, nonmetastatic Ewing's sarcoma of bone: a long-term follow-up of the First Intergroup study. J Clin Oncol 8:1664–1674

Oberlin O, Habrand JL, Zucker JM et al (1992) No benefit of ifosfamide in Ewing's sarcoma: a nonrandomized study of the French Society of Pediatric Oncology. J Clin Oncol 10:1407–1412

Ochs JJ, Freeman AI, Douglass HO et al (1978) cis-Dichlorodiammineplatinum (II) in advanced osteogenic sarcoma. Cancer Treat Rep 62:239–245

Oldham RK, Pomeroy TC (1972) Treatment of Ewing's sarcoma with adriamycin (NSC-123127). Cancer Chemother Rep 56:635–639

Paulussen M, Ahrens S, Dunst J et al (2001) Localized Ewing tumor of bone: final results of the cooperative Ewing's Sarcoma Study CESS 86. J Clin Oncol 19:1818–1829

Phillips RF, Higinbotham NL (1967) The curability of Ewing's endothelioma of bone in children. J Pediatr 70:391–397. doi:10.1016/S0022-3476(67)80136-7

Picci P, Bacci G, Campanacci M et al (1985) Histologic evaluation of necrosis in osteosarcoma induced by chemotherapy. Regional mapping of viable and nonviable tumor. Cancer 56:1515–1521

Pinkel D (1962) Cyclophosphamide in children with cancer. Cancer 15:42–49

Provisor A, Ettinger L, Nachman J et al (1997) Treatment of nonmetastatic osteosarcoma of the extremity with preoperative and postoperative chemotherapy: a report from the Children's Cancer Group. J Clin Oncol 15:76–84

Rosen G (1985) Preoperative (neoadjuvant) chemotherapy for osteogenic sarcoma: a ten year experience. Orthopedics 8:659–664

Rosen G, Wollner N, Tan C et al (1974) Disease-free survival in children with Ewing's sarcoma treated with radiation therapy and adjuvant four-drug sequential chemotherapy. Cancer 33:384–393

Rosen G, Caparros B, Mosende C et al (1978) Curability of Ewing's sarcoma and considerations for future therapeutic trials. Cancer 41:888–899

Rosen G, Caparros B, Huvos AG et al (1982) Preoperative chemotherapy for osteogenic sarcoma: selection of postoperative adjuvant chemotherapy based on the response of the primary tumor to preoperative chemotherapy. Cancer 49:1221–1230

Saeter G, Alvegård TA, Elomaa I et al (1991) Treatment of osteosarcoma of the extremities with the T-10 protocol, with emphasis on the effects of preoperative chemotherapy with single-agent high-dose methotrexate: a Scandinavian Sarcoma Group study. J Clin Oncol 9:1766–1775

Saylors RL, Stine KKC, Sullivan J, et al. (2001) Cyclophosphamide plus topotecan in children with recurrent or refractory solid tumors: a Pediatric Oncology Group phase II study. J Clin Oncol 19:3463–3469

Scheef W, Klein HO, Brock N et al (1979) Controlled clinical studies with an antidote against the urotoxicity of oxazaphosphorines: preliminary results. Cancer Treat Rep 63:501–505

Schwartz HS, Sodergren JE, Sternberg SS, Philips FS (1966) Actinomycin D: effects on Ridgway osteogenic sarcoma in mice. Cancer Res 26:1873–1879

Schwartz HS, Sodergren JE, Ambaye RY (1968) Actinomycin D: drug concentrations and actions in mouse tissues and tumors. Cancer Res 28:192–197

Smeland S, Müller C, Alvegard TA et al (2003) Scandinavian Sarcoma Group Osteosarcoma Study SSG VIII: prognostic factors for outcome and the role of replacement salvage chemotherapy for poor histological responders. Eur J Cancer 39:488–494

Smith MA, Ungerleider RS, Horowitz ME, Simon R (1991) Influence of doxorubicin dose intensity on response and outcome for patients with osteogenic sarcoma and Ewing's sarcoma. J Natl Cancer Inst 83:1460–1470

Souhami RL, Craft AW, Van der Eijken JW et al (1997) Randomised trial of two regimens of chemotherapy in operable osteosarcoma: a study of the European Osteosarcoma Intergroup. Lancet 350:911–917. doi:10.1016/S0140-6736(97)02307-6

Sutow WW (1968) Vincristine (NSC-67574) therapy for malignant solid tumors in children (except Wilms' tumor). Cancer Chemother Rep 52:485–487

Sutow W, Sullivan M (1962) Cyclophosphamide therapy in children with Ewing's sarcoma. Cancer Chemother Rep 23:55–60

Sutow WW, Vietti TJ, Fernbach DJ et al (1971) Evaluation of chemotherapy in children with metastatic Ewing's sarcoma and osteogenic sarcoma. Cancer Chemother Rep 55:67–78

Sutow WW, Sullivan MP, Wilbur JR, Cangir A (1975) Study of adjuvant chemotherapy in osteogenic sarcoma. J Clin Pharmacol 15:530–533. doi:10.1002/j.1552-4604.1975.tb01476.x

Taylor W, Ivins J, Dahlin D et al (1978) Trends and variability in survival from osteosarcoma. Mayo Clin Proc 53:695–700

Taylor W, Ivins J, Pritchard D et al (1985) Trends and variability in survival among patients with osteosarcoma: a 7-year update. Mayo Clin Proc 60:91–104

Thompson J, George EO, Poquette CA et al (1999) Synergy of topotecan in combination with vincristine for treatment of pediatric solid tumor xenografts. Clin Cancer Res 5:3617–3631

Turc-Carel C, Philip I, Berger M-P et al (1983) Chromosomal translocations in Ewing's sarcoma. N Engl J Med 309:496–498. doi:10.1056/NEJM198308253090817

Van Dalen EC, Caron HN, Dickinson HO, Kremer LCM (2005) Cardioprotective interventions for cancer patients receiving anthracyclines. Cochrane Database Syst Rev (2):CD003917

Von Hoff DD (1979) Risk factors for doxorubicin-induced congestive heart failure. Ann Intern Med 91:710

Wagner L, McAllister N (2007) Temozolomide and intravenous irinotecan for treatment of advanced Ewing sarcoma. Pediatr Blood 48:132–139. doi:10.1002/pbc

Wagner LM, Crews KR, Iacono LC et al (2004) Phase I trial of temozolomide and protracted irinotecan in pediatric patients with refractory solid tumors. Clin Cancer Res 10:840–848. doi:10.1158/1078-0432.CCR-03-0175

Weinfeld MS, Dudley HR Jr (1962) Osteogenic sarcoma a follow-up study of the ninety-four cases observed at the Massachusetts general hospital from 1920 to 1960. J Bone Joint Surg 44:269–276

Whang-Peng J, Triche TJ, Knutsen T et al (1984) Chromosome translocation in peripheral neuroepithelioma. N Engl J Med 311:584–585. doi:10.1056/NEJM198408303110907

Winkler K, Beron G, Kotz R et al (1983) Adjuvant chemotherapy in osteosarcoma – effects of cisplatinum, BCD, and fibroblast interferon in sequential combination with HD-MTX and adriamycin. Preliminary results of the COSS 80 study. J Cancer Res Clin Oncol 106(Suppl):1–7

Winkler K, Beron G, Kotz R et al (1984) Neoadjuvant chemotherapy for osteogenic sarcoma: results of a Cooperative German/Austrian study. J Clin Oncol 2:617–624

Winkler K, Beron G, Delling G et al (1988) Neoadjuvant chemotherapy of osteosarcoma: results of a randomized cooperative trial (COSS-82) with salvage chemotherapy based on histological tumor response. J Clin Oncol 6:329–337

Winkler K, Bielack S, Delling G et al (1990) Effect of intraarterial versus intravenous cisplatin in addition to systemic doxorubicin, high-dose methotrexate, and ifosfamide on histologic tumor response in osteosarcoma (study COSS-86). Cancer 66:1703–1710

Womer R, Daller R, Fenton JG, Miser J (2000) Granulocyte colony stimulating factor permits dose intensification by interval compression in the treatment of Ewing's sarcomas and soft tissue sarcomas in children. Eur J Cancer 36:87–94. doi:10.1016/S0959-8049(99)00236-1

Womer RB, West DC, Krailo MD et al (2012) Randomized controlled trial of interval-compressed chemotherapy for the treatment of localized Ewing sarcoma: a report from the Children's Oncology Group. J Clin Oncol 30:4148–4154. doi:10.1200/JCO.2011.41.5703

Radiation Management

Ashley Sekhon, Karl Haglund, and Michael Guiou

Contents

7.1	**Ewing Sarcoma**	110
7.1.1	Introduction	110
7.1.2	Indications for Radiotherapy	111
7.1.3	Volumes	112
7.1.4	Dose and Fractionation	113
7.1.5	Techniques: 3DCRT, IMRT, Proton/Ion	115
7.1.6	Site-Specific Considerations	116
7.1.7	Quality	117
7.1.8	Metastatic Disease	117
7.1.9	Side Effects	118
7.2	**Osteosarcoma**	119
7.2.1	Indications	120
7.2.2	Future Directions	121
References		122

A. Sekhon, MD • K. Haglund, MD, PhD
M. Guiou, MD (✉)
Department of Radiation Oncology,
The Ohio State University Comprehensive
Cancer Center, 410 West 10th Avenue,
Columbus, OH 43210, USA
e-mail: Ashley.sekon@osumc.edu;
Karl.haglund@osumc.edu;
Michael.guiou@osumc.edu

Abstract

In 1921 when James Ewing first described the case of a "round cell sarcoma" discovered in the radius of a 14-year-old girl, he was surprised to see the rapid resolution of tumor following application of radium (Ewing 1921). "The prompt recession under radium was also quite unlike our experience with osteogenic sarcoma. With the recession of the tumor the shaft was well restored and normal function regained. The patient left the hospital with instructions to return weekly for observation, which was continued for several months." Since that time, radiation therapy has played an integral role in the management of Ewing sarcoma. A report on 50 children treated at Massachusetts General Hospital between 1930 and 1952 documented sustained 5-year local control in 15 of 22 patients who received wide-field irradiation (Wang and Schulz 1953). Cure was achieved in four of these individuals. This was in contrast to those who underwent primary surgical resection, where only 1 of 10 patients was alive 5 years later. The authors emphasized the radiosensitive nature of the tumor, favoring radiotherapy over a potentially mutilating surgery. Indeed in an era where limitations in surgical technique permitted only radical resection or amputation, radiation alone comprised the standard of care for localized disease (Shankar et al. 1999; Donaldson 1980; Bacci et al. 1989;

© Springer International Publishing Switzerland 2015
T.P. Cripe, N.D. Yeager (eds.), *Malignant Pediatric Bone Tumors - Treatment & Management*,
Pediatric Oncology, DOI 10.1007/978-3-319-18099-1_7

Evans et al. 1991; Jenkin 1991; Kinsella et al. 1991). However, in light of considerable advances in orthopedic surgery and effective multi-agent chemotherapy over the past several decades, the precise role of radiotherapy in a multidisciplinary setting continues to evolve, and the optimal approach to ensuring local control remains controversial (Shankar et al. 1999; Burgert et al. 1990; Pisters et al. 2007; Grier et al. 2003; McGovern and Mahajan 2012; Dunst et al. 1995).

7.1 Ewing Sarcoma

7.1.1 Introduction

In 1921 when James Ewing first described the case of a "round cell sarcoma" discovered in the radius of a 14-year-old girl, he was surprised to see the rapid resolution of tumor following application of radium (Ewing 1921). "The prompt recession under radium was also quite unlike our experience with osteogenic sarcoma. With the recession of the tumor the shaft was well restored and normal function regained. The patient left the hospital with instructions to return weekly for observation, which was continued for several months." Since that time, radiation therapy has played an integral role in the management of Ewing sarcoma. A report on 50 children treated at Massachusetts General Hospital between 1930 and 1952 documented sustained 5-year local control in 15 of 22 patients who received wide-field irradiation (Wang and Schulz 1953). Cure was achieved in four of these individuals. This was in contrast to those who underwent primary surgical resection, where only 1 of 10 patients was alive 5 years later. The authors emphasized the radiosensitive nature of the tumor, favoring radiotherapy over a potentially mutilating surgery. Indeed in an era where limitations in surgical technique permitted only radical resection or amputation, radiation alone comprised the standard of care for localized disease (Shankar et al. 1999; Donaldson 1980; Bacci et al. 1989; Evans et al. 1991; Jenkin 1991; Kinsella et al. 1991). However, in light of considerable advances in orthopedic surgery and effective multi-agent

chemotherapy over the past several decades, the precise role of radiotherapy in a multidisciplinary setting continues to evolve, and the optimal approach to ensuring local control remains controversial (Shankar et al. 1999; Burgert et al. 1990; Pisters et al. 2007; Grier et al. 2003; McGovern and Mahajan 2012; Dunst et al. 1995).

There have been multiple factors leading to a relative increase in the use of surgery as a local therapy (Shankar et al. 1999; Pisters et al. 2007; Halperin 2005). Perhaps most importantly, the introduction of limb-salvage procedures and advancements in various reconstruction techniques have resulted in excellent local control with preservation of mobility and function (Leitman and Michael 2010) (see Chap. 9). Furthermore, the routine use of cytotoxic chemotherapy often produces a significant decrease in extraosseous disease extent, rendering tumors more resectable (Halperin 2005). While Ewing sarcoma is widely recognized as a radiosensitive tumor, the local failure rate when treating with radiation alone remains 10–25 % (Dunst and Schuck 2004). This potential for disease recurrence compounded by concern for long-term sequelae, particularly secondary malignancy, has promoted surgery as the primary form of local therapy in a majority of multi-institutional clinical trials (Burgert et al. 1990; Dunst et al. 1995; Oberlin et al. 2001; Schuck et al. 2003; Paulussen et al. 2001; Donaldson et al. 1998).

Comparisons between surgery and radiation in all published analyses are thus retrospective in nature, largely related to local culture and practices and thus difficult to interpret. The majority of randomized clinical trials have focused on modifications in chemotherapy regimens (Grier et al. 2003; Perez et al. 1981). The most widely employed local management strategy has been risk-adapted, and frequently dependent upon specific characteristics of each patient's disease (Donaldson 2004). Review of these studies suggests that patients for whom definitive radiation was recommended more commonly presented with lesions at inaccessible sites (i.e., proximal/pelvic lesions), greater overall tumor volume, or with a suboptimal response to systemic therapy. Patients with marginal or intralesional resection, or those with a poor pathologic response to induction chemotherapy, comprised a "high risk" group that received post-operative radiotherapy. A number of reports have recognized such clinical characteristics as negative prognostic indicators (Donaldson et al. 1998; Schuck et al. 2002).

Multivariate analysis from the European Cooperative Ewing's Sarcoma Study (CESS) 86 found both tumor size >200 mL and poor histologic response to be significantly correlated with inferior outcomes (Dunst et al. 1995). Patients considered to be poor responders had the highest rates of metastatic relapse (52 %) and overall failures (62 %). Although the risk of isolated local failure was higher in patients receiving radiation alone versus those who underwent resection (7 % vs. 0 %), it was reinforced that this difference likely represented an underlying selection bias. Even then the overall frequency of relapse was not influenced by the type of local treatment, with rates of 30 % following definitive radiotherapy, 26 % after radical surgery, and 34 % with combined local therapies.

In a multi-institutional cooperative group study led by the Pediatric Oncology Group (POG), initial tumor site was determined to be strongly correlated with event-free survival (EFS) (Donaldson et al. 1998). Patients with distal extremity and central disease fared relatively well with a 5-year EFS of 65 % and 63 %, respectively, whereas patients with pelvic and sacral primary tumors did poorly with a 5-year EFS of only 24 %. Those with proximal extremity disease had an intermediate EFS of 46 %. When the form of local therapy utilized was further examined, pelvic primaries comprised 20 % of the radiotherapy group and only 8 % of the surgery group ($p=0.03$). This distribution was in comparison to either central or distal disease, which comprised 40 % of the radiotherapy group versus 76 % of the surgery group.

The most reliable means of truly determining the efficacy of surgery compared to radiation is in the context of a randomized trial (Donaldson et al. 1998). However such a study is unlikely to be feasible in the management of Ewing sarcoma. In each patient there exists the potential need for all three therapies to ensure optimal outcome. Local therapy is individualized and influenced by several factors including patient age, potential morbidity, tumor site and size, response to che-

Table 7.1 Local control – Ewing sarcoma

Group	Era	n	Dose (Gy)	5-year overall LC (%)	LC with RT alone
IESS-I	1973–1978	331	45–65	85	
IESS-II	1978–1982	214	50–55	90	
SJCRH	1978–1988	43	30–60	68	58
CESS-81	1981–1986	32	46–60	74	53
U of Fl	1982–1987	39	50–60	85	
POG 8346	1983–1988	104	55.8		65
CESS-81	1986–1991	44	60	93	86
MSKCC	1990–2004	60	36–60	77[a]	7[a]

Abbreviations: *IESS* Intergroup Ewing Sarcoma Study, *SJCRH* St. Jude Children's Research Hospital, *CESS* Cooperative Ewing Sarcoma Study, *U of Fl* University of Florida, *POG* Pediatric Oncology Group, *MSKCC* Memorial Sloan Kettering Cancer Center, *n* number of patients, *Gy* gray, *LC* local control, *RT* radiation therapy
[a]Reported as 3-year local control

motherapy, and institutional policy (Schuck et al. 2002). Regardless of selection biases, multidisciplinary therapy has led to the continued improvement in both local control and survival of children and adolescents diagnosed with Ewing sarcoma (Table 7.1). In this respect, surgery and radiation serve to complement one another as local therapies. The ultimate goal remains to maximize therapeutic outcomes while still preserving function, decreasing morbidity, and minimizing late effects of treatment when possible.

7.1.2 Indications for Radiotherapy

In a combined retrospective analysis of local therapy in the CESS 81 and 86 as well as the European Intergroup Ewing's Sarcoma Study 92 (EICESS 92), Schuck et al. examined indications for radiation in 1,058 patients with non-metastatic Ewing tumor (Schuck et al. 2003). As in other studies, definitive radiotherapy was the preferred modality when surgery would only allow for intralesional resection or a debulking procedure. The primary criteria for post-operative radiation were resection status and poor pathologic tumor response. Not surprisingly, it was found that the addition of radiation improved local control in those with intralesional or marginal resections regardless of histologic response. However, patients deemed poor pathologic responders after wide resection experienced superior outcomes when treated with post-operative radiotherapy (local relapse of 5 % vs. 12 %), though the comparison is limited due to small patient numbers. Local control and EFS were equivalent in patients receiving radiation alone as compared with intralesional resection and adjuvant radiation, further solidifying the use of definitive radiation in poor surgical candidates. The EICESS 92 trial also permitted pre-operative radiotherapy in patients with <50 % reduction in the soft tissue tumor component. While there was no apparent improvement in EFS, the local relapse rate was only 5.3 % in this population, arguing for the use of neoadjuvant radiotherapy if function-preserving surgery with narrow margins is anticipated.

Current treatment guidelines call for postoperative radiation in the setting of residual gross or microscopic disease, and where there has been a suboptimal response to induction chemotherapy. This level of response has classically been defined as ≥10 % viable tumor cells in the surgical specimen. Based on the findings above some argue for the use of adjuvant radiotherapy, albeit to a lower total dose, in cases of gross total resection with adequate margins but a poor pathologic response (Donaldson 2004). This philosophy selects for a single "low risk" subgroup of patients who are precluded from radiotherapy due to both a satisfactory histologic response to chemotherapy and an appropriate margin status (>1 cm). Although variation in institutional practices exists, radiation is generally excluded when a wide resection has been achieved regardless of histologic response.

The appropriate timing for radiation delivery is not well defined, with prior studies initiating treatment anywhere from 9 to 18 weeks post-induction chemotherapy (Dunst et al. 1995; Schuck et al. 2003; Donaldson et al. 1998). Due to a number of confounding factors, it is difficult to determine how a potential delay in radiation may have affected long-term outcomes. Nonetheless it appears that a prolonged time to local therapy overall may lead to inferior outcomes due to possible interval development of drug resistance (Donaldson 2004). Regarding post-operative radiotherapy, European investigators found patients treated within a 60-day period following surgery experienced local control rates of 98 % versus 92 % for patients treated at later time points (Schuck et al. 2002). This difference was not statistically significant, nor did it influence survival. Current Children's Oncology Group (COG) protocols generally require the incorporation of definitive radiotherapy when indicated at 12–13 weeks into systemic therapy, and 8 weeks post-surgical resection.

7.1.3 Volumes

For decades, radiation volumes for Ewing sarcoma encompassed the entire bone. This approach was prompted by several early reports implicating the propensity of Ewing tumors to spread along the medullary cavity of the bone (Phillips and Sheline 1969). A subsequent publication by Suit emphasized the rarity of local disease recurrence outside of the involved primary site (Suit 1964). This observation led to gradual reductions in field size with resultant equivalent local control. In the St. Jude Children's Research Hospital experience, 94.7 % (18/19) of recurrences were confined to the irradiated bone (Arai et al. 1991). The radiation target volume was defined as the pre-chemotherapy osseous tumor in addition to the post-induction residual soft tissue extent with a 3 cm margin. The authors concluded that the lack of marginal failures indicated a reduction of irradiation volume was possible without incurring significant risk.

Similarly, the POG 8346 trial sought to determine if a more tailored radiation field was equivalent to standard whole bone radiation (Donaldson et al. 1998). Patients undergoing radiotherapy were prospectively randomized to either receive standard field treatment (SFRT), consisting of 39.6 Gy to the whole bone with a 16.2 Gy boost to the initial tumor plus a 2 cm margin, or involved field radiation (IFRT) to the initial tumor and a 2 cm margin with 55.8 Gy. Unfortunately the randomization portion of the study was discontinued prematurely due to poor accrual. However of the 40 patients randomized, there was no observed difference in 5-year EFS with SFRT versus IFRT (37 % vs. 39 % EFS). The remainder of the 94 patients received IFRT. The majority of local failures were central, within the radiotherapy port (62 %).

The precise definition of target volumes in radiation is crucial to successful execution. There are three main volumes in radiation planning. The gross tumor volume (GTV) consists of visible tumor present on physical exam and/or imaging. The second volume, the clinical target volume (CTV), contains the GTV plus a margin to include potential localized subclinical disease spread. The final treatment volume is known as the planning target volume (PTV). This is an expansion from the CTV to allow for uncertainties inherent in the technology, such as day-to-day minor variations in setup and patient movement.

Current radiotherapy contouring guidelines for Ewing sarcoma define GTV1 as the pre-treatment osseous and soft tissue disease (Donaldson 2004). In tumors that exhibit an infiltrative component into a body cavity (e.g., thorax, abdomen), the GTV1 may be modified to exclude the portion extending into the cavity if there has been a response to chemotherapy such that normal tissues have returned to their baseline position. A 1.5 cm margin is added to GTV1 to create CTV1. The expansion from CTV1 to PTV1 is institution specific, but typically is within the range of 0.5–1 cm.

For unresected tumors, GTV2 is the boost volume, and is defined as the pre-treatment boney abnormalities and residual soft tissue disease following induction chemotherapy. For inadequately resected tumors, GTV2 is the area of gross or microscopic residual disease, or the site of a close margin. A 1 cm margin is added to create the CTV2. Again, a 0.5–1 cm margin is added to the CTV2 to form the PTV2.

7.1.4 Dose and Fractionation

Given the high rate of in-field failure, studies have explored the utility of dose escalation. To date, the data is conflicting. The first Intergroup Ewing Sarcoma Study (IESS-I) did not demonstrate a dose response between 30 and 60 Gy (Razek et al. 1980). Local control was achieved in 6/6 (100 %) patients treated with 30–39.9 Gy, 37/43 (86 %) with 40–49.9 Gy, 80/91 (88 %) with 50–59.9 Gy, and 50/53 (94 %) with $\geq$60 Gy. Likewise, a retrospective review in an era of more modern radiation technique using 3D conformal and IMRT planning (see section on "Technique") at Memorial Sloan Kettering Cancer Center (MSKCC) did not show a radiation dose response (Trang et al. 2006). Patients who received doses <55 Gy and $\geq$55 Gy experienced 3-year LC of 78 % and 73 %, respectively ($p = 0.518$).

Investigators at St. Jude Children's Research Hospital found that lower doses of 30–36 Gy to tumors <8 cm in greatest dimension with an objective response to induction chemotherapy provided 5-year local control rate of 90 % ($n = 9/10$) (Arai et al. 1991). This rate was in comparison to a local control rate of 52 % ($n = 11/21$) in tumors $\geq$8 cm treated with identical doses. However, an update from the same institution by Krasin et al. showed higher rates of local recurrence in children with <8 cm tumors who received doses <40 Gy (19 % $\pm$ 9 %), with no local failures occurring with doses $\geq$40 Gy (Krasin et al. 2004). This difference approached statistical significance ($p = 0.084$). A recent paper published by Paulino et al. showed similar results. For tumors $\leq$8 cm, the 5-year local control rate was 50 % when treated with <49 Gy, versus 94.1 % when treated with doses $\geq$49 Gy. In tumors >8 cm, a radiation dose <54 Gy resulted in a 5-year local control rate of only 26.7 % compared to 85.7 % when treated with doses $\geq$54 Gy (Paulino et al. 2007a).

The recommended dose in definitive management of localized Ewing tumors is 55–60 Gy fractionated into 1.5–1.8 Gy doses. Such irradiation is typically delivered as 45 Gy to GTV1 with a 10.8 Gy boost to a reduced volume (GTV2) (Table 7.2). As suggested by Donaldson, a boost to a total dose of 60 Gy may be in order when there is <50 % soft tissue regression following induction chemotherapy (Donaldson 2004). In the adjuvant setting, gross residual disease or tumors with poor pathologic response should be treated to 55.8 Gy. Microscopic disease should receive a total dose of 50.4 Gy. Some

Table 7.2 Radiation recommendations

Setting	Volume	Margin (CTV + PTV)	Dose (Gy)	Total dose (Gy)
Definitive	GTV1	2–2.5 cm	45	55.8
	GTV2	1.5–2 cm	10.8	
Gross residual disease	GTV1	2–2.5 cm	45	55.8
	GTV2	1.5–2 cm	10.8	
Microscopic disease	GTV1	2–2.5 cm	45	50.4
	GTV2	1.5–2 cm	5.4	
≥10 % viable tumor cells			55.8	55.8

Abbreviations: *GTV* gross tumor volume, *CTV* clinical target volume, *PTV* planning tumor volume, *Gy* gray

institutions will also deliver 45 Gy to widely resected tumors with a poor response to chemotherapy (Donaldson 2004). It is important to note that substantial dose limitations exist depending upon the primary tumor site and adjacent critical strictures. For example, vertebral body tumors are traditionally treated to a maximal dose of 45 Gy with conventional fractionation due to the proximity of the spinal cord. Alternatively, the pre-chemotherapy osseous tumor and soft tissue disease plus a 2 cm margin can be treated to 45 Gy, and a boost dose to a total of 50.4 Gy can be given to the pre-chemotherapy osseous tumor and post-chemotherapy soft tissue extent with a 2 cm margin.

When the heart is located within the treatment field for thoracic and chest wall lesions, the Children's Oncology Group (COG) recommends that no more than 50 % of the heart be included, and that the maximum dose is ≤30.6 Gy. Similarly, 50 % of the liver should not receive >30 Gy. These normal tissue tolerance guidelines may require further modification in the presence of more intensive chemotherapeutic regimens.

The study of radiation dose is certainly crucial as late effects of radiotherapy have been documented with higher doses (Jentzsch et al. 1981; Paulino 2004; Kuttesch et al. 1996). One potential means of achieving a higher effective dose without the associated late morbidity is with an altered fractionation scheme. Hyperfractionation is the delivery of a total dose of radiation in a greater number of treatments (i.e., fractions), with a smaller dose per treatment. Accelerated fractionation refers to total dose delivery over a

shorter time course, and serves to compensate for tumor repopulation that may occur when reducing the dose per fraction. Whereas conventional radiotherapy is typically given once daily, hyperfractionated regimens are generally delivered twice daily with an interval of at least 6 h between each treatment to reduce acute toxicity.

Many rapidly growing tumors remain sensitive to radiation even at lower fraction doses. Conversely, normal tissues that demonstrate a delayed response to radiation damage, also known as late-responding tissues (e.g., lung, kidney, spinal cord), are less sensitive to these smaller doses per fraction. Therefore accelerated hyperfractionation in certain malignancies can enhance the therapeutic ratio by reducing potential late effects while still allowing for optimal tumor control.

Historically, numerous Ewing's sarcoma patients have been treated with accelerated hyperfractionation (Marcus et al. 1991; Bolek et al. 1996; Elomaa et al. 2000). Indelicato et al. proposed three theoretical advantages to this regimen (Indelicato et al. 2008). Firstly, the shortened treatment course allows for minimization of repopulation in a rapidly growing tumor. Secondly, Ewing sarcoma is a class of tumors (small round blue cell) that demonstrates high radiosensitivity; therefore, good cell kill is observed even with a smaller fraction size. Accelerated hyperfractionation schedules permit an increase in total dose in a given period of time and theoretically improve chances of local control. Finally it is well known that hyperfractionation can decrease late effects to nearby normal tissue. This final advantage serves as an undeniable benefit in the pediatric population.

Following the above premises, Italian SE-91 investigators are examining accelerated hyperfractionation as part of multimodal therapy in Ewing tumors, with the goal of improving overall and event-free survival (Rosito et al. 1999). The preliminary 3-year local control rate of 93–94 % with either definitive or adjuvant radiation is promising. However the data regarding utilization of conventional fractionation in comparison to a hyperfractionated regimen is mixed. In CESS 86, all patients treated with definitive or post-operative radiotherapy were randomized to either receive conventionally fractionated radiation alone or a hyperfractionated split course concurrent with systemic therapy (Dunst et al. 1995). The latter consisted of 1.6 Gy given twice daily with an interfraction interval of at least 6 h in two series of 22.4 Gy each when in an adjuvant setting. Definitive treatment involved two series of 22.4 Gy and a 16 Gy boost series. According to the authors, the primary objective of hyperfractionation was to administer radiation without an interruption in chemotherapy. Ultimately the type of fractionation (conventional vs. hyperfractionation) had no impact on local control (82 % vs. 86 %), relapse-free survival (53 % vs. 58 %), or overall survival (63 % vs. 65 %) in definitively treated patients. The same held true for post-operative cases. There was also no difference in the frequency of radiation-related complications amongst the two groups.

The University of Florida experience (Bolek et al. 1996; Indelicato et al. 2008) differed somewhat from these findings, as twice daily fractionation resulted in less range of motion loss, fibrosis, and limb length discrepancy. There was an increase in the likelihood of pathologic fracture in children treated with conventional fractionation as well, although this variation could be attributed to the comparatively larger field sizes and difference in radiation energies. Still, there was no statistically significant difference in 5-year local control rates between the two treatment groups. With these findings in mind, perhaps the most compelling reason for the use of hyperfractionation is the potential reduction in radiation-induced late sequelae.

7.1.5 Techniques: 3DCRT, IMRT, Proton/Ion

Radiation technique has made remarkable advancements over the years by incorporating improvements in imaging and computing power. The emergence of computed tomography (CT) and magnetic resonance imaging (MRI) has been particularly transformative, as all modern therapeutic radiation requires accurate delineation of not only the intended target volumes, but also the normal structures that must be avoided (McGovern and Mahajan 2012). External beam radiation (EBRT) refers to the delivery of radiation to a patient at a distance from an external source.

Forms of EBRT vary through the application of diverse computer technologies. Traditionally, three-dimensional conformal radiotherapy (3DCRT) has been used in the treatment of Ewing's sarcoma. This method incorporates computer assisted planning, allowing for field design and beam placement for an individual target based on diagnostic imaging. Normal tissue can additionally be strategically blocked using multi-leaf collimation (MLC) built into linear accelerators. Conversely, IMRT employs computer based inverse planning algorithms where MLCs are used to generate intensity maps within a given radiation field by integrating parameters set by the planner to meet the objectives of a given treatment plan.

Due to its high level of precision and conformity, IMRT is a technique that is widely applied in the adult population. Theoretically, IMRT would be especially advantageous in pediatric patients where the concomitant sparing of neighboring organs at risk is just as imperative as ensuring adequate dose to the tumor itself. Yet the history of IMRT use in children is markedly different than that of adults for a number of reasons. Among these are increased fraction time, necessity for exact immobilization, and fear for secondary malignancy induction due to low dose spillage in surrounding tissues (Hall and Wuu 2003; Hall 2006; Schneider et al. 2006). In a single institution review of IMRT use in select pediatric cases, Sterzing et al. concluded the benefits of optimal disease control outweighed the risk of possibly increased rates of secondary malignancies (Sterzing et al. 2009). This finding was particularly true in cases of re-irradiation, where treatment with 3DCRT would have undoubtedly led to unacceptable morbidity. Authors from MSKCC argue the actual probability of secondary malignancy with IMRT is unlikely, given the literature has shown radiation-induced tumors to be dose dependent (Trang et al. 2006). In a study comparing the two techniques, Mansur et al. actually found that overall peripheral dose was similar between 3DCRT and IMRT plans for five pediatric patients with malignancies of the brain and skull base (Mansur et al. 2007).

Reports on IMRT planning in Ewing's sarcomas are rare. However the implementation of this technique may prove useful in treatment of pelvic tumors, where the close proximity of disease to the bowel, bladder, or rectum presents appreciable challenges to eradication with either radiation or surgery. This was the basis of an eight patient analysis completed by Mounessi and colleagues (Mounessi et al. 2013). All patients were diagnosed with a pelvic Ewing's sarcoma, and underwent planning with both 3DCRT and IMRT techniques. Results demonstrated IMRT to be superior in terms of conformity, resulting in a decrease of normal tissue exposure to high dose levels. There was a trade-off to this normal tissue sparing, however, as the dose homogeneity was lower with IMRT due to prioritizing of PTV coverage and organ sparing. There were also statistically significant higher volumes of normal tissue receiving low doses (2 Gy) of radiation in IMRT plans compared to 3DCRT. The authors concluded the enhanced therapeutic ratio provided by IMRT outweighed the potential risk of secondary malignancy. A recent publication from MSKCC also examined the utility of IMRT dose painting in a small group of Ewing sarcoma patients with pulmonary metastasis. There were no local failures, and an overall decreased mean dose to the esophagus, heart, spinal cord, and liver when compared to conventional methods (Yang et al. 2013). Although the data surrounding IMRT use in Ewing tumors is currently limited, there clearly appears to be an emerging role for this technique in the management of pediatric malignancies.

Charged particle therapy (proton and carbon ion) has been gaining popularity in the past several years, and has specifically piqued the interest of clinicians practicing in the field of pediatric oncology. This is due to the ability of particle therapy to deposit maximum dose at a defined depth with a sharp fall-off – a phenomenon known as the Bragg peak. Consequently, the dose exiting the body is essentially eliminated. Furthermore, there is a decreased dose entering the body as compared with photons. The end result is a highly conformal coverage of the radiotherapy target, but decreased dose to all other structures (Halperin 2005). The potential benefits of these radiotherapy modalities are obvious in the pediatric population, where concerns for normal tissue exposure and late sequelae

are high. Currently charged particle therapy is most commonly applied in treatment of spinal sarcomas, malignancies of the head and neck, or CNS disease (Delaney et al. 2009). Clinical outcome studies thus far have confirmed a reduction in radiation-related toxicities without sacrificing tumor control, but more long-term follow-up is needed in order to validate the alleged benefits of particle therapy (McGovern and Mahajan 2012).

7.1.6 Site-Specific Considerations

Certain precautions should be taken when treating Ewing tumors at specific sites in order to ensure safe and effective treatment that also attenuates the potential for toxicity. For example, avoiding circumferential irradiation in extremity lesions is necessary to reduce the likelihood of fibrosis and edema. Furthermore, the probability of limb length discrepancies and growth aberrations can be reduced with exclusion of at least one epiphyseal plate when possible. Distal extremity tumors located at the feet or hands may require the use of tissue compensation, such as water or rice baths, to ensure homogeneous coverage of the radiotherapy target. Another option to achieving dose homogeneity in distal extremity tumors is application of a single-photon beam incident on the contralateral surface of the hand or foot combined with an ipsilateral electron field (Halperin 2005).

Rib lesions, also known as Askin tumors, pose unique challenges, given their large size and frequent extension to the pleural surfaces. As mentioned previously, the radiation volume and dose may be limited by nearby organs such as the heart or liver. In patients with cytologically positive effusions, inclusion of the pleural cavity in the treatment volume is recommended due to the high likelihood of local relapse. In general, when the vertebral bodies are included in the treatment field, the entire width should be encompassed so as to prevent radiation-induced scoliosis.

Finally, immobilization techniques including vacuum bags or thermoplastic masks are crucial to daily reproducibility during treatment. The actual delivery of conformal radiation can be further augmented with the use of image guided radiotherapy, which corrects for interfraction setup variations through employment of in-room or on-board imaging techniques such as cone-beam CT.

7.1.7   Quality

Given routine use of 3DCRT and IMRT for Ewing sarcoma, accurate target delineation becomes exceedingly important. Such precision has been greatly facilitated by the integration of CT and MRI into treatment planning, so much so that current COG guidelines require at least one of these modalities be completed for all Ewing sarcoma patients at the time of diagnosis (Meyer et al. 2008). In terms of radiotherapy, the additional impact of central quality review cannot be overlooked. For example, in the CESS 81 trial poor outcomes in patients treated with either definitive or post-operative radiotherapy (local failure rates of 47 % and 20 %, respectively) were partly attributed to poor quality control; 90 % of patients with protocol deviations experienced local relapse (Dunst et al. 1991). This finding prompted investigators involved in CESS 86 to implement a central radiation review (Dunst et al. 1995). With improved radiotherapy quality control, there was considerable improvement in local control (local failure rates of 14 % and 5 % in definitive and post-operative cases, respectively). The improvement was particularly evident with pelvic lesions and large tumors (>100 mL), with the likelihood of local relapse on CESS 81 of 40 % and 36 %, respectively, versus 10 % and 7 % on CESS 86.

Overwhelming disparities in local control rates were also found in the POG 8346 trial based on deviations in target volumes or dose distribution (Donaldson et al. 1998). Patients with no protocol deviations had a local control rate of 80 %, whereas those with either minor or major deviations had local control rates of 48 % and 16 %, respectively.

7.1.8   Metastatic Disease

The tendency for Ewing sarcoma to metastasize early, often exclusively to the lungs, stimulated interest in the use of prophylactic pulmonary radiotherapy. A complicating factor with lung irradiation is that pulmonary parenchymal tolerance can be exceeded before reaching tumoricidal doses (Whelan et al. 2002). Therefore administering radiation at a time point when only subclinical disease is present would require lower doses (and subsequently cause less toxicity) to achieve the same level of pulmonary control. This thinking was the premise behind the incorporation of prophylactic bilateral whole lung irradiation (WLI) in IESS-I (Nesbit et al. 1981). Patients with localized disease were randomized to one of three adjuvant treatment arms: standard vincristine, actinomycin D, and cyclophosphamide (VAC) chemotherapy, VAC plus adriamycin (VACA), or VAC plus prophylactic WLI. Long-term follow-up demonstrated an increased frequency of pulmonary metastasis after prophylactic WLI (20 %) as compared to VACA (15 %, $p = 0.35$) (Nesbit et al. 1990). There was also a statistically significant 5-year relapse-free survival advantage with VACA (60 %) over VAC plus WLI (44 %, $p < 0.05$) and VAC alone (24 %, $p < 0.001$). A similar improvement in 5-year OS was demonstrated with VACA versus VAC plus WLI (65 % vs. 44 %, $p = 0.001$), suggesting that the addition of adriamycin was superior to adjuvant prophylactic WLI.

Despite its lack of utility in the prophylactic setting, WLI has found a role in treatment of patients who present with overt pulmonary metastasis at the time of diagnosis, as supported by a retrospective review of 30 patients on the CESS trials (Dunst et al. 1993). At the time of the analysis, nine of the ten patients treated with WLI were in complete remission. A strong dose response was also observed, with relapsed patients having received significantly lower doses (12–16 Gy) than complete responders (18–21 Gy; $p = 0.028$). The authors concluded bilateral lung irradiation improved survival in patients with pulmonary spread.

A survival benefit with WLI to 14–18 Gy in patients with disseminated Ewing tumors was also shown on the EICESS trial (Bolling et al. 2008). This improvement held true whether patients had isolated pulmonary involvement or combined pulmonary and osseous disease. Of course, these findings must be interpreted with caution as the selection of therapy was in a non-randomized setting with a small number of patients. Results from the COG's recent prospective randomized trial comparing bilateral WLI to a high-dose chemotherapy regimen using busulfan and melphalan will help clarify this issue.

The use of radiotherapy to extra-pulmonary metastatic sites has not yet been as thoroughly examined. Paulino et al. reported promising results in their study of patients with metastatic disease who received not only local treatment of their primary tumor, but also radiation to areas of distant osseous spread (Paulino et al. 2013). Of the six long-term survivors, all patients had irradiation to all bony sites of involvement. Interestingly, on multivariate analysis, only the use of local therapy to the primary site was found to be prognostic of both overall and progression-free survival, thus highlighting the importance of aggressive treatment to the primary tumor even in metastatic cases.

Finally, radiation has been widely accepted as an effective means of palliation, including children and adolescents with disseminated Ewing sarcoma. Investigators from Duke University demonstrated an overall response rate of 84 % in patients treated with palliative doses (median dose of 30 Gy) to osseous, pulmonary, and intracranial disease (Koontz et al. 2006). In a population with an estimated median survival of 1–2 years, the ability to provide adequate symptom relief without a protracted treatment course is undoubtedly a valuable tool.

7.1.9 Side Effects

Pediatric radiation has evolved tremendously since the time of James Ewing and the discovery of Ewing sarcoma. However, reports on the relationship between radiation dose and volume and the resultant side effects using contemporary techniques have been lacking. A majority of the available analyses involve patients treated in the 1970s–1980s using lower energies, higher doses, and larger fields based on 2D imaging – methods that would currently be described as obsolete.

Consequently these results should be interpreted with caution. Nevertheless, it is unlikely that even with such noteworthy advances in imaging and technique that long-term toxicities from radiotherapy can be completely avoided.

Chronic side effects from radiotherapy to pediatric bone malignancies are variable, and ultimately depend upon the prescribed dose as well as location of disease. Following treatment of the extremity, mild to moderate limb atrophy and fibrosis are often reported up to 10 years later based on objective assessment scales (Paulino 2004). In a retrospective study from the University of Iowa, the degree of limb length discrepancy was more profound at ages <10. Extremity mobility and function were preserved with no or minimal detectable impairment in 87 % of patients (Paulino et al. 2007b). Conversely, toxicity results from the POG 8346 trial demonstrated only 61 % of those treated with either definitive or adjuvant radiotherapy were free from any orthopedic complications 5 years later (Donaldson et al. 1998). A number of smaller series have shown a majority of patients (90 %) with a median follow-up of 3–5 years experience either excellent or very good limb function (Bertucio et al. 2001). The development of fractures post-radiotherapy is also a concern, although investigators at the University of Florida found that this risk significantly diminished with the application of a hyperfractionated regimen (Indelicato et al. 2008). The probability of scoliosis can be significantly reduced by treating the entire width of the vertebral body, as previously mentioned. Peripheral neuropathy and vascular complications are uncommon (Paulino 2004).

The most concerning sequela of radiation is the development of secondary malignancy. Modern retrospective reviews have shown the etiology of secondary neoplasms in Ewing sarcoma is complex, and at least partially explained by the interplay of alkylating chemotherapy and irradiation (Donaldson et al. 1998; Tucker et al. 1987). There is a wide range of incidences and cumulative risk estimates reported in the literature. Kuttesh et al. and coworkers examined 266 Ewing sarcoma survivors in the USA, and found the risk of developing a second malignancy to be 3 % after 10 years, and 6.5 % after 20 years (Elomaa et al. 2000). The risk doubled between 15 and 25 years after treatment. The incidence was dose dependent, with no secondary tumors occurring at doses <48 Gy. An analysis of secondary neoplasms in patients treated with definitive or adjuvant radiotherapy in the CESS trials revealed an increasing risk of 1–3 % after 10 years and 3–6 % after 15 years. Secondary malignancies accounted for 1 % (3/328) of deaths, all of which were caused by acute myeloid leukemia (Dunst et al. 1998). That said, the authors recognized the follow-up period was relatively short with regard to the induction of secondary solid tumors. In the most recent update from the Childhood Cancer Survivor Study of 2,434 5-year survivors of pediatric bone and soft tissue tumors, the 30-year cumulative incidence of subsequent neoplasm for survivors of osteosarcoma was 6 % as compared to 10.1 % for Ewing sarcoma (Friedman et al. 2010). While the true incidence of radiation-induced secondary tumors is unclear, it is likely in the range of 4–8 % when moderate-dose conformal radiotherapy is given (Shankar et al. 1999; Donaldson et al. 1998).

The systematic implementation of multidisciplinary treatment for children and adolescents with Ewing sarcoma has resulted in dramatic improvements in outcomes. Whereas at one point in time the outlook for these patients was dismal (5-year OS 5–10 %), more recent publications from various institutions reveal 5-year disease-free, event-free, and relapse-free survival rates between 60 and 69 % (Donaldson 2004). Local control rates are equally encouraging, ranging from 74 to 93 %. Given this progress, the current impetus of ongoing pediatric cancer trials is to reduce treatment-related toxicity without sacrificing a high cure rate. This goal relies on the continued consideration of individual patient characteristics, such as patient age, primary tumor size and location, and potential long-term morbidity, to ensure that the most appropriate sequence and combination of therapies is used. Within the field of radiation oncology, we can look forward to more conformal and precise treatment delivery, thereby improving upon the quality of life post-therapy.

7.2 Osteosarcoma

Osteosarcoma was recognized early in the nineteenth century as a relatively uncommon, but particularly lethal malignancy that primarily affected adolescents and young adults (Sweetnam 1968). As with other extremity tumors, the established treatment at that time involved amputation or disarticulation. Despite excellent local control rates, 80 % of patients, even those with seemingly localized disease, rapidly developed pulmonary metastasis and died within the first 2 years of diagnosis (Cade 1955). Renowned British physician Sir Stanford Cade appropriately summarized these results while presenting at a conference on bone malignancies by stating, "If you do not operate they die; if you do operate they die just the same."

The lack of improvement in survival even with disfiguring and morbid surgery led to the search for alternative therapies, including radiation. In his paper on the primary management of osteosarcoma, Cade argued palliation and tumor shrinkage could be achieved using radiotherapy alone (Cade 1955). Subsequent disease control for several months thereby naturally selected a favorable subgroup of patients who could then receive amputation with a decreased risk of distant metastases and prolonged survival. This approach allowed for a large number of patients to be spared a mutilating surgical procedure. Furthermore, the 5-year survival rates of 15–20 % with radiotherapy were equivalent to those accomplished by immediate surgical ablation (Allen and Stevens 1973; Poppe et al. 1968; Jenkin et al. 1972; Lee and MacKenzie 1964; Flatman 1976). Such a rational and humane approach to osteosarcoma treatment, also known as the Cade technique, prevailed for several years until the systematic integration of chemotherapy with limb-salvage surgery was found to produce incomparable long-term disease-free survival in 60–70 % of osteosarcoma patients (Carrle and Bielack 2006; Link et al. 1986; Bacci et al. 2002; Bielack et al. 1996; Fuchs et al. 1998; Meyers et al. 2005; Smeland et al. 2004). Today the mainstay of care consists of intensive multi-agent chemotherapy combined with surgical resection.

7.2.1 Indications

Radiotherapy plays a relatively minor role in the contemporary management of osteosarcoma due in part to the fact that osteosarcoma has traditionally exhibited only modest radiosensitivity (Mahajan et al. 2008; Anderson 2003; Machak et al. 2003; DeLaney et al. 2005a). A number of series report the presence of viable tumor cells in surgical specimens after doses as high as 60–70 Gy (Sweetnam 1968; Lee and MacKenzie 1964; Machak et al. 2003; de Moor 1975). In contrast, a direct relationship between dose and percent tumor necrosis has also been shown (Gaitan-Yanguas 1981). Researchers proposed that the efficacy of conventionally fractionated radiation was limited by both tumor cell repair of sublethal radiation injury, and decreased sensitivity due to a comparatively high fraction of hypoxic tumor cells (Goffinet et al. 1975; van Putten 1968; Weichselbaum et al. 1977). In an effort to overcome these barriers, radiation was combined with various radiosensitizers, such as 5-bromodeoxyuridine (BUdR) (Kinsella and Glastein 1987; Martinez et al. 1985). This thymidine analog is able to capture radiation-produced electrons when it is incorporated into DNA, ultimately forming damaging radicals that cause strand breaks. While durable local control was reported in seven of nine patients treated with BUdR and radiation, the tissue toxicity was felt to be excessive, causing this particular combination of therapies to fall out of favor.

Review of the literature suggests radiation may contribute to local control when combined with surgery and/or chemotherapy in a select group of patients. In many cases of pelvic, axial skeleton, base of skull, or head and neck tumors, satisfactory resection with acceptable margins can present a challenge (DeLaney et al. 2005a). Even with disease confined to the extremity, Picci et al. found an increase in local recurrence following limb salvage surgery with less than wide surgical margins and a poor response to chemotherapy (Picci et al. 1997). In patients with "good" tumor necrosis, the development of local relapse occurred at a median of 13 months, in comparison to 9 months in those with "fair" necrosis ($p=0.001$). The Cooperative

Osteosarcoma Study Group (COSS) reported a 5-year overall survival rate of 0 % in subtotally resected or unresectable pelvic osteosarcomas (Ozaki et al. 2003). This rate was improved to 29 % with the addition of radiotherapy ($p=0.003$). A similar survival trend was noted by the COSS in an analysis of patients with vertebral lesions when radiation was incorporated into the treatment algorithm (Ozaki et al. 2002).

The benefit of radiotherapy was further illustrated by a study from Massachusetts General Hospital (MGH) where 41 patients with either unresectable disease or an inadequate margin status (defined as close or positive) were given definitive radiotherapy to a median dose of 66 Gy (DeLaney et al. 2005a). Patients with spinal, pelvic, trunk, or recurrent extremity lesions received a combination of pre-operative radiation of 20 Gy to help prevent tumor auto-transplantation at surgery, followed by completion of the prescribed course post-operatively. Post-operative radiation alone was delivered to primary tumors of the extremity, and lesions of the head and neck or base of skull. The gross tumor volume (GTV) encompassed the site of gross tumor involvement with a 1 cm margin, and clinical tumor volume (CTV) included the GTV along with any tissues at risk of microscopic disease, plus a 2 cm margin. The 5-year local control and overall survival rates were 68 % ± 8.3 % and 71.5 % ± 8 %, respectively. Not surprisingly, the extent of resection was predictive of outcomes, with superior survival in patients with gross total resection (74.45 % ± 9.1 %) as compared to those with subtotal resection or biopsy only (74.1 % ± 16 %, 25 % ± 21.65 %, respectively).

Similarly, a publication by Machak et al. reported a local control rate at 5 years of 56 % in 31 extremity osteosarcoma patients who had refused surgery, and were therefore treated with radiation to a median dose of 60 Gy after induction chemotherapy (Machak et al. 2003). Among the 11 patients with a favorable clinical response to chemotherapy, no local failures were seen. Carceres et al. also observed a high response rate in patients with limb osteosarcomas who received chemotherapy and 60 Gy of radiation (Carceres et al. 1984). In 12 of 15 (80 %) treated patients, post-treatment biopsy was actually negative for

Table 7.3 Local control – osteosarcoma

References	Era	n	Dose (Gy)	Modality	Overall LC (%)	LC with RT alone
Ozaki et al.	1979–1998	11	30–56	Photon	≤27.4	
Delaney et al.	1980–2002	41	44–80	Photon/proton	68	
Ciernak et al.	1983–2009	55	50.4–≥70	Proton	85	
Machak et al. (2003)	1986–1999	31	40–68	Photon		56 %
Kamada et al. (2002)	1996–1999	58	52.8–73.6	Carbon ion		76

Abbreviations: *n* patient number, *Gy* gray, *LC* local control, *RT* radiation therapy

disease. Thus, in situations where wide resection is not technically feasible, positive or close surgical margins exist, disease is located at sites of high risk of local relapse (e.g., spine, pelvis, head and neck, skull), or the patient prefers a nonsurgical option, the addition of radiotherapy can serve to improve outcomes.

7.2.2 Future Directions

Despite the historically poor response of osteosarcomas to external beam radiotherapy, research efforts within the field of radiation have sought to develop innovative techniques to not only improve disease control, but also optimize palliation. Extracorporeal irradiation, first described in 1968, is a biological limb reconstruction that involves en bloc tumor resection, irradiation of the resected pathological bone, and reimplantation of the irradiated bone (Hong et al. 2001; Yamamoto et al. 2002). The use of irradiated bone provides anatomical precision, avoids immunological rejection, and reduces the risk of post-operative infection. Additionally, samarium lexidronam is a bone-seeking radiopharmaceutical that has been suggested as a novel means of palliation in osteosarcoma (Anderson and Nunez 2007).

Perhaps the largest body of research, however, has been dedicated to the utilization of charged particle therapy. The major emphasis for proton therapy in clinical research has involved dose escalation for tumors in which local control with conventional radiotherapy is suboptimal (Delaney et al. 2005b). Accordingly, recent reports have demonstrated the efficacy of charged particle radiotherapy for patients with osteosarcoma (Ciernik et al. 2011; Matsunobu et al. 2012; Kamada et al. 2002). As previously mentioned, the rationale for the use of charged particles rather than photons is the superior dose distribution, characterized by a lower dose region in normal tissue proximal to the tumor, a uniform high-dose region within the tumor, and very minimal dose beyond the tumor itself. A study from MGH demonstrated impressive 3- and 5-year local control rates of 82 % and 72 %, respectively, in patients with unresectable or partially resected disease who were treated with proton therapy (Ciernik et al. 2011). The mean dose was 68.4 Gy, with 50.1 % of the patients receiving a total dose ≥70 Gy. Investigators from Chiba, Japan, have reported encouraging data using heavy ion-based particle treatment. In 58 osteosarcoma patients treated with carbon ions as monotherapy, the local control rate was 65 % after 5 years with an OS rate of 29 % (Kamada et al. 2002). Overall, results from particle-based radiotherapies yield high control rates that far exceed the results obtained from conventional radiation in osteosarcoma (Table 7.3).

Even with a proton beam, it is difficult to deliver tumoricidal doses to the dura when it is involved by spinal or paraspinal disease without going above spinal cord tolerance (Delaney et al. 2005b). A strategy developed by Delaney et al. utilizes a custom-designed yttrium-90 plaque to boost the dural surface intraoperatively (Delaney et al. 2003). The applicator reportedly allows for 100 % of the dose to reach the dura, while only 8 % of dose is present at a depth of 4 mm. Consequently, 10–15 Gy can be delivered to the dura with minimal dose to the cord surface, and essentially no dose to the center or contralateral aspect of the cord. With a median follow-up of 2 years, no acute toxicities or treatment-related neurological sequelae have been reported with dural plaque brachytherapy.

In summary, the introduction of a multimodal approach to osteosarcoma consisting primarily of multi-agent chemotherapy and surgical resection has dramatically improved the outcome in a disease that was once felt to be universally lethal. Whereas conventional radiotherapy has proven to be valuable in select cases of incompletely resected or unresectable tumors, the most exciting advances in radiation oncology involve the incorporation of charged particles. Both proton and carbon ion-based therapies offer the prospect of an increase in achievable dose to the tumor volume with concomitant reduction in normal tissue toxicity. Such advances will hopefully result in meaningful clinical gains in osteosarcoma treatment in the future.

References

Allen CF, Stevens KR (1973) Preoperative irradiation for osteogenic sarcoma. Cancer 31:1364–1366

Anderson PM (2003) Effectiveness of radiotherapy for osteosarcoma that responds to chemotherapy. Mayo Clin Proc 78:145–146

Anderson P, Nunez R (2007) Samarium lexidronam (153sm-edtmp): skeletal radiation for osteoblastic bone metastases and osteosarcoma. Expert Rev Anticancer Ther 7:1517–1527

Arai Y, Kun LE, Brooks T et al (1991) Ewing's sarcoma: local tumor control and patterns of failure following limited-volume radiation therapy. Int J Radiat Oncol Biol Phys 21:1501–1508

Bacci G, Toni A, Avella M et al (1989) Long-term results in 144 Ewing's sarcoma patients treated with combined therapy. Cancer 63:1477–1486

Bacci G et al (2002) Italian Sarcoma Group/Scandinavian Sarcoma Group high dose ifosfamide in combination with high dose methotrexate, adriamycin and cisplatin in neo-adjuvant treatment of extremity osteosarcoma: preliminary results of an Italian Sarcoma Group/Scandinavian Sarcoma Group pilot study. J Chemother 14:198–206

Bertucio CS, Wara WM, Matthay KK et al (2001) Functional and clinical outcomes of limb-sparing therapy for pediatric extremity sarcomas. Int J Radiat Oncol Biol Phys 49:763–769

Bielack SS, Kempf-Bielack B, Winkler K (1996) Osteosarcoma: relationship of response to preoperative chemotherapy and type of surgery to local recurrence. J Clin Oncol 14:683–684

Bolek TW, March RB Jr, Mendenhall NP et al (1996) Local control and functional results after twice-daily radiotherapy for Ewing's sarcoma of the extremities. Int J Radiat Oncol Biol Phys 35:687–692

Bolling T, Schuck A, Paulussen M et al (2008) Whole lung irradiation in patients with exclusively pulmonary metastases of Ewing tumors. Toxicity analysis and treatment results of the EICESS-92 trial. Strahlenther Onkol 184(4):193–197

Burgert EO Jr, Nesbit ME, Garnsey LA et al (1990) Multimodal therapy for management of non-pelvic localized Ewing's sarcoma of bone: intergroup study IESS-II. J Clin Oncol 8:1514–1524

Cade S (1955) Osteogenic sarcoma: a study based on 133 patients. J R Coll Surg Edinb 1:79–111

Carceres E et al (1984) Local control of osteogenic sarcoma by radiation and chemotherapy. Int J Radiat Oncol Biol Phys 10:35–39

Carrle D, Bielack SS (2006) Current strategies of chemotherapy in osteosarcoma. Int Orthop 30(6):445–451

Ciernik F et al (2011) Proton-based radiotherapy for unresectable or incompletely resected osteosarcoma. Cancer 117(19):4522–4530

de Moor NG (1975) Osteosarcoma: a review of 72 cases treated by megavoltage radiation therapy, with or without surgery. S Afr J Surg 13:137–146

Delaney TF et al (2003) Intraoperative dural irradiation by customized 192iridium and 90yttrium brachytherapy plaques. Int J Radiat Oncol Biol Phys 57:239–245

DeLaney TF et al (2005a) Radiotherapy for local control of osteosarcoma. Int J Radiat Oncol Biol Phys 61:492–498

Delaney TF et al (2005b) Advanced-technology radiation therapy in the management of bone and soft tissue sarcomas. Cancer Control 12(1):27–35

Delaney TF, Liebsch NJ, Pedlow FX et al (2009) Phase II study of high-dose photon/proton radiotherapy in the management of spine sarcomas. Int J Radiat Oncol Biol Phys 74(3):732–739

Donaldson SS (1980) A story of continuing success – radiotherapy for Ewing's sarcoma. Int J Radiat Oncol Biol Phys 7:279–281

Donaldson SS (2004) Ewing sarcoma: radiation dose and target volume. Pediatr Blood Cancer 42:471–476

Donaldson SS, Torrey M, Link MP et al (1998) A multidisciplinary study investigating radiotherapy in Ewing's sarcoma: end results of POG #8346. Pediatric Oncology Group. Int J Radiat Oncol Biol Phys 42(1):125–135

Dunst J, Schuck A (2004) Role of radiotherapy in Ewing tumors. Pediatr Blood Cancer 42:465–470

Dunst J, Sauer R, Burgers JM et al (1991) Radiation therapy as a local treatment in Ewing's sarcoma. Results of the Cooperative Ewing's Sarcoma Studies CESS 81 and CESS 86. Cancer 67(11):2818–2825

Dunst J, Paulussen M, Jurgens H (1993) Lung irradiation for Ewing's sarcoma with pulmonary metastases at diagnosis: results of the CESS-studies. Strahlenther Onkol 169(10):621–623

Dunst J, Jurgens H, Sauer R et al (1995) Radiation therapy in Ewing's sarcoma: an update of the CESS 86 trial. Int J Radiat Oncol Biol Phys 32(4):919–930

Dunst J, Ahrens S, Paulussen M et al (1998) Second malignancies after treatment for Ewing's sarcoma: a report of the CESS-studies. Int J Radiat Oncol Biol Phys 42(2):379–384

Elomaa I, Blomqvist C, Saeter G et al (2000) Fiver-year results in Ewing's sarcoma: the Scandinavian Sarcoma Group experience with the SSG IX protocol. Eur J Cancer 36:875–880

Evans RG, Nesbit ME, Gehan EA et al (1991) Multimodal therapy for management of localized Ewing's sarcoma of pelvic and sacral bones: a report from the Second Intergroup Study (IESS-II). J Clin Oncol 9:1173–1180

Ewing J (1921) Diffuse endothelium of bone. Proc NY Pathol Soc 21:17–24

Flatman GE (1976) Osteosarcoma: the contribution of radiotherapy. Proc R Soc Med 69(8):549–551

Friedman DL, Whitton J, Leiserning W et al (2010) Subsequent neoplasms in 5-year survivors of childhood cancer: the Childhood Cancer Survivors Study. J Natl Cancer Inst 102:1083–1095

Fuchs N et al (1998) Long-term results of the Cooperative German-Austrian Swiss Osteosarcoma Study Group's protocol COSS-86 of intensive multi drug chemotherapy and surgery for osteosarcoma of the limbs. Ann Oncol 9:893–899

Gaitan-Yanguas M (1981) A study of the response to osteogenic sarcoma and adjacent normal tissues to radiation. Int J Radiat Oncol Biol Phys 7:593–595

Goffinet DR et al (1975) Combined radiosensitizer infusion and irradiation in osteogenic sarcomas. Radiology 117:211–214

Grier HE, Krailo MD, Tarbell NJ et al (2003) Addition of ifosfamide and etoposide to standard chemotherapy for Ewing's sarcoma and primitive neuroectodermal tumor of bone. N Engl J Med 348:694–701

Hall EJ (2006) Intensity-modulated radiation therapy, protons, and the risk of second cancers. Int J Radiat Oncol Biol Phys 65:1–7

Hall EJ, Wuu CS (2003) Radiation-induced second cancers: the impact of 3D-CRT and IMRT. Int J Radiat Oncol Biol Phys 56:83–88

Halperin EC (2005) Ewing Sarcoma. In: Halperin EC, Constine L, Tarbell N (eds) Pediatric radiation oncology. Lippincott Williams & Wilkins, Philadelphia, pp 291–318

Hong A et al (2001) Extracorporeal irradiation for malignant bone tumors. Int J Radiat Oncol Biol Phys 50:441–447

Indelicato DJ, Keole SR, Shahlaee AH et al (2008) Definitive radiotherapy for Ewing tumors of extremities and pelvis: long-term disease control, limb function, and treatment toxicity. Int J Radiat Oncol Biol Phys 72(3):871–877

Jenkin RDT (1991) Long-term follow-up of Ewing's sarcoma of bone. Int J Radiat Oncol Biol Phys 20:639–641

Jenkin RD, Allt WE, Fitzpatrick PJ (1972) Osteosarcoma: an assessment of management with particular reference to primary irradiation and selective delayed amputation. Cancer 30(2):393–400

Jentzsch K, Binder H, Cramer H et al (1981) Leg function after radiotherapy for Ewing's sarcoma. Cancer 47:1267–1278

Kamada T et al (2002) Efficacy and safety of carbon ion radiotherapy in bone and soft tissue sarcomas. J Clin Oncol 20:4466–4471

Kinsella TJ, Glastein E (1987) Clinical experience with intravenous radio sensitizers to unresectable sarcoma. Cancer 59:908–915

Kinsella TJ, Miser JS, Waller B et al (1991) Long-term follow-up Ewing's sarcoma of bone treated with combined modality therapy. Int J Radiat Oncol Biol Phys 20:389–395

Koontz BF, Clough RW, Halperin EC (2006) Palliative radiation therapy for metastatic Ewing sarcoma. Cancer 106(8):1790–1793

Krasin M, Rodriguez-Galindo C, Billups CA et al (2004) Definitive irradiation in multidisciplinary management of localized Ewing sarcoma family of tumors in pediatric patients: outcome and prognostic factors. Int J Radiat Oncol Biol Phys 60:830–838

Kuttesch JF, Wexler LH, Marcus RB et al (1996) Second malignancies after Ewing's sarcoma. J Clin Oncol 14:2812–2825

Lee ES, MacKenzie DH (1964) Osteosarcoma: a study of the value of preoperative megavoltage radiotherapy. Br J Surg 51:252–274

Leitman SA, Michael JJ (2010) Bone sarcomas: overview of management, with a focus on surgical treatment considerations. Cleve Clin J Med 77:S8–S12

Link MP et al (1986) The effect of adjuvant chemotherapy on relapse-free survival in patients with osteosarcoma of the extremity. N Engl J Med 314:1600–1606

Machak GN et al (2003) Neoadjuvant chemotherapy and local radiotherapy for high-grade osteosarcoma of the extremities. Mayo Clin Proc 78:147–155

Mahajan A et al (2008) Multimodality treatment of osteosarcoma: radiation in a high-risk cohort. Pediatr Blood Cancer 50:976–982

Mansur DB, Klein EE, Maserang BP (2007) Measured peripheral dose in pediatric radiation therapy: comparison of intensity-modulated and conformal techniques. Radiother Oncol 82:179–184

Marcus RB Jr, Cantor A, Heare TC et al (1991) Local control and function after twice-a-day radiotherapy for Ewing's sarcoma of bone. Int J Radiat Oncol Biol Phys 21:1509–1515

Martinez A et al (1985) Intra-arterial infusion of radio sensitizer (BUdR) combined with hypofractionated irradiation and chemotherapy for primary treatment of osteogenic sarcoma. Int J Radiat Oncol Biol Phys 11:123–128

Matsunobu A et al (2012) Impact of carbon ion radiotherapy for unresectable osteosarcoma of the trunk. Cancer 118:4555–4563

McGovern SL, Mahajan A (2012) Progress in radiotherapy for pediatric sarcomas. Curr Oncol Rep 14:320–326

Meyer JS, Nadel HR, Marina N et al (2008) Imaging guidelines for children with Ewing sarcoma and osteosarcoma: a report from the Children's Oncology Group Bone Tumor Committee. Pediatr Blood Cancer 51:163–170

Meyers PA et al (2005) Osteosarcoma: a randomized, prospective trial of the addition of ifosfamide and/or muramyl tripeptide to cisplatin, doxorubicin, and high-dose methotrexate. J Clin Oncol 23:2004–20011

Mounessi FS, Lehrich P, Haverkamp U et al (2013) Pelvis Ewing sarcomas: three-dimensional conformal vs. intensity-modulated radiotherapy. Strahlenther Onkol 189:308–314

Nesbit ME Jr, Perez CA, Tefft M et al (1981) Multimodal therapy for the management of primary, nonmetastatic

Ewing's sarcoma of bone: an Intergroup study. Natl Cancer Inst Monogr 56:255–262

Nesbit ME Jr, Gehan EA, Burgert EO Jr et al (1990) Multimodal therapy for the management of primary, nonmetastatic Ewing's sarcoma of bone: a long-term follow-up of the First Intergroup study. J Clin Oncol 8(10):1664–1674

Oberlin O, Le Deley MC, Bui BN et al (2001) Prognostic factors in localized Ewing's tumors and peripheral neuroectodermal tumors: the third study of the French Society of Paediatric Oncology (EW88 study). Br J Cancer 85(11):1646–1654

Ozaki T et al (2002) Osteosarcoma of the spine: experience of the Cooperative Osteosarcoma Study Group. Cancer 92:1069–1077

Ozaki T et al (2003) Osteosarcoma of the pelvis: experience of the Cooperative Osteosarcoma Study Group. J Clin Oncol 21(2):334–341

Paulino AC (2004) Late effects of radiotherapy for pediatric extremity sarcomas. Int J Radiat Oncol Biol Phys 60:265–274

Paulino AC, Nguyen TX, Mai WY et al (2007a) Dose response and local control using radiotherapy in non-metastatic Ewing sarcoma. Pediatr Blood Cancer 49:145–148

Paulino AC, Nguyen TX, Mai WY (2007b) An analysis of primary site control and late effects according to local control modality in non-metastatic Ewing sarcoma. Pediatr Blood Cancer 48:423–429

Paulino AC, Mai WY, Teh BS (2013) Radiotherapy in metastatic Ewing sarcoma. Am J Clin Oncol 36(3):283–286

Paulussen M, Ahrens S, Dunst J et al (2001) Localized Ewing tumor of bone: final results of the cooperative Ewing's sarcoma study CESS 86. J Clin Oncol 19(6):1818–1829

Perez CA, Tefft M, Nesbit M et al (1981) The role of radiation therapy in the management of non-metastatic Ewing's sarcoma of bone. Report of the Intergroup Ewing's Sarcoma Study. Int J Radiat Oncol Biol Phys 7:141–149

Phillips RF, Sheline GE (1969) Radiation therapy of malignant bone tumors. Radiology 92:1537–1545

Picci P et al (1997) Risk factors for local recurrences after limb-salvage surgery for high-grade osteosarcomas of the extremities. Ann Oncol 8:899–903

Pisters PW, O'Sullivan B, Maki RG (2007) Evidence-based recommendations for local therapy for soft tissue sarcomas. J Clin Oncol 25(8):1003–1008

Poppe E, Liverud K, Efskind J (1968) Osteosarcoma. Acta Chir Scand 134:549–556

Razek A, Perez CA, Tefft M et al (1980) Local control related to radiation dose, volume, and site of primary lesion in Ewing's sarcoma. Cancer 46:516–521

Rosito P, Mancini AF, Rondelli R et al (1999) Italian Cooperative Study for the treatment of children and young adults with localized Ewing sarcoma of bone: a

preliminary report of 6 years of experience. Cancer 86:421–428

Schneider U, Lomax A, Premier P et al (2006) The impact of IMRT and proton radiotherapy on secondary cancer incidence. Strahlenther Onkol 182:647–652

Schuck A, Rube C, Konemann S et al (2002) Postoperative radiotherapy in the treatment of Ewing tumors: influence of the interval between surgery and radiotherapy. Strahlenther Onkol 178:25–31

Schuck A, Ahrens S, Paulussen M et al (2003) Local therapy in localized Ewing tumors: resultsof 1058 patients treated in the CESS 81, CESS 86, and EICESS 92 Trials. Int J Radiat Oncol Biol Phys 55(1):168–177

Shankar AG, Pinkerton CR, Atra A, et al. (1999) Local therapy and other factors influencing site of relapse in patients with localized Ewing's saroma. Eur J Cancer 35(12):1698–1704

Smeland S et al (2004) Chemotherapy in osteosarcoma: the Scandinavian Sarcoma Groups experience. Acta Orthop Scand Suppl 75:92–98

Sterzing F, Stoiber EM, Nill S et al (2009) Intensity modulated radiotherapy (IMRT) in treatment of children and adolescents – a single institution's experience and a review of the literature. Radiat Oncol 4(37):1–10

Suit HD (1964) Intact tumor cells in irradiated tissue. Arch Pathol 78:648–651

Sweetnam R (1968) Osteosarcoma: Hunterian Lecture delivered at the Royal College of Surgeons of England. Ann R Coll Surg 44(1):38–58

Trang HL, Meyers PA, Wexler LH et al (2006) Radiation therapy for Ewing's sarcoma: results Memorial Sloan-Kettering in the modern era. Int J Radiat Oncol Biol Phys 64(2):544–550

Tucker MA, D'Angio GJ, Boice JD et al (1987) Bone sarcomas linked to radiotherapy in children. N Engl J Med 317:588–593

van Putten LM (1968) Tumor deoxygenation during fractionated radiotherapy: studies with a transplantable mouse osteosarcoma. Eur J Cancer 4:172–182

Wang CC, Schulz MD (1953) Ewing's sarcoma – a study of fifty cases treated at the Massachusetts General Hospital, 1930–1950 inclusive. N Engl J Med 248:571–576

Weichselbaum R, Little JB, Nove J (1977) Response of human osteosarcoma in vitro to irradiation: evidence for unusual cellular repair activity. Int J Radiat Biol Relat Stud Phys Chem Med 31:295–299

Whelan JS, Burcombe RJ, Janinis J et al (2002) A systematic review of the role of pulmonary irradiation in the management of primary bone tumours. Ann Oncol 13(1):23–30

Yamamoto T et al (2002) Osteosarcoma of the distal radius treated by Intraoperative extracorporeal irradiation. J Hand Surg [Am] 17:160–164

Yang JC, Wexer LH, Meyers PA et al (2013) Intensity-modulated radiotherapy with dose-painting pediatric sarcomas with pulmonary metastases. Pediatr Blood Cancer 60(10):1616–1620

Histological Response and Biological Markers

8

Kellie B. Haworth and Bhuvana A. Setty

Contents

8.1   **Introduction**... 126

8.2   **Histological Response**................................. 126
8.2.1   Definition and Characterization of
        Histological Response.............................. 127
8.2.2   Prognostic Indications of Histological
        Response in Osteosarcoma...................... 128
8.2.3   Prognostic Indications of Histological
        Response in Ewing Sarcomas................. 129
8.2.4   Alternative Methods of Determining
        Histological Response.............................. 130

8.3   **Biological Markers**...................................... 130
8.3.1   The REMARK Criteria............................. 130
8.3.2   Biological Markers in Osteosarcoma........... 131
8.3.3   Biological Markers in Ewing Sarcoma......... 133

Conclusions.. 135

References.. 136

Abstract

The optimization of treatment strategies for patients with bony tumors has proven to be elusive. Though patients with localized disease have achieved increased survival rates with the most recent therapeutic revolutions of dose escalation and interval compression, prognosis continues to remain significantly poor for those patients with metastatic disease. Stratification of bone tumor patients into risk categories is one method to target more intensified treatment regimens for patients with historically worse outcomes, while sparing patients with lower-risk disease from toxicities associated with highly aggressive therapies. Strategies to risk stratify these patients must involve incorporation of their tumor biology, including the presence or absence of significant biological markers, and their interval responses to treatment. The prognostic implications of biological markers and the histological response to neoadjuvant chemotherapy for bone tumors have been extensively studied. As further designations of risk groups for patients evolve, it has become apparent that these are crucial factors to consider.

K.B. Haworth (✉) • B.A. Setty
Division of Hematology/Oncology/BMT,
Nationwide Children's Hospital,
700 Children's Drive, Columbus, OH 43205, USA
e-mail: Kellie.haworth@nationwidechildrens.org;
Bhuvana.setty@nationwidechildrens.org

© Springer International Publishing Switzerland 2015
T.P. Cripe, N.D. Yeager (eds.), *Malignant Pediatric Bone Tumors - Treatment & Management*,
Pediatric Oncology, DOI 10.1007/978-3-319-18099-1_8

8.1 Introduction

Advancements in treatment outcomes of patients with bone tumors have been scarce in the past several decades, despite considerable efforts to intensify therapies for these patients. Though current 5-year overall survival (OS) for patients with localized Ewing sarcoma and osteosarcoma is approximately 70 %, in vast contrast, those patients presenting with metastases at diagnosis exhibit 5-year OS rates of approximately 30 % for both diseases (http://www.cancer.org/cancer/ osteosarcoma/detailedguide/osteosarcoma-survival-rates). Given these statistics and the current employment of multimodal therapies that include highly aggressive chemotherapeutic regimens, it is evident that new approaches are drastically necessary. The search for new methodologies to attack bony tumors poses a challenge. The most recent clinical improvements were seen in the 1990s after the implementation of dose escalation and dose interval compression. Theses advances in therapeutic intensification have unfortunately also resulted in significant increases in chemotherapy-induced toxicities for these patients.

Oncological practitioners strive to further define risk categories for patients, with an overall goal to optimize therapeutic approaches and minimize treatment-related toxicities. The strategic objective is to target patients who have high-risk disease with more intensive treatments, while sparing those with low-risk disease from therapies which have the potential to induce both acute and lifelong side effects. The most currently relevant risk stratification approaches include tailoring treatment according to patient responses while identifying and utilizing diagnostic and prognostic biomarkers. The ultimate result is, to an extent, the personalization of therapy for each individual patient.

Several prognostic indicators have been proposed for many bone tumors, with a select few exhibiting enough compelling data to warrant therapeutic changes. Historically relevant markers have since been determined to be no longer significant due to the improvement in outcomes associated with more aggressive and technically skilled therapeutic approaches. For example, the presence of a pathological fracture was previously considered to be an indicator of worse prognosis and thus was an indication for amputation. Recent studies suggest that such a finding has no significant correlation with patient survival outcomes given the emergence of advanced limb salvage procedure techniques (Chandrasekar et al. 2011; Xie et al. 2012; Zuo et al. 2013). The histological subtype and features of bony tumors, once believed to have a significant impact on survival, were studied in two consecutive trials of the European Osteosarcoma Intergroup and have proven to play a very small role in the overall outcome of patients (Hauben et al. 2002). Substantial literature supports various clinical–pathological features to be indicators of high-risk disease and therefore negative prognostic features, such as primary tumor site (axial versus appendicular location), increasing tumor size, decreased necrosis after neoadjuvant chemotherapy, and increased patient age. However, none of these have been found to be as clinically significant as the presence of metastatic disease (Bacci et al. 2004a, b; Cotterill et al. 2000; Lee et al. 2010; Lin et al. 2007; Martin and Brennan 2003; Oberlin et al. 2001; Paulussen et al. 2001a, b; Rodriguez-Galindo et al. 2008; Sauer et al. 1987). Thus, ongoing Children's Oncology Group (COG) clinical trials for bone tumors risk-stratify patients only by the presence or absence of metastases.

Indicators which have been studied and maintained as predictive of prognosis in patients with bone tumors include tumor size at diagnosis, the presence and extent of metastatic spread, the feasibility of total surgical resection or local control, the anatomic site of the primary tumor (in the case of Ewing sarcoma) (Biswas et al. 2014; Qureshi et al. 2013), and the histological response of the tumor to neoadjuvant chemotherapy (Wunder et al. 1998).

8.2 Histological Response

The current value of determining a patient's response to initial chemotherapy has proven useful for prognostication purposes but not for therapeutic decision-making. Recent COG trials for treatment of bone tumors have not identified success with intensification of treatment based upon therapeutic response thus far. Evaluation of the postchemotherapy histological response is presently being employed as a prognostic indicator for both osteosarcoma and Ewing sarcoma. Unfortunately, oncologists have been unable to exploit this insightful feature into the translation of improved therapies.

8.2.1 Definition and Characterization of Histological Response

The extent of chemotherapy-induced tumor necrosis upon examination of resection specimens defines "histological response." Historically, the quantification of a tumor's response to chemotherapy was first discovered to be a significant prognostic factor in osteosarcoma. This finding was further explored in other bony tumor types and later accepted as a significant feature in Ewing sarcoma as well. The prognostic indicators of histological response for both osteosarcoma and Ewing sarcoma have been repeatedly demonstrated in several studies conducted by various national cooperative groups. Other types of bone tumors have not incorporated histological response as a standardized predictive feature, though individual reports of using the established grading scales in other tumor types exist (Coffin et al. 2005).

A means to measure the therapeutic response through a grading system was first proposed in 1979 for osteosarcoma and has been further modified and reiterated by several authors since then (Huvos 1988; Picci et al. 1994; Raymond et al. 1987; Rosen et al. 1979; Salzer-Kuntschik et al. 1983; Wold 1998). Extrapolation of the original grading systems used in osteosarcoma was later applied to Ewing sarcoma, and further development of classifications specific for this disease ensued (Wunder et al. 1998). For both diseases, "good response" is generally defined as the presence of greater than 90 % tumor necrosis, with an "intermediate response" ranging from 50–60 to 90 % necrosis and "poor response"

described as less than 50–60 % necrosis, though various grading schemes currently exist (see Tables 8.1 and 8.2).

Table 8.1 Histologic response grading systems for treated osteosarcomas

Reference	Response grade	Response grade definition
Huvos (1988), Provisor et al. (1997)	I	Viable; little to no chemotherapeutic effect
	II	Partially necrotic
	III	Largely necrotic
	IV	Totally necrotic; no histologic evidence of viable tumor within specimen
Rosen et al. (1979)	I	Little to no chemotherapeutic effect
	II	Partial response, <50 % necrosis, some viable tumor remaining
	III	>90 % tumor necrosis, foci of viable tumor remaining
	IV	No viable-appearing tumor cells
Raymond et al. (1987)		Percentage of necrosis estimated
Picci et al. (1994)	Good	>90 % necrosis
	Fair	60-90 % necrosis
	Poor	<60 % necrosis
Wold (1998)** **Used in COG clinical trials	I	No chemotherapeutic effect
	II	Some necrosis
	A	50 % viable tumor remaining
	B	5–50 % viable tumor remaining
	III	Scattered foci; <5 % viable tumor remaining
	IV	No viable tumor remaining
Salzer-Kuntschik et al. (1983)	I	No viable-appearing tumor cells
	II	Single viable tumor cells or 1 viable cell cluster, <0.5 cm
	III	<10 % Viable tumor remaining
	IV	10–50 % Viable tumor remaining
	V	>50 % Viable tumor remaining
	VI	No chemotherapeutic effect

Adapted from Coffin et al. (2005), Lowichik et al. (2000)

Table 8.2 Histologic response grading systems applied to treated Ewing sarcomas/PNETs

Reference	Response grade	Response grade definition
Huvos (1988)	I	Viable; little to no chemotherapy effect
	II	Partially necrotic
	III	Largely necrotic
	IV	Totally necrotic; no histologic evidence of viable tumor within specimen
Salzer-Kuntschik et al. (1983)	I	No viable appearing tumor cells
	II	Single vital tumor cells or 1 vital cell cluster, <0.5 cm
	III	Vital tumor, <10 %
	IV	Vital tumor, 10–50 %
	V	Vital tumor, >50 %
	VI	No effect of chemotherapy
Picci et al. (1993, 1997)	I	1+ macroscopic nodule of viable tumor (>one 10× field) or Scattered microscopic nodules in summation (>one 10× field)
	II	Isolated microscopic nodules of viable tumor cells in summation (<one 10× field)
	III	No viable tumor cell nodules; scattered individual tumor cells permitted

Adapted from Coffin et al. (2005), Lowichik et al. (2000)

8.2.2 Prognostic Indications of Histological Response in Osteosarcoma

The phenomenon of prognostic histological response has been observed for osteosarcoma in pediatric patients as well as the adolescent and young adult (AYA) population alike. It has been recognized in several studies that pediatric patients with osteosarcoma who have a good histological response have significantly higher survival rates (5-year overall survival (OS) rate of approximately 76 %, 5-year event-free survival (EFS) rate of approximately 73 %), as compared to patients with less than 90 % postchemotherapy tumor necrosis, who have an OS of 48 % and EFS of 44 % (Bacci et al. 2001, 2002a, 2006b; Ferrari et al. 2001; Goorin et al. 2003; Halperin 2011). Utilizing cutoffs for postsurgery necrosis of 95 % or greater in those 18 years or older, a good response has been correlated to increased overall survival in the AYA population (Janeway et al. 2012).

With hopes to use histological response in order to determine an appropriate subsequent treatment course for patients with bone tumors, several clinical trials incorporated the determination of histological response and consequent patient risk stratification with therapeutic modulation into their protocols. However, a majority of the clinical trials failed to show significant improvement in patient outcomes using this as a risk stratification method. For instance, in the three neoadjuvant chemotherapeutic osteosarcoma studies performed at the MD Anderson Cancer Center, Treatment and Investigation of Osteosarcoma (TIOS) I-III, the preoperative chemotherapeutic response was used to plan postoperative treatment. The postchemotherapy percentage of tumor necrosis (using cutoff of 90 % or greater) was found to significantly correlate with relapse and the development of pulmonary metastases ($p = 0.01$) (Hudson et al. 1990). As another example, one of the principal objectives of the study CCG-782 was to use histological response of the primary tumor after neoadjuvant chemotherapy to determine the postoperative chemotherapy regimen. This study defined a cutoff of less than 95 % tumor necrosis as poor responders who demonstrated significantly higher risk for an adverse event as compared to good responders (relative risk 0.23, $p < 0.0001$) (Miser et al. 1993). In the POG 8561 trial, patients who had less than 10 % viable tumor after induction with chemotherapy were shown to have significantly improved EFS (73 %) when compared with patients with poor response. It was concluded, however, that better response did not translate into survival benefit (Goorin et al. 2003). The Cooperative Osteosarcoma Study Group study COSS-82 explored reduced intensity of preoperative chemotherapy and the salvage of poor responders (defined as less than

90 % tumor necrosis) and concluded that changing drugs for salvage failed to improve survival outcomes (Winkler et al. 1993). EURAMOS, a joint protocol of the world's leading multi-institutional osteosarcoma groups (Children's Oncology Group (COG), Cooperative Osteosarcoma Study Group (COSS), European Osteosarcoma Intergroup (EORTC/MRC), Scandinavian Sarcoma Group (SSG)), aimed to optimize the treatment of osteosarcoma patients through its collaboration. The EURAMOS-1 trial took into account the strong prognostic value of tumor response to preoperative chemotherapy and divided patients accordingly. Postoperative therapy was determined by the histological response of the tumor, with poor responders (defined as less than 90 % necrosis) stratified to receive intensified chemotherapy, while good responders were introduced to biological agents. Details of this study are described in Chap. 6. More recently, in cases of resectable osteosarcoma, the COG study AOST0331 sought to optimize treatment strategies based upon histological response to preoperative chemotherapy (www. clinicaltrials.gov, NCT00134030). In a recent meta-analysis of therapeutic regimens for localized high-grade osteosarcoma, it was concluded that the salvage of poor responders by changing drugs or intensifying treatment postoperatively does not prove to be efficacious (Anninga et al. 2011). It has also been shown that response to preoperative chemotherapy is more important than primary metastases in predicting survival for patients with osteosarcoma of the extremities (Bielack et al. 2002). Recent results of COG AOST0331/EURAMOS-1 have shown no benefit to intensified therapy for poor responders with localized osteosarcoma (http://www.ssg-org.net/wp-content/uploads/2011/03/EURAMOS-1-Poor-Response-Randomisation1.pdf).

8.2.3 Prognostic Indications of Histological Response in Ewing Sarcomas

As in osteosarcoma, poor histological response has been demonstrated to be an independent adverse prognostic factor for EFS in Ewing sarcoma patients (Bacci et al. 2004b). These patients exhibit drastic differences in relapse-free survival according to their histological response (Qureshi et al. 2013). Preoperative chemotherapeutic response has been reported to be the single-most predictive indicator of event-free survival in postoperative Ewing sarcoma patients (Wunder et al. 1998). In addition, histological response was determined to have the largest impact in the prediction of local recurrence of Ewing sarcoma after surgical treatment of the primary tumor, with central site of disease as a second independent predictive factor (Lin et al. 2007). Significant correlations between histological response to chemotherapy and primary tumor location, presence of metastases, and histological features relating to patient survival have been demonstrated (Coffin et al. 2005).

Also similar to what is seen in osteosarcoma, studies of the treatment of Ewing sarcoma patients based upon their histological response have yielded varying results. According to the French Society of Pediatric Oncology's study, EW88, which used a threshold of 95 % tumor necrosis as a good response in localized Ewing sarcoma patients, further therapeutic trials were recommended based on histological response or tumor volume according to the method used for local control (Lopez Guerra et al. 2012; Oberlin et al. 2001). The German Cooperative Ewing Sarcoma Study, CESS 86, demonstrated poor histological response as a negative predictor of EFS. The study also noted that 52 % of patients survived after risk-adapted therapy (Paulussen et al. 2001a). It has since been demonstrated that the outcome of nonmetastatic Ewing sarcoma bone tumors is influenced by several variables in addition to histological response. It has been proposed that criteria to stratify Ewing sarcoma patients according to risk of relapse include all variables that show prognostic significance, such as gender, age, volume of tumor, type of local treatment, type of chemotherapy, the presence of distant recurrences, and serum LDH level, as opposed to being based on a single prognostic factor (Bacci et al. 2006a; Lopez Guerra et al. 2012).

8.2.4 Alternative Methods of Determining Histological Response

Recent advances in radiological technologies have led to the exploration of radiographic determinants for histological response to neoadjuvant chemotherapy. ^{18}F-fluorodeoxy-D-glucose (FDG)-positron emission tomography (PET) SUV_{max} is surging as a correlative predictor of histological response (Dutour et al. 2009; Kim et al. 2011). ^{18}F-FDG PET is a noninvasive imaging modality that predicts histological response to chemotherapy of various malignancies (Kim et al. 2011). 18 F-FDG PET SUV_{max} has been reported to correlate with histological response in osteosarcoma and may even predict response earlier than histological analysis (Dutour et al. 2009). It has also been reported that the relative responses in SUV from prechemotherapy (SUV1) to postchemotherapy (SUV2) as calculated by SUV(2:1) [(SUV1-SUV2)/SUV1] $\geq$0.5 and SUV2 $\leq$ 2.5 are related to favorable histological responses to chemotherapy, with sensitivity of SUV(2:1) at 0.5 and SUV2 at 2.5 of 93 % and 88 % and specificity at 88 % and 78 %, respectively (Kim et al. 2011). Metabolic tumor volume (MTV) measured by ^{18}F-FDG PET can also predict outcome of osteosarcoma of the extremities (Byun et al. 2013). MTV has been reported to be an independent predictor of metastasis in this group of patients, and the combination of MTV with histological response predicted survival more accurately than chemotherapeutic response alone (Byun et al. 2013). The change in SUV_{max} between baseline and post-treatment imaging is not significantly associated with histological response for either Ewing sarcoma or osteosarcoma. ^{18}F-FDG PET responses to neoadjuvant chemotherapy are different for Ewing sarcoma and osteosarcoma (Gaston et al. 2011). Observed differences between the groups include the overall MTV, likely secondary to a difference in the distribution of the injected ^{18}F-FDG dose within the primary tumor. Therefore, a 50 % reduction in MTV, associated with favorable histological response in osteosarcoma, was found to incorrectly predict good responders in Ewing sarcoma.

An increase of the Ewing sarcoma cutoff values to a 90 % MTV reduction was necessary for it to be associated with a favorable outcome (Gaston et al. 2011). These data suggest that response to chemotherapy as reflected by changes in PET characteristics should be interpreted differently in the two sarcoma types (Gaston et al. 2011).

8.3 Biological Markers

In addition to histological response induced by neoadjuvant chemotherapy, other prognostic indicators have emerged for malignant bone tumors. The presence of certain molecular or genetic features has been described to be an important prognostic marker, and new data arise regularly from preclinical studies with newly proposed markers such as those described below (Hingorani et al. 2013; Kobayashi et al. 2010; Limmahakhun et al. 2011; van Doorninck et al. 2010). The utilization of biomarkers and the ongoing discovery of new potential therapeutic targets have led researchers and clinicians one step closer in the approach toward patient risk stratification and personalized targeted therapeutic strategies. With the steady emergence of various molecules being touted as potential "biomarkers," a set of guidelines, the REMARK criteria, has also been developed to elucidate their clinical usefulness. As a translational approach, biological markers have been categorized according to their utility and may be considered as either diagnostic, prognostic, or potential therapeutic targets (further discussed in Chap. 15).

8.3.1 The REMARK Criteria

"Personalized medicine," involving the notion of individualized treatment plans according to the individual patient's disease and outcome, is the ultimate goal for the treatment of patients with cancer including those with bone tumors. Biomarkers are being studied to guide decision-making toward a rational and directed approach. Along these lines, there has been an emergence of numerous proposed biomarkers. Without a standardized approach, however, which path to choose is unclear. Therefore, the precise definition of what qualifies as a "biomarker" has been developed, along with guidelines as to how that biomarker should be validated and applied in clinical protocols. A biomarker must provide a distinct risk:benefit ratio to enable clinical decision-making, be easily available, be cost effective, and be capable of being performed with available technologies.

Progressions in laboratory techniques and expansions of tumor tissue banking have led to more studies that include aims to explore potential biomarkers. However, conflicting results have often arisen. As a result, level of evidence (LOE) measures were created originally by the American Society of Clinical Oncology and have been further modified (Hayes et al. 1996; Simon et al. 2009). Reporting Recommendations for Tumor Marker Prognostic Studies (REMARK) guidelines were published by the National Cancer Institute in 2005 and recently updated in 2012. These guidelines require studies of biomarkers to meet specific criteria in order to be considered adequate, including clearly describing characteristics and treatment modalities for all patients and specimens involved, use of reproducible methodologies including disclosure of assay methods and detailed study design, and involving a clear biostatistical strategy. Data should be clearly reported, with analyses showing the relation of the marker to standard prognostic variables. The criteria also highlight the significance of reporting study limitations and implications for future research and clinical value (Altman et al. 2012; McShane et al. 2005).

8.3.2 Biological Markers in Osteosarcoma

Osteosarcoma is characterized by complex karyotypic abnormalities without chromosomal translocations or distinct patterns. Numerous genes have been shown to contribute to osteosarcoma tumorigenesis. Although continual progress has been made in detecting genetic alterations in osteosarcoma, to date no distinctive molecular marker has been proven to have better prognostic implications than the clinical markers which are currently employed. Nonetheless, the search continues to identify markers that may be utilized to guide therapeutic modifications. Some of the well-known biomarkers are discussed below.

DMP-1 Dentin Matrix Protein 1 (DMP-1) has been proposed to be a diagnostic marker of bone-forming tumors. It is highly expressed in osteocytes and found in dentin and bone. Expression has been reported in osteosarcoma, with negative stains in other bony neoplasms such as Ewing sarcoma, chondrosarcoma, leiomyosarcoma, fibrosarcoma, and giant cell tumor of bone (Kashima et al. 2013). As there are more definitive pathological techniques and stains to distinguish osteosarcomas, the role of DMP-1 remains unclear.

Oncogenes and Tumor Suppressor Genes Several oncogenes and tumor suppressor genes have been implicated to have prognostic significance in osteosarcoma. The ongoing COG biology study, AOST06B1, examines the potential roles of RB/p53, ERBB2, MDM2, p16, and p21, LOH at 3q and 18q, the amplification or overexpression of C-sis, Gli, and C-fos, the presence of the SV-40T-antigen sequence, and Myc/Ras pathway (Martin et al. 2014; Patino-Garcia et al. 2003).

RB1 One of the earliest associations of tumor suppressor genes with osteosarcoma was found in patients who survived bilateral retinoblastoma. Loss of heterozygosity (LOH) of the retinoblastoma gene RB1 was identified to be associated with the development of osteosarcoma and can be found in a high percentage of patients with osteosarcoma. Studies investigating correlation of outcome with RB1 gene status have shown mixed results, and significant association has not been identified in more recent studies (Kong and Hansen 2009; Patino-Garcia et al. 2003).

p53 and MDM2 Osteosarcoma is one of the most common tumors associated with patients with Li–Fraumeni syndrome (Kong and Hansen 2009). As a result, cell cycle regulators such as p53 and its related proteins p16 and p21 are suspected to serve as prognostic indicators in osteosarcoma (Diller et al. 1990; Fu et al. 2013; McIntyre et al. 1994; Miller et al. 1996a; Scholz et al. 1992; Ueda et al. 1993). p53 has been highlighted as an effective biomarker for the prediction of survival in patients with osteosarcoma (Fu et al. 2013). Amplification of MDM2, a negative regulator of p53, has also been observed in metastatic or recurrent osteosarcomas and is thought to potentially play a role as an indirect pathway to p53 inactivation (Ladanyi et al. 1993a; Miller et al. 1996b; Patino-Garcia et al. 2003). Studies investigating the function of TP53 in projecting osteosarcoma outcomes have shown that the functional status of p53 is not associated with response to chemotherapy, but mutant p53 status has been reported to be associated with slight decrease in overall survival (Kong and Hansen 2009).

HER2/Neu The proto-oncogene HER2/Neu, erbB-2, is a member of the epidermal growth factor receptor family and is variably expressed in osteosarcoma cells (Kong and Hansen 2009). Expression of HER2/erbB-2 has been reported to correlate with survival in osteosarcoma (Gorlick et al. 1999; Morris et al. 2001; Onda et al. 1996). Targeted therapy against erbB2, however, was proven to be ineffective for treatment of osteosarcoma (Kong and Hansen 2009).

LOH of 3q and 18q Loss of heterozygosity in 3q and 18q has been frequently observed in osteosarcoma (Kong and Hansen 2009; Kruzelock et al. 1997). These locations may contain other tumor suppressor genes which have not yet been identified. They are currently both under review as potential prognostic indicators in the COG biology committee, although there is no published literature directly correlating loss of heterozygosity at either locus with patient outcomes.

Myc and Ras A small percentage of osteosarcoma patients have been reported to have Myc amplification (Barrios et al. 1993; Ladanyi et al. 1993b). The amplification of C-myc is implicated in osteosarcoma pathogenesis, with studies demonstrating enhanced invasion characteristics of osteosarcoma cell lines with its amplification via the MEK-ERK pathway (Han et al. 2012). Amplification of c-myc has been correlated with a worse prognosis and decreased 3-year overall survival for osteosarcoma patients (Wu et al. 2012). Interestingly, it has also been reported that c-myc amplification occurs most frequently alongside of RB1 alterations, indicating that these may together play a role in the pathogenesis and progression of osteosarcoma (Ozaki et al. 1993). Ras gene mutations have been identified in several cancer types, but their role in osteosarcoma has not yet been determined (Antillon-Klussmann et al. 1995; Barrios et al. 1993; Nardeux et al. 1987).

C-sis and C-fos C-sis encodes a chain of the platelet-derived growth factor, PDGF, and it has been identified as amplified in human osteosarcoma cells, as well as in spontaneous canine osteosarcomas (Graves et al. 1984; Kochevar et al. 1990). C-fos plays a role in normal bone metabolism, and osteosarcoma develops in transgenic mice which overexpress c-fos (Wu et al. 1990). Human osteosarcoma patients have been found to overexpress c-fos as well, though it is yet unclear whether or not it relates to prognosis (under study by COG).

Genes Related to Interactions with the Environment Other potential prognostic indicators in osteosarcoma include the expression of genes related to environmental interactions, such as metalloproteinase (MMP), c-MET, insulin-like growth factor-1 (IGF-1), Ezrin, and Survivin. The metalloproteinases are thought to be responsible for lysing extracellular matrix proteins and therefore possibly play a role in invasion and metastasis (Kong and Hansen 2009). The c-met oncogene codes for hepatocyte growth factor (HGF) receptor. Stimulation of c-met induces cellular responses which include cell division, and overexpression of c-met has been correlated with poor outcomes in adult tumors. C-met is highly expressed in 60 % of human osteosarcoma, but it has not yet been studied as a prognostic indicator (Ferracini et al. 1995). Since peak incidence of osteosarcoma coincides with periods of rapid bone growth, it is possible that hormones which influence growth contribute to its development. Insulin-like growth factor 1 is regulated by growth hormone and has been demonstrated to function in the growth, turnover, and metabolism of normal bone. Osteosarcoma cell lines have displayed IGF-1 dependence in culture, and several drugs that inhibit growth hormone are being examined for the treatment of a variety of cancers (Burrow et al. 1998; Jentzsch et al. 2014; MacEwen et al. 2004). Ezrin (VIL2), an actin-cytoskeleton cross-linker, is thought to be essential for metastasis. In a limited sample of pediatric osteosarcoma patients, Ezrin expression was shown to be associated with favorable outcome (Kong and Hansen 2009; Zhang et al. 2014). Survivin (BIRC5) is a member of the Inhibitor of Apoptosis (IAP) family of proteins. It binds caspase-3 and -7 and was found to be expressed in osteosarcoma tumors but not in normal tissues, and its expression has been correlated with increased malignancy and metastasis (Hingorani et al. 2013; Kong and Hansen 2009).

Chromosomes Markers associated with chromosome function such as telomerase and tumor cell ploidy are also being studied as potential prognostic indicators for osteosarcoma. Telomerase serves as a regulator of the number of replications a cell may undergo (Wen et al. 2002), and it is hypothesized that it may play a role in the progression of tumors. Telomerase expression has been negatively correlated with prognosis in several adult cancers including osteosaracoma (Kong and Hansen 2009; Nakashima et al. 2003; Sanders et al. 2004). Though ploidy has been previously investigated as a prognostic indicator in prior osteosarcoma studies, it is being re-examined in the context of current clinical trials (Bauer et al. 1989; Gebhardt et al. 1990).

Drug Resistance Genes The MDR1 gene encodes P-glycoprotein, a transmembrane protein responsible for the efflux of numerous chemotherapeutic agents including doxorubicin. Multidrug resistance protein (MRP) is a family member of P-glycoprotein and is responsible for efflux of doxorubicin and etoposide (Grant et al. 1994; Loe et al. 1996). Methotrexate transport and metabolism via the dihydrofolate reductase enzyme has been shown to play a significant role in treatment of osteosarcoma. Increased expression of glutathione S-transferase P1 (GSTP1), a phase II detoxification enzyme, has been associated with significantly higher relapse rate and a worse clinical outcome in osteosarcoma (Kong and Hansen 2009). It was found to be upregulated in osteosarcoma cells when treated with doxorubicin or cisplatin.

Bone Turnover Markers Markers for bone turnover have also been studied as potential prognostic indicators for osteosarcoma. Serological markers like alkaline phosphatase have been reported to be predictive of time to recurrence for osteosarcoma patients (Bacci et al. 2002b). Higher levels are associated with earlier relapses of the disease (Kong and Hansen 2009). It has been proposed that alkaline phosphatase may be useful in the monitoring and assessment of efficacy of therapy in pediatric osteosarcoma (Ambroszkiewicz et al. 2006, 2010a, b).

Indications of bone marrow recovery after chemotherapy may be of prognostic value in osteosarcoma as well. The time for recovery of lymphocytes has been reported to be a significant indicator of outcomes in osteosarcoma patients. Using a threshold absolute lymphocyte count of ≥ 800 cells/µl on day 14, researchers were able to distinguish significant differences in overall survival based upon "early" versus "late" lymphocyte recovery, with a reported 5 year OS of 92.3 % versus 33.3 %, respectively. Risk stratification and subsequent therapy based on the threshold absolute lymphocyte count on day 14 may thus be a rational strategy that could be tested in a clinical trial (Moore et al. 2010).

8.3.3 Biological Markers in Ewing Sarcoma

Several studies of prognostic biomarkers in Ewing sarcoma have yielded the emergence of four main categories which adhere to REMARK criteria, including *EWSR1* translocation type, cell cycle proteins, copy number alterations (CNAs), and subclinical disease measurement (Pinto et al. 2011; van Maldegem et al. 2012; Wagner et al. 2012), among others.

EWS Translocation A translocation involving the EWSR1 gene on chromosome 22 is the molecular hallmark of Ewing sarcomas. Typically, the 5′ of *EWSR1* is fused to the 3′ of an *ETS* gene family member, most commonly *FLI1* on chromosome 11, t(11;22)(q24;q12). The EWS-FL1 fusion protein was the first sarcoma gene to be cloned and represents a dominant oncogene. This translocation has been further categorized into the more frequently occurring Type 1, involving exon 6, and Type 2, involving exon 5. The remaining minority of cases are comprised of the 3′ translocation companion with various *ETS* family genes (Sankar and Lessnick 2011), including ERG on chromosome 21 in 10 %, EWS-ETV1 (<1 %), EWS-ETV4 (<1 %), EWS-FEV (<1 %).

The fusion type may have prognostic relevance in Ewing sarcoma (Halperin 2011). Correlations between prognosis and fusion type were initially reported from retrospective studies conducted in the late 1990s, with reports of patients with type-1 fusion having significantly improved overall survival compared to those with other fusion types. In other reports, lower relapse rates were associated with type-1 fusion in patients with localized disease. Both Euro-EWING and COG subsequently evaluated outcomes and fusion status, with results that were not supportive of the original findings (Le Deley et al. 2010; Shukla et al. 2013). In the Euro-EWING trial, there was no difference exhibited in the distribution of sex, age, tumor volume, tumor site, disease extension, or histological response between the four fusion type groups. The study concluded that EWS fusion type was not prognostically significant for risk of disease progression or relapse (Le Deley et al. 2010).

Cell Cycle Proteins Cell cycle regulation markers have been shown to have clinical significance in Ewing sarcomas (Lopez-Guerrero et al. 2011).

Genetic alterations in the RB pathway have been described in Ewing sarcoma, including deletions of both RB1 and CDKN2A (INK4A/ARF) (Huang et al. 2005; Kovar et al. 1997; Mackintosh et al. 2012). Numerous retrospective studies have shown correlations between patient outcome and alterations in CDKN2A (Kovar et al. 1997). In 2013, the COG Ewing Sarcoma Biology Committee found strong evidence to support CDKN2A loss as a strong negative prognostic marker (Shukla et al. 2013).

The mutational status of p53 has also been assessed in retrospective studies as a potential prognostic biomarker in Ewing sarcoma (Yang et al. 2014). p53 overexpression has been associated with advanced disease at time of diagnosis, poorer treatment response, and inferior overall survival, independent of site, local treatment, or extent of tumor necrosis (Abudu et al. 1999; Yang et al. 2014). High p53 expression has also been reported to be the strongest prognostic factor correlating with decreased overall survival (de Alava et al. 2000). p53 mutations and/or CDKN2A deletions are associated with poor response to chemotherapy (Huang et al. 2005). A significant association exists between increased p53 expression and metastatic disease and poorer progression-free survival and disease-specific survival in patients with localized disease (Lopez-Guerrero et al. 2011).

Copy Number Alterations Copy number alterations (CNAs) and genomic instability have been repeatedly reported in Ewing sarcoma (Jahromi et al. 2012; Shukla et al. 2013). The most commonly reported alterations in Ewing sarcoma are trisomy 8, trisomy 12, and gain of 1q (Shukla et al. 2013). Alterations that correlated with outcome are 1p36.3 loss (Hattinger et al. 1999), 1q21-q22 gain (Armengol et al. 1997; Kullendorff et al. 1999; Mackintosh et al. 2012; Tarkkanen et al. 1999), 6p21.1 gain (Tarkkanen et al. 1999), 8 gain (Armengol et al. 1997; Jahromi et al. 2012; Tarkkanen et al. 1999; Zielenska et al. 2001), 12 gain (Armengol et al. 1997; Tarkkanen et al. 1999; Zielenska et al. 2001), 16q loss (Jahromi et al. 2012; Ozaki et al. 2001), 20 gain (Jahromi et al. 2012; Roberts et al. 2008), or other combinations

(Ferreira et al. 2008; Jahromi et al. 2012; Kullendorff et al. 1999; Ozaki et al. 2001; Roberts et al. 2008; Savola et al. 2009; Zielenska et al. 2001). Independent studies have identified chromosomal copy number alterations as accepted prognostic indicators. The COG Ewing Sarcoma Biology Committee recommends that tumor and germline DNA be collected from all Ewing sarcoma patients registered on future therapeutic studies so that CNAs and other genetic mutations can be evaluated as prognostic and predictive biomarkers (Shukla et al. 2013). The COG has also discussed prospective incorporation of copy number alterations in its upcoming relapsed/refractory Ewing sarcoma trial (Shukla et al. 2013).

Subclinical Disease Measurement Minimal residual disease (MRD) has been well established as a crucial part of pediatric acute lymphoblastic leukemia therapeutic decision-making (Biondi et al. 2000; Borowitz et al. 2008). COG protocols for leukemia have integrated standardized timing and methodologies for MRD, and it is considered to be a prognostic indicator for risk stratification. Utilization of MRD as a means of subclinical disease detection and prognostic correlation in Ewing sarcoma has yet to be validated, and current methodologies for this incorporate RT-PCR and flow cytometry. These studies are designed to identify pathognomonic fusion transcripts in blood and/or bone marrow as evidence of occult micrometastatic or persistent disease. The COG Ewing Sarcoma Biology Committee is unconvinced that RT-PCR-based assays will be clinically optimal for prognostication and treatment stratification (Shukla et al. 2013). Although potentially significant, the technicalities and logistics regarding tissue collection and performance of RNA-based studies on blood and bone marrow specimens make RT-PCR analysis of subclinical disease less realistic for routine clinical practice (Shukla et al. 2013). More recently, flow cytometry detecting CD99 has been used in attempt to identify subclinical disease in Ewing sarcoma (Ash et al. 2011; Dubois et al. 2010). Studies have also reported high tumoral CD56 expression as a significant poor prognostic factor (Ash et al. 2011). Planned COG studies are now

underway to validate these findings in newly diagnosed patients (AEWS07B1) and in patients with recurrent disease (AEWS07B1 and ADVL1221) (Shukla et al. 2013).

Other Potential Prognostic Indicators Numerous other potential prognostic markers for Ewing sarcoma have been studied and correlated with significant outcome differences. A majority of these, unfortunately, do not fulfill REMARK criteria for reporting and will require further validation (Shukla et al. 2013). Promising candidates include 9p21 status, heat shock proteins (HSP), telomerase, interleukins, tumor necrosis factor (TNF), VEGF and members of its pathway, lymphocyte count, and Ki-67 status (Scotlandi et al. 1995; van Maldegem et al. 2012). Epithelial mesenchymal transition (EMT) markers are also proposed as potential markers for prognostic significance. These include desmoplakin, pGSK3b, ZO-1, Snail, and CK8/18 (Machado et al. 2012). Further validation of these is required.

Hepatoma-derived growth factor (HDGF) has been shown to be upregulated in Ewing sarcoma and has been reported to be significantly correlated with tumor volume, metastases at diagnosis, low overall survival rate, and low disease-free survival rate (Yang et al. 2013). It has also been reported to improve prognostic stratification for patients with Ewing family tumors when combined with p53 expression status (Yang et al. 2014).

As also explored in osteosarcoma, BIRC5, or Survivin, is a poor prognostic marker for Ewing sarcoma as well. Preclinical studies have shown BIRC5 to be overexpressed in Ewing sarcomas, and high expression is described as an independent prognostic indicator of worse outcomes (Hingorani et al. 2013). Further studies are needed to validate these findings.

Conclusions

The stratification of patients with bone tumors into high- or low-risk categories may ultimately result in the optimization of therapeutic regimens for these patients. Qualifying a patient as a "good" or "poor" responder to neoadjuvant chemotherapy might direct the administration of more or less intensified chemotherapeutic regimens, though recent clinical trials have shown that histologic response currently offers prognostic value rather than therapeutic guidance. In addition to the post-chemotherapy histologic response, a large number of prognostic indicators exist for bone malignancies. The utilization of these markers to contribute to patient risk stratification and personalized targeted therapeutic strategies is under evaluation. Biologic markers, whether diagnostic, prognostic, or potential therapeutic targets, require standardized evaluation and reporting in order to successfully interpret their practicality, and the guidelines proposed within the REMARK criteria were put forth for this reason. Several established biomarkers exist for the most common pediatric bone tumors, osteosarcoma and Ewing sarcoma, with numerous reported novel prognostic indicators on the horizon.

As the field continues to develop and evolve, oncologists consistently strive to further define risk categories for patients, with the aim of optimizing therapeutic strategies and minimizing long-term toxicities of chemotherapy. Methods of risk stratification include tailoring treatment according to patient responses and the identification of diagnostic and prognostic biomarkers. As the search for new methods to cure bony malignancies persists, the detection of further prospective therapeutic targets continues to show promise and anticipation in the eventual improvement in survival rates for these patients.

References

Abudu A, Mangham DC, Reynolds GM, Pynsent PB, Tillman RM, Carter SR, Grimer RJ (1999) Overexpression of p53 protein in primary Ewing's sarcoma of bone: relationship to tumour stage, response and prognosis. Br J Cancer 79(7-8):1185–1189. doi:10.1038/sj.bjc.6690190

Altman DG, McShane LM, Sauerbrei W, Taube SE (2012) Reporting Recommendations for Tumor Marker Prognostic Studies (REMARK): explanation and elaboration. PLoS Med 9(5), e1001216. doi:10.1371/journal.pmed.1001216

Ambroszkiewicz J, Gajewska J, Klepacka T, Bilska K, Wozniak W, Laskowska-Klita T (2006) Biochemical bone turnover markers in patients with conventional and nonconventional osteosarcoma. Pol Merkur Lekarski 21(124):330–334

Ambroszkiewicz J, Gajewska J, Klepacka T, Chelchowska M, Laskowska-Klita T, Wozniak W (2010a) Clinical utility of biochemical bone turnover markers in children and adolescents with osteosarcoma. Adv Med Sci 55(2):266–272. doi:10.2478/v10039-010-0043-2

Ambroszkiewicz J, Gajewska J, Klepacka T, Chelchowska M, Laskowska-Klita T, Wozniak W (2010b) A comparison of serum concentrations of biochemical bone turnover markers in patients with osteosarcoma with good and poor prognosis. Pol Merkur Lekarski 29(169):19–26

Anninga JK, Gelderblom H, Fiocco M, Kroep JR, Taminiau AHM, Hogendoorn PCW, Egeler RM (2011) Chemotherapeutic adjuvant treatment for osteosarcoma: where do we stand? Eur J Cancer 47(16):2431–2445, doi: http://dx.doi.org/10.1016/j.ejca.2011.05.030

Antillon-Klussmann F, Garcia-Delgado M, Villa-Elizaga I, Sierrasesumaga L (1995) Mutational activation of ras genes is absent in pediatric osteosarcoma. Cancer Genet Cytogenet 79(1):49–53, doi: 016546089400115R [pii]

Armengol G, Tarkkanen M, Virolainen M, Forus A, Valle J, Bohling T, Asko-Seljavaara S, Blomqvist C, Elomaa I, Karaharju E, Kivioja AH, Siimes MA, Tukiainen E, Caballín MR, Myklebost O, Knuutila S (1997) Recurrent gains of 1q, 8 and 12 in the Ewing family of tumours by comparative genomic hybridization. Br J Cancer 75(10):1403–1409

Ash S, Luria D, Cohen IJ, Goshen Y, Toledano H, Issakov J, Yaniv I, Avigad S (2011) Excellent prognosis in a subset of patients with Ewing sarcoma identified at diagnosis by CD56 using flow cytometry. Clin Cancer Res 17(9):2900–2907. doi:10.1158/1078-0432.CCR-10-3069

Bacci G, Ferrari S, Bertoni F, Picci P, Bacchini P, Longhi A, Donati D, Forni C, Campanacci L, Campanacci M (2001) Histologic response of high-grade nonmetastatic osteosarcoma of the extremity to chemotherapy. Clin Orthop Relat Res (386):186–196

Bacci G, Ferrari S, Longhi A, Picci P, Mercuri M, Alvegard TA, Saeter G, Donati D, Manfrini M, Lari S, Briccoli A, Forni C (2002a) High dose ifosfamide in combination with high dose methotrexate, adriamycin and cisplatin in the neoadjuvant treatment of extremity osteosarcoma: preliminary results of an Italian Sarcoma Group/Scandinavian Sarcoma Group pilot study. J Chemother 14(2):198–206. doi:10.1179/joc.2002.14.2.198

Bacci G, Longhi A, Ferrari S, Lari S, Manfrini M, Donati D, Forni C, Versari M (2002b) Prognostic significance of serum alkaline phosphatase in osteosarcoma of the extremity treated with neoadjuvant chemotherapy: recent experience at Rizzoli Institute. Oncol Rep 9(1):171–175

Bacci G, Ferrari S, Longhi A, Donati D, Barbieri E, Forni C, Bertoni F, Manfrini M, Giacomini S, Bacchini P (2004a) Role of surgery in local treatment of Ewing's sarcoma of the extremities in patients undergoing adjuvant and neoadjuvant chemotherapy. Oncol Rep 11(1):111–120

Bacci G, Forni C, Longhi A, Ferrari S, Donati D, De Paolis M, Barbieri E, Pignotti E, Rosito P, Versari M (2004b) Long-term outcome for patients with non-metastatic Ewing's sarcoma treated with adjuvant and neoadjuvant chemotherapies. 402 patients treated at Rizzoli between 1972 and 1992. Eur J Cancer 40(1):73–83

Bacci G, Longhi A, Ferrari S, Mercuri M, Versari M, Bertoni F (2006a) Prognostic factors in non-metastatic Ewing's sarcoma tumor of bone: an analysis of 579 patients treated at a single institution with adjuvant or neoadjuvant chemotherapy between 1972 and 1998. Acta Oncol 45(4):469–475. doi:10.1080/02841860500519760

Bacci G, Longhi A, Versari M, Mercuri M, Briccoli A, Picci P (2006b) Prognostic factors for osteosarcoma of the extremity treated with neoadjuvant chemotherapy: 15-year experience in 789 patients treated at a single institution. Cancer 106(5):1154–1161. doi:10.1002/cncr.21724

Barrios C, Castresana JS, Ruiz J, Kreicbergs A (1993) Amplification of c-myc oncogene and absence of c-Ha-ras point mutation in human bone sarcoma. J Orthop Res 11(4):556–563. doi:10.1002/jor.1100110410

Bauer HC, Kreicbergs A, Silfversward C, Tribukait B (1989) Ploidy and morphology in osteosarcoma. Anal Quant Cytol Histol 11(2):96–103

Bielack SS, Kempf-Bielack B, Delling G, Exner GU, Flege S, Helmke K, Kotz R, Salzer-Kuntschik M, Werner M, Winkelmann W, Zoubek A, Jürgens H, Winkler K (2002) Prognostic factors in high-grade osteosarcoma of the extremities or trunk: an analysis of 1,702 patients treated on neoadjuvant cooperative osteosarcoma study group protocols. J Clin Oncol 20(3):776–790

Biondi A, Valsecchi MG, Seriu T, D'Aniello E, Willemse MJ, Fasching K, Pannunzio A, Gadner H, Schrappe M, Kamps WA, Bartram CR, van Dongen JJ, Panzer-Grumayer ER (2000) Molecular detection of minimal residual disease is a strong predictive factor of relapse in childhood B-lineage acute lymphoblastic leukemia with medium risk features. A case control study of the International BFM study group. Leukemia 14(11):1939–1943

Biswas B, Rastogi S, Khan SA, Mohanti BK, Sharma DN, Sharma MC, Mridha AR, Bakhshi S (2014) Outcomes and prognostic factors for Ewing-family tumors of the extremities. J Bone Joint Surg Am 96(10):841–849. doi:10.2106/JBJS.M.00411

Borowitz MJ, Devidas M, Hunger SP, Bowman WP, Carroll AJ, Carroll WL, Linda S, Martin PL, Pullen DJ, Viswanatha D, Willman CL, Winick N, Camitta BM (2008) Clinical significance of minimal residual disease in childhood acute lymphoblastic leukemia and its relationship to other prognostic factors: a Children's Oncology Group study. Blood 111(12):5477–5485. doi:10.1182/blood-2008-01-132837

Burrow S, Andrulis IL, Pollak M, Bell RS (1998) Expression of insulin-like growth factor receptor, IGF-1, and IGF-2 in primary and metastatic osteosarcoma. J Surg Oncol 69(1):21–27. doi:10.1002/(SICI)1096-9098(199809)69:1<21::AID-JSO5>3.0.CO;2-M [pii]

Byun BH, Kong CB, Park J, Seo Y, Lim I, Choi CW, Cho WH, Jeon DG, Koh JS, Lee SY, Lim SM (2013) Initial metabolic tumor volume measured by 18F-FDG PET/CT can predict the outcome of osteosarcoma of the extremities. J Nucl Med 54(10):1725–1732. doi:10.2967/jnumed.112.117697

Chandrasekar CR, Grimer RJ, Carter SR, Tillman RM, Abudu AT, Jeys LM (2011) Outcome of pathologic fractures of the proximal femur in nonosteogenic primary bone sarcoma. Eur J Surg Oncol 37(6):532–536. doi:10.1016/j.ejso.2011.02.007

Coffin CM, Lowichik A, Zhou H (2005) Treatment effects in pediatric soft tissue and bone tumors: practical considerations for the pathologist. Am J Clin Pathol 123(1):75–90

Cotterill SJ, Ahrens S, Paulussen M, Jurgens HF, Voute PA, Gadner H, Craft AW (2000) Prognostic factors in Ewing's tumor of bone: analysis of 975 patients from the European Intergroup Cooperative Ewing's Sarcoma Study Group. J Clin Oncol 18(17): 3108–3114

de Alava E, Antonescu CR, Panizo A, Leung D, Meyers PA, Huvos AG, Pardo-Mindán FJ, Healey JH, Ladanyi M (2000) Prognostic impact of P53 status in Ewing sarcoma. Cancer 89(4):783–792

Diller L, Kassel J, Nelson CE, Gryka MA, Litwak G, Gebhardt M, Bressac B, Ozturk M, Baker SJ, Vogelstein B et al (1990) p53 functions as a cell cycle control protein in osteosarcomas. Mol Cell Biol 10(11):5772–5781

Dubois SG, Epling CL, Teague J, Matthay KK, Sinclair E (2010) Flow cytometric detection of Ewing sarcoma cells in peripheral blood and bone marrow. Pediatr Blood Cancer 54(1):13–18. doi:10.1002/pbc.22245

Dutour A, Decouvelaere AV, Monteil J, Duclos ME, Roualdes O, Rousseau R, Marec-Berard P (2009) 18F-FDG PET SUVmax correlates with osteosarcoma histologic response to neoadjuvant chemotherapy: preclinical evaluation in an orthotopic rat model. J Nucl Med 50(9):1533–1540. doi:10.2967/jnumed.109.062356

Ferracini R, Di Renzo MF, Scotlandi K, Baldini N, Olivero M, Lollini P, Cremona O, Campanacci M, Comoglio PM (1995) The Met/HGF receptor is over-expressed in human osteosarcomas and is activated by either a paracrine or an autocrine circuit. Oncogene 10(4):739–749

Ferrari S, Bertoni F, Mercuri M, Picci P, Giacomini S, Longhi A, Bacci G (2001) Predictive factors of disease-free survival for non-metastatic osteosarcoma of the extremity: an analysis of 300 patients treated at the Rizzoli Institute. Ann Oncol 12(8):1145–1150

Ferreira BI, Alonso J, Carrillo J, Acquadro F, Largo C, Suela J, Teixeira MR, Cerveira N, Molares A, Goméz-López G, Pestaña A, Sastre A, Garcia-Miguel P, Cigudosa JC (2008) Array CGH and gene-expression profiling reveals distinct genomic instability patterns associated with DNA repair and cell-cycle checkpoint pathways in Ewing's sarcoma. Oncogene 27(14):2084–2090. doi:10.1038/sj.onc.1210845

Fu HL, Shao L, Wang Q, Jia T, Li M, Yang DP (2013) A systematic review of p53 as a biomarker of survival in patients with osteosarcoma. Tumour Biol 34(6):3817–3821. doi:10.1007/s13277-013-0966-x

Gaston LL, Di Bella C, Slavin J, Hicks RJ, Choong PF (2011) 18F-FDG PET response to neoadjuvant chemotherapy for Ewing sarcoma and osteosarcoma are different. Skeletal Radiol 40(8):1007–1015. doi:10.1007/s00256-011-1096-4

Gebhardt MC, Lew RA, Bell RS, Baldini N, Litwak G, Mankin HJ (1990) DNA ploidy as a prognostic indicator in human osteosarcoma. Chir Organi Mov 75(1 Suppl):18–21

Goorin AM, Schwartzentruber DJ, Devidas M, Gebhardt MC, Ayala AG, Harris MB, Helman LJ, Grier HE, Link MP (2003) Presurgical chemotherapy compared with immediate surgery and adjuvant chemotherapy for nonmetastatic osteosarcoma: Pediatric Oncology Group Study POG-8651. J Clin Oncol 21(8):1574–1580. doi:10.1200/JCO.2003.08.165

Gorlick R, Huvos AG, Heller G, Aledo A, Beardsley GP, Healey JH, Meyers PA (1999) Expression of HER2/erbB-2 correlates with survival in osteosarcoma. J Clin Oncol 17(9):2781–2788

Grant CE, Valdimarsson G, Hipfner DR, Almquist KC, Cole SP, Deeley RG (1994) Overexpression of multidrug resistance-associated protein (MRP) increases resistance to natural product drugs. Cancer Res 54(2):357–361

Graves DT, Owen AJ, Barth RK, Tempst P, Winoto A, Fors L, Hood LE, Antoniades HN (1984) Detection of c-sis transcripts and synthesis of PDGF-like proteins by human osteosarcoma cells. Science 226(4677):972–974

Halperin EC (2011) Pediatric radiation oncology, 5th edn. Lippincott, Williams & Wilkins, Philadelphia

Han G, Wang Y, Bi W (2012) C-Myc overexpression promotes osteosarcoma cell invasion via activation of MEK-ERK pathway. Oncol Res 20(4):149–156

Hattinger CM, Rumpler S, Strehl S, Ambros IM, Zoubek A, Potschger U, Gadner H, Ambros PF (1999) Prognostic impact of deletions at 1p36 and numerical aberrations in Ewing tumors. Genes Chromosomes Cancer 24(3):243–254

Hauben EI, Weeden S, Pringle J, Van Marck EA, Hogendoorn PC (2002) Does the histological subtype of high-grade central osteosarcoma influence the response to treatment with chemotherapy and does it affect overall survival? A study on 570 patients of two consecutive trials of the European Osteosarcoma Intergroup. Eur J Cancer 38(9):1218–1225

Hayes DF, Bast RC, Desch CE, Fritsche H Jr, Kemeny NE, Jessup JM, Locker GY, Macdonald JS, Mennel RG, Norton L, Ravdin P, Taube S, Winn RJ (1996) Tumor marker utility grading system: a framework to evaluate clinical utility of tumor markers. J Natl Cancer Inst 88(20):1456–1466

Hingorani P, Dickman P, Garcia-Filion P, White-Collins A, Kolb EA, Azorsa DO (2013) BIRC5 expression is a poor prognostic marker in Ewing sarcoma. Pediatr Blood Cancer 60(1):35–40. doi:10.1002/pbc.24290

Huang HY, Illei PB, Zhao Z, Mazumdar M, Huvos AG, Healey JH, Wexler LH, Gorlick R, Meyers P, Ladanyi M (2005) Ewing sarcomas with p53 mutation or p16/p14ARF homozygous deletion: a highly lethal subset associated with poor chemoresponse. J Clin Oncol 23(3):548–558. doi:10.1200/JCO.2005.02.081

Hudson M, Jaffe MR, Jaffe N, Ayala A, Raymond AK, Carrasco H, Wallace S, Murray J, Robertson R (1990) Pediatric osteosarcoma: therapeutic strategies, results, and prognostic factors derived from a 10-year experience. J Clin Oncol 8(12):1988–1997

Huvos AG (1988) Surgical pathology of bone sarcomas. World J Surg 12(3):284–298

Jahromi MS, Putnam AR, Druzgal C, Wright J, Spraker-Perlman H, Kinsey M, Zhou H, Boucher KM, Randall RL, Jones KB, Lucas D, Rosenberg A, Thomas D, Lessnick SL, Schiffman JD (2012) Molecular inversion probe analysis detects novel copy number alterations in Ewing sarcoma. Cancer Genet 205(7-8):391–404. doi:10.1016/j.cancergen.2012.05.012

Janeway KA, Barkauskas DA, Krailo MD, Meyers PA, Schwartz CL, Ebb DH, Seibel NL, Grier HE, Gorlick R, Marina N (2012) Outcome for adolescent and young adult patients with osteosarcoma: a report from the Children's Oncology Group. Cancer 118(18):4597–4605. doi:10.1002/cncr.27414

Jentzsch T, Robl B, Husmann M, Bode-Lesniewska B, Fuchs B (2014) Worse prognosis of osteosarcoma patients expressing IGF-1 on a tissue microarray. Anticancer Res 34(8):3881–3889, doi: 34/8/3881 [pii]

Kashima TG, Dongre A, Oppermann U, Athanasou NA (2013) Dentine matrix protein 1 (DMP-1) is a marker of bone-forming tumours. Virchows Arch 462(5):583–591. doi:10.1007/s00428-013-1399-z

Kim DH, Kim SY, Lee HJ, Song BS, Cho JB, Lim JS, Lee JA (2011) Assessment of chemotherapy response using FDG-PET in pediatric bone tumors: a single institution experience. Cancer Res Treat 43(3):170–175. doi:10.4143/crt.2011.43.3.170

Kobayashi E, Masuda M, Nakayama R, Ichikawa H, Satow R, Shitashige M, Honda K, Yamaguchi U, Shoji

A, Tochigi N, Morioka H, Toyama Y, Hirohashi S, Kawai A, Yamada T (2010) Reduced argininosuccinate synthetase is a predictive biomarker for the development of pulmonary metastasis in patients with osteosarcoma. Mol Cancer Ther 9(3):535–544. doi:10.1158/1535-7163.MCT-09-0774

Kochevar DT, Kochevar J, Garrett L (1990) Low level amplification of c-sis and c-myc in a spontaneous osteosarcoma model. Cancer Lett 53(2-3):213–222

Kong C, Hansen MF (2009) Biomarkers in osteosarcoma. Expert Opin Med Diagn 3(1):13–23. doi:10.1517/17530050802608496

Kovar H, Jug G, Aryee DN, Zoubek A, Ambros P, Gruber B, Windhager R, Gadner H (1997) Among genes involved in the RB dependent cell cycle regulatory cascade, the p16 tumor suppressor gene is frequently lost in the Ewing family of tumors. Oncogene 15(18):2225–2232. doi:10.1038/sj.onc.1201397

Kruzelock RP, Murphy EC, Strong LC, Naylor SL, Hansen MF (1997) Localization of a novel tumor suppressor locus on human chromosome 3q important in osteosarcoma tumorigenesis. Cancer Res 57(1):106–109

Kullendorff CM, Mertens F, Donner M, Wiebe T, Akerman M, Mandahl N (1999) Cytogenetic aberrations in Ewing sarcoma: are secondary changes associated with clinical outcome? Med Pediatr Oncol 32(2):79–83

Ladanyi M, Cha C, Lewis R, Jhanwar SC, Huvos AG, Healey JH (1993a) MDM2 gene amplification in metastatic osteosarcoma. Cancer Res 53(1):16–18

Ladanyi M, Park CK, Lewis R, Jhanwar SC, Healey JH, Huvos AG (1993b) Sporadic amplification of the MYC gene in human osteosarcomas. Diagn Mol Pathol 2(3):163–167

Le Deley MC, Delattre O, Schaefer KL, Burchill SA, Koehler G, Hogendoorn PC, Lion T, Poremba C, Marandet J, Ballet S, Pierron G, Brownhill SC, Nesslböck M, Ranft A, Dirksen U, Oberlin O, Lewis IJ, Craft AW, Jürgens H, Kovar H (2010) Impact of EWS-ETS fusion type on disease progression in Ewing's sarcoma/peripheral primitive neuroectodermal tumor: prospective results from the cooperative Euro-E.W.I.N.G. 99 trial. J Clin Oncol 28(12):1982–1988. doi:10.1200/JCO.2009.23.3585

Lee J, Hoang BH, Ziogas A, Zell JA (2010) Analysis of prognostic factors in Ewing sarcoma using a population-based cancer registry. Cancer 116(8):1964–1973. doi:10.1002/cncr.24937

Limmahakhun S, Pothacharoen P, Theera-Umpon N, Arpornchayanon O, Leerapun T, Luevitoonvechkij S, Pruksakorn D (2011) Relationships between serum biomarker levels and clinical presentation of human osteosarcomas. Asian Pac J Cancer Prev 12(7):1717–1722

Lin PP, Jaffe N, Herzog CE, Costelloe CM, Deavers MT, Kelly JS, Patel SR, Madewell JE, Lewis VO, Cannon CP, Benjamin RS, Yasko AW (2007) Chemotherapy response is an important predictor of local recurrence

in Ewing sarcoma. Cancer 109(3):603–611. doi:10.1002/cncr.22412

Loe DW, Deeley RG, Cole SP (1996) Biology of the multidrug resistance-associated protein, MRP. Eur J Cancer 32A(6):945–957

Lopez Guerra JL, Marquez-Vega C, Ramirez-Villar GL, Cabrera P, Ordonez R, Praena-Fernandez JM, Ortiz MJ (2012) Prognostic factors for overall survival in paediatric patients with Ewing sarcoma of bone treated according to multidisciplinary protocol. Clin Transl Oncol 14(4):294–301. doi:10.1007/s12094-012-0798-y

Lopez-Guerrero JA, Machado I, Scotlandi K, Noguera R, Pellin A, Navarro S, Serra M, Calabuig-Fariñas S, Picci P, Llombart-Bosch A (2011) Clinicopathological significance of cell cycle regulation markers in a large series of genetically confirmed Ewing's sarcoma family of tumors. Int J Cancer 128(5):1139–1150. doi:10.1002/ijc.25424

Lowichik A, Zhou H, Pysher TJ, Smith L, Lemons R, Coffin CM (2000) Therapy associated changes in childhood tumors. Adv Anat Pathol 7(6):341–359

MacEwen EG, Pastor J, Kutzke J, Tsan R, Kurzman ID, Thamm DH, Wilson M, Radinsky R (2004) IGF-1 receptor contributes to the malignant phenotype in human and canine osteosarcoma. J Cell Biochem 92(1):77–91. doi:10.1002/jcb.20046

Machado I, Lopez-Guerrero JA, Navarro S, Alberghini M, Scotlandi K, Picci P, Llombart-Bosch A (2012) Epithelial cell adhesion molecules and epithelial mesenchymal transition (EMT) markers in Ewing's sarcoma family of tumors (ESFTs). Do they offer any prognostic significance? Virchows Arch 461(3):333–337. doi:10.1007/s00428-012-1288-x

Mackintosh C, Ordonez JL, Garcia-Dominguez DJ, Sevillano V, Llombart-Bosch A, Szuhai K, Scotlandi K, Alberghini M, Sciot R, Sinnaeve F, Hogendoorn PC, Picci P, Knuutila S, Dirksen U, Debiec-Rychter M, Schaefer KL, de Alava E (2012) 1q gain and CDT2 overexpression underlie an aggressive and highly proliferative form of Ewing sarcoma. Oncogene 31(10):1287–1298. doi:10.1038/onc.2011.317

Martin RC 2nd, Brennan MF (2003) Adult soft tissue Ewing sarcoma or primitive neuroectodermal tumors: predictors of survival? Arch Surg 138(3):281–285

Martin JW, Chilton-MacNeill S, Koti M, van Wijnen AJ, Squire JA, Zielenska M (2014) Digital expression profiling identifies RUNX2, CDC5L, MDM2, RECQL4, and CDK4 as potential predictive biomarkers for neoadjuvant chemotherapy response in paediatric osteosarcoma. PLoS One 9(5), e95843. doi:10.1371/journal.pone.0095843

McIntyre JF, Smith-Sorensen B, Friend SH, Kassell J, Borresen AL, Yan YX, Russo C, Sato J, Barbier N, Miser J et al (1994) Germline mutations of the p53 tumor suppressor gene in children with osteosarcoma. J Clin Oncol 12(5):925–930

McShane LM, Altman DG, Sauerbrei W, Taube SE, Gion M, Clark GM (2005) REporting recommendations for tumor MARKer prognostic studies (REMARK). Nat Clin Pract Urol 2(8):416–422

Miller CW, Aslo A, Campbell MJ, Kawamata N, Lampkin BC, Koeffler HP (1996a) Alterations of the p15, p16, and p18 genes in osteosarcoma. Cancer Genet Cytogenet 86(2):136–142. doi:0165-4608(95)00216-2 [pii]

Miller CW, Aslo A, Won A, Tan M, Lampkin B, Koeffler HP (1996b) Alterations of the p53, Rb and MDM2 genes in osteosarcoma. J Cancer Res Clin Oncol 122(9):559–565

Miser JS, Pritchard DJ, Rock MG, Shives TC, Gilchrist GS, Smithson WA, Arndt CA, Edmonson JH, Schaid DJ (1993) Osteosarcoma in adolescents and young adults: new developments and controversies. The Mayo Clinic studies. Cancer Treat Res 62:333–338

Moore C, Eslin D, Levy A, Roberson J, Giusti V, Sutphin R (2010) Prognostic significance of early lymphocyte recovery in pediatric osteosarcoma. Pediatr Blood Cancer 55(6):1096–1102. doi:10.1002/pbc.22673

Morris CD, Gorlick R, Huvos G, Heller G, Meyers PA, Healey JH (2001) Human epidermal growth factor receptor 2 as a prognostic indicator in osteogenic sarcoma. Clin Orthop Relat Res (382):59–65

Nakashima H, Nishida Y, Sugiura H, Katagiri H, Yonekawa M, Yamada Y, Iwata H, Nagasaka T, Ishiguro N (2003) Telomerase, p53 and PCNA activity in osteosarcoma. Eur J Surg Oncol 29(7):564–567. doi:S0748798303001173 [pii]

Nardeux PC, Daya-Grosjean L, Landin RM, Andeol Y, Suarez HG (1987) A c-ras-Ki oncogene is activated, amplified and overexpressed in a human osteosarcoma cell line. Biochem Biophys Res Commun 146(2):395–402. doi:0006-291X(87)90542-0 [pii]

Oberlin O, Deley MC, Bui BN, Gentet JC, Philip T, Terrier P, Carrie C, Mechinaud F, Schmitt C, Babin-Boillettot A, Michon J (2001) Prognostic factors in localized Ewing's tumours and peripheral neuroectodermal tumours: the third study of the French Society of Paediatric Oncology (EW88 study). Br J Cancer 85(11):1646–1654. doi:10.1054/bjoc.2001.2150

Onda M, Matsuda S, Higaki S, Iijima T, Fukushima J, Yokokura A, Kojima T, Horiuchi H, Kurokawa T, Yamamoto T (1996) ErbB-2 expression is correlated with poor prognosis for patients with osteosarcoma. Cancer 77(1):71–78. doi:10.1002/(SICI)1097-0142(19960101)77:1<71::AID-CNCR13>3.0.CO;2-5 [pii] 10.1002/(SICI)1097-0142(19960101)77:1<71::AID-CNCR13>3.0.CO;2-5

Ozaki T, Ikeda S, Kawai A, Inoue H, Oda T (1993) Alterations of retinoblastoma susceptible gene accompanied by c-myc amplification in human bone and soft tissue tumors. Cell Mol Biol (Noisy-le-Grand) 39(2):235–242

Ozaki T, Paulussen M, Poremba C, Brinkschmidt C, Rerin J, Ahrens S, Hoffmann C, Hillmann A, Wai D, Schaefer KL, Boecker W, Juergens H, Winkelmann W, Dockhorn-Dworniczak B (2001) Genetic imbalances revealed by comparative genomic hybridization in Ewing tumors. Genes Chromosomes Cancer 32(2):164–171

Patino-Garcia A, Pineiro ES, Diez MZ, Iturriagagoitia LG, Klussmann FA, Ariznabarreta LS (2003) Genetic and epigenetic alterations of the cell cycle regulators and tumor suppressor genes in pediatric osteosarcomas. J Pediatr Hematol Oncol 25(5):362–367

Paulussen M, Ahrens S, Dunst J, Winkelmann W, Exner GU, Kotz R, Amann G, Dockhorn-Dworniczak B, Harms D, Müller-Weihrich S, Welte K, Kornhuber B, Janka-Schaub G, Göbel U, Treuner J, Voûte PA, Zoubek A, Gadner H, Jurgens H (2001a) Localized Ewing tumor of bone: final results of the cooperative Ewing's Sarcoma Study CESS 86. J Clin Oncol 19(6):1818–1829

Paulussen M, Frohlich B, Jurgens H (2001b) Ewing tumour: incidence, prognosis and treatment options. Paediatr Drugs 3(12):899–913

Picci P, Rougraff BT, Bacci G, Neff JR, Sangiorgi L, Cazzola A, Baldini N, Ferrari S, Mercuri M, Ruggieri P et al (1993) Prognostic significance of histopathologic response to chemotherapy in nonmetastatic Ewing's sarcoma of the extremities. J Clin Oncol 11(9):1763–1769

Picci P, Sangiorgi L, Rougraff BT, Neff JR, Casadei R, Campanacci M (1994) Relationship of chemotherapy-induced necrosis and surgical margins to local recurrence in osteosarcoma. J Clin Oncol 12(12):2699–2705

Picci P, Bohling T, Bacci G, Ferrari S, Sangiorgi L, Mercuri M, Ruggieri P, Manfrini M, Ferraro A, Casadei R, Benassi MS, Mancini AF, Rosito P, Cazzola A, Barbieri E, Tienghi A, Brach del Prever A, Comandone A, Bacchini P, Bertoni F (1997) Chemotherapy-induced tumor necrosis as a prognostic factor in localized Ewing's sarcoma of the extremities. J Clin Oncol 15(4):1553–1559

Pinto A, Dickman P, Parham D (2011) Pathobiologic markers of the ewing sarcoma family of tumors: state of the art and prediction of behaviour. Sarcoma 2011:856190. doi:10.1155/2011/856190

Provisor AJ, Ettinger LJ, Nachman JB, Krailo MD, Makley JT, Yunis EJ, Huvos AG, Betcher DL, Baum ES, Kisker CT, Miser JS (1997) Treatment of nonmetastatic osteosarcoma of the extremity with preoperative and postoperative chemotherapy: a report from the Children's Cancer Group. J Clin Oncol 15(1):76–84

Qureshi SS, Kembhavi S, Vora T, Ramadwar M, Laskar S, Talole S, Kurkure P (2013) Prognostic factors in primary nonmetastatic Ewing sarcoma of the rib in children and young adults. J Pediatr Surg 48(4):764–770. doi:10.1016/j.jpedsurg.2012.07.049

Raymond AK, Chawla SP, Carrasco CH, Ayala AG, Fanning CV, Grice B, Armen T, Plager C, Papadopoulos NE, Edeiken J et al (1987) Osteosarcoma chemotherapy effect: a prognostic factor. Semin Diagn Pathol 4(3):212–236

Roberts P, Burchill SA, Brownhill S, Cullinane CJ, Johnston C, Griffiths MJ, McMullan DJ, Bown NP,

Morris SP, Lewis IJ (2008) Ploidy and karyotype complexity are powerful prognostic indicators in the Ewing's sarcoma family of tumors: a study by the United Kingdom Cancer Cytogenetics and the Children's Cancer and Leukaemia Group. Genes Chromosomes Cancer 47(3):207–220. doi:10.1002/gcc.20523

Rodriguez-Galindo C, Navid F, Liu T, Billups CA, Rao BN, Krasin MJ (2008) Prognostic factors for local and distant control in Ewing sarcoma family of tumors. Ann Oncol 19(4):814–820. doi:10.1093/annonc/mdm521

Rosen G, Marcove RC, Caparros B, Nirenberg A, Kosloff C, Huvos AG (1979) Primary osteogenic sarcoma: the rationale for preoperative chemotherapy and delayed surgery. Cancer 43(6):2163–2177

Salzer-Kuntschik M, Delling G, Beron G, Sigmund R (1983) Morphological grades of regression in osteosarcoma after polychemotherapy – study COSS 80. J Cancer Res Clin Oncol 106(Suppl):21–24

Sanders RP, Drissi R, Billups CA, Daw NC, Valentine MB, Dome JS (2004) Telomerase expression predicts unfavorable outcome in osteosarcoma. J Clin Oncol 22(18):3790–3797. doi:10.1200/JCO.2004.03.043 22/18/3790 [pii]

Sankar S, Lessnick SL (2011) Promiscuous partnerships in Ewing's sarcoma. Cancer Genet 204(7):351–365. doi:10.1016/j.cancergen.2011.07.008

Sauer R, Jurgens H, Burgers JM, Dunst J, Hawlicek R, Michaelis J (1987) Prognostic factors in the treatment of Ewing's sarcoma. The Ewing's Sarcoma Study Group of the German Society of Paediatric Oncology CESS 81. Radiother Oncol 10(2):101–110

Savola S, Klami A, Tripathi A, Niini T, Serra M, Picci P, Kaski S, Zambelli D, Scotlandi K, Knuutila S (2009) Combined use of expression and CGH arrays pinpoints novel candidate genes in Ewing sarcoma family of tumors. BMC Cancer 9:17. doi:10.1186/1471-2407-9-17

Scholz RB, Kabisch H, Weber B, Roser K, Delling G, Winkler K (1992) Studies of the RB1 gene and the p53 gene in human osteosarcomas. Pediatr Hematol Oncol 9(2):125–137. doi:10.3109/08880019209018328

Scotlandi K, Serra M, Manara MC, Maurici D, Benini S, Nini G, Campanacci M, Baldini N (1995) Clinical relevance of Ki-67 expression in bone tumors. Cancer 75(3):806–814

Shukla N, Schiffman J, Reed D, Davis IJ, Womer RB, Lessnick SL, Lawlor ER (2013) Biomarkers in Ewing sarcoma: the promise and challenge of personalized medicine. A Report from the Children's Oncology Group. Front Oncol 3:141. doi:10.3389/fonc.2013.00141

Simon RM, Paik S, Hayes DF (2009) Use of archived specimens in evaluation of prognostic and predictive biomarkers. J Natl Cancer Inst 101(21):1446–1452. doi:10.1093/jnci/djp335

Tarkkanen M, Kiuru-Kuhlefelt S, Blomqvist C, Armengol G, Bohling T, Ekfors T, Virolainen M, Lindholm P, Monge O, Picci P, Knuutila S, Elomaa I (1999) Clinical correlations of genetic changes by comparative genomic hybridization in Ewing sarcoma and related tumors. Cancer Genet Cytogenet 114(1):35–41

Ueda Y, Dockhorn-Dworniczak B, Blasius S, Mellin W, Wuisman P, Bocker W, Roessner A (1993) Analysis of mutant P53 protein in osteosarcomas and other malignant and benign lesions of bone. J Cancer Res Clin Oncol 119(3):172–178

van Doorninck JA, Ji L, Schaub B, Shimada H, Wing MR, Krailo MD, Lessnick SL, Marina N, Triche TJ, Sposto R, Womer RB, Lawlor ER (2010) Current treatment protocols have eliminated the prognostic advantage of type 1 fusions in Ewing sarcoma: a report from the Children's Oncology Group. J Clin Oncol 28(12):1989–1994. doi:10.1200/JCO.2009.24.5845

van Maldegem AM, Hogendoorn PC, Hassan AB (2012) The clinical use of biomarkers as prognostic factors in Ewing sarcoma. Clin Sarcoma Res 2(1):7. doi:10.1186/2045-3329-2-7

Wagner LM, Smolarek TA, Sumegi J, Marmer D (2012) Assessment of minimal residual disease in ewing sarcoma. Sarcoma 2012:780129. doi:10.1155/2012/780129

Wen J, Wang L, Zhang M, Xie D, Sun L (2002) Repression of telomerase activity during in vitro differentiation of osteosarcoma cells. Cancer Invest 20(1):38–45

Winkler K, Bielack SS, Delling G, Jurgens H, Kotz R, Salzer-Kuntschik M (1993) Treatment of osteosarcoma: experience of the Cooperative Osteosarcoma Study Group (COSS). Cancer Treat Res 62: 269–277

Wold LE (1998) Practical approach to processing osteosarcomas in the surgical pathology laboratory. Pediatr Dev Pathol 1(5):449–454

Wu JX, Carpenter PM, Gresens C, Keh R, Niman H, Morris JW, Mercola D (1990) The proto-oncogene c-fos is over-expressed in the majority of human osteosarcomas. Oncogene 5(7):989–1000

Wu X, Cai ZD, Lou LM, Zhu YB (2012) Expressions of p53, c-MYC, BCL-2 and apoptotic index in human osteosarcoma and their correlations with prognosis of patients. Cancer Epidemiol 36(2):212–216. doi:10.1016/j.canep.2011.08.002

Wunder JS, Paulian G, Huvos AG, Heller G, Meyers PA, Healey JH (1998) The histological response to chemotherapy as a predictor of the oncological outcome of operative treatment of Ewing sarcoma. J Bone Joint Surg Am 80(7):1020–1033

Xie L, Guo W, Li Y, Ji T, Sun X (2012) Pathologic fracture does not influence local recurrence and survival in high-grade extremity osteosarcoma with adequate surgical margins. J Surg Oncol 106(7):820–825. doi:10.1002/jso.23150

Yang Y, Li H, Zhang F, Shi H, Zhen T, Dai S, Kang L, Liang Y, Wang J, Han A (2013) Clinical and biological significance of hepatoma-derived growth factor in Ewing's sarcoma. J Pathol 231(3):323–334. doi:10.1002/path.4241

Yang Y, Zhen T, Zhang F, Dai S, Kang L, Liang Y, Xue L, Han A (2014) p53 and hepatoma-derived growth factor expression and their clinicopathological association with Ewing family tumour. J Clin Pathol 67(3):235–242. doi:10.1136/jclinpath-2013-201705

Zhang Y, Zhang L, Zhang G, Li S, Duan J, Cheng J, Ding G, Zhou C, Zhang J, Luo P, Cai D, Kuang L, Zhou Y, Tong L, Yu X, Zhang L, Xu L, Yu L, Shi X, Ke A (2014) Osteosarcoma metastasis: prospective role of ezrin. Tumour Biol 35(6):5055–5059. doi:10.1007/s13277-014-1799-y

Zielenska M, Zhang ZM, Ng K, Marrano P, Bayani J, Ramirez OC, Sorensen P, Thorner P, Greenberg M, Squire JA (2001) Acquisition of secondary structural chromosomal changes in pediatric ewing sarcoma is a probable prognostic factor for tumor response and clinical outcome. Cancer 91(11):2156–2164

Zuo D, Zheng L, Sun W, Hua Y, Cai Z (2013) Pathologic fracture does not influence prognosis in stage IIB osteosarcoma: a case-control study. World J Surg Oncol 11:148. doi:10.1186/1477-7819-11-148

Surgical Approach: Limb Salvage Versus Amputation

Vincent Y. Ng and Thomas J. Scharschmidt

Contents

9.1   **Introduction**.   144
9.1.1   Timing of Local Control   144
9.1.2   Role of Skeletal Maturity   145

9.2   **Indications and Contraindications
        for Limb Salvage**.   145

9.3   **Reconstructive Options**   145
9.3.1   Autograft.   146
9.3.2   Allografts   146
9.3.3   Metallic Prosthesis   147
9.3.4   Combination (Alloprosthetic
        Composite)   148

9.4   **Amputation**   149
9.4.1   Indications   149
9.4.2   Risks/Benefits/Alternatives.   150
9.4.3   Rehabilitation and Prosthetics   150

9.5   **Surgical Techniques**   150
9.5.1   Ray Resection and Partial
        Hand Amputation   150
9.5.2   Transradial and Transhumeral
        Amputation.   151
9.5.3   Shoulder Disarticulations
        and Forequarter Amputations   151
9.5.4   Below Knee Amputation   151
9.5.5   Above Knee Amputation (AKA)   152
9.5.6   Hip Disarticulation   153
9.5.7   Pediatric Amputations   153

9.6   **Summary**   154

References.   154

V.Y. Ng, MD
Division of Musculoskeletal Oncology,
Department of Orthopaedics,
University of Maryland Medical Center,
22 S Greene Street, Baltimore,
MD 21201, USA

T.J. Scharschmidt, MD (✉)
Division of Musculoskeletal Oncology,
Department of Orthopaedics,
The Ohio State University,
1074 OSU CarePoint East,
543 Taylor Avenue, Columbus,
OH 43203, USA
e-mail: Thomas.scharschmidt@osumc.edu

Abstract

Major advances have been made in the last 30 years in the treatment of pediatric bone sarcomas. Chemotherapy has been credited with the largest advance in overall survival (from 20–30 % to 60–70 %), but increased expertise in surgical techniques, advanced imaging, and reconstructive options have also had major impact in the area of limb salvage (Weisstein et al. 2005). The surgical decisions in this setting are complex with many intricacies that come in to play. Treatment algorithms should be prioritized by the patient's overall survival first, then the salvage of the limb. Two key principles must always be remembered: the limb salvage procedure should not result in a worse survival for the patient and the function of the limb should be acceptable. Consideration of limb function, appearance, and length must

© Springer International Publishing Switzerland 2015
T.P. Cripe, N.D. Yeager (eds.), *Malignant Pediatric Bone Tumors - Treatment & Management*,
Pediatric Oncology, DOI 10.1007/978-3-319-18099-1_9

be included in the decision of whether to attempt limb salvage versus amputation. Social and financial factors also play a role. The interests and potential future vocation of the patient must be considered, which may not be known in the young patient (Choong and Sim 1997). The goal of this chapter is to outline the approach and surgical considerations when deciding limb salvage and amputation in the setting of pediatric bone sarcoma.

9.1 Introduction

Major advances have been made in the last 30 years in the treatment of pediatric bone sarcomas. Chemotherapy has been credited with the largest advance in overall survival (from 20–30 % to 60–70 %), but increased expertise in surgical techniques, advanced imaging, and reconstructive options have also had major impact in the area of limb salvage (Weisstein et al. 2005). The surgical decisions in this setting are complex with many intricacies that come in to play. Treatment algorithms should be prioritized by the patient's overall survival first, then the salvage of the limb. Two key principles must always be remembered: the limb salvage procedure should not result in a worse survival for the patient and the function of the limb should be acceptable. Consideration of limb function, appearance, and length must be included in the decision of whether to attempt limb salvage versus amputation. Social and financial factors also play a role. The interests and potential future vocation of the patient must be considered, which may not be known in the young patient (Choong and Sim 1997). The goal of this chapter is to outline the approach and surgical considerations when deciding limb salvage and amputation in the setting of pediatric bone sarcoma.

General principles of the resection for limb salvage include an extensile longitudinal approach that allows for resection of the biopsy tract and adequate exposure of the adjacent neurovascular bundles. The goal of resection is to perform a "wide resection," which by definition leaves a cuff of normal tissue around the mass. Reconstruction options for large skeletal defects must be available, and adequate soft tissue cover-

age for closure is of vital importance (DiCaprio and Friedlaender 2003).

9.1.1 Timing of Local Control

The timing, when local control in the form of surgical resection is performed, should be individualized based on the patient presentation, diagnosis, and stage of disease. Most centers utilize standard protocols from co-operative groups, such as Children's Oncology Group (COG), which generally call for a period of neoadjuvant chemotherapy prior to surgical resection of the mass. Interestingly, this approach was constructed as the concept of limb salvage was being developed. Before modern modular prosthetic components were available for widespread use, when a patient required a megaprothesis for limb salvage there was often a delay of 6–12 weeks for the device companies to manufacture the implant required. Chemotherapy was initiated during this delay and several advantages of this approach were discovered. First, micrometastatic disease is treated immediately, potentially decreasing early development of drug-resistant clones (Jaffe 2014). Secondly, the period of neoadjuvant treatment allows the surgeon to appropriately plan the procedure and have multiple discussions with the family regarding treatment options. Third, the initial response to chemotherapy may affect the local control approach. Patients may see their tumor progress, shrink, or they may develop metastatic disease, all of which could change options available for surgery. And lastly, systemic treatment up front allows histologic evaluation of the resected tumor, and the percent of tumor necrosis in the case of osteosarcoma correlates with overall survival (Fig. 9.1).

One additional scenario that deserves discussion is the presence of pathological fracture. The occurrence of a pathologic fracture, either at presentation or during induction chemotherapy, was traditionally treated with immediate amputation. However, it has now been established that although overall survival is worse in these patients (55 % compared to almost 80 %), limb salvage can still be performed in select cases in which negative surgical margins can be achieved (Scully et al. 2002).

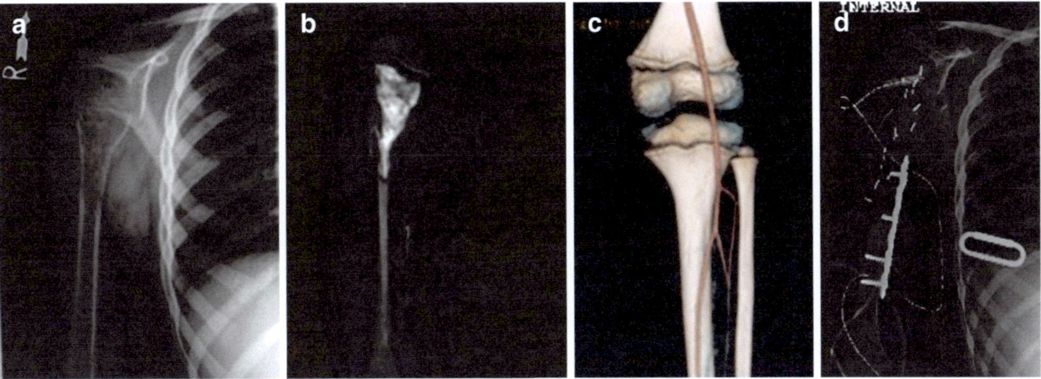

Fig. 9.1 Pre-operative x-ray (**a**) and MRI (**b**) demonstrating an aggressive sarcoma of the proximal humerus in a 5-year-old boy. A vascularized fibula (**c**) was harvested and used to reconstruct the proximal humerus (**d**)

9.1.2 Role of Skeletal Maturity

One of the major differences when considering limb salvage versus amputation in the pediatric population is the growth potential in terms of skeletal maturity. Skeletal maturity (as defined by closure of the growth plates) is gender dependent but is generally not reached until the age of 16–18 years. The most common locations for the development of osteosarcoma include the areas of rapid bone growth (distal femur, proximal tibia, proximal humerus). Therefore, the younger the child is at the time of diagnosis, the more growth that must be accounted for in the surgical decision and reconstruction. In general, the younger (and smaller) the patient, the more difficult limb salvage is to achieve and the worse the morbidity (Guillon et al. 2011). Additional factors that play a role in the decision to perform limb salvage in the skeletally immature patient include size of the resection and tumor, size of available implants, other reconstructive options, size of soft tissue envelope, and potential for lengthening after index procedure.

9.2 Indications and Contraindications for Limb Salvage

With current treatment approaches, limb salvage can generally be offered in 90 % of cases (Wilkins et al. 2005). General indications include isolated disease, a good response to chemotherapy, and no involvement of the adjacent neurovascular structure. There are really no absolute contraindications to limb salvage, but the overall function of the limb should always be considered and several relative contraindications have been defined. These contraindications to limb salvage include progression during chemotherapy, encasement of neurovascular structures, the very skeletally immature patient, and sometimes pathologic fracture resulting in a high degree of local tissue contamination. Another consideration should be minimizing the time to resumption of chemotherapy after the local control surgery. Outcome data suggest that systemic therapy should be resumed within 6 weeks of surgery to maximize survival for the patient. Therefore, attempts to minimize infection and wound complications should be paramount. Judicious use of flaps for wound coverage, minimizing operative time, and pre-surgical optimization of blood counts should all be employed to minimize the time the patient will be off systemic treatment.

9.3 Reconstructive Options

Once the decision to proceed with limb salvage has been made, there are multiple potential options available for the reconstruction. When the tumor is present in an expendable bone, local control can be achieved with resection without reconstruction. Locations amenable to this

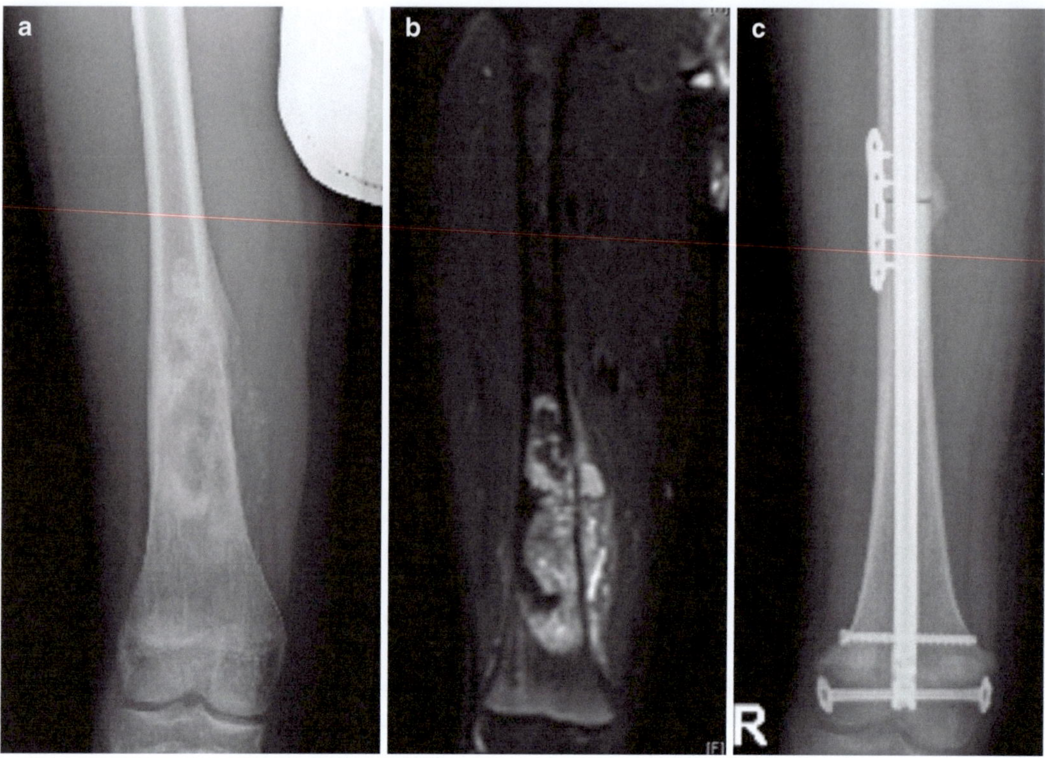

Fig. 9.2 Pre-operative x-ray (**a**) and MRI (**b**) showing an osteosarcoma of the distal femur. Intercalary physeal sparing allograft was used to reconstruct the defect (**c**)

include the fibula, portions of the pelvis and sacrum, and portions of the ulna. Outside of these select areas reconstruction is usually required.

9.3.1 Autograft

The use of autografts in reconstruction for structural defects is fairly limited. The most common indication utilizes the fibula, either in a vascularized or non-vascularized fashion. The mid-portion of the fibula can serve as a structural strut, and has been described in combination with an allograft to promote healing (Li et al. 2011). Vascularized fibular graft has also been described for reconstruction of intercalary resections of long bones (tibia, femur, humerus) (Chen et al. 2007). Another potential indication exists in the very young child (<8 years old) with a malignant proximal humerus tumor. Skeletal growth is an issue, and the proxi-

mal fibular epiphysis can be harvested on a vascularized pedicle for reconstruction in an attempt to maintain some growth in the limb (Fig. 9.2).

9.3.2 Allografts

Prior to the advent and development of metallic prosthesis in the last 30 years, allograft reconstruction was the mainstay of treatment for pediatric sarcoma patients. Allografts have been used longer than any other reconstruction method. Osteoarticular allografts were used extensively for reconstruction involving the joint and allow a strong repair for ligaments and other soft tissue. Unfortunately, very few of the chondrocytes survive the preservation and sterilization process, so the natural course is for the joint surface to degenerate over time. Osteoarthritis develops in the first 5–10 years in 15 % of patients (Mankin

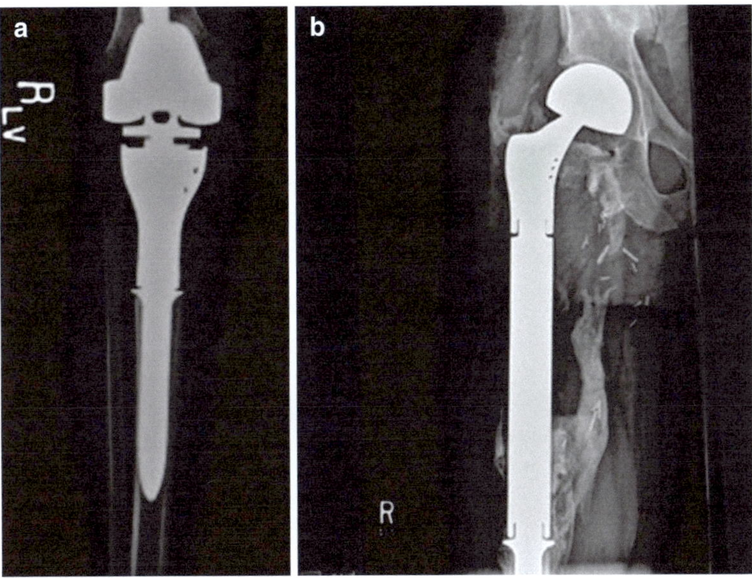

Fig. 9.3 Examples of modular prosthesis. A proximal tibia (**a**) and proximal femur (**b**) is shown. Heterotopic ossification is commonly seen after the reconstruction, seen particularly well in (**b**)

et al. 1996). Thus, metallic solutions have largely replaced this reconstruction when tumor resection requires the joint to be removed, although it can still be employed in select circumstances (Muscolo et al. 2008).

The major usage of structural allografts occurs in intercalary resections and reconstructions (Fig. 9.3). This technique can be employed in cases where the tumor is limited to the diaphysis and the physis can be spared. The allograft is usually stabilized and protected with either a plate or rod, which minimizes the potential for fracture of the allograft (Miller and Virkus 2010). The ability to spare the joint allows functional outcomes to be maximized for these patients.

The modes of failure associated with allograft reconstruction include infection, fracture, and non-union. Up to 50 % of patients can be expected to experience one of these complications, and the rate of early complication is high (Mankin et al. 1996).

9.3.3 Metallic Prosthesis

The advent and development of metallic "mega"-protheses has replaced the utilization of allografts in most circumstances. Modern systems offer

tremendous modularity that allows the surgeon to

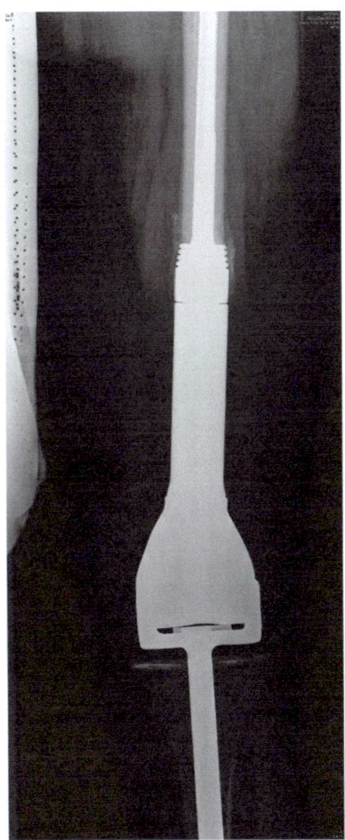

Fig. 9.4 Plain radiograph showing reconstruction with a non-invasive expandable prosthesis in a 8 years old patient. The prosthesis can be lengthened in the office using an electromagnetic coil

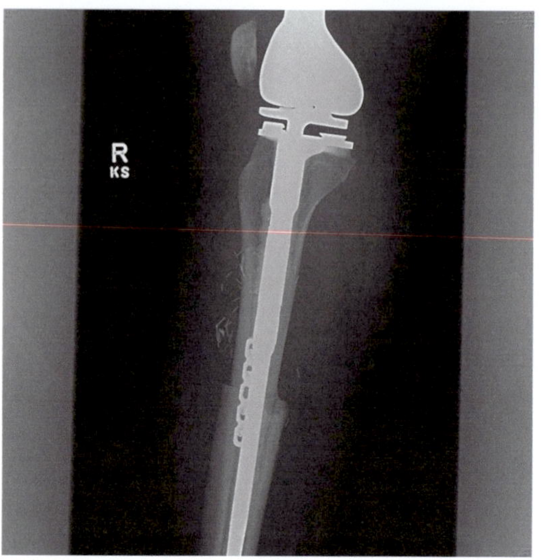

Fig. 9.5 Lateral radiograph of a knee showing an example of an allograft-prosthestic combination reconstruction that was utilized after resection of the proximal tibia for osteosarcoma. An allograft proximal tibia with extensor mechanism attached is used to reconstruct the bone defect and a metallic prosthetic knee is placed in combination for joint reconstruction

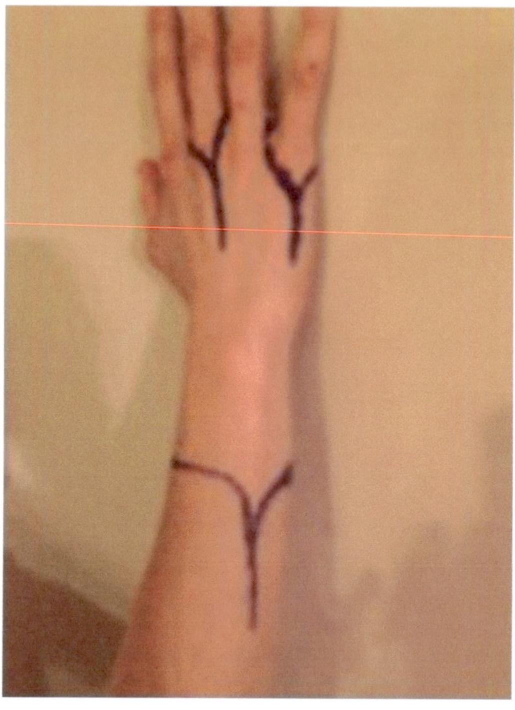

Fig. 9.6 Incisions for transradial amputation and ray resections

reconstruct almost any length of skeletal defect intra-operatively (Fig. 9.4). Immediate range of motion and weight bearing can often be allowed with these constructs. In addition, there is a lower risk of infection and non-union when compared to allografts, and there is no risk of disease transmission. These devices can also be used for salvage after failure of a prior allograft (Foo et al. 2011). Also available are expandable prostheses, which allow growth of the limb in the child in either an invasive or non-invasive manner (Fig. 9.5). The development of expandable options was a tremendous advance in the realm of limb salvage for young patients (Beebe et al. 2010). The child usually undergoes lengthening every 1 cm or so. Lengthening in larger increments can cause increased pain and neuropraxia. Despite high interest and emotional acceptance with these devices, studies have not shown superiority to limb salvage versus amputation (Henderson et al. 2012).

The main modes of failure for metallic prosthesis include loosening and infection. Either of these can be disastrous for the patient and can lead to extensive revision or even to amputa-

tion. The 10-year survival for these devices is around 60 % (Morgan et al. 2006). Location plays a role in the durability of the reconstruction, with proximal humeral and proximal femur doing the best (77 % at 10 years), distal femur next (65 % at 10 years), and proximal tibia prostheses faring the worst (50 % at 10 years) (Damron 1997).

9.3.4 Combination (Alloprosthetic Composite)

Combining both an allograft and a prosthetic in a reconstruction is performed in an attempt to capture the benefits and avoid the pitfalls of each of the respective methods. The composite reconstruction can help restore bone stock and provide strong ligamentous attachments with the allograft portion, while the prosthetic portion avoids the cartilage degradation associated with osteoarticular allografts (Fig. 9.6).

9.4   Amputation

Amputation is one of the oldest surgical procedures known to man. The most common indications for amputation are: infection, ischemia, trauma, and malignancy. With improved antibiotics, revascularization procedures, soft tissue reconstruction, and limb-salvage techniques, fewer patients require amputation today than ever before. Nevertheless, sometimes amputation is the more prudent option in terms of either time for recovery or risk of complications. In these instances, it is important for surgeons to emphasize to patients that amputation represents the beginning of a new life rather than the culmination of previous treatment failures (Figs. 9.7 and 9.8).

9.4.1   Indications

Approximately 13,000 Americans live with lower extremity amputations due to malignancy (Ziegler-Graham et al. 2008). With the advent of modern chemotherapy, survival rates have

Table 9.1 Considerations impacting surgical choice for malignant bone tumors

Patient factors	Oncologic factors
Risk tolerance for recurrence	Responsiveness to adjuvant treatment
Occupation	Local aggressiveness
Ability to undergo rehabilitation	Stage of disease
Age	Single lesion or multifocal lesion
Cosmesis	
Treatment factors	**Anatomic factors**
Prior treatment sequellae	Size of lesion
Chemoresponsiveness	Proximity to critical structures
Radiation responsiveness	Extent of contamination
	Ability to achieve negative or wide margins

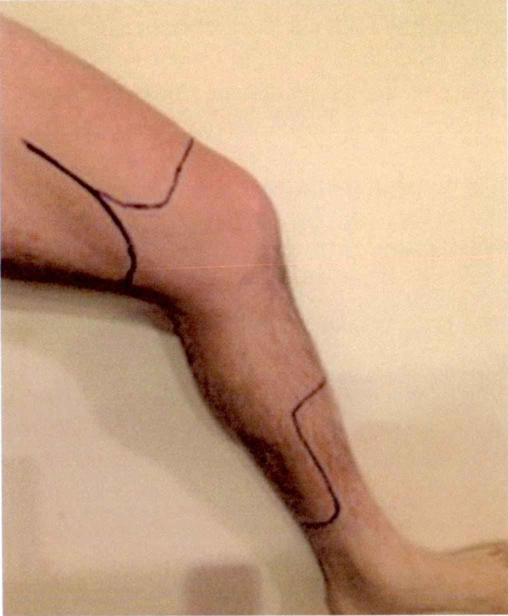

Fig. 9.7 Incisions for above- and below-knee amputations

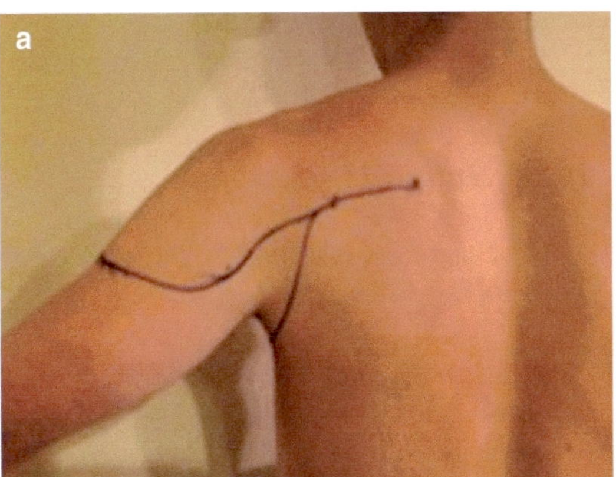

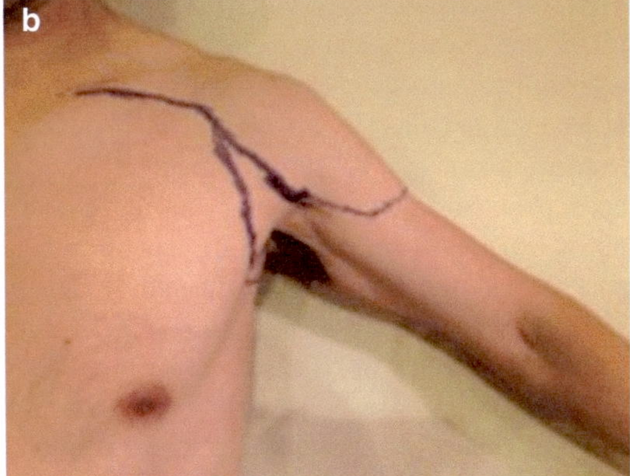

Fig. 9.8 Incision for shoulder disarticulation or forequarter amputation. (**a**) Posterior incision (**b**) Anterior incision

improved from approximately 20 % prior to the 1970s to nearly 70 % for primary bone sarcomas (Ng et al. 2013). Effective imaging technology and radiation techniques have allowed most patients with soft tissue sarcomas to preserve their limb without significant increases in local recurrence rates or overall mortality.

The threshold to perform an amputation for tumor varies widely amongst institutions. Every situation is unique and should be evaluated on a case-by-case basis. There are numerous important factors to consider (Table 9.1).

On a fundamental level, it is important to note that the oncologic role of surgical resection or amputation for an extremity-based primary lesion is local control. If metastases are already present, eradicating local sites of tumor is less essential, particularly if they are minimally symptomatic and if there is not a reasonable chance of long-term survival with systemic therapy. For non-metastatic cases, achieving local control is necessary for long-term survival. However, it is unclear what additional risk of metastasis is incurred with local recurrence of tumor followed by timely re-resection or amputation. If the surgeon and patient are relatively risk-tolerant and there are effective adjuvant modalities, limb-salvage may be attempted in even high-risk cases, with the philosophy that amputation can always be performed later in the event of local recurrence.

9.4.2 Risks/Benefits/Alternatives

With loss of a limb, patients lose function and cosmesis. The impact upon the patient depends on the availability of an effective prosthesis, the patient's occupation and lifestyle, and the specific body part lost. Approximately 90–100 % of patients experience phantom-limb sensations and more than 50 % experience some degree of phantom-limb pain (Krane and Heller 1995). Phantom pain is most prevalent at 6–18 months following surgery and decrease with time (Bosmans et al. 2010).

Amputation has several advantages over limb-salvage. Typically, it has a lower rate of complications such as fracture, infection, wound healing issues, and neurovascular injury. Amputations can usually be performed more rapidly than limb-salvage surgery and may be preferable in medi-

cally comorbid patients. In theory one might think the local recurrence rate would be lower due to wider margins, but the data suggest that limb-salvage is equally effective at local control.

Surgical limb-salvage options include Van Nes rotationplasty for distal femoral or proximal tibial malignancies (Cammisa et al. 1990) and vascular bypass for tumors encasing critical vessels. Sacrifice of either the femoral or sciatic nerve in the lower extremity is acceptable and can be compensated with bracing. Loss of both major nerves, however, renders the limb functionally incapacitated. In the upper extremity, tendon transfers, nerve transplants, and specialized procedures such as opponensplasty can reduce the morbidity of major tumor resections.

9.4.3 Rehabilitation and Prosthetics

The rehabilitation process for amputees begins pre-operatively rather than post-operatively. Prosthetic education and psychosocial support play a large role in patient satisfaction. Many young patients seek and ultimately utilize the latest technology in prosthetics, but for the first 9–12 months of recovery, a more basic prosthesis is often used. Numerous prosthetic adjustments are necessary to optimize fitting and comfort while the stump is healing and attaining a steady state. Although a full discussion of the available prosthetics for all amputation levels is beyond the scope of this chapter, it is important that the surgeon be familiar with the basic principles of prosthetic compatibility and have a close working relationship with a reliable prosthetist.

9.5 Surgical Techniques

9.5.1 Ray Resection and Partial Hand Amputation

The extent of the amputation is largely dependent on the extent of the malignant process. For amputations involving border digits, a teardrop-shaped incision is performed with the apex proximally and along the ulnar or radial side of the hand. The incision is carried through the webspace and the proper digital neurovascular bundle to the adjacent finger is preserved if possible. For a complete ray resection, the metacarpal is disarticulated at the carpometacarpal joint. If more than one border ray is resected, one side of the palmar vascular arches will likely need to be ligated. The vascularity to the hand is not jeopardized because there are two arches (deep and superficial) and each have dual blood supplies (radial and ulnar arteries). Oftentimes with border ray resections, a flap such as a reverse radial forearm flap is needed for soft tissue coverage.

For amputations involving central digits only, a dorsally-based racquet-shaped incision is used. The adjacent proper digital neurovascular bundles are preserved if possible. The intermetacarpal ligament from adjacent digits should be repaired to improve stability of the hand. A closing wedge osteotomy of the distal row of carpal bones at the base of the resected rays can be performed in order to close down the space between the adjacent digits and prevent dropping of small objects.

9.5.2 Transradial and Transhumeral Amputation

The transradial and transhumeral amputations are relatively straightforward procedures. In all instances, maximal length of the stump should be preserved. A fishmouth incision is used. The fascia and muscles are transected as distally as possible to provide ample bony coverage. All neurovascular structures are transected separately. Nerves should be transected under tension and allowed to retract. Using drillholes, the anterior and posterior compartment musculature are myodesed to the end of the bone. A tension-free fascial closure should be endeavored in all cases. Because the skin is highly mobile and well-vascularized in the upper extremity, elevating large subcutaneous flaps to achieve skin coverage is rarely an issue.

9.5.3 Shoulder Disarticulations and Forequarter Amputations

The patient is positioned lateral. An incision is performed in line with the clavicle and carried down into a deltopectoral approach. This incision is carried laterally and posteriorly following the distal border of the deltoid muscle. Posteriorly, this incision is carried in line along the spine of the scapula. To create a fishmouth incision, a second limb of the incision is carried down the lateral chest wall and curved posteriorly to join the first incision.

A standard deltopectoral approach is performed and the deltoid insertion is subperiosteally elevated off the humerus. The pectoralis major, latissimus dorsi and teres major insertions are released off the humerus. The conjoint tendon origin and pectoralis minor insertion on the coracoid process are released. This muscular exposure should reveal the brachial plexus and axillary artery clearly. If more proximal control of the vessels is necessary, these structures should be identified deep to the clavicle. The lateral two-thirds of the clavicle is subperiosteally skeletonized. The clavicle is carefully transected and the lateral two-thirds is removed. The neurovascular bundle is seen clearly emerging from the chest cavity and running over the first rib into the arm.

If the scapula is to be removed, it can be easily dissected posteriorly by raising large subcutaneous flaps and releasing its muscular attachments off the chest wall. If the scapula is to be maintained, the shoulder can be disarticulated at the glenoid, maintaining the acromion for better cosmesis. The deltoid flap is very well-perfused and can simply be folded over the soft tissue defect for closure.

9.5.4 Below Knee Amputation

In an ideal situation, the tibial osteotomy is planned at approximately 15 cm distal to the knee joint line. A long posterior flap approximately 15 cm long is utilized in which the medial edge of the flap is along the posteromedial border of the tibia and the lateral edge of the flap is in line with the fibula. The anterior soft tissue flap is angled 90° from the posterior flap rather than a fishmouth to reduce dog-ears and redundant skin during closure.

After incising the skin, the fascia is incised slightly distally to ensure a tension-free fascial closure. The muscles of the anterior compartment are transected at the same level as the planned tibial osteotomy. The anterior neurovascular bundle is identified. The nerve is transected sharply under tension to allow it to retract, and the artery and vein are ligated separately. Next, the peroneal muscles are transected at the same level.

If a standard below the knee amputation is being performed, the tibia is then osteotomized at the planned level and the fibula osteotomized slightly proximally. If an Ertl or transosseous bone bridge is planned, a sleeve of periosteum should be raised off the tibia distal to the planned resection level and the fibula should be transected about 6–8 cm distal to the tibial level.

The proximal end of the osteotomized distal tibia should be lifted anteriorly, and the deep posterior compartment muscles subperiosteally elevated off the amputated tibia and fibula to the level of the long posterior flap at which point they should be transected. The posterior tibial and fibular vessels can be clamped at this level for temporary control. The deep posterior compartment and soleus muscles are resected, leaving only the gastrocnemius muscles on the posterior flap. The neurovascular structures are transected and ligated at the level of the tibial osteotomy.

If no bone-bridge is planned, the edges of the cut bone should be smoothed down and drill holes placed in the anterior and medial aspects of the tibia. If the patient is skeletally immature, an uncontaminated metatarsal or phalangeal head and neck harvested from the amputated foot can be pressfit into the open canal of the osteotomized tibia to reduce the risk of overgrowth. If a bone-bridge is intended, a high-speed burr should be used to create a slot in the tibia to accept a segment of fibula to be placed between the remaining fibula and the tibia. This segment can be secured with heavy non-absorbable suture through drill holes, an Endobutton®, or screws (Ng and Berlet 2010). A flap of periosteum can be sutured over the fibular segment to improve osseous union.

For closure, non-absorbable suture is run through the gastrocnemius muscle and used to secure it over the front of the tibia through drillholes. The posterior and anterior fascia are sutured together for a tension-free closure. Nylon sutures are used for skin closure. To remove redundant skin and eliminate dog-ears, triangles of skin are removed from each side at the ends of the incision as the wound is progressively closed. A well-padded posterior splint is applied to keep the knee in extension and prevent flexion contractures.

9.5.5 Above Knee Amputation (AKA)

The level of an AKA is largely determined by the location of the pathology, but as a general rule, as much length as possible should be preserved. A fishmouth incision is planned with equal sized anterior or posterior flaps. Depending on the skin available, medial-lateral flaps can be successful as well. The "angle" at the corners of the fishmouth should be very acute to allow preservation of maximal skin. In fact, a guillotine amputation may be performed initially, and once the rest of the limb has been removed, the skin flaps can be fashioned from the guillotined stump by essentially removing dog-ears.

The quadriceps musculature is transected at the level of the anterior flap. The periosteum is subperiosteally elevated back to the level of the bone resection. In order to have enough soft tissues for closure, the femoral osteotomy should be at least 10–12 cm proximal to the extent of the flaps. Approximately 8–10 cm proximal to the superior pole of the patella, the femoral vessels may be found directly posterior to the medial intermuscular septum, diving into the adductor hiatus. These vessels should be carefully dissected and ligated.

After performing the femoral osteotomy, as much length as possible for the adductor musculature should be preserved. The hamstrings are transected at the level of the posterior flap and the sciatic nerve sharply transected under tension. Drillholes should be placed anteriorly and laterally. Large non-absorbable suture should be used to affix the adductors and hamstrings to the femur. The quadriceps are folded over the top and sutured to the hamstrings. If the patient is skeletally immature, a harvested uncontaminated metatarsal or phalangeal head and neck can be pressfit into the end of the femur to reduce overgrowth. The skin is closed with nylons and the stump is wrapped in a well-padded dressing.

9.5.6 Hip Disarticulation

Achieving soft tissue coverage for hip disarticulations and hemipelvectomies can be challenging depending on the location and size of the tumor. The main two workhorse flaps for coverage are anterior and posterior.

For a standard posterior flap hip disarticulation, the patient is positioned supine with a bump under the ipsilateral trunk and a teardrop shaped incision is made with the apex or corner starting near the anterior superior iliac spine. The posterior aspect of the incision wraps around distal to the gluteal musculature. The femoral triangle is explored and the main vessels are ligated separately. All of the anterior and medial compartment muscles are transected near their origin. A circumferential hip capsulotomy is performed and the femur is disarticulated. The gluteal muscles are released at their insertions and are separated from the hamstrings and vastus lateralis. The sciatic nerve is transected proximally under tension. The superior and inferior gluteal vessels are preserved as they are the blood supply for the posterior flap. The posterior flap is folded anteriorly and used to cover the resultant soft tissue defect.

For a standard anterior flap hip disarticulation, the patient is positioned lateral, but held in place loosely by a beanbag such that he or she can be rolled posteriorly to a more supine position for the anterior dissection. The medial incision starts just medial to the femoral vessels proximally and is extended to the medial knee. The greater saphenous vein is ligated and the spermatic cord is protected in males. The femoral vessels are identified, but the integrity of the femoral sheath is maintained. The quadriceps muscles are transected just proximal to the knee and subperiosteally elevated off the anterior femur. The superficial femoral artery is identified and ligated at the level of the adductor hiatus. The lateral incision is performed slightly posterior to the lateral intermuscular septum. As the anterior flap is elevated, the medial plane of dissection is carried out between the vastus medialis and femoral vessels anteriorly and the adductor musculature posteriorly. The sartorius muscle may be sutured over the femoral sheath to help provide coverage posteriorly. The deep femoral artery is ligated as it travels directly posterior to the femur and the multiple perforator vessels are cauterized as they travel laterally. As the flap is elevated proximally and anteriorly, the lateral circumflex vessels and its branches are protected because they are a main blood supply to the anterior flap.

The proximal lateral portion of the incision is angled posteromedially towards the posterior sacral iliac spine at the tip of the greater trochanter, similar to a posterolateral approach to the hip. The muscular insertions are subperiosteally elevated off the proximal femur and a circumferential capsulotomy is performed. The ligamentum teres is transected and the femur is disarticulated. The anterior flap is brought posteriorly to cover the resultant soft tissue defect.

9.5.7 Pediatric Amputations

Special considerations are required for amputations in patients less than 10 years old compared to adolescents and adults (Rab 2001; Cummings and Kapp 1992). First, all physes should be preserved if possible to allow for continued longitudinal growth of the stump. An acceptable length femoral stump in an 8-year old child may not be adequate to support a prosthesis once the patient grows into a full-grown adult due to the loss of the distal physis which provides the majority of femoral length. Second, disarticulations are advantageous in pediatric amputations because it prevents terminal overgrowth, allows for an end-bearing stump, and retains adequate shape to the stump as the child grows. In adults, disarticulations are bulbous and difficult to fit for prostheses. In children, transosseous amputations tend to become conical and rotationally unstable for prostheses while disarticulations develop into well-shaped stumps. Third, preservation of the proximal fibula, even if very short, is advantageous for below-knee amputations. The additional width of the stump allows for more effective prosthetic fitting. Fourth, parents should be forewarned that terminal overgrowth is very common, particularly in transhumeral and below-knee amputations, and that multiple revisions of bony prominences may be necessary. The exact mechanism is unclear and there is no highly reliable method to prevent it. Fifth, superior healing capacity in children allow for success in using creative wound closure techniques that would likely not work in adults. Retaining maximal bone length is recommended despite tenuous soft tissue coverage is recommended, even if the use of split-thickness skin grafts is necessary.

9.6 Summary

The surgical management of pediatric bone sarcomas remains a challenge. Limb-sparing surgery can be achieved in 90 % of cases, but only in cases where survival of the patient is not diminished compared to amputation and where the reconstructed limb affords a good functional outcome. Many options exist for the reconstruction and are tailored to the individual patient. Amputation is still the best option for some patients and with the progress made in prosthesis design and durable and functional outcome can be achieved in many patients.

References

Beebe K, Benevenia J, Kaushal N et al (2010) Evaluation of a noninvasive expandable prosthesis in musculoskeletal oncology patients for the upper and lower limb. Orthopedics 33:396

Bosmans JC, Geertzen JH, Post WJ et al (2010) Factors associated with phantom limb pain: a 3 1/2 year prospective study. Clin Rehabil 24:444–453

Cammisa FPJ, Glasser DB, Otis JC et al (1990) The Van Nes tibial rotationplasty. A functionally viable reconstructive procedure in children who have a tumor of the distal end of the femur. J Bone Joint Surg Am 72:1541–1547

Chen CM, Disa JJ, Lee HY et al (2007) Reconstruction of extremity long bone defects after sarcoma resection with vascularized fibula flaps: a 10-year review. Plast Reconstr Surg 119:915–924; discussion 925–926

Choong PF, Sim FH (1997) Limb-sparing surgery for bone tumors: new developments. Semin Surg Oncol 13:64–69

Cummings DR, Kapp SL (1992) Lower-limb pediatric prosthetics: general considerations and philosophy. J Pediatr Orthop 4:196

Damron TA (1997) Endoprosthetic replacement following limb-sparing resection for bone sarcoma. Semin Surg Oncol 13:3–10

Dicaprio MR, Friedlaender GE (2003) Malignant bone tumors: limb sparing versus amputation. J Am Acad Orthop Surg 11:25–37

Foo LS, Hardes J, Henrichs M et al (2011) Surgical difficulties encountered with use of modular endoprosthesis for limb preserving salvage of failed allograft reconstruction after malignant tumor resection. J Arthroplasty 26:744–750

Guillon MA, Mary PM, Brugiere L et al (2011) Clinical characteristics and prognosis of osteosarcoma in young children: a retrospective series of 15 cases. BMC Cancer 11:407

Henderson ER, Pepper AM, Marulanda G et al (2012) Outcome of lower-limb preservation with an expandable endoprosthesis after bone tumor resection in children. J Bone Joint Surg Am 94:537–547

Jaffe N (2014) Historical perspective on the introduction and use of chemotherapy for the treatment of osteosarcoma. Adv Exp Med Biol 804:1–30

Krane EJ, Heller LB (1995) The prevalence of phantom sensation and pain in pediatric amputees. J Pain Symptom Manag 10:21–29

Li J, Wang Z, Pei GX et al (2011) Biological reconstruction using massive bone allograft with intramedullary vascularized fibular flap after intercalary resection of humeral malignancy. J Surg Oncol 104:244–249

Mankin, HJ, Gebhardt, MC, Jennings, LC et al (1996) Long-term results of allograft replacement in the management of bone tumors. Clin Orthop Relat Res (324):86–97

Miller BJ, Virkus WW (2010) Intercalary allograft reconstructions using a compressible intramedullary nail: a preliminary report. Clin Orthop Relat Res 468:2507–2513

Morgan HD, Cizik AM, Leopold SS et al (2006) Survival of tumor megaprostheses replacements about the knee. Clin Orthop Relat Res 450:39–45

Muscolo DL, Ayerza MA, Aponte-Tinao L et al (2008) Allograft reconstruction after sarcoma resection in children younger than 10 years old. Clin Orthop Relat Res 466:1856–1862

Ng VY, Berlet GC (2010) Evolving techniques in foot and ankle amputation. J Am Acad Orthop Surg 18:223–235

Ng VY, Scharschmidt TJ, Mayerson JL et al (2013) Incidence and survival in sarcoma in the United States: a focus on musculoskeletal lesions. Anticancer Res 33:2597–2604

Rab GT (2001) Principles of amputation in children. In: Chapman MW (ed) Chapman's orthopaedic surgery, 3rd edn. Lippincott Williams & Wilkins, Philadelphia

Scully SP, Ghert MA, Zurakowski D et al (2002) Pathologic fracture in osteosarcoma: prognostic importance and treatment implications. J Bone Joint Surg Am 84-A:49–57

Weisstein JS, Goldsby RE, O'donnell RJ (2005) Oncologic approaches to pediatric limb preservation. J Am Acad Orthop Surg 13:544–554

Wilkins RM, Camozzi AB, Gitelis SB (2005) Reconstruction options for pediatric bone tumors about the knee. J Knee Surg 18:305–309

Ziegler-Graham K, Mackenzie EJ, Ephraim PL et al (2008) Estimating the prevalence of limb loss in the United States: 2005 to 2050. Arch Phys Med Rehabil 89:422–429

Rehabilitation Following Orthopaedic Surgery in Children with Bone Tumors

10

Michelle A. Miller and Nathan Rosenberg

Contents

10.1	**Functional Assessment**	156
10.2	**Pre-surgical Treatment**	156
10.3	**Post-surgical Rehabilitation**	156
10.3.1	Ablation	156
10.3.2	Limb Salvage	161
10.3.3	School and Community Re-entry	163
10.4	**Functional Impairments Related to Chemotherapy**	167
10.5	**Aging Following Limb Salvage or Acquired Amputation**	168
References		169

Abstract

Bone tumors and associated interventions can lead to a decrease in a child's function in areas of mobility and activities of daily living. The degree of impairment can vary from complete dependence for these activities to subtle biomechanical changes that limit extracurricular participation. Rehabilitation efforts are directed at restoration of function and quality of life in children with new functional impairments. This chapter discusses the initial functional evaluation, the functional impact of different surgical interventions, the functional impact of chemotherapy and radiation, and functional considerations as the child ages. Some of the available rehabilitation options including prosthetics, bracing, therapy, and equipment are reviewed as well as the recommended education for families and patients regarding the rehabilitation process.

Bone tumors and associated interventions can lead to a decrease in a child's function in areas of mobility and activities of daily living. The degree of impairment can vary from complete dependence for these activities to subtle biomechanical changes that limit extracurricular participation. Rehabilitation efforts are directed at restoration of function and quality of life in children with new functional impairments.

M.A. Miller, MD (✉) • N. Rosenberg, MD
Department of Physical Medicine,
Nationwide Children's Hospital, 700 Children's
Drive, Columbus, OH 43205, USA
e-mail: Michelle.miller@nationwidechildrens.org;
Nathan.rosenberg@nationwidechildrens.org

© Springer International Publishing Switzerland 2015
T.P. Cripe, N.D. Yeager (eds.), *Malignant Pediatric Bone Tumors - Treatment & Management*,
Pediatric Oncology, DOI 10.1007/978-3-319-18099-1_10

10.1 Functional Assessment

Prior to the initiation of treatment, a history and physical examination pertaining to function should be obtained to determine if any pre-existing impairments exist. This assessment includes an evaluation of the child's capabilities in regards to mobility (transfers, standing, sitting, rolling, kneeling, walking, and running), basic activities of daily living (ADLs – grooming, toileting, dressing, and bathing), and higher level ADLs (cooking, household chores, education, driving and employment). A strength and range of motion examination including an assessment of core strength will help determine which rehabilitation interventions may be beneficial prior to surgery, chemotherapy or radiation.

Similarly, a complete assessment of function, range of motion, and strength should be completed after any surgical intervention. A detailed understanding of the surgical intervention including the site, any compromise of the neurovascular or muscular systems, and the time needed for wound and/or bone healing is necessary. Timing and plans for chemotherapy and/or radiation should also be reviewed.

For example, the time until first prosthetic fitting after surgery in an uncomplicated situation is regularly greater than 2 months (So et al. 2014). This estimation does not take into account the time required after a prosthesis is obtained for adjustments of the prosthesis and gait training. Such a time course often comes as a surprise to patients who anticipate a quicker return to ambulation. For this reason, detailed education regarding prosthetic devices, assistive devices and bracing sets appropriate expectations and helps facilitate subsequent adjustment. Functional impairment after limb salvage surgery also persists for many months and frequently many years following surgery (Marina et al. 2013). Even though an intact limb is present, patients exhibit loss of strength, decreased range of motion and associated biomechanical gait changes. Aggressive therapy early during the limb salvage treatment course has been associated with better outcomes (Ham et al. 1998). For these reasons, anticipatory guidance and physiatrist assessment should be provided both before and after surgical intervention to ensure that the maximum functional potential is reached.

10.2 Pre-surgical Treatment

Although rehabilitation specialists may not always be consulted prior to surgery, and most of their efforts are usually focused on post-surgical recovery a "prehabilitation" course including a focused strength and range of motion program can be beneficial in reducing post-surgical functional complications. Additionally, a thorough social history can be helpful in determining whether amputation or limb salvage is most appropriate. Successful utilization of a prosthetic limb requires a great deal of patience, social support and availability of financial resources (Horgan and Maclachlan 2004). Home accessibility and the ability to attend frequent prosthetist and outpatient therapy appointments should be considered.

Providing anticipatory guidance prior to surgical intervention can be beneficial for patients, families and caregivers. A thorough description of prospective timelines for functional progression helps with planning and with reducing anxiety.

10.3 Post-surgical Rehabilitation

Post-surgical rehabilitation treatment should be individualized based on the tumor location, the surgical intervention, the developmental level of the child, planned radiation or chemotherapy, comorbidities, and the child's and family's goals. Common sequelae after surgery may include phantom sensation, phantom pain or neuropathic pain, musculoskeletal pain, loss of range of motion, weakness, and delayed wound healing. Surgical interventions may be roughly divided into ablation and limb-salvage procedures.

10.3.1 Ablation

The term "ablation" includes amputations and rotationplasty of the knee which are described in detail in Chap. 9. The most common areas of involvement are the proximal humerus, the pelvis, the proximal femur, the distal femur and the proximal tibia. Amputations at these levels include the forequarter, shoulder disarticulation, proximal transhumeral, hemipelvectomy, transfemoral, knee disarticulation, and transtibial locations, respectively. The decision to proceed with amputation or limb salvage requires careful consideration with regard to tumor treatment and remission, function, and patient and family preferences. The initial goals following surgery are pain management, edema control, wound healing, prevention of contracture formation and initiation of radiation and/or chemotherapies.

Phantom sensation and phantom pain are common when the nerves must be sacrificed or are compromised during an amputation. Phantom sensation is the feeling that the limb or part of the limb is still present. For example, a child may complain that their ankle itches on the side of a transfemoral amputation. Having the child scratch the corresponding area on the unaffected limb may help alleviate the feeling noted. Gentle reassurance and education for the child and family regarding this phenomenon is all that is typically necessary.

Phantom pain is thought to be due to hyperexcitability of the severed or injured nerve. It presents as burning, cramping or aching dysesthetic pain in the amputated portion of the limb and is more intense at night (Dillingham et al. 2002). Multiple interventions have been described in the literature for relief including medications such as gabapentin, anticonvulsants, tricyclic antidepressants, and nerve blocks. Modalities such as transcutaneous nerve stimulation may be helpful as well as massage and different types of tactile stimuli to desensitize the limb. The desensitization techniques should optimally be performed for 20–30 min three times a day as tolerated by the skin and scar (Ganz et al. 2008). Phantom pain should be differentiated from stump pain due to a neuroma or scar entrapment of the nerve. The pain is similar in nature, but is often elicited by tapping over the affected nerve. Anesthetic blocks in the area and scar massage may be helpful. Musculoskeletal pain is typically managed with scheduled opiates or nonsteroidal anti-inflammatory drugs (NSAIDs). However, it should be remembered that NSAIDs may delay bone healing, which is especially relevant

with rotationplasty and limb salvage surgery. Controlling the pain and residual limb edema facilitates range of motion exercises and manipulation of the residual limb. These activities help prevent contracture formation. Contractures are not fully reversible and significantly impair long term function. It is critical to begin mobilization as early as possible.

Preparation of the residual limb for a prosthetic device begins as soon after surgery as possible. The goal is to have a limb which is tapered with a cylindrical shape; has a mobile, nonadherent, well-placed suture line; and is tolerant of external pressure. These features may be achieved with a removable, rigid or semi-rigid postoperative dressing, ace wrapping or shrinkers (see Figs. 10.1 and 10.2). These pressure dressings help to decrease edema and pain. The skin should be checked frequently for any signs of breakdown or infection and the dressings must be changed frequently as the limb remodels. Care must be taken when applying ace wraps so that there is a gradient with the highest pressure distally and the lowest proximally. Typically, shrinkers are not used until the surgical incision is well-healed and staples/sutures are removed

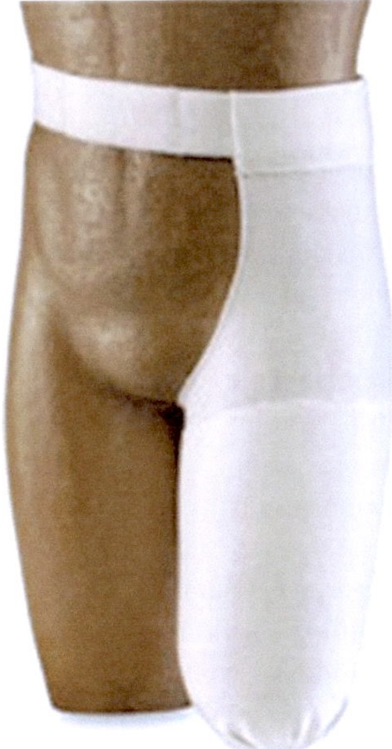

Fig. 10.1 Fabric shrinker for a transfemoral amputation. There is a pressure gradient to move the fluid from the distal tip proximally

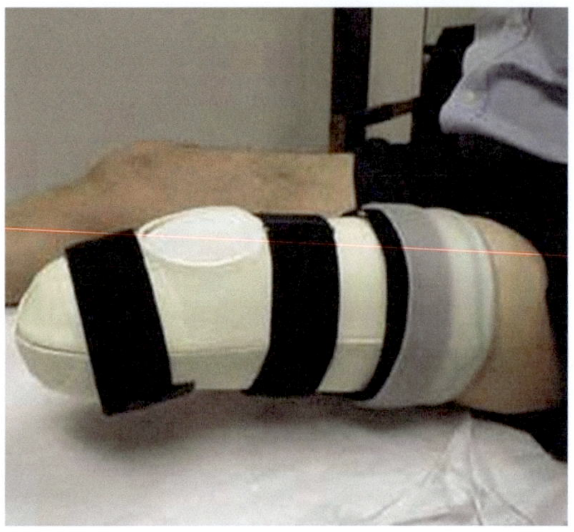

Fig. 10.2 A removable semi-rigid post-operative dressing. This is placed immediately post-operatively to assist with wound healing, molding of the residual limb, pain, and early mobilization

because there is significant shear across the incision when donning or doffing the shrinker.

Preprosthetic training begins as soon as surgical clearance is given and continues until prosthetic fitting is completed. Prosthetic fabrication and fitting ideally should be completed within 4–8 weeks after surgery. Early prosthetic fitting in the upper limb is important, because prosthetic acceptance declines if fitting is delayed beyond the third postoperative month (Fleming et al. 1999). Unfortunately, prosthetic fitting is often delayed in the oncology population due to delayed wound healing secondary to radiation and chemotherapies. So et al. reported a median of 230.5 days until definitive prosthetic fitting in their study of children who had rotationplasty of the knee and required chemotherapy (So et al. 2014). Preprosthetic training helps the child and family transition to prosthetic use and maintains motivation.

Amputation results in a loss of body symmetry, which creates imbalances around the shoulder girdle in transhumeral amputees and around the pelvis with lower limb amputees. Balance in sitting, standing and walking must be relearned. In addition, there may be muscle imbalances around the proximal joint depending on the level of the amputation.

In the upper limb this imbalance results in shoulder elevation and scapula rotation on the affected side. In the lower limb, the anterior superior iliac spine is higher on the affected side and the center of gravity is laterally displaced over the unaffected side. Abnormal and compensatory patterns of movement must be evaluated and adjusted as needed. Patients begin to relearn body position with observing and correcting static postures in the mirror. The amputee is encouraged to use muscle memory to relearn correct postural and limb positioning control (Ganz et al. 2008). As residual limb mobilization progresses, training is focused on recognizing the abnormal postures and positioning that occur with basic ADLs and mobility.

In upper limb amputees, ADLs are mastered with one hand and, when appropriate, with the use of adaptive equipment such as a reacher, sock aide, long handled sponge, and a rocker knife to cut meat. The child progresses from independence with basic hygiene to the advanced ADLs as age appropriate. Hand dominance is retrained when necessary, especially with handwriting and keyboarding. Repetitive tasks can be used for strengthening. These tasks include fine motor exercises with pegs, beads and theraputty, as well as gross motor exercises with equipment and mirrors. Isometric exercises are effective in creating muscle bulk for stabilization of the limb in the socket of the prosthesis if the residual limb is long enough. The stability of the prosthesis depends on both the bulk of the stabilizing musculature and the child's ability to voluntarily vary residual limb configuration. Because balance is the often disrupted in a new amputee, the goals should include strengthening of the trunk, core, and lower limbs using isometric exercise and aerobic training. For the child with a transhumeral amputation, active assisted range of motion (AAROM) should be done daily at the shoulder. For the child with a transfemoral amputation, maintaining range of motion at the hip is critical and for the child with a transtibial amputation, range of motion must be aggressively pursued at the hip and the knee. The knee is typically kept in full extension except when in therapy. The loss of range of motion and subsequent contracture has significant impact on the fit of the prosthesis and the function of that limb. Bed mobility and getting up from the bed to a chair should begin on post-op day 1. A physical therapist can then begin working on sitting, standing,

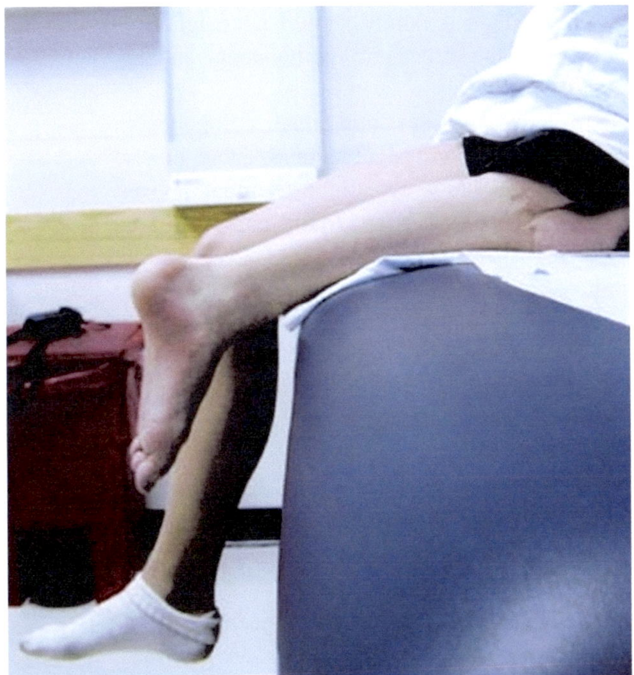

Fig. 10.3 A rotationplasty uses the intact foot and ankle to create a functional knee join

and ambulation skills. For the lower limb amputee, training is also needed in the use of a wheelchair and any assistive devices such as a walker or crutches. In addition, a tub bench is generally recommended for showering, given the residual balance difficulties and levels of fatigue.

Children with tumor involvement of the knee may decide to undergo rotationplasty in which the tibia with the attached foot and ankle are rotated 180° and attached to the femur (see Fig. 10.3). The ankle then takes on the role of the knee joint. The upper leg initially must be immobilized to allow healing of the osteotomy site. Range of motion at the ankle to increase plantar flexion and muscle re-education of the ankle is started once there is adequate soft tissue healing. To achieve "knee" extension, the child must plantarflex the ankle and to achieve "knee" flexion, the child must dorsiflex the ankle. Full weight-bearing may be initiated once there is complete healing of the osteotomy site. The initial prosthesis often allows room for the foot to extend outside of the socket and bypasses the knee so that knee flexion is not allowed. As the flexibility of the ankle improves, the foot can be contained within the prosthesis (So et al. 2014). Over time, patients can learn these skills quite effectively and even be able to run.

Describing the planned prosthesis, premyoelectric testing and training, and defining the prosthetic expectations of the child and family are all important tasks for the team during the pre-prosthetic period. If a myoelectric prosthesis is being considered, early site testing and training are needed. The residual limb is evaluated by a specially trained occupational therapist for the best sites for placement of the electrodes. The occupational therapist needs to work closely with the physician and prosthetist in the design of the socket and optimal electrode site placement. Motor training is done to increase muscle activity at specific sites using biofeedback. This training may be very difficult in the short trans-humeral amputee due to the paucity of muscle and may change if there is muscle atrophy from radiation therapy. Once isolated movements are mastered, proportional control of the muscle is learned, which controls the speed and force of the prosthetic movements. Advances in prosthetic design have improved hand functionality through myoelectric control with individual actuation of the fingers. In addition, research continues in developing an interface between the brain and the prosthesis which can bypass the need for muscle activation of the electrodes.

The child and family should be taught the names of the prosthetic components in the planned prosthesis.

Teaching includes individual components, such as the figure-of-eight harness, cable, elbow unit or elbow hinge, wrist unit, terminal device, hook or hand, socket, knee unit, and foot. The type of suspension should be reviewed and the indications for socks to improve fit and allow for growth in the socket. Once the prosthesis arrives, these areas should be reviewed as well as the expectations of the child/adolescent with a new limb loss and the family. Often these expectations for function are unrealistic, especially in the upper limb. It is helpful to reinforce the supportive roles the prosthesis will play in cosmesis, gross task and object stabilization, push, and assistive function. A child's acceptance of the prosthesis is significantly impacted by the family's opinion of the prosthesis. In addition, care for the residual limb, care for the prosthesis, and potential pitfalls with the prosthesis such as pistoning and misalignment should be reviewed with the child and family.

Each prosthesis is unique and customized to the individual's needs and body habitus. There are four categories of upper limb prosthetic systems: the passive system, the body-powered system, the externally powered system, and the hybrid system. There are two categories of lower limb prosthetic systems: the passive system and the body-powered system. Each child's functional goals, extra-curricular activities and lifestyle, geographic location, anticipated environmental exposures, access to prosthetists for maintenance, and financial resources need to be considered in choosing a system. A passive system is primarily cosmetic and often used with forequarter amputees as a stabilizer, for example. A passive system is fabricated for the child who does not have enough strength or movement to control a prosthesis or uses a prosthesis only for cosmesis. A body-powered system prosthesis uses the child's residual limb strength and range of motion to control the prosthesis. An externally powered system uses an outside power source such as a battery to operate the prosthesis. A hybrid system combines the body-powered system and the externally powered sys-

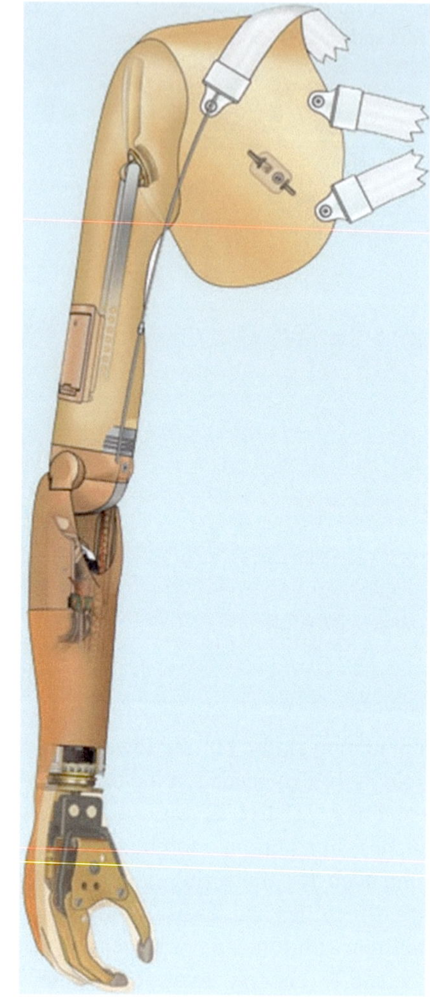

Fig. 10.4 An example of a hybrid system is a body-powered elbow joint with an externally powered terminal device

tem. An example of a hybrid system is a body-powered elbow joint with an externally powered terminal device (see Fig. 10.4).

A short transhumeral amputation which occurs proximal to the insertion of the deltoid muscle is a prosthetic challenge. Body-powered control is achieved by scapular motion with assistance from the humerus. In this case, strength and leverage are reduced and cable-powered prosthetic control is severely limited. Up to 5 in. of total excursion of scapular motion is required to open the terminal device with the elbow in the fully flexed position (Bray 1989). A transhumeral prosthesis uses two control cables. One of these cables flexes the elbow and operates the terminal device. The other cable is used to lock and unlock the elbow. Shoulder flexion applies tension to the cable, causing the elbow to flex and the terminal device to open or close depending on how it is set up. To lock the elbow in flexion, the shoulder joint must be extended and abducted at the same time. A "figure-of-eight" body harness can be worn with a transhumeral prosthesis so that the contralateral shoulder can assist to operate the cables and give the child more power and control of the prosthesis.

The cables are eliminated in myoelectric prostheses. They are more comfortable, have a more natural appearance, and provide more precise hand functions with much less effort as compared to body-powered prostheses. However, they tend to be heavier. Suction suspension is possible for the transhumeral level if the residual limb is long enough. The subsequent decrease in harnessing decreases the load on the contralateral axilla. This can reduce the pressure on the contralateral brachial plexus and joints, enhance proprioception, and improve myoelectric contact. Research is now investigating prosthetic implants similar to the dental implants currently in use which would eliminate the need for harnessing and external suspension systems. Suction suspension is usually not possible in residual limbs with recent skin grafts, excessively bulbous distal ends, excessive redundant tissue, or significant adherent distal scarring which is painful.

Lower limb prostheses are not as complex since the fine motor manipulation required of the upper limb is not a factor in the lower limb. However, due to the weight-bearing and constant impact forces through the lower limb, the prosthesis and the joints must be durable, lightweight, and have adequate suspension. Table 10.1 lists some of the prostheses available for the different levels of amputation seen in the population. Functionally, children with a rotationplasty or a transtibial amputation do very well. Energy expenditure to walk the same distance as peers without an amputation increases by only 7 %. This increases to 25 % in the transfemoral group (Waters and Mulroy 1999). With age, the energy expenditure differ-ence will increase between the amputee group and the non-amputee group.

10.3.2 Limb Salvage

Limb-sparing procedures have become possible because of advances in imaging, reconstructive surgery, microsurgery, chemotherapy and radiation therapy. As these procedures became more widely utilized by the 1970s, they replaced surgical amputation in preference (Marcove et al. 1970). Upper and lower limb characteristics are different and must be kept in mind when considering the optimal surgical intervention. Since the upper limb is non–weight-bearing and tumors typically present in the proximal humerus for example, distal function can be maintained even with significant sensory impairment following a limb-sparing procedure. Interestingly, the literature does not show a significant difference in quality of life or functional outcomes between limb salvage and ablative surgery groups with malignant bone tumors of the lower limb (Bekkering et al. 2012).

Research has demonstrated that the 70–85 % of malignant tumors treated by limb salvage do not have a significantly different oncologic result (Van Hoesel et al. 2003). The goal is to preserve function, prevent tumor recurrence, improve cosmesis, and enable the rapid administration of chemotherapy or radiation therapy. Initial endoprosthetics replaced the involved bone entirely. Advances in technology now offer expandable and modular options. These are particular helpful in children who are still growing.

The complication rate is much higher after limb salvage than after amputation in the oncology population and must be a factor in their rehabilitation plan. Early complications include infection, wound necrosis, and nerve injury. Late complications include aseptic loosening, prosthetic fracture and dislocation, and graft nonunion (Benevenia et al. 2004).

Frieden et al. reported that early mobilization and gait training in addition to periodic hospitalizations for lengthening of the prosthesis were some of the important factors for successful rehabilitation (Freiden et al. 1993). In 2013, Shehadeh et al.

Table 10.1 Prosthetic options for the different levels of amputation

Level of amputation	Prosthesis	Functional capabilities	Other considerations
Forequarter	Sculpted insert	None	Provides symmetry at the shoulders to improve fit and drape of clothing
Forequarter/shoulder disarticulation	Lightweight passive prosthesis	None	Provides balance to the trunk and cosmesis
Forequarter/shoulder disarticulation	Hybrid forequarter prosthesis	Myoelectrics may control the elbow and/or the hand or a cable system may be used to control the hand (terminal device)	Very heavy and bulky The size of the socket needed for suspension tends to trap heat in the trunk.
Proximal transhumeral	Myoelectric prosthesis	Myoelectrics give elbow flexion and extension and can power the hand for grip, pronation and supination. Shoulder flexion and extension are often limited by the length of the amputation and if the deltoid is present and usable	Very heavy and bulky
Proximal transhumeral	Body powered prosthesis	Uses a cable system (often 2 cables) to control the elbow and the terminal device	Lighter than the myoelectrics, but requires good contralateral strength
Proximal transhumeral	Hybrid prosthesis	Provides battery powered elbow flexion and extension. The individual will open and close the terminal device using contralateral shoulder movements with a cable system	Often combines a myoelectric elbow with and a cable driven terminal device
Hemipelvectomy	Hemipelvectomy socket with anterior hip joint, knee joint and SACH (solid ankle cushion heel) foot	Provides support for standing, transfers and walking	Alignment must be carefully adjusted to prevent the prosthetic knee from buckling. Prosthetic side should be shorter in length to allow for clearance when swinging the leg in walking
Transfemoral	Quadrilateral or Ischial containment socket with prosthetic knee and either an energy storing foot or a SACH foot	Can walk independently though speed will be decreased	Energy expenditure may increase from 25–87 % for walking
Knee disarticulation	Socket with a prosthetic knee and either an energy storing foot or a SACH foot	Walks without difficulty, though cadence may be asymmetric, Walking speed will be slower.	Knee height may be difficult to match due to the size of the prosthetic knee
Transtibial (below knee)	BKA prosthesis with either an energy storing foot or a SACH foot	Walks without difficulty, but mild increase in energy expenditure of 7 %	Active children tend to prefer the energy storing foot which provides better push off

The child's size and strength will determine if myoelectric prostheses are an option. The myoelectric prosthesis is heavy and bulky as well as expensive published a standardized approach to rehabilitation of the individual undergoing limb sparing surgery for sarcomas (Shehadah et al. 2013). He noted improvement in patient outcome as measured by the Musculoskeletal Tumor Society-International Symposium on the Limb Salvage (MSTS-ISOL) scoring system. Although the MSTS has some limitations in evaluating function and physical activity, a standardized approach to therapy based on the surgery performed and the site and size of the tumor is warranted.

For the child who has undergone surgical intervention involving the proximal humerus or the shoulder girdle, initial treatment should include immobilization of the shoulder to allow the grafts and prosthetic to heal. Exercises for the hand and active assisted range of motion (AAROM) of the elbow can be initiated. Full elbow extension should be avoided to protect the insertions of the elbow flexor musculature. Strengthening and active range of motion (AROM) of the trunk and the non-operative limbs should also be instituted to prevent deconditioning. Performing basic ADLs such as brushing teeth, combing hair and washing the face with the unaffected upper limb can bring some normalcy and independence to the daily routine. Functional activities such as feeding oneself, handwriting and keyboarding as well as fine motor skills should be assessed and occupational therapy initiated if there are deficits and especially if the dominant hand is affected. After post-op day 10, the sling can be removed to allow for gentle Codman exercises. Active hand and elbow strengthening should proceed, but postpone full elbow extension exercises until after week 4. If there has been scapular replacement, then commence scapulothoracic movement exercises after week 4. ADLs such as dressing and bathing should be addressed within the second week post-op. Modifications in technique can be taught and the need for adaptive equipment such as a reacher or a long handled sponge assessed. If the wound has not healed sufficiently or other medical concerns such as an accessed port arise, bathing in a tub or shower may need to be postponed. The sling may be discontinued after week 6 and AAROM of the shoulder begun (Shehadah et al. 2013). Serletti et al. using the Enneking Outcome Measurement Scale, reported the functional outcome as "excel-lent" or "good" in greater than 70 % of the patients who had reconstruction after resection of limb sarcomas (Serletti et al. 1998).

In the lower limb, a similar progression with initial immobilization of the affected joint followed by strengthening and weight bearing is indicated. Tables 10.2, 10.3, and 10.4 list the progression in assessment, rehabilitation and education for the lower limb sparing surgical procedures. Multiple studies have demonstrated long term impairments in the child's gait, strength, ADL performance, and ability to progress from sit to stand (Gerber et al. 2006; Beebe et al. 2009). The deficits in strength were oftentimes noted in bilateral limbs and did not necessarily involve the operative field area. Gait speed was significantly slower and there was increased time spent in stance phase on the side which had not had surgery. Range of motion tended to be reduced at the hip and knee in children with tumors presenting in the distal femur and proximal tibia (Beebe et al. 2009). This finding supports the need for ongoing functional assessments and therapeutic interventions. In a separate study of physical activity, Götte et al. noted significantly lower physical activity in children with bone tumors hospitalized for chemotherapy compared to children with other types of cancer. They spent the majority of their time in bed while in the hospital. An exercise program was recommended during these hospital stays to improve wellness and prevent deconditioning and secondary complications (Götte et al. 2014).

10.3.3 School and Community Re-entry

Careful planning and education regarding school and community re-entry should be completed prior to discharge from the hospital. Chemotherapy and risk of infection may preclude a child from attending school routinely. It is strongly recommended that the child have some interaction with his or her peers for socialization and emotional support. This may be through on line schooling, video conferencing or sharing of written work. Often, the child will benefit from tutors from the school in the home setting when they are not able to attend. Some school districts may also provide

Table 10.2 Rehabilitation following pelvic resection (Shehadah et al. 2013)

	Goals	Post-op day 1–3	Post-op day 3 to week 6	Post-op >6 weeks	Family education
Pelvic resection of the iliac bone (Type I)	Heal abdominopelvic musculature under minimal tension Minimal decrease in hip function with normal knee and ankle function Independent with basic ADLs	Keep the ipsilateral lower limb suspended in 30° hip flexion and abduction Consult PT and OT for upper limb range of motion and positioning	Fit with hip abductor brace placing ipsilateral lower limb fixed in 30° hip abduction Weight-bearing as tolerated (WBAT) for all transfers and ambulation Propel wheelchair AROM of knee and ankle with strengthening Work on ADLs and assess for adaptive equipment Generalized strengthening for the upper limbs and unaffected lower limb	Discontinue hip abduction brace and start active hip abductor strengthening Continue to assess and strengthen the ipsilateral knee and ankle musculature and the contralateral lower limb musculature Use assistive device for ambulation until hip abduction strength is regained	Bracing needs and requirements Precautions for range of motion Wound healing Signs and symptoms of neuropathy Adaptive equipment Energy expenditure and fatigue School and community reentry
Pelvic resection of the acetabulum with reconstruction (Type II)		Keep the ipsilateral lower limb suspended in 30° hip flexion and abduction Consult PT and OT for upper limb range of motion and positioning	Fit with hip abductor brace placing ipsilateral lower limb in fixed 30° hip abduction and 0–60° hip flexion Touch-toe weight-bearing (TTWB) in brace for transfers and ambulation. If hip abductor muscles are intact, then may be partial weight-bearing (PWB) with the brace AROM and strengthening of the ipsilateral knee and ankle musculature Work on ADLs and assess for adaptive equipment Generalized strengthening for the upper limbs and unaffected lower limb	Discontinue hip abduction brace and start active hip abductor and flexor strengthening Advance to WBAT for ambulation with an assistive device	Adaptive recreation and leisure interests
Pelvic resection of the pubic bone (Type III)		Consult PT and OT for upper limb, knee, and ankle range of motion May start bed-to-chair transfers	WBAT for transfers and ambulation with an assistive device After 7 days, begin active hip range of motion and strengthening on the ipsilateral side Work on ADLs and assess for adaptive equipment Generalized strengthening for the upper limbs and unaffected lower limb	Continue to work on strengthening and conditioning of all muscle groups	

Table 10.3 Rehabilitation following proximal and distal femur replacement (Shehadah et al. 2013)

	Goals	Post-op day 1–3	Post-op day 4 to week 6	Post-op >6 weeks	Family education
Proximal or total femur resection and replacement	Prevent hip dislocation Independent with ambulation but uses a wheelchair for longer distances Independent with basic ADLs	Immobilize knee with a rigid knee immobilizer or long leg cast for total femur Keep leg suspended in 30° of abduction and flexion Consult PT and OT Start basic ADLs in bed Begin AAROM ankle and exercises	May discontinue the knee immobilizer for the total femur at week 2 and begin active assisted knee flexion exercises Work on abductor strengthening of the affected limb Ambulate with an assistive device, TTWB on the affected limb and in a brace which is locked into 30° of abduction and allows only 0-60° of flexion Work on ADLs and assess for adaptive equipment Generalized strengthening for the upper limbs and unaffected lower limb	May remove hip brace once active hip abduction is demonstrated and begin full weight-bearing Continue to assess and strengthen the ipsilateral distal musculature and the contralateral lower limb musculature Wean away from an assistive device for ambulation	Bracing needs and requirements Precautions for range of motion at the hip and knee Wound healing Signs and symptoms of neuropathy Adaptive equipment Energy expenditure and fatigue School and community reentry Adaptive recreation and leisure skills
Distal Femur resection	Active knee movement of 0–90° Independent with ambulation Independent with basic ADLs	Use knee immobilizer Keep leg elevated for edema control Start isometric exercises for the quadriceps and hamstrings Consult PT and OT May start bed-to-chair transfers but non-weight bearing through the affected limb	If cemented prosthesis, begin WBAT with knee immobilizer If prosthesis is not cemented, then PWB with the knee immobilizer Begin isometric quadriceps strengthening At week 2, begin knee AAROM if the skin is healed D/C knee brace when patient is able to do a straight leg raise (SLR) against gravity Begin hamstring strengthening at week 2 and full weight-bearing Assess ADLs at the wheelchair and standing levels Order adaptive equipment as needed such as a reacher, long-handled sponge, or shoe horn Generalized strengthening for the upper limbs and unaffected lower limb	Concentric and eccentric knee strengthening Aggressive range of motion of the knee Continue to assess and strengthen the ipsilateral distal musculature and the contralateral lower limb musculature Wean away from an assistive device for ambulation	Same as above If knee flexion is less than 60° at 6 months post-op, may need manipulation under anesthesia or surgical release

Table 10.4 Rehabilitation following proximal tibia replacement (Shehadah et al. 2013)

	Goals	Post-op day 1–5	Post-op day 5 to week 6	Post-op >6 weeks	Family education
Proximal tibia resection and replacement	Full active knee extension without any extension lag Independent with all ambulation Independent with basic ADLs	Immobilize knee with a rigid knee immobilizer or long leg cast Keep leg elevated to control for swelling Consult PT and OT Allow weight-bearing on leg as tolerated Work on transfers to and from the wheelchair Propel wheelchair Start basic ADLs at the wheelchair level or in bed Begin AAROM ankle exercises	Keep knee in immobilizer to allow for healing Work on isometric quadriceps strengthening of the affected limb Ambulate with an assistive device, bearing weight through the leg as tolerated Work on ADLs and assess for adaptive equipment Generalized strengthening for the upper limbs and unaffected lower limb	Begin passive and gentle AAROM of the affected knee with goal of 90° Continue to assess and strengthen the ipsilateral hip musculature and the contralateral lower limb musculature Begin concentric and eccentric strengthening of the quadriceps and hamstrings once cleared by the surgeon Wean away from an assistive device for ambulation	Bracing needs and requirements Precautions for range of motion Wound healing Signs and symptoms of neuropathy Adaptive equipment Energy expenditure and fatigue School and community reentry

therapy services while the child is on home instruction such as speech therapy, occupational therapy and physical therapy to work on school-related ADLs and mobility. The impairments are assessed through a multi-factored evaluation (MFE) completed by the school and any accommodations are written in an Individualized Education Plan (IEP) which is discussed with and agreed upon by the school and the family. Typical accommodations may include extra time for test taking and completing homework, a scribe or copy of class notes if handwriting is impaired, an extra set of books to be kept at home, extra time to get from class to class, adaptive physical education, assistance in the cafeteria, use of the elevator in a multi-level building and accessible transportation with door to door service. When the child returns to school, a wheelchair for longer distances may be indicated due to fatigue and/or weakness. In the classroom, they may be able to maneuver with a walker, crutches or independent of an assistive device. If possible, a trip to the school prior to starting classes can alleviate anxiety and help with learning how to navigate within the school setting. In addition, a chance to interact with peers and tell their story can help alleviate the awkwardness of explaining where they have been and any differences which their peers may notice. See Chap. 12 for a more detailed discussion of the psychosocial needs of children with malignant bone tumors.

When feasible, community outings while in the hospital are helpful in teaching children and adolescents how to navigate different terrains, cross streets, maneuver through the public, and advocate for themselves. The first time out with a wheelchair or assistive device can be very difficult. In addition, any physical changes such as an amputation or hair loss can be devastating to the individual. Therapeutic recreation (TR) specialists and psychology are particularly helpful in these areas. In addition, TR specialists should also investigate the child's leisure and recreational interests. There may be certain restrictions initially, but many activities can be adapted. Providing a list of recreational options, resources, and education regarding adapted sports is beneficial for both the child and family.

10.4 Functional Impairments Related to Chemotherapy

Chemotherapy is nearly universally utilized in bone tumors and side effects from these treatments can lead to functional impairments. Vincristine has been shown to cause an axonal sensorimotor peripheral neuropathy that often manifests first with ankle dorsiflexion weakness and foot drop. In the setting of lower limb amputation, foot drop and sensory impairment in the unaffected limb can lead to much greater mobility impairment. The intact limb has greater weight bearing requirements than the prosthetic limb and provides essential sensory feedback in the form of proprioception and light touch sensation. A similar effect is seen in gait training after limb salvage surgery given the increased requirements on the intact limb and associated weakness and sensory impairment. Bracing with an ankle-foot orthosis (AFO) to provide support and promote heel strike is often necessary. Additional peripheral neuropathy symptoms such as neuropathic pain, hand weakness and constipation secondary to autonomic neuropathy can also be seen with vincristine therapy. These can all limit mobility and age appropriate participation in activities of daily living.

Cisplatin has been associated with hearing loss (Podratz et al. 2011) and sensory peripheral neuropathy. Hearing loss can lead to delays in speech and language development in younger patients. The sensory peripheral neuropathy is due to induction of apoptosis in dorsal root ganglion sensory neurons. Symptoms can worsen after Cisplatin has been discontinued in a phenomenon known as "coasting." Despite having adequate strength for ambulation, patients with sensory peripheral neuropathy can have profoundly impaired gait secondary to loss of proprioception for limb position and poor light touch sensation.

Doxorubicin can lead to decreased left ventricular function and chronic cardiomyopathy, which can cause poor endurance and exercise tolerance. Amputee gait requires significantly increased energy as compared to non-amputees and cardiomyopathy can limit walking distances. For those patients with higher levels of function, cardiomyopathy may limit sports participation.

10.5　Aging Following Limb Salvage or Acquired Amputation

A number of chronic complications can present after the initial phase of rehabilitation is complete. When amputations are performed in the skeletally immature child, alterations in bony growth can present obstacles. Terminal overgrowth occurs when bone is transected through the metaphysis or diaphysis. The distal aspect of the long bone that was transected continues to grow and often becomes quite sharp. This can lead to soft tissue pain, poor prosthesis fit requiring socket modifications, bursa formation and even piercing of the skin. Surgical intervention is required in approximately one half of these cases (O'Neal et al. 1996). As the child continues to grow, additional resection procedures may be needed. Each procedure leads to relative shortening of the residual limb and decreased production of mechanical torque during ambulation or upper limb activities. For these reasons, joint disarticulation is sometimes preferred as the epiphysis is preserved and terminal overgrowth does not occur.

Linear growth in a child with amputation will eventually produce significant leg length discrepancy unless prosthetic adjustments are made. This leg length discrepancy leads to altered gait mechanics and decreased efficiency. While prosthetic components can be somewhat modified for growth, limits are quickly reached and frequent fabrication of new prostheses are required during the growing years. Endoprosthetic components are typically adjusted when a 1 cm limb length discrepancy is noted.

In prosthetic gait, weight is shifted to the intact limb in a greater proportion (Norvell et al. 2005), leading to greater forces on joints in that limb. Higher rates of knee osteoarthritis have been observed in the contralateral limb of amputees compared to rates in the general population (Norvell et al. 2005). Anticipatory guidance and screening exams should be provided including discussions regarding proper prosthetic alignment, maintaining a healthy body mass index and potential use of handheld assistive devices such as canes.

Long-term follow-up in patients who have been treated for bone tumors provides data regarding function, level of education attained, employability and income. Marina et al. reported functional outcomes in survivors of extremity sarcoma after 20 years or greater using data from the Childhood Cancer Survivor Study. It was demonstrated that long term limitations in activities such as carrying groceries up stairs and walking short community distances became more prevalent as patients aged. These activity limitations were more common for patients with lower limb amputations than upper limb amputations. Higher level lower limb amputation was also associated with increased activity limitation. Patients with upper limb amputations were less likely to graduate college than those with lower limb amputations. Those patients with limb sparing surgery had the highest college graduation rates. Patients with amputation had higher unemployment rates than those not treated with amputation. These rates remained fairly stable as patients aged. It was also found the annual income of less than $20,000 was most common in patients with lower limb amputation and the proportion of patients in this income class increased with age.

While survival rates for bones tumors have increased in the past 30 years (Esiashvili et al. 2008; Ognjanovic et al. 2009), there remains a subset of patients for whom it is clear that there is a poor prognosis for survival. Despite decreased expected life span, a focus on function and quality of life during this time period remains paramount. The rehabilitation team can be helpful in determining patient and family functional goals and in helping to set realistic expectations. One must consider the amount of effort and time required to achieve certain functional goals. Those goals that have not been achieved such as efficient ambulation or upper limb prosthetic mastery can improve short-term quality of life but often come at a cost. The energy, time and potential frustration required to achieve these goals may outweigh their benefits. For example, manual wheelchair use may be preferable to lower limb prosthetic ambulation given decreased energy consumption and less time required for training. Each case must be considered separately in order to properly apply the values of the child and family to their unique medical and psychosocial setting.

References

Beebe K, Song KJ, Ross E et al (2009) Functional outcomes after limb-salvage surgery and endoprosthetic reconstruction with an expandable prosthesis: a report of 4 cases. Arch Phys Med Rehabil 90:1039–1047

Bekkering WP, Vliet Vlieland TPM, Fiocca M et al (2012) Quality of life, functional ability and physical activity after different surgical interventions for bone cancer of the leg: a systematic review. Surg Oncol 21:e39–e47

Benevenia J, Blackskin MF, Patterson FR (2004) Complications after limb salvage surgery. Curr Probl Diagn Radiol 33:1–15

Bray JJ (1989) Prosthetic principles: upper extremity amputations (fabrication and fitting principles), 3rd edn. Prosthetics Orthotics Education Program, University of California Press, Los Angeles

Dillingham TR, MacKenzie EJ, Pezzin LE (2002) Limb amputation and limb deficiency: epidemiology and recent trends in the United States. South Med J 95:875–883

Esiashvili N, Goodman M, Marcus RB Jr (2008) Changes in incidence and survival of Ewing sarcoma patients of the past 3 decades. J Pediatr Hematol Oncol 30:425–430

Fleming LL, Malone JM, Robertson J (1999) Immediate, early and late post-surgical management of upper limb amputation. Prosthet Orthot Int 23:55–58

Freiden RA, Ryniker D, Kenan S et al (1993) Assessment of patient function after limb-sparing surgery. Arch Phys Med Rehabil 74(1):38–43

Ganz O, Gulick K, Smurr LM et al (2008) Managing the upper extremity amputee: a protocol for success. J Hand Ther 21:160–176

Gerber LH, Huffman K, Chaudhry U et al (2006) Functional outcomes and life satisfaction in long-term survivors of pediatric saromas. Arch Phys Med Rehabil 87:1611–1617

Götte M, Kesting S, Winter C et al (2014) Comparison of self-reported physical activity in children and adolescents before and during cancer treatment. Pediatr Blood Cancer 61:1023–1028

Ham SJ, van der Graaf WTA, Pras E et al (1998) Soft tissue sarcoma of the extremities. A multi-modality diagnostic and therapeutic approach. Cancer Treat Rev 24:373–391

Horgan O, Maclachlan M (2004) Psychosocial adjustment to lower-limb amputation: a review. Disabil Rehabil 26(14/15):837–850

Marcove RC, Miké V, Hajek JV et al (1970) Osteogenic sarcoma under the age of twenty-one. A review of one hundred and forty-five operative cases. J Bone Joint Surg Am 52:411–423

Marina N, Hudson MM, Jones KE et al (2013) Changes in health status among aging survivors of pediatric upper and lower extremity sarcoma: a report from the childhood cancer survivor study. Arch Phys Med Rehabil 94:1062–1073

Norvell DC, Czerniecki JM, Reiber GE et al (2005) The prevalence of knee pain and symptomatic knee osteoarthritis among veteran traumatic amputees and non-amputees. Arch Phys Med Rehabil 86:487–493

O'Neal ML, Bahner R, Ganey T et al (1996) Osseous overgrowth after amputation in adolescents and children. J Pediatr Orthop 16(1):78–84

Ognjanovic S, Linabery AM, Charbonneau B et al (2009) Trends in childhood rhabdomyosarcoma incidence and survival in the United States, 1975–2005. Cancer 115:4218–4226

Podratz JL, Knight AM, Ta LE et al (2011) Cisplatin induced mitochondrial DNA damage in dorsal root ganglion neurons. Neurobiol Dis 41(3):661–668

Serletti M, Carras AJ, O'Keefe RJ et al (1998) Functional outcome for soft tissue reconstruction for limb salvage after sarcoma surgery. Plast Reconstr Surg 102:1576–1583

Shehadah A, El Dahleh M, Salem A et al (2013) Standardization of rehabilitation after limb salvage surgery for sarcomas improves patients' outcomes. Hematol Oncol Stem Cell Ther 6(3–4):105–111

So NF, Andrews KL, Anderson K et al (2014) Prosthetic fitting after rotationplasty of the knee. Am J Phys Med Rehabil 93(4):328–334

Van Hoesel R, Veth R, Bökkerink JP et al (2003) Limb salvage in musculoskeletal oncology. Lancet Oncol 4:343–350

Waters RL, Mulroy S (1999) The energy expenditure of normal and pathologic gait. Gait Posture 9(3):207–231

Paula M. Sanborn

Contents

11.1 **Introduction** 172

11.2 **Role of the Oncology Nurse
Navigator**.......................... 172
11.2.1 Multidisciplinary Team Coordination and
Communication 174

11.3 **Diagnostic Workup**.................. 174
11.3.1 New Patient Intake Process 174
11.3.2 Education on Diagnosis
and Central Line.................... 175

11.4 **Treatment Initiation**................. 177
11.4.1 Patient and Family Teaching 177
11.4.2 Patient Calendar..................... 177
11.4.3 Home Medication Teaching............. 178
11.4.4 Managing Treatment Side Effects 180
11.4.5 Tracking Evaluation and Schedules....... 190
11.4.6 Referrals........................... 190
11.4.7 Home Care Coordination 191

11.5 **Transitioning to Survivorship** 192
11.5.1 Primary Care Physician Coordination 192
11.5.2 Tracking Regular Surveillance
Appointments...................... 192
11.5.3 Survivorship Care Plans and Cancer
Treatment Summary.................. 193

11.5.4 Prevention of Secondary Cancers......... 197
11.5.5 Late Effects of Treatment of the Bone
Tumor Patient...................... 197

Conclusion 198

References.............................. 200

Abstract

As patients and their families are facing a pediatric cancer diagnosis, they will be asked to navigate a complex healthcare system while coordinating their multiple treatment plans their child will face. The oncology nurse navigator (ONN) plays a vital role in caring for and navigating the bone tumor patient and their family from the very onset of diagnosis through the continuum of care. The Oncology Nurse Navigator serves as a single point of contact for patients and families, providing education regarding their disease process, treatment and side effects management and helping them become experts in their cancer care from diagnosis to survivorship. The ONN creates multidisciplinary team coordination and communication, facilitating and acting as a liaison with the healthcare team on behalf of the patient and family.

P.M. Sanborn, BSN
Division of Hematology/Oncology/BMT,
Nationwide Children's Hospital,
700 Children's Drive, Columbus, OH 43205, USA
e-mail: Paula.sanborn@nationwidechildrens.org

© Springer International Publishing Switzerland 2015
T.P. Cripe, N.D. Yeager (eds.), *Malignant Pediatric Bone Tumors - Treatment & Management*,
Pediatric Oncology, DOI 10.1007/978-3-319-18099-1_11

11.1 Introduction

When a child is diagnosed with cancer, it often produces an overwhelming emotional response that tends to run the gamut of emotions from shock and denial to anger and anxiety. But that is usually just the beginning and parents don't realize the magnitude of the journey on which they are about to embark with their child. A multitude of medical tests and consultations are typically needed to determine a definitive diagnosis, an accurate staging, and a course of treatment. There will be numerous cycles of treatment and evaluations that encompass clinic appointments, infusion appointments, and many faces and names to remember. Even as patients and their families are facing one of the greatest challenges of their lives, they will be asked to navigate a complex healthcare system while coordinating the multiple treatment plans their child will face (Wilcox and Bruce 2010). The oncology nurse navigator (ONN) plays a vital role in caring for and navigating the bone tumor patient and family from the very onset of diagnosis. The ONN provides comfort and support, as well as reinforces and explains the information provided by the physician (Pearson 2009). The ONN becomes the single point of contact from the first day they are contacted by the bone tumor team throughout the disease continuum, providing patients and families with a familiar individual which can help reduce their anxieties. The ONN can provide necessary educational information to the patient and family over time, allowing them to truly understand and process all the information as it is received (Pedersen and Hack 2010).

> Finding out your child has cancer is a terrifying experience. Your world as you know it stops. Having a nurse navigator along our journey helped us through each day. If I had a question, day or night, she was there. The always calming advice she gave or the nudge I needed to get my child to the ER when I was trying to decide if she needed to go, might have saved her from serious health issues. The love that came from her heart, the smiles that she shared and the compassion showed through when she left the room, and my daughter would say, "mom, I love her so much." Our Nurse Navigator made our daughter's day brighter. We are thankful for that. Without her, I couldn't have

managed to keep track of all of her treatments, appointments, medications, and all the information needed to care for my daughter without her help. The daily calendars she made for us showed us the way. She was our safe place. She provided us with the education and understanding along the way and even today as we face each day trying to live our lives beyond cancer. She carried us through some of the darkest days of our lives and we are eternally grateful. She will be in our hearts forever, along with many others we met along the way in our cancer journey. (Mother of 16 yo osteosarcoma patient)

11.2 Role of the Oncology Nurse Navigator

The ONN serves as a single point of contact for patients and their families throughout their entire cancer care experience and, most importantly, is an advocate and personal care coach on the patient's behalf (Francz 2014). The navigator functions as an advocate for the patient and provides education to the patient and their family regarding their disease process, treatment and side effect management, and treatment options. Navigators facilitate communication and act as a liaison with the healthcare team on behalf of the patient (Francz 2014; New 2014).

The patient navigation concept was introduced by Harold P. Freeman, MD, and implemented in 1990 at Harlem Hospital in New York (Wilcox and Bruce 2010). The goal of the program was to reduce or eliminate cancer disparities in the poor and underserved populations that bear a heavier burden of cancer (Wilcox and Bruce 2010; Brown et al. 2012; Pedersen and Hack 2010). Freeman's original patient navigator program launched a national movement (Wilcox and Bruce 2010). Many different types of oncology nurse navigator programs exist such as disease specific or general. The oncology nurse navigator's degree of educational preparation varies at each individual program's needs (Wilcox and Bruce 2010).

In 2012, the American College of Surgeons Commission on Cancer (CoC) released new standards that reflected the goal of ensuring patient-centered care. One of these new standards that will be initiated in 2015 requires that accredited cancer centers have a patient navigation process in place (Society 2013).

The Oncology Nursing Society (ONS) recognized the need to clarify the role and core competencies for the many oncology nurses who identified their primary role function as navigation of the oncology patient. Out of this need, the ONS developed Oncology Nurse Navigator Core Competencies that are intended to describe the fundamental knowledge and skills that an ONN should possess. These competencies are meant to reflect many practices and settings across the cancer continuum and were released in 2013 by the ONS (Society 2013).

The Oncology Nurse Navigator Core Competencies include four competency categories:

Category 1: Professional Role: The ONN demonstrates professionalism within both the workplace and community through respectful interactions and effective teamwork. He or she works to promote and advance the role of the ONN and takes responsibility to pursue professional growth and development.

Category 2: Education: The ONN provides appropriate and timely education to patients, families, and caregivers to facilitate understanding and support informed decision making.

Category 3: Coordination of Care: The ONN facilitates the appropriate and efficient delivery of healthcare services, both within and across systems, to promote optimal outcomes while delivering patient-centered care.

Category 4: Communication: The ONN demonstrates interpersonal communication skills that enable exchange of ideas and information effectively with patients, families, and colleagues at all levels. This includes writing, speaking, and listening skills.

These detailed competencies can be viewed at: https://www.ons.org/sites/default/files/ONNCompetencies_rev.pdf

The oncology nurse navigator role simplifies the complicated healthcare journey for the pediatric cancer patient and their parents.

Benefits of ONN Role to Pediatric Cancer Patients and Their Families

- Serves as a single point of access for all patients and families. The navigator remains an ongoing, consistent point of contact for patients and families through the full continuum of care.
- Supports patients as they move throughout their pediatric cancer journey, from diagnosis to treatment and through follow-up care. Activities include facilitating communication between inpatient and outpatient settings, specialty consultations, research, test scheduling, and palliative or hospice care if necessary. These services result in fewer delays in treatments, improved communication between the care team, and less confusion for patients and their families.
- Provides valuable education to patients and families regarding treatment, nutrition, and financial psychosocial support.
- Helps to decrease hospitalizations, including ER visits associated with complications in care, by identifying complications sooner and directing earlier interventions at the clinical level.
- Assures access to established community resources including support groups, housing assistance, transportation, and financial assistance.
- Assures access to assistance regarding access to financial resources for patients and their families with treatment-related costs, including drugs.
- Provides emotional support that parents need during and after treatment and assures connection to supportive and psychosocial programs and initiatives.
- Works closely with the research team to identify research protocols, assures adherence to the protocols, and reinforces information

about clinical trials with the patient and family.

- Serves as a liaison with primary care physician.

11.2.1 Multidisciplinary Team Coordination and Communication

The ONN is instrumental in communicating across all barriers of the bone tumor patient's healthcare team. The navigator's role not only assists the patient and family but also members of the team that may include the primary oncologist, advanced practice nurse, surgeon, orthopedic oncologist, social workers, psychologist, physical therapist, inpatient and outpatient nurses, radiation oncology team, home care nurses, palliative care team, school liaison, research team, discharge planners, and other healthcare specialists. The navigator communicates patient information through all team members to provide seamless care for the patient and family. Enhanced communication among healthcare providers builds relationships within the team and directly enhances patient care as all work together to meet individual patient needs (Wilcox and Bruce 2010). These can be accomplished during bone tumor biweekly to weekly meetings where patients are discussed among the team, identifying any barriers to care and addressing needs. Research protocols are also discussed in these team meetings. Another source of communication is through email and the electronic medical record (EMR). Most EMR systems allows for routing of patient encounters by phone or patient clinic visits. These encounters can be flagged for importance and follow-up needed by a team member. The ONN routes telephone encounters to team members as they occur showing clear documentation of patient information so team members can be kept up to date with patient care concerns or issues.

11.3 Diagnostic Workup

11.3.1 New Patient Intake Process

If the new bone tumor patient is diagnosed through an inpatient hospitalization, the inpatient team notifies the bone tumor team. The bone tumor team including the oncologist, practitioner, and ONN meet with the patient and family during their inpatient stay and discuss treatment and arrange the diagnostic workup while they are admitted. The new patient referral may also come from an orthopedic oncologist, neurosurgeon, or general surgeon. The referral is usually started by a call from the surgeon to one of the bone tumor oncologists or directly to the oncology nurse navigator when the patient is in the surgeon's office. The ONN retrieves all patient information including demographics, insurance information, office visit note, and pathology report and arranges for pathology slides and all scans completed to be sent to the primary oncologist's institution. The patient information is reviewed with the oncologist and a diagnosis is determined. A review of open bone studies or standard treatment regimens is completed with the oncology practitioner for required scans for staging. The ONN contacts the family after verification that the diagnosis has been discussed with the family from the original surgeon's office. The ONN introduces herself to the family, giving them her contact number to call with any questions and concerns.

Following this initial intake process, the patient and families' ability to travel to the institution and their work schedules are assessed by the ONN prior to arranging their staging scans, medical tests for pretreatment, and initial appointment with the oncology team. The ONN answers any questions by phone and explains to the patient and family the purpose and procedures of all required tests prior to their arrival to the institution. The ONN acts as a new resource for the patient, and family. The ONN listens, debriefs, offers support, and provides information until their first appointment with the oncologist. If the new bone tumor patient is a male teen, based on the family's level of understanding by the ONN, fertility preservation is discussed prior to the initial appointment, and if requested by the family, a referral to a facility that specializes in sperm analysis and enables cryopreservation and long-term storage is made (see Chap. 5). Appointments are made for required staging scans, electrocardiogram (EKG), and echocardiograms for pre-anthracycline screening, as well as audiograms for pre-cisplatin, and first consultation appointment with the oncology team. If applicable, a urine collection kit is given for a 12 hour creatinine clearance evaluation along with instructions to bring this specimen to their surgery appointment. The ONN reviews with the patient and family the instructions of how to collect and store. By bringing this specimen with them, it facilitates initiation of chemotherapy after the central line is placed and decreases the hospital stay. Insurance information is relayed to the prior authorization team and patient registration to assure timely prior authorization for new patient scans and appointments. After review of patient information with the oncologist, if appropriate, the ONN contacts the research team if the patient is eligible for an open study. The goal of the team is to initiate therapy within 5–7 days of the initial referral.

11.3.2 Education on Diagnosis and Central Line

During the patient and family's first appointment with the oncologist, the family is given a teaching notebook. The Children's Oncology Group Family Notebook is utilized as the teaching guide for our patients and their families (Murphy 2011). The notebook is tagged by the ONN with specific information such as central line, bone marrow aspirate and biopsy, spinal tap, blood counts, and diagnosis description. Team member cards as well as a sheet documenting all team member names and phone numbers are placed in the notebook. *Helping Hands* (see Fig. 11.1) for each chemotherapy drug and diagnosis pamphlets are placed in the notebook. After the oncologist discusses treatment, the ONN stays with the patient and family and answers questions, reviews with the patient what type of central line catheter they will receive will look like, and explains how it is accessed and utilized for treatment. The ONN verifies that the family has the ONN's contact information in case they have further questions or concerns.

The physical and emotional care information that the family receives at the initial appointments can become very overwhelming. It's the role of the ONN to assess absorption of information given at this initial appointment and continually update and reteach families about their child's disease and treatment throughout the care continuum (Heiney and Wells 1995). Families are asked to bring their notebook for all admissions to enable teaching throughout treatment.

The bone tumor social worker is also notified of the initial appointment and meets with the family, completing an initial distress screening, and gives them her contact information.

After the patient leaves their initial oncology appointment, a referral is made to pediatric surgery for central line placement, and biopsy procedure is discussed with the surgeon by the primary oncologist. If indicated, a referral is made to the hematology/oncology procedure schedulers to add a bone marrow aspirate/biopsy/spinal tap to the central line surgery date. All efforts are made to combine all initial surgical procedures.

From the first appointment with the bone tumor team, family-centered care is initiated. The foundation of family-centered care is the understanding that the family is the true expert in the care of their child and the primary source of strength and support (Pearson 2009). It is through constant contact with the oncology team through the ONN that helps prepare and support the bone tumor patient and their family to be experts in their cancer care (Pearson 2009; Kelly and Porock 2005; Wilcox and Bruce 2010).

NATIONWIDE CHILDREN'S
When your child needs a hospital, everything matters.™

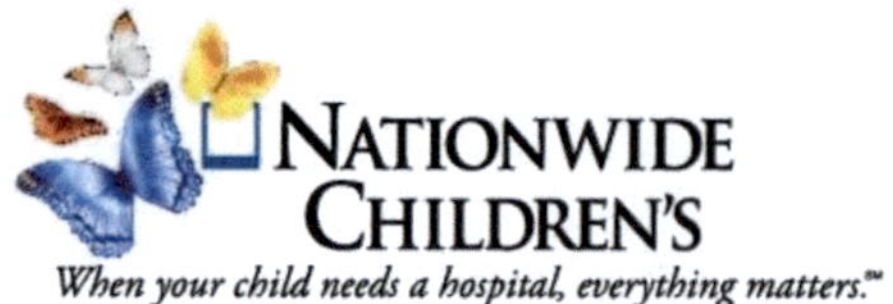

Helping Hand™

Doxorubicin, Adriamycin®, ADR, DOX (For Hematology/Oncology Patients)

Doxorubicin (dox-oh-RUE-beh-sin) is a chemotherapy medicine prescribed by your child's doctor. It is given by IV infusion over 20 to 30 minutes or as a continuous IV infusion for several days (Picture 1).

Picture 1 Receiving IV chemotherapy.

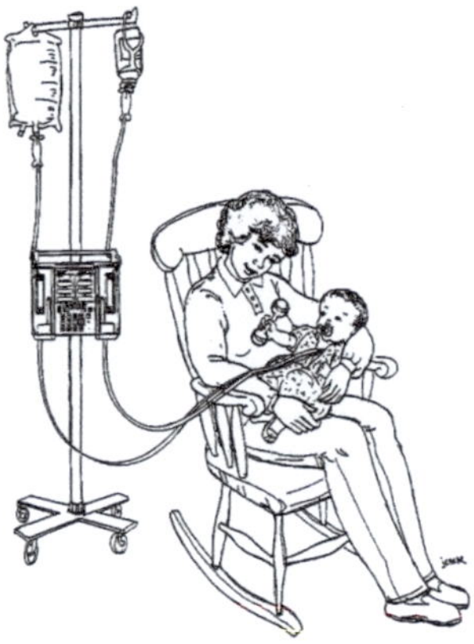

Dosage

- The amount of doxorubicin prescribed will depend on your child's diagnosis, current weight, height, blood counts and heart tests (EKG, ECHO).
- Doxorubicin is given on the days marked on the chemotherapy roadmap (schedule).

Possible Side Effects

- Nausea and vomiting may occur in patients receiving doxorubicin. This usually lasts up to 24 hours after the medicine is given.
- Heart muscle damage may occur with doxorubicin.
- Mouth sores may occur 3 to 10 days after receiving doxorubicin.
- Ulcers (sores) in the throat or stomach may occur. They may cause pain with swallowing, heartburn, abdominal pain, diarrhea and blood in stools.
- Urine color may turn pink or orange-red up to 48 hours after doxorubicin is given. This is from the medicine, not from blood in the urine.
- Hair loss may occur 2 or more weeks after treatment begins. It is not permanent.
- Low blood counts occur 7 to 10 days after treatment.
- Your child might have tissue damage, irritation or burning of the skin surrounding tissue **if** the medicine leaks out of the vein while it is being given. This is not likely if your child has a central venous catheter (PICC, SIP, CVC).
- Increased skin redness at previous radiation therapy sites may occur.

HH-V-42 10/90, Revised 7/03

Fig. 11.1 Teaching tools

11.4 Treatment Initiation

11.4.1 Patient and Family Teaching

Prior to initiation of chemotherapy, the ONN meets with the family and patient and reviews all chemotherapy drugs, utilizing our institution's teaching tools called *Helping Hands*, the APHON drug handouts, and the Children's Oncology Group Family Teaching Notebook. This handbook can be located at: http://www.childrensoncologygroup.org/index.php/cog-family-handbook. All side effects are reviewed and a "when to call and who to call" tool with side effects is communicated to the family. The ONN reviews the discharge summary with the patient and family prior to discharge with each new chemotherapy drug, reinforcing side effects that may occur with each new drug. This tool also documents how to reach the ONN during office hours and the numbers to contact the oncology fellow on call after office hours and on the weekends. The ONN communicates with family members that this document may be good to keep on the refrigerator as a reference for anyone that may be responsible for the care of the patient. For the bone tumor patient receiving doxorubicin, the ONN discusses the EKG and echocardiogram and reviews with them when it will be repeated during treatment to assess for potential side effects. Knowing up front that these will be completed again tends to alleviate the anxiety that may occur if they arrive for their next chemotherapy admission that includes doxorubicin and they are getting an EKG and echocardiogram. Parents tend to think something is wrong, not that it is being completed to evaluate for side effects. Repeat audiograms for the patient receiving cisplatin are also explained. If applicable, treatment schemas are given to families to help them understand the timing of admissions and chemotherapy. Many patients and families utilize the schema to document chemotherapy treatments, as they mark off each one. This gives them something to look forward to as they can visualize an end to their child's therapy.

On the patient's second admission or visit for chemotherapy, the ONN reviews all lab values with the patient and family, including chemistries, complete blood count (CBC), and their urinalysis. During this time, she teaches the patient and family about their absolute neutrophil count (ANC), showing them how to calculate it as well as how it relates to the signs and symptoms of neutropenia. For those patients receiving highly emetic chemotherapy regimens, the ONN reviews closely the value of the BUN and creatinine that is completed and explains its ability to determine hydration status.

11.4.2 Patient Calendar

An ongoing calendar is created by the ONN and given monthly to help the patient and their family with grasping where they need to be. This calendar has become an effective teaching tool in helping patients and families understand their treatment schedule. Families frequently express that the calendar is used to guide them in making other family member appointments and schedules. Several families have stated that it is kept posted on the refrigerator at home so that everyone in the family knows the schedule. For the osteosarcoma patient receiving methotrexate, this calendar also instructs them when to hold or give their weekend Bactrim doses. The ONN also documents when counts are low and recovering on the calendar (see Fig. 11.2). Because it is an editable word document, the calendar allows for delays and can be updated accordingly. The calendar is often shared with other team members such as psychology and social work so they are aware of the patient's upcoming appointments. The ONN also uses this calendar to teach delayed emesis medication teaching, when to start and stop their medications. If pegfilgrastim, filgrastim, or home care visits are being utilized, this is documented on the calendar as well.

It is essential that families understand the basics of their child's disease; what to expect from their chemotherapy, biotherapy, radiation, and/or surgery; how to recognize adverse side effects; what is considered an emergency; and how to seek help (Lahl et al. 2008). They also need to understand all required tests and

Sun	Mon	Tue	Wed	Thu	Fri	Sat
Aug 31 *Bactrim twice a day*	**1** Admit for Methotrexate at 9:00am in the Infusion Center	**2**	**3**	**4** Discharge when Methotrexate level is low enough	**5**	**6** HOLD BACTRIM
7 HOLD BACTRIM	**8** Admit for Methotrexate at 9:00am in the Infusion Center	**9**	**10**	**11** Discharge when Methotrexate level is low enough	**12**	**13** HOLD BACTRIM
14 HOLD BACTRIM	**15** Admit for Cisplatin/ Doxorubicin at 9:00am in the Infusion Center	**16**	**17** Discharge after hydration completed and Neulasta injection completed	**18** *Take Zofran/Decadron twice a day*	**19** *Take Zofran/Decadron twice a day*	**20** *Take Zofran/Decadron twice a day* *Bactrim twice a day*
21 *Take Zofran/Decadron twice a day* *Bactrim twice a day*	**22** Clinic apt at 9:30am for labs and a physical *STOP taking Decadron and change Zofran dose to as needed for nausea*	**23** ***blood counts getting low***	**24**	**25** Check labs at a close to home center or local lab	**26** *Orthopedic Oncologist apt at 9:30am* ***blood counts getting lower***	**27** *Bactrim twice a day*
28 *Bactrim twice a day*	**29** Check labs at a close to home center or local lab ***blood counts starting to improve***	**30**	**Oct 1**	**2** Check labs at a close to home center or local lab ***blood counts higher ***	**3** *Pain Clinic apt at 10:30am*	**4** *Bactrim twice a day*

Fig. 11.2 Patient treatment calendar

how to prepare for these tests, procedures, and blood work, in their role in delivering supportive care. Each family is unique and it is the responsibility of the ONN to effectively teach the patient and family by using verbal, written, and visual information that best meets their learning needs. The initial teaching is overwhelming, but the ONN has learned to go through teaching slowly, utilizing review and ongoing reinforcement, while allowing avail-ability for questions. Most families are able to rise to the challenge (Lahl et al. 2008; Garcia 2014).

11.4.3 Home Medication Teaching

Prior to discharge, the ONN meets with the patient and family and reviews all home medications on their "Andrew's medication list." Each

<u>**Andrew's meds**</u>

Sucralfate (CARAFATE) 100mg/ml oral suspension
<u>Purpose</u>: for oral and esophageal irritation, pain.
<u>Dose</u>: 1,000mg, Take 10 ml by mouth every 6 hours for 14 days.

Gabepentin (NEURONTIN) 100mg oral capsule
<u>Purpose</u>: Neuropathic pain
<u>Dose</u>: 300mg, Take 3 capsules by mouth 3 times daily.

Oxycodone(ROXICODONE) 5mg oral tablet
<u>Purpose</u>: pain
<u>Dose</u>: 7.5mg, Take 1.5 tablets by mouth every 4 hours *as needed* for breakthrough pain.

Zofran ODT (Ondansetron) 4mg oral tablet, rapid dissolve
<u>Purpose</u>: anti-nausea
<u>Dose</u>: Take 1 tablet by mouth every 8 hour. Take 1.5 tablets twice a day for 2 days after Cisplatin. May take up to every 6 hours *as needed* for nausea

Zantac (Ranitidine) 75mg tablet
<u>Purpose</u>: helps reduce acid reflux or heartburn
<u>Dose</u>: 150mg, take 2 tablets twice daily

Phenergan (Promethazine) 12.5mg oral tablet
<u>Purpose</u>: Anti-nausea medication
<u>Dose</u>: 12.5mg: Take 1 tablet by mouth every six hours *as needed* for nausea. This medication may make you drowsy.

Bactrim (TMP-SMZ) 80-400mg oral tablet
<u>Purpose</u>: Prevent PCP pneumonia in patients receiving chemotherapy
<u>Dose</u>: 120mg: Take 1.5tablets twice daily on *Saturday and Sunday only*. Do NOT take on weekends after you receive Methotrexate.

Miralax (Polyethylene glycol) 17 gram oral powder
<u>Purpose</u>: Laxative and stool softener
<u>Dose</u>: 17grams: Take 17grams by mouth as directed one time daily for constipation.

Lidocaine-Prilocaine (EMLA) 2.5-2.5% topical cream
<u>Purpose</u>: Numbs the port site prior to access
<u>Dose</u>: 2.5grams: Apply topically to port site 1 hour prior to access.

Meds to avoid: No motrin, naprosyn, or aspirin products. For non-narcotic pain relief use Tylenol only. **Do NOT use Tylenol for fevers without calling the hematology clinic or hematologist on call first**

Fig. 11.3 Sample home medication list

home medication name, dose, schedule, and purpose is listed on their medication list and reviewed (see Fig. 11.3). If the ONN realizes that the family is overwhelmed and anxious about the home medications, he/she will create a "MyMedSchedule" from the website: https://secure.medactionplan.com/mymedschedule/index.htm. This is a free application that allows a medication list with schedules that can be created, listing all medications hourly for the family. This application also shows a picture of the medication and can be created in English and Spanish. It also can be utilized as an app on a smartphone with medication due alerts and refill reminders. There are several other sites that can be utilized for medication teaching. Pill boxes can also be used for adherence to drug regimens. All prescriptions are verified with the bone tumor practitioner prior to discharge. The discharge instructions and follow-up are created by the ONN during each admission or visit to the clinic. The discharge instructions are reviewed with the patient and family. The instructions include side effects of each chemotherapy drugs they received and signs and symptoms of neutropenia, anemia, and thrombocytopenia, and who to call and when to call is clearly documented in the discharge plan. The ONN utilizes the electronic medical record to create "smart phrases" for each visit for chemotherapy. The smart phrases contain the discharge instructions and are shared with other team members to promote consistency in the information given to families.

11.4.4 Managing Treatment Side Effects

11.4.4.1 Nausea and Vomiting

Nausea and vomiting are two of the most common side effects of chemotherapy and radiation treatment. Nausea and vomiting can be anticipatory, acute, or delayed (Lahl et al. 2008; Rheingans 2008) There is a variety of techniques to control nausea and vomiting. The most common treatment is the utilization of antiemetics. Treatment for nausea and vomiting occurs before, during, and after chemotherapy administration. Several categories of antiemetics are used in children and young adults with cancer (Lahl et al. 2008). There are also non-pharmacological techniques that can be used to aid in nausea and vomiting depending on their age. Utilizing an engaged psychosocial team that consists of child life (play) therapists, music therapists, massage therapists, and psychologists may help the patient using music, play, distraction, guided imagery or exercise to help them overcome their nausea and vomiting (Lahl et al. 2008).

Each patient's antiemetic regimen is determined by the emetic potential of the chemotherapy or radiation treatment (see Table 11.1). Prevention of nausea and vomiting is always the goal for patients. Staying ahead of the nausea and vomiting produces better outcomes and a better quality of life for the patient. The ONN teaches the patient and family that treatment of nausea and vomiting is comparable to effective pain control. If you don't stay prepared and ahead of it, it can spiral out of control and become difficult to gain relief. If nausea and vomiting is not well controlled on the first experience with chemotherapy, patients are more likely to experience

Table 11.1 Emetogenic risk of therapies used for malignant bone tumors

High risk	Moderate risk	Low risk	Minimal risk
Carboplatin	Cyclophosphamide <1 g/m^2	Docetaxel	Bevacizumab
Cisplatin	Cyclophosphamide (oral)	Doxorubicin (liposomal)	Dexrazoxane
Cyclophosphamide >1 g/m^2	Daunorubicin	Etoposide	Sorafenib
Dactinomycin	Doxorubicin	Gemcitabine	Sunitinib
Methotrexate >12 g/m^2	Etoposide	Methotrexate >50 to 250 mg/m^2	Temsirolimus
	Ifosfamide	Nilotinib	Vincristine
	Irinotecan	Paclitaxel	Vinorelbine
	Methotrexate >250 mg to 12 g/m^2	Topotecan	
	Temozolomide		
	Vinorelbine		
Multiple agent risk			
Cyclophosphamide+ Doxorubicin			
Cyclophosphamide+ Etoposide			
Doxorubicin + ifosfamide			
Doxorubicin+ Methotrexate			
Etoposide + ifosfamide			

anticipatory nausea and vomiting (Baggott and Association of Pediatric Oncology Nurses (U.S.) 2002).

For delayed emesis, patients and families are instructed to utilize Zofran and Decadron twice a day for 4 days after receiving chemotherapy drugs that are highly or moderately emetic regardless if they feel nauseated or not. They are also instructed to utilize Phenergan or Ativan as a breakthrough medication. Each patient's gastrointestinal responses need to be evaluated individually with each chemotherapy administration so their needs can be assessed prior to discharge and through post-discharge calls from the ONN. Guidelines established by the National Comprehensive Cancer Network (NCCN) – *NCCN Clinical Practice Guidelines in Oncology for Antiemesis* and the Pediatric Oncology Group of Ontario (POGO) and *the POGO Guidelines for the Classification of the Acute Emetogenic Potential of Antineoplastic Medication in Pediatric Cancer Patients* – are both resources utilized by the bone tumor team in their approach to the prevention of nausea and vomiting in children receiving antineoplastic agents.

Anticipatory nausea and vomiting (ANV) can occur any time after the first treatment, or sometimes even prior to the first treatment. The incidence and severity are influenced by the patient's expectations of what is to come, as well as anxiety about nausea and vomiting. ANV most often begins within 2 hours before treatment and is most severe at the time of administration (Baggott and Association of Pediatric Oncology Nurses (U.S.) 2002). Managing ANV is crucial in controlling the patient's nausea and vomiting throughout their treatment. The patient's environment is important in determining the relative factors to their ANV. Psychogenic factors such as walking into the hospital, smelling particular odors, or the sight of a syringe can trigger nausea (Garcia 2014). Lorazepam administered at bedtime the night before chemotherapy treatment and again the following morning can diminish the distress and reduce the incidence and severity of anticipatory nausea and vomiting (Baggott and Association of Pediatric Oncology Nurses (U.S.) 2002).

Triaging nausea and vomiting from home can become frustrating for the patient and family. The ONN instructs the family and patient who are experiencing gastrointestinal toxicities to avoid foods that are high in sugar, processed foods, and fried or greasy foods. They are instructed to eat small meals that are easily digested (crackers, rice, toast, potatoes, or chicken) every 3–4 hours and to avoid the kitchen area or areas where there may be strong food odors. Pushing fluid intake in small quantities every 20–30 minutes, eating popsicles, slushies, or water are also techniques taught to the caregivers. Families are also instructed to utilize nonpharmocological interventions such as distraction, play, music therapy, and guided imagery while at home. The ONN teaches the patient and family to monitor for signs of dehydration such as few or no tears when crying, a dry or pasty mouth, cracked lips, sunken eyes, lack of energy, increased sleeping, dry skin, and concentrated, dark urine (Murphy 2011). If they have been unable to keep fluids down for 24 hours, are more lethargic, are urinating less, or are vomiting their medications, they are brought in to the infusion clinic or emergency department for evaluation.

11.4.4.2 Anorexia

Anorexia and cachexia are two of the most common nutritional side effects from cancer and its treatment. Factors contributing to anorexia may include nausea, vomiting, taste aversion from the chemotherapy or radiation treatments, anxiety, depression, mucositis, increased sensitivities to odors, and environmental changes (Lahl et al. 2008). Evaluation of the bone tumor patient's weight and oral intake at each visit is crucial during treatment. The patient's nutritional status is evaluated at the beginning of therapy by placing a consult to Clinical Nutrition Services. This nutritional screening is an ongoing process that must take into account patient weights, food intake, treatment that affects nutrition, functional status, physical examination, and lab results indicating nutritional biomarkers such as albumin and prealbumin levels. The initiation of Clinical Nutrition Services early in treatment aids in preventing malnutrition (Baggott and Association of

Pediatric Oncology Nurses (U.S.) 2002). Nutrition management may include diet modifications, oral supplements, enteral feedings, parenteral nutrition, and/or medications to stimulate the appetite (Baggott and Association of Pediatric Oncology Nurses (U.S.) 2002).

11.4.4.3 Mucositis

Mucositis is caused by acute changes in the epithelium of the oral cavity resulting in the death or rapidly dividing epithelia cells (Eilers and Million 2007). Chemotherapeutic agents inhibit the growth and maturation of oral mucosal cells and disrupt the primary mucosal barrier in the mouth and throat. These changes can occur as early as 2–3 days after the administration of chemotherapy and peak in severity 7–10 days later, typically showing resolution within 2 weeks (Wohlschlaeger 2004). Chemotherapeutic agents that produce mucositis are listed in Table 11.2.

Table 11.2 Agents causing mucositis

Alkylating agents	Busulfan
	Cyclophosphamide
	Ifosfamide
	Melphalan
	Procarbazine
	Temozolomide
	Thiotepa
Anthracyclines	Daunomycin
	Doxorubicin
	Idarubicin
	Mitoxantrone
Antimetabolites	Cytarabine
	5-Fluorouracil
	Hydroxyurea
	Mercaptopurine
	Methotrexate
	Thioguanine
Antineoplastic antibiotics	Bleomycin sulfate
	Dactinomycin
Nitrosoureas	Carmustine
	Lomustine
Plant alkaloids	Etoposide
	Paclitaxel
	Vinblastine
	Vincristine

Oral mucositis is a frequent and potentially severe complication following chemotherapy and radiation. Not only is mucositis painful, but it can also cause impaired nutrition, infection, and treatment delays (Baggott and Association of Pediatric Oncology Nurses (U.S.) 2002; Eilers and Million 2007; Wohlschlaeger 2004). Mucositis has the potential to directly impact a patient's quality of life. If it is severe, it may prevent adequate oral intake of food and fluids and the ability to take oral medications. It may sometimes lead to costly and unwanted hospitalization for parenteral nutrition, intravenous medications, and intravenous pain management (Wohlschlaeger 2004).

Due to the frequency of mucositis, teaching oral care to the patient and family prior to the beginning of their first chemotherapy treatment is a nursing priority. Patient education and participation are crucial since most patients are discharged after the completion of chemotherapy, and the monitoring and management of oral care and mucositis takes place at home (Eilers and Million 2007; Baggott and Association of Pediatric Oncology Nurses (U.S.) 2002). It is the ONN's role to provide and supervise ongoing care and the triage of any complications after discharge. It is the goal of the ONN to manage the patient at home and avoid rehospitalization.

The first step of mouth care involves a thorough assessment by the medical team and a consult to dentistry prior to initiating treatment. Ongoing oral mucosa assessment with each treatment admission and prior to discharge allows the medical team to identify early oral lesions (Wohlschlaeger 2004). The second step is assessing their current, pretherapy oral care regimen and addressing any teaching needs or concerns. Next, the ONN instructs the family on a daily oral care regimen that includes brushing teeth four times a day, after meals and before bedtime with a soft toothbrush. Special instructions are given to patients who drink a lot of high-sugar sports drinks, requesting they brush after eating foods high in sugar. Mouthwashes can be used, but they should not contain alcohol. Parents and patients are taught to inspect their mouth daily for any signs of mucositis. They are instructed to

Table 11.3 Food considerations regarding mucositis

General guidelines	Recommended	Not recommended
1. Small pieces of food	1. Tepid or cool liquids	1. Spicy, salty, bitter foods
2. Use straw with liquids	2. Puddings, Jell-O	2. Dry foods (crackers, toast, chips)
3. Nutritional supplements (e.g., boost, scandishake, ensure)	3. Cottage cheese, soft cheeses	3. Oranges, grapefruits, citrus fruits
4. Topical analgesics prior to eating	4. Bananas, peaches, applesauce	4. Chewing gum, candy
5. Mouthwash following meals	5. Milkshakes, smoothies	
6. Avoid hot foods	6. Popsicles, ice cubes, Italian water ice	

look at the entire mouth: the lips, gums, tongue, side of the tongue, under the tongue, cheeks, roof of the mouth, and around the teeth. Avoiding spicy, bitter, salty, or acidic foods is another precaution for the patient (see Table 11.3). Keeping the mouth moist by eating popsicles, ice chips, slushies, smoothies, or cool fluids may also help with oral mucositis.

Once the mucositis appears, pain is usually the first limiting symptom. The patient and family are instructed to continue with their current oral care regimen but may add sodium bicarbonate rinses (mixture of one fourth teaspoon salt, one fourth teaspoon baking soda, 4 oz of water), saline rinses or sterile water rinses every 1–2 hours, lip lubrication, and a mouthwash such as Philadelphia Mouthwash, containing a mixture of magnesium aluminum hydroxide, diphenhydramine, viscous lidocaine ,and water, that acts as a numbing agent to help with swallowing (Murphy 2011). They are instructed to take a pain reliever and then 20 minutes later use the Philadelphia Mouthwash to attempt at eating, drinking, or taking their oral medications throughout the day (Murphy 2011). Patients and families are instructed to call if they are unable to eat or drink secondary to the pain. While triaging the patient, the ONN assesses for hydration status; requesting volume of fluid intake, what does their urine look and how often have they urinated, is it less? Also, asking if the oral secretions are thick, are there a lot of oral secretions, any hoarseness or a "muffled" voice, any bleeding or nausea and vomiting, and lastly any airway stridor. If any signs of a compromised airway are identified within triage, the patient is asked to come in for evaluation, either to the outpatient clinic area or the emergency room. After evaluation by the medical team, the patient may begin antimicrobial treatment.

11.4.4.4 Fatigue

Defining fatigue has been a challenge, but ongoing pediatric fatigue research suggests that both children from 7 to 12 years of age and adolescents from age 13 to 18 years of age can effectively describe fatigue in terms of physical and mental symptoms (Baggott and Association of Pediatric Oncology Nurses (U.S.) 2002). Younger children described fatigue as a sad or mad face stating they feel tired or weak. Teens elaborated more, describing not only physical symptoms of sleepiness, nausea, dizziness, and a weakening of their body but also being mentally tired, feeling "not themselves," and feeling sorry for themselves (Baggott and Association of Pediatric Oncology Nurses (U.S.) 2002). Contributing factors for younger children were associated with getting treatment, having pain, having low blood counts (anemia), changes in their sleep patterns, not being as physically active as they were pretreatment, and environmental factors while being in the hospital, such as interrupted sleep, or hearing noises and seeing lights on in the hallways. The adolescent patient identified the contributing factors relating to their fatigue as environmental: hearing noises, being in the hospital, going for treatment, nurses making noise, and young children making noise. They also related fatigue to personal/behavioral factors such as changing usual sleep patterns, changing sleep positions due to their disease or central line, doing too many things, being bored, having fears and anxieties, and being worried (Baggott and Association of Pediatric Oncology Nurses (U.S.) 2002).

Treatment strategies are varied, but regardless of the age of the patient, they all begin with a thorough assessment of the patient, including what they consider their causes of their fatigue (Lahl et al. 2008; Murphy 2011). The medical team can look for correctable causes such as anemia, pain, dehydration, or poor nutrition and work to alleviate or improve these conditions. A distinction is needed between fatigue and depression along with evaluating the patient's pattern of activity during treatment (Baggott and Association of Pediatric Oncology Nurses (U.S.) 2002). The younger children identified that taking time out for short naps during the day, having visitors, and doing fun activities helped with their feelings of fatigue. Having an extensive psychosocial program that includes music therapy, art therapy, play therapy, and massage therapy can all contribute to helping with distraction and "fun activities" as mentioned by the younger children. The adolescent patient identified alleviating factors for their fatigue as going outdoors, having protected rest time, having fun with friends, taking naps, resting, and keeping busy. They also mentioned that treatments such as getting medications for sleep, having physical therapy, and getting a blood transfusion helped with fatigue symptoms (Baggott and Association of Pediatric Oncology Nurses (U.S.) 2002).

As healthcare professionals, we need to give the patients and families the permission to rest while they are in the hospital, letting them know that it's okay to post a "nap time" or "rest time" on the door of their hospital room. For the many "technologically wired-in" patients that we care for, it's also often about evaluating sleep hygiene. Making sure that all electronics are turned off at night so they can sleep well is a first step in evaluating sleep hygiene. Many times our patients cannot attend school full time, but allowing them to go for half days or even a few hours when their counts are good makes a huge difference in their attitude. Discussing their daily routines at home, cutting back on long naps during the day to manage better sleep patterns at night, and making a routine each day are other ways to combat

fatigue. Creating nutritional plans and accessing the oncology dietician to help in creating adequate dietary needs with the goal of maximizing wellbeing can give energy to the patient experiencing fatigue. Maintaining adequate nutrition throughout the day is imperative for the patient experiencing fatigue. Instructing patients and families to eat small, high-calorie, high-protein snacks every 3–4 hours may help sustain the patient's energy level (LaTour 2014). Exercise as a response to fatigue has shown significant strides in overcoming the symptoms of fatigue (Griffie and Godfroy 2014). Collaboration with the multidisciplinary team to keep the patient active during admits and while at home is another key to overcoming fatigue (Griffie and Godfroy 2014).

11.4.4.5 Pain

Pain is often the most common side effect for the bone tumor patient. If it is not well controlled, it can significantly impact the patient's quality of life. For pain that is associated with tumor growth and sometimes even the occurrence of a pathological fracture, over-the-counter acetaminophen or ibuprofen become insufficient in controlling the pain. Medications that combine an analgesic and oral opioid are frequently the next step. The most effective intervention for relief of tumor pain is to initiate treatment as soon as possible (Pearson 2009) (see Table 11.4).

Initial pain assessment should include a self-report (location, character, time of worst and least pain, factors that improve and aggravate pain, and intensity utilizing a pain rating scale), parent input, observation of behavior, physical examination, and physiological measures/diagnostic results (Pearson 2009). Assessments in the future will often be compared to this initial baseline pain assessment. If pain resolves itself quickly after treatment begins, it is indicative of a positive response to therapy. If pain increases while receiving chemotherapy, either at the tumor site or other areas, it is troublesome in that it may indicate a lack of response to treatment. Frequently, imaging or pathology may confirm this concern. A sudden onset of acute pain without accompanying trauma may indicate a pathological fracture (Pearson 2009).

Table 11.4 Sources of pain in patients undergoing bone tumor therapy

	Treatment related	Surgery related	Procedure related
Bone (primary or metastatic): bone marrow Central nervous system Neuropathic Somatic or visceral	*Chemotherapy*: Mucositis Peripheral neuropathy Aseptic bone necrosis Myalgias or arthralgias Extravasation injuries Bone pain Typhlitis Pancreatitis Constipation or bowel obstruction *Radiation therapy*: Mucositis Radiation dermatitis Myelopathy Radiation fibrosis Osteoradionecrosis Radiation-induced peripheral nerve tumors Radiation burns	Acute postoperative *Post-thoracotomy syndrome*: numbness or neuropathic pain that can occur after thoracic surgeries	Finger stick Venipuncture Intravenous cannulation Implanted central venous catheter Venous access device removal Suture removal Bone marrow aspiration Bone marrow biopsy Lumbar puncture LP-related headache or backache

Managing the bone pain that commonly accompanies pegfilgrastim or filgrastim can sometimes be worrisome to the patient and family if they were not aware of the possibility that it may occur. Many times they are immediately concerned and anxious that this "new pain" is indicative of metastasis or treatment not working. The first step in alleviating this worry is to review with the patient and family the purpose and side effects of these drugs, giving them a medication reference handout to review prior to their first treatment with pegfilgrastim or filgrastim. They are instructed to start taking acetaminophen (after taking their temperature prior to each dose) or utilize their prescribed pain medication scheduled to stay ahead of the bone pain. If their home pain regimen does not control the bone pain associated with pegfilgrastim, they are sometimes admitted or brought into the outpatient infusion clinic for intravenous pain medications. For those patients who experience significant bone pain with their pegfilgrastim treatment, the medical team may add the antihistamine, loratadine. Loratadine is given prior to the pegfilgrastim injection and then daily until count recovery occurs.

Postsurgical pain is expected and involves the consultation of the inpatient anesthesia or pain team to initiate and manage intravenous and epidural pain medications. This team rounds on the patient daily and is the continuous medical contact for nursing staff during their surgical admit for pain control. For the local control procedures such as limb salvage and amputation, incorporating physical therapy and a rehabilitation program mandates good pain control. The need to continually evaluate the effectiveness of treatment cannot be overemphasized (Pearson 2009). The nurses play an intricate role in assuring the timing of pain medications coincides with the physical therapy and rehabilitation plan (Pearson 2009). For those patients recovering from post thoracotomy, deep breathing and coughing exercises are also managed more effectively if the patient has adequate pain control.

Progressive disease pain is a multifaceted problem and requires consulting with other specialists such as radiation therapists with radiosensitizing chemotherapy, radiofrequency, ablation, cryoablation, nerve blocks, as well as pain medications to manage progressive disease pain and promote quality of life (Pearson 2009). The bone tumor team works closely with the palliative care team at our institution, consulting them early on in the treatment regimen to foster relationships among the palliative team and the patient and family. They are introduced as symptom management experts, and the bone tumor team regularly meets with the palliative care team and combines patient appointments to offer comprehensive care to the patient and family.

Neuropathic pain and neuropathy are common symptoms of the pediatric bone tumor patient's treatment. The patient and family are advised prior to treatment that neuropathy may occur. Presentation may include a burning pain, numbness, and tingling that often start in the feet, hands, or fingertips, not being able to feel hot or cold, more sensitive to touching things, poor coordination, muscle weakness, cramping, or twitching (Baggott and Association of Pediatric Oncology Nurses (U.S.) 2002). The medical team continually evaluates for signs and symptoms of neuropathy during treatment. It may lead to dose adjustments in chemotherapy regimens due to neuropathy. The medical team may utilize anticonvulsants such as gabapentin to help with pain management. Physical therapy is often consulted as well. Some other nonpharmocological treatments that may help alleviate the pain are relaxation therapy, massage therapy, acupuncture, or devices that affect nerve signals (Baggott and Association of Pediatric Oncology Nurses (U.S.) 2002).

Referring our patients to an outpatient pain clinic is another option to help the patient manage acute to chronic pain. The Pain Services Clinic at our institution provides a comprehensive assistance to patients with complex and/or long-term pain-related problems. The clinic is in an integrated, interdisciplinary model where rehabilitation and facilitation of normal developmental trajectory are the primary goals. The services provided include comprehensive biopsychosocial assessment, pharmacological and regional anesthetic management, individual and family therapy, biofeedback, breathing, relaxation and imagery training, and counseling regarding management of patient/family psychosocial disorders related to acute and chronic pain, physical and or occupational therapy, massage, and acupuncture. The ONN facilitates referral and helps the patient manage outpatient appointments to the pain clinic during treatment.

Navigating the bone tumor patient through their pain can be challenging. With the integration of the electronic medical record (EMR) that allows the ONN to view all patient appointments, discharge summaries, and medication records, it has become much easier to review current pain medications with the patient and family. The first step in triaging pain is assessing the pain by asking for the location, quality, intensity, and duration of the pain. The ONN also assesses for aggravating or relieving factors and cognitive response to pain (Baggott and Association of Pediatric Oncology Nurses (U.S.) 2002). For children who are unable to fully verbalize their pain, a FACES pain scale is included in their teaching notebook, and the family is asked to have the patient rate their pain utilizing this scale (see Fig. 11.4). The ONN reviews current medications the patient is taking and formulates a plan with the patient and family utilizing current prescriptions and requests a callback later in the day for follow-up to monitor if there has been any relief. If the current pain regimen is not managing the patient's pain, the ONN documents in the patient EMR and notifies the practitioner for possible change in regimen or the evaluation to be seen by a practitioner. Each triage and evaluation by the ONN is unique and individualized. Sometimes patients and families just need a review and guidance of taking their pain medications as prescribed, often fearful of addiction. The ONN

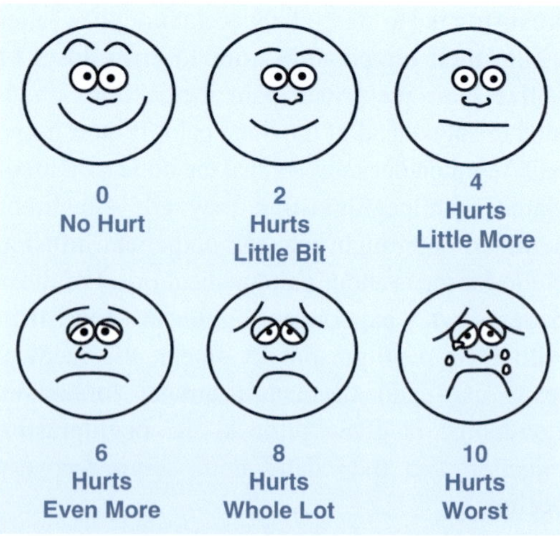

Fig. 11.4 Wong-Baker FACES® pain rating scale

offers support and guidance to the patient and family which typically involves listening to their concerns (Black and Caufield 2007). Anxiety, nausea, constipation, lack of sleep, dehydration, anemia, or fatigue can all increase a patient's level of pain (Baggott and Association of Pediatric Oncology Nurses (U.S.) 2002). It's the responsibility of the ONN to be able to listen and rule out any or all of the above during phone triage.

Lastly, pain is not managed by just the medical team in pediatric institutions. It involves a multidisciplinary, multi-team approach that includes a wide variety of team members from child life specialists, music therapists, art thera-pists, volunteers, nurses, technicians, massage therapist, acupuncturists, psychologists, palliative care team members, hospice team members, pastoral services, and, lastly, the patient and family. Team members get to know the patient and utilize their professional skills to help the patient deal with their pain in many ways other than just utilizing pain medications. The patient and family can take these new interventions and apply them while at home. Their pain is managed through other nonpharmacological and cognitive-behavioral intervention (Baggott and Association of Pediatric Oncology Nurses (U.S.) 2002) (see Table 11.5).

Table 11.5 Pain management strategies

Type	Recommended ages	Indications	Contraindications
Heat	6 months or older	Relieves muscle pain and joint stiffness, relaxes muscles, eases spasms	Contraindicated on irradiated tissue or over tumor sites
Cold	6 months or older	Injury, bruising, muscle spasms, headaches	Contraindicated on tissue damaged by radiation and patients with peripheral vascular disease
Massage	All ages	Achy muscles, muscle spasms, tense muscles, soothing and relaxing for the body and mind	None
TENS (transcutaneous electrical nerve stimulation)	3 years and older	Headaches, muscle aches and spasms, bone metastasis, neuropathy, phantom limb pain	Caution in those patients with epilepsy, cardiac problems, or pacemakers
Acupuncture or acupressure	All ages	Acute pain, headaches, musculoskeletal pain, persistent, recurrent, or chronic pain	To be performed only by a trained acupuncturist
Relaxation	7 years and older	Acute pain, persistent achy pain, chronic pain, abdominal or limb pain	None
Music	All ages	Acute, chronic, and procedural pain	None
Breathing	3 years and older	Nonacute pain, persistent achy pain, chronic pain, abdominal or limb pain, pain associated with tension or anxiety	None
Blowing away pain	1 year and older	Acute, brief pain, procedural pain	None
Biofeedback	3 years and older	Migraine and muscle tension headaches, persistent muscle pain	None
Imagery	3 years and older	Acute, chronic, and procedural pain	Patient with severe emotional problems or psychiatric illness, or history of hallucinations
Hypnosis	3 years and older	Acute, chronic, and procedural pain	Patient with severe emotional problems or psychiatric illness, or history of hallucinations
Distractions	10 months and older	Treatment-related pain, acute and chronic pain	None

11.4.4.6 Fever

Management of the pediatric bone tumor patient with fever and neutropenia differs greatly from that of other patients with fever. Due to the high mortality rate associated with untreated infection, all fevers experienced by children with neutropenia are considered due to a life-threatening infection until proven otherwise (Baggott and Association of Pediatric Oncology Nurses (U.S.) 2002; Mize et al. 2014). From the initial contact with the patient and family, the ONN reviews a "who to call and when to call" guideline sheet with family. Fever greater than 100.5 °F (38.05 °C) or higher is located at the top of this list and is documented in every discharge summary and teaching document for the family. The ONN provides the family with a thermometer and assures that the family is proficient in monitoring for temperatures. When triaging the patient over the phone, the ONN gathers pertinent information regarding the physical status of the patient such as alertness, paleness, any change in color to feet or hands, any duskiness to lips or mouth, looking for any changes in circulation, any respiratory difficulties, changes in pain, diarrhea, pain or burning with urination, persistent cough, rash, sore throat, chills or shaking, stiff neck, any bleeding or bruising, and any exposures to infectious illnesses. If the triage performed exhibits any emergent issues, the family is asked to hang up and call 911. If they live a distance from the institution and the patient's temperature is greater than 102° and exhibits any one of the alerted assessment, they are asked to go to the closest local hospital and to have the ED staff contact the fellow or attending on call at our institution. If no other symptoms persist and the patient is stable, they are directed to come to the hospital for evaluation and to pack a bag because depending on their degree of neutropenia, they may be admitted. The ONN alerts the ED intake of the patient diagnosis, where they are in their therapy, and any complications or pertinent information so that the patient is alerted as a fever and neutropenic cancer patient and does not have to wait long in the ED intake process. The ONN then communicates the patient information to the inpatient team and the primary team. For the patients whose fevers are greater than 101.5°, the family is instructed to give the patient a dose of acetaminophen prior to leaving for the hospital so that temperature status can be managed. Most bone tumor patients currently in treatment have their labs checked twice a week either at an outside lab or at the hospital laboratory, allowing the primary team to monitor where they are in their blood count recovery. Since the ONN retrieves these counts and communicates the results to the patient and family, she is usually aware of neutropenia status of the patient when the patient calls with a fever. Once again, the EMR serves as an ideal, comprehensive tool in managing the bone tumor patients. Each institution utilizes fever and neutropenia precautions differently. Some institutions maintain a fever as 101 °F.

11.4.4.7 Neutropenia

Managing neutropenia at home can be worrisome for patients and families. Prior to discharge after their first chemotherapy treatment, the ONN reviews neutropenia cautions with the family, teaching them about their complete blood count and what it includes. The COG Family Handbook is utilized for complete blood count teaching. The ANC is explained and reviewed with them, letting them know that each time they have their labs drawn, we will be able to determine their child's ability to fight infections by calculating the ANC with them. If their ANC is less than 500, they are at higher risk of infection, and it is at this time when they should be cautious to wear a mask when outside the home, avoid crowds, and monitor daily for temps (Murphy 2011; Baggott and Association of Pediatric Oncology Nurses (U.S.) 2002). Making the child feel isolated or alone due to not being able to have friends over or attend school can be avoided by monitoring the ANC. The ONN instructs families to avoid any sick contacts, purchase alcohol-based hand sanitizer, and place it by the front door and in the kitchen, requesting that all visitors utilize the hand sanitizer when visiting the home. The ONN gives the family boxes of pediatric and adult masks to wear when the patient is neutropenic or a family member is ill. Encouraging the patient and entire family to adapt to regular handwashing is the most effective way to prevent the spread of infection in the home (Murphy 2011; Baggott and Association of Pediatric Oncology Nurses (U.S.) 2002). The family is instructed to keep other sick children directly away from the bone tumor patient, making sure they do not share drinks or food. When the patient's ANC has recovered, it is okay to go out, visit friends, and sometimes even go to school for a few hours, first checking with the school nurse or office to make sure there is not a lot of illness in the school. Any friends coming to visit should be screened for exposures to any illnesses, or if they have a fever, runny nose, cough, diarrhea, or rash, they should not visit. Personal hygiene and good, consistent dental hygiene are important before, during, and after treatment (Baggott and Association of Pediatric Oncology Nurses (U.S.) 2002; Murphy 2011).

One of the most common questions we receive is if the patient can keep or get a new pet. For the patients who have a pet, they are asked to avoid any stool and urine from animals. They are also instructed not to clean the cages of pets in the home. Pets in the home should be well cared for, clean, and immunized (Murphy 2011).

Patients are also instructed to avoid mowing grass or plowing fields; avoid barns and farming; no digging in sand or dirt; no swimming in creeks, rivers, or lakes; avoid people with chickenpox or shingles; no drinking of raw milk; no eating raw or uncooked meat or eggs; and no raw cookie dough. Patients are instructed to wear a mask when they are coming and leaving the hospital or if they are walking around the hospital. They are also instructed to wear a mask for precaution when they are around a construction area or if they are out in an area where they are mowing the grass or plowing fields (Murphy 2011).

Managing neutropenia prophylactically by the medical team starts with the patient taking Bactrim on the weekends to prevent *Pneumocystis jiroveci* pneumonia (Mize et al. 2014). Depending on recurrent fungal and viral infections that the patient might experience, the medical team may place a patient on prophylactic antifungals or antivirals during neutropenic times in their therapy (Mize et al. 2014). Currently in the United States,

all influenza injectable vaccines are a "killed virus." In the neutropenic or immunocompromised patient, it is recommended that the pediatric cancer patient receive the injectable vaccine, but they should not receive the "live virus" that is in the commonly used influenza nasal spray vaccine (Mize et al. 2014). The entire family of a pediatric bone tumor patient is recommended to receive the injectable influenza vaccine.

11.4.4.8 Constipation

In the complex treatment of the pediatric bone tumor patient, constipation is usually a multifactorial problem (Baggott and Association of Pediatric Oncology Nurses (U.S.) 2002). Constipation may be related to narcotic analgesic or vinca alkaloids that have a neurotoxic effect on the smooth muscle of the gastrointestinal tract causing decreased peristaltic activity, decreased oral intake secondary to nausea and vomiting, decreased activity, or secondary to abdominal surgery (Baggott and Association of Pediatric Oncology Nurses (U.S.) 2002). It is important to perform a baseline assessment and history of the patient's bowel habits prior to beginning treatment. Prophylactic stool softeners and/or laxatives, a diet high in fiber, and adequate fluid intake may help prevent or alleviate constipation during treatment (Baggott and Association of Pediatric Oncology Nurses (U.S.) 2002; Lahl et al. 2008). Nonpharmaceutical actions to help prevent constipation include encouraging physical activity, providing privacy, and diet (Lahl et al. 2008; Baggott and Association of Pediatric Oncology Nurses (U.S.) 2002). Teaching the family that a diet that consists of a variety of fruits and vegetables, whole grain breads and cereals, and high-fiber snack foods such as fig bars, date or raisin bars, and oatmeal cookies may help in the prevention of constipation is essential. The ONN also reinforces with the patient and family that they should notify the medical team immediately if the patient experiences any pain, tearing, or burning during bowel movements due to the potential of infection secondary to neutropenia. The ONN works with the patient and family to adequately adjust their stool softeners and diet to prevent constipation.

11.4.4.9 Diarrhea

Diarrhea in the bone tumor patient is most often related to their treatment or medications, but this first needs to be triaged and assessed. The ONN reviews the patient medication history of any antibiotics, changes in diet, ill contacts at home, or any antineoplastic medications they may be receiving that cause diarrhea (Baggott and Association of Pediatric Oncology Nurses (U.S.) 2002). The first step to diarrhea management is to monitor the amount and volume, teaching the family to document how many stools they are having daily. Much like evaluating for dehydration in the patient experiencing nausea and vomiting, the ONN teaches the family to look for signs and symptoms such as decreased urine output, no tears with crying, dry, pasty oral mucosa, increased lethargy, and dry skin. For patients being treated with antibiotics, stool cultures may be sent. For the patients receiving chemotherapy agents causing diarrhea, utilizing loperamide around the clock until no stooling has occurred for 12 hours can help stop the diarrhea. Also, avoiding foods containing milk products, tea, coffee, and drinks with caffeine will help with the diarrhea. They are instructed to drink plenty of water, sports drinks, or electrolyte-containing drinks, to drink broth or clear soup, to avoid taking any stool softeners, and to eat foods such as bananas, rice, apple sauce, chicken, white toast, or canned fruits. For those patients receiving irinotecan, the medical team may initiate the use of cefixime and charcoal tablets to aid in decreasing diarrhea during treatment.

11.4.5 Tracking Evaluation and Schedules

Tracking evaluations and schedules for all on and off therapy bone tumor patients requires a detailed patient list within the electronic medical record (EMR). One technique is to create a patient list within the EMR system at our institution listed as "sarcoma patients." Through the EMR system, the patient list is created containing the following properties: patient name, medical record number, age/sex, last admission date, new results, last discharge date, DOB, room number, last weight in kilograms, and expected admission date. When the ONN opens their desktop, this is the list that automatically opens up, allowing her to see where her patients are, if they are admitted, have results, or have been discharged recently from another department. This list has also been made available to all bone tumor team members including phone nurses who cover the ONN's role while she is not in the office. The ONN also keeps a file of each patient's treatment schema that enables her to create calendars for patients, know upcoming treatments, and monitor for upcoming scan schedules. The ONN is able to utilize the EMR "chart review" section to monitor upcoming appointments. For off therapy patients, these charts are forwarded into the ONN's "inbasket" where they sit with instructions in the routing or plan of care note documented by the practitioner when the patient is due for their next follow-up scans. This basket is reviewed daily by the ONN, and weekly scans are ordered and appointments scheduled. The ONN utilizes the plan of care documentation from oncology appointments with the practitioners and also utilizes the online COG protocol guidelines for monitoring/evaluations for patients who were on study. The sarcoma team (bone tumor team) meets every 2 weeks and discusses patients; reviewing scans and plan of treatments are discussed. This also gives opportunity to follow up with the practitioners about plans for evaluation. A member of the research team attends this meeting which allows collaboration for any concerns or questions about evaluation timing.

11.4.6 Referrals

Surgery and radiation referrals can be challenging if they are outside the institution. Our institution utilizes an outside radiation facility for both photon and proton radiation. Depending on the institution, the patient information requested varies. The ONN has a list of contacts for several proton and photon radiation centers in the Midwest and Northeastern United States. Documenting all contact information including emails and phone numbers in the patient's chart in telephone encounters allows other team members to easily retrieve contact numbers. Since most of the centers are teaching institutions, they require all requested information be faxed or mailed to them along with a copy of the patient's scans. Through trial and error, the ONN has found that sending the package including all paperwork and the disc of scans together works most effectively. For most of our patients receiving photon therapy at the cancer center close to our institution, the referral process involves contacting the intake coordinator with patient information and obtaining a patient appointment that can be communicated to the primary team and to the patient and family, coordinating it along with their inpatient admissions and clinic appointments. A disc of scans is couriered to the cancer center in the same day, and all information is faxed to the intake coordinator. If the cancer center we are referring our patients to utilizes the same EMR system, it allows us to access the patient chart at these institutions to monitor their appointments and progress while receiving radiation treatments. Consent to access this system in EPIC is called "Care Everywhere" is required to be signed by the parent or guardian. The radiation staff notifies the ONN of the treatment plan and schedule for the patient so that schedules can be coordinated.

Surgery referrals are made for line placement or surgical procedures. If the surgeon is at our institution, the process of referral is easy. For scheduling purposes, the referral is made in the EMR system, but the ONN also emails or contacts the surgeon's scheduling staff to answer any questions or concerns. The emails are documented in the patient's EMR so that all team members are aware of the referral follow-up. The ONN often communicates by email or phone encounters to surgeons and the surgeon's scheduling staff, informing them of where the patients are in their treatment plan so that collaboration

for local control with their office can begin. Our institution has comprehensive specialty clinics in which the oncologist and the surgeon see patients collaboratively, creating seamless communication between specialties. Examples of a few of these clinics that the bone tumor patient may be seen in are the orthopedic oncology clinic and surgical oncology clinics. For surgery referrals outside our institution, the process can be challenging. After all documents, scans, and pathology are sent, it can be difficult to retrieve follow-up plans and return communication from outside institutions. Persistence in calling the office typically prevails, but this can be time consuming.

11.4.7 Home Care Coordination

Home care coordination is organized with the discharge planner and case management for our division. We communicate daily about our shared patients and notify each other of any changes in the plan of care. A weekly list of patient chemotherapy treatments is sent to the schedulers for our infusion center. The ONN sends this email to the discharge planner, notifying her of any upcoming admits, and documents any home care needs on this email. The ONN coordinates and assures home care orders are signed by the attending oncologist and sent to the home care company in a timely manner. If the outpatient pharmacy or home care infusion pharmacy has questions, they contact the ONN for clarification or directions in delays of treatment. Some home care coordination involves palliative care or hospice care. This coordination can include nurses, aides, chaplain services, massage therapy, or recreation therapy, depending on the demographics of the family. For hospice care, the ONN, who has known the patient and family from diagnosis, continues to support them until end of life. Most of this support provided from the ONN is through listening or answering any questions or concerns they may have about what to expect at the end of life for their child.

11.5 Transitioning to Survivorship

Transitioning bone tumor patients from treatment to off therapy can be an ambivalent experience for the patient and family. They have just spent the last several months navigating appointments, admissions, fevers, medications, and side effects with their bone tumor team, and suddenly they are instructed they do not need to come back for 3 months. They are excited to have finished the race but anxious about the future and worry for relapse. The bone tumor team has become their tour guide in the day-to-day adventures of treatment, learning to trust and depend on them. When treatment ends, they become fearful about terminating the relationship they have become so dependent upon. The oncology team supports the patient and family during this time, helping them transition from almost daily conversations with the oncology team to fostering relationships with a primary care physician.

11.5.1 Primary Care Physician Coordination

Once the central line is removed, the patient and family are referred to their pediatrician or primary care physician (PCP) for routine colds and fevers in between follow-up appointments with the bone tumor team. Transitioning care to the PCP needs to include excellent communication between the oncology team and the PCP. For some patients, who did not have an established pediatrician or primary care physician prior to diagnosis, they may consider the oncology team as their primary care physician (PCP). Finding a primary care physician can be difficult. The best advice when it comes to finding a new PCP is asking friends and family who their physician is and do they like them? Why do they like their PCP? If finding a PCP through family and friends does not work, most insurance companies have a number you can call, and someone will help you find a PCP in your area. Most of these companies also have websites that allow you to navigate several physicians in your area. The ONN often times brings up websites with the patients and family and helps them initiate the process. The ONN can sometimes contact the new PCP and discuss a new patient appointment with the office staff which often produces an earlier appointment for the patient. The ONN also sends a treatment summary or care plan to the PCP once medical release is completed, making sure the PCP has access to the oncology team as needed. We are fortunate that we have a large teaching medical center close by and they have a residents' clinic that our patients can be referred to for follow-up care. By sending our patients to this facility, it allows the bone tumor team access to their electronic medical record. There are also several websites and apps for smartphone users that can link you to a new PCP. See below for list:

www.ehealthinsurance.com/individual-health.../
    choosing-pcp/
https://www.medmutual.com/.../Choosing-a-
    Primary-Care-Physician.aspx
www.bcbs.com/blog/five-tips-for-choosing-a-
    PCP.html
www.zocdoc.com/primary-care-doctors
www.bcbsm.com/index/.../choose-or-change-
    pcp-online.html
mmeht.org/FindingPhysician.htm
https://www.cchplink.com/providersite/secure/
    findadoctor.aspx
www.aetna.com/about-aetna-insurance/sas/
    mobile/ (a smartphone app)

11.5.2 Tracking Regular Surveillance Appointments

Tracking regular off therapy surveillance appointments is not complicated for the ONN, but it can be time consuming. Utilizing the EMR system to help track patient appointments and last scans is essential. This task can become difficult if the practitioner does not complete their last visit note in a timely manner. The ONN reviews all bone tumor patient's last visit notes for the practitioner's impression and plan documented in the history and physical. Through this documentation, the ONN keeps a spreadsheet that allows her to document last scan dates, next due date for scans, last EKG and echocardiogram, and how many months they are off therapy. By utilizing the EMR chart review, the ONN is able to follow up on all scans ordered or not ordered by the practitioner. Children's Oncology Group treatment protocols are accessed for guidelines of recommended evaluations needed for each follow-up visit.

11.5.3 Survivorship Care Plans and Cancer Treatment Summary

The Institute of Medicine (IOM) and the National Research Council published *From Cancer Patient to Cancer Survivor: Lost in Transition in 2005.* The authors created a number of recommendations. One of these recommendations was that survivorship should be viewed as a separate phase of cancer care and that when a patient completes their primary treatment they should be provided with a comprehensive care summary and follow-up plan written by the primary oncology team who coordinated their oncology treatment. This care summary and follow-up is now referred to as a survivorship care plan (LaTour 2014; McClellan et al. 2013; Hewitt 2006).

This need was also reinforced in 2012 when the American College of Surgeon's Commission on Cancer (CoC) created new standards that require all hospitals that are accredited by the CoC to complete a survivorship care plan (SCP) that is clearly and effectively explained for all patients completing treatment.

CoC Standard 3.3 Survivorship Care Plan The cancer committee develops and implements a process to disseminate a comprehensive care summary and follow-up plan to patients with cancer who are completing cancer treatment. The process is monitored, evaluated, and presented at least annually to the cancer committee and documented in minutes (LaTour 2014).

The cancer treatment summary is the first and most essential part of this new standard. Upon discharge from cancer treatment, including treatment of recurrences, every patient should be given a record of all care received and important disease characteristics (see Table 11.6).

The Children's Oncology Group Long-Term Follow-Up Guidelines for Survivors of Childhood, Adolescent, and Young Adult Cancers have two templates available in electronic format at www.survivorshipguidelines.org (See Fig. 11.5). It is also suggested that the SCP be provided to the patient's primary care provider. This plan will inform the patient and the PCP of the long-term effects of cancer and treatment and identify and provide guidance on follow-up care, prevention, and health maintenance for the survivor (Horowitz et al. 2009; McClellan et al. 2013).

The *Passport for Care* application for survivors of childhood cancer is being developed in collaboration with the Children's Oncology Group to address healthcare information needs of long-term survivors (See Fig. 11.6). The Passport for Care (PFC) is an Internet-based tool devel-

Table 11.6 Essential elements of treatment summary

Diagnostic tests performed and results	Tumor characteristics (site(s), stage and grade, hormonal status, marker information)
Dates of treatment initiation and completion	Psychosocial, nutritional, and other supportive services provided
Surgery dates	Full contact information on treating institutions and key individual providers
Chemotherapy including agents used, treatment regimen, total dosage, identifying number and title of clinical trials	Identification of a key point of contact and coordinator of continuing care
Radiotherapy	
Transplant	
Hormonal therapy	
Indicators of treatment response and toxicities experienced during treatment	

oped to provide survivors and their PCP with individualized, accurate, and timely healthcare information related to the treatment they received. The PFC provides them with summaries of their cancer history and treatment. This information drives algorithms to produce individualized monitoring and management recommendations derived from the Children's Oncology Group (COG) long-term follow-up guidelines (Horowitz et al. 2009).

Where the treatment summary provides the details about the type of treatment received as well as any complications or side effects that the patient experienced, the survivorship care plan provides information about the plan for follow-up to include screening recommenda-

SUMMARY OF CANCER TREATMENT
(Comprehensive)

DEMOGRAPHICS			
Name: (last, first, middle)	**Sex:** (M/F)	**Date of Birth:**	**COG Reg #:**
Address: (number, street, city, state/province, postal code, country)			
Phone:	**SS#**	**Race/Ethnicity:** (see list #1)	
Alternate contact:		**Relationship:**	**Phone:**

CANCER DIAGNOSIS	
Diagnosis: (see list #2)	
Date of Diagnosis: **Age at Diagnosis:** **Date Therapy Completed:**	
Sites involved/stage /diagnostic details:	**Laterality:**(Right/Left/NA)
Hereditary/congenital history: (see list #3)	
Pertinent past medical history:	
Treatment Center:	**Medical Record #:**
MD/APN Contact Information:	

RELAPSE(S) ☐ Yes   ☐ No   *If yes, provide information below*

Date:	Site(s):	Laterality: (Right/Left/NA)	Date Therapy Completed:

SUBSEQUENT MALIGNANT NEOPLASM(S) ☐ Yes   No ☐ *If yes, provide information below*

Date:	Type: (see list #4)	
Stage/Site(s):		Date Therapy Completed:

CANCER TREATMENT SUMMARY				
PROTOCOL(S) ☐ Yes ☐ No *If yes, provide information below*				
Acronym/Number	**Title/Description**	**Initiated**	**Completed**	**On-Study**

CHEMOTHERAPY ☐ Yes ☐ No *If yes, complete chart below*		
Drug Name	**Route**	**Additional Information†**
(see list # 5)	(see list #6)	(see list #7)

Fig. 11.5 Cancer treatment summary

SUMMARY OF CANCER TREATMENT (continued)

RADIATION Yes ☐ No ☐					*If yes, complete chart below*						
Site/Field	Laterality	Start Date	Stop Date	Fractions	Dose per Fraction (Gy)*	Initial Dose (Gy)*	Boost Site	Boost Dose (Gy)*	Total Dose (including boost) (Gy)*	Type
(see list #8)							(see list #9)			(see list #10)
Radiation oncologist:						Institution:				

*Note: To convert cGy or rads to Gy, divide dose by 100 (example: 2400 cGy = 2400 rads = 24 Gy)

HEMATOPOIETIC CELL TRANSPLANT Yes ☐ No ☐			*If yes, complete chart below*	
Type	Source	Date of Infusion	Conditioning Regimen	Institution/Treating MD
(see list #11) Tandem? ☐ Yes ☐ No	(see list #12)		(see list #13)	

GVHD prophylaxis/treatment (For transplant patients only) ☐ Yes ☐ No *If yes, complete chart below*		
Type	First Dose	Last Dose
(see list #14)		

Was this patient ever diagnosed with **chronic** graft-versus-host disease (cGVHD)?   Yes ☐ No ☐

SURGERY Yes ☐ No ☐		*If yes, complete chart below*		
Date	Procedure	Site (if applicable)	Laterality (if applicable)	Surgeon/Institution
	(see list #15)			

OTHER THERAPEUTIC MODALITIES ☐ Yes ☐ No		*If yes, complete chart below*
Therapy	Route	Cumulative Dose (if known)
(see list # 16)	(see list #6)	(see list #7)

COMPLICATIONS/LATE EFFECTS ☐ Yes ☐ No			*If yes, complete chart below*
Problem	Date onset	Date resolved	Status
(see list #17)			(Active/Resolved)

Adverse Drug Reactions/Allergies ☐ Yes ☐ No		*If yes, complete chart below*	
Drug	Reaction	Date	Status
			(Active/Resolved)

Additional Information/Comments ☐ Yes ☐ No	*If yes, provide information below*

Summary prepared by: (name/title/institution)	Date prepared:
Summary updated by: (name/title/institution)	Date updated:

Fig. 11.5 (continued)

tions and possible late side effects. Teaching the patient and family about late effects should not start at the end of therapy, but at the beginning of treatment and throughout the continuum of care. Handing the patient and family an end of treatment summary and a notebook full of handouts is not the most effective teaching method. Setting aside an end of therapy appointment to review all treatment received and the SCP is most effective for the patient and family, providing a quiet time to review information. When the survivor is ready to transition from active treatment to follow-up, it is essential that they know who is primarily responsible for their future care. Utilizing technology is another effective tool for teaching about late effects of treatment.

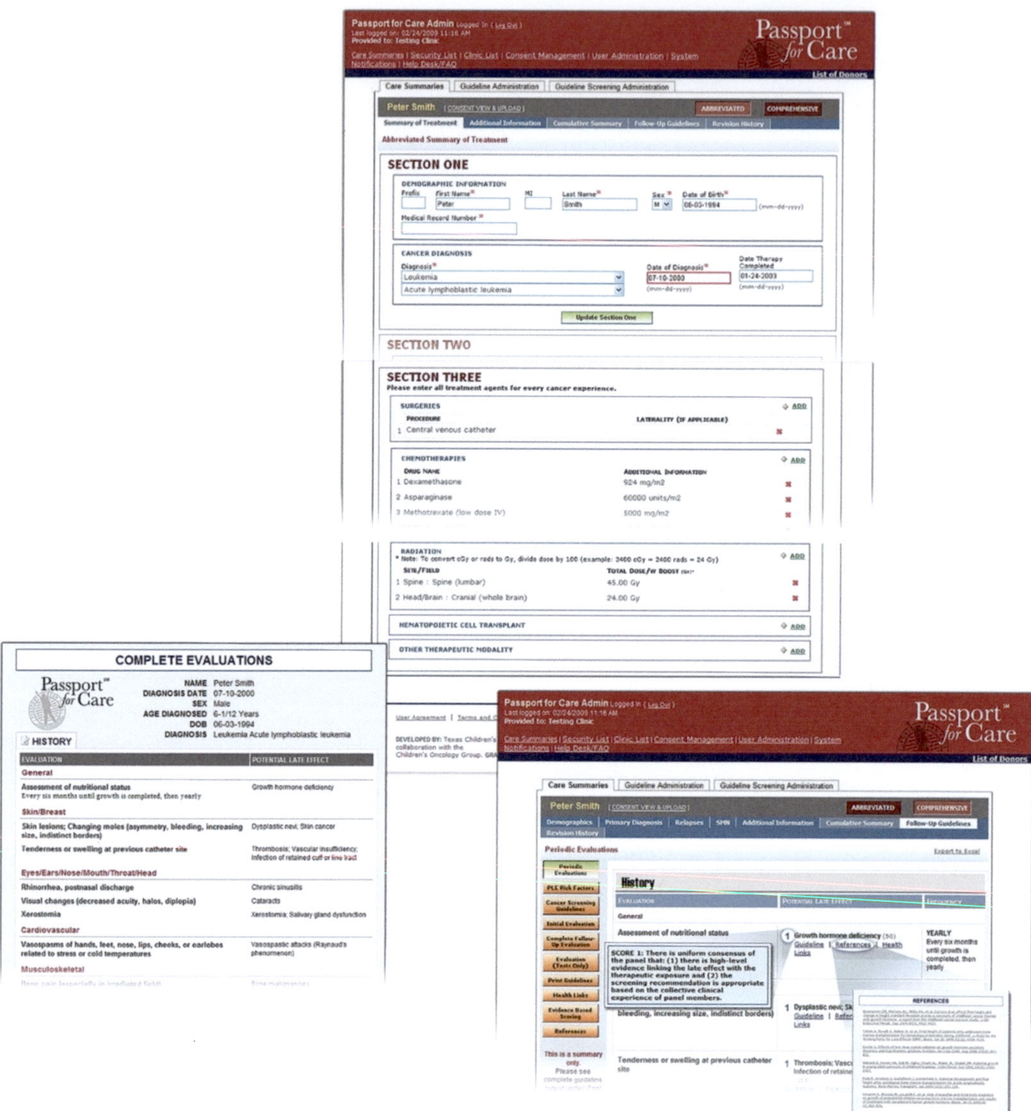

Fig. 11.6 Passport for Care

PFC is one example of how a patient and family can utilize Web-based sites to review information. Livestrong has utilized the website http://www.livestrongcareplan.org/, where patients can go online and develop their care plans and a tool that allows them to print a copy for their PCP. In the world where most patients and families have smartphones, there are apps like the AYA Healthy Survivorship that allows the survivor to keep track of their plan, screening and late effects as well as contact a community of survivors (http://www.curesearch.org/Article View2.aspx?id=10091). Searching "cancer" or "cancer care" in the apps template will lead the survivor to several tools they can utilize. The Institute of Medicine has declared a minimum standards of care be included in the survivorship care plan (see Table 11.7).

Table 11.7 Survivorship care plan

Diagnostic tests performed and results	Tumor characteristics (site(s), stage and grade, hormonal status, marker information)
Dates of treatment initiation and completion	Psychosocial, nutritional, and other supportive services provided
Surgery dates	Full contact information on treating institutions and key individual providers
Chemotherapy including agents used, treatment regimen, total dosage, identifying number and title of clinical trials	Identification of a key point of contact and coordinator of continuing care
Radiotherapy	
Transplant	
Hormonal therapy	
Indicators of treatment response and toxicities experienced during treatment	

Each institution has to determine the process of completing and reviewing these cancer treatment summaries and the survivorship care plans with their patients. The follow-up component offers an opportunity to identify which provider is responsible for care in the future and helps the patient understand who to call and when to call. Nurses serving as navigators can identify the patient's PCP and be sure the contact information is included with the patient electronic medical record. With multiple survivorship models now in use, studies have confirmed that there is no one way to provide survivorship care (LaTour 2014). What is important is that an SCP discussion occurs consistently and with one member of the healthcare team whom the patient identifies as a primary contact (LaTour 2014).

11.5.4 Prevention of Secondary Cancers

As the bone tumor team transitions the patient into survivorship, discussing and screening for secondary cancers is imperative. Studies have shown that as a childhood cancer survivor becomes older, they have a slightly higher risk of developing a second cancer compared to people their same age in the general population (Hudson and Hester 2013; McClellan et al. 2013). Contributors to this risk are the person's age during cancer therapy, treatment they received, and their genetic and family history (Hudson and Hester 2013). At the end of therapy, the bone tumor team and ONN review the patient's risk of developing a secondary cancer by reviewing the cancer treatment summary and family history. In some cases, early or more frequent screening may be recommended to ensure early detection. Reinforcing the importance of follow-up appointments is essential for this screening process. Teaching the patient and family to practice health maintenance behaviors such as regular checkups, developing a relationship with a primary care provider who knows their cancer treatment summary, risks of late complications, and recommended screening evaluations will improve the chances of catching problems at an earlier, treatable stage (McClellan et al. 2013; Hudson and Hester 2013). Patients are encouraged to report any new or persistent symptoms to the healthcare provider (see Table 11.8).

The ONN and bone tumor team instructs the patient at end of therapy on behaviors that can reduce their risk of getting a secondary cancer (see Table 11.9).

11.5.5 Late Effects of Treatment of the Bone Tumor Patient

Beyond monitoring for recurrence, caring for the childhood cancer survivor must include evaluation of potential long-term effects, health education, and promotion of health screening (Lahl et al. 2008). The late effects of the bone tumor patient are directly related to their treatment modalities, and the nurse must continue to support and assure adequate appointment follow-up for these patients that are at risk. The bone tumor

Table 11.8 Guideline of symptoms to report during follow-up

Easy bruising or bleeding	Changes in moles	Persistent abdominal pain	Persistent cough or hoarseness
Paleness of the skin	Sores that do not heal	Blood in the stools	Shortness of breath
Excessive fatigue	Lumps	Blood in the urine	Bloody sputum
Bone pain	Difficulty swallowing	Painful urination or defecation	Discolored areas or sores in the mouth that do not heal
Vision changes	Changes in bowel habits		Persistent headaches
Persistent early morning vomiting			

Table 11.9 Behavior modifications following cancer therapy

Avoid cancer-promoting behaviors	Drink alcohol in moderation	Diet and exercise	Get vaccinated
Do not smoke Do not chew tobacco Avoid secondhand smoke Protect the skin from sun exposure Avoid tanning beds	Limit the use of alcohol	Reduce daily fat intake to 30 % or less of calorie intake Eat foods high in fiber Eat a diet high in cruciferous vegetables (cabbage, brussels sprouts, broccoli, cauliflower) Avoid or limit daily intake of processed or preserved foods such as pickled, salt-cured, or lunch meats Eat a diet high in vitamin C and A such as fresh citrus fruits, melons, green and yellow vegetables	Human papillomavirus (HPV) vaccine Hepatitis B vaccine

team must work as a team to manage these patients by offering resources and education related to their disease history, treatments, and possible health deficits (Lahl et al. 2008; McClellan et al. 2013). To improve knowledge and understanding of late effects, it's imperative that late effects of treatment received are taught and reinforced throughout the pediatric bone tumor patient's treatment (Cherven et al. 2014). Creating an "end-of-therapy" appointment with the practitioner and clinician to discuss the treatment summary and survivorship care plan and reinforce the possibility of late effects creates an opportunity to assess for learning deficits with the patient and family (see Table 11.10).

Conclusion

In today's healthcare environment of cancer care complexity, the ONN role can provide a practical solution to maintain safe, individualized, coordinated care that doesn't leave the pediatric bone tumor patient and family feeling like they are just a number within the healthcare system (Howitt 2011). By initiating a relationship at diagnosis and continuing this partnership with the patient and family into survivorship, the ONN knows the child/adolescent and family well because of the long-term nature of their relationship (Howitt 2011).

Table 11.10 Long-term effects of cancer therapy

System	Causative agents	Potential effects	Interventions
Genitourinary	Cyclophosphamide Ifosfamide Radiation Cisplatin Carboplatin Methotrexate	Hemorrhagic cystitis Bladder fibrosis Kidney dysfunction	Education about reporting hematuria Maintain adequate hydration Monitor blood pressure Referral to urologist
Cardiovascular	Anthracyclines	Cardiomyopathy Exercise intolerance Hypertension	Routine tests: echocardiogram (total dose dependent) Education: dietary management Exercise program Avoid alcohol and tobacco Avoid heavy lifting Electrolyte supplementation
Reproductive and endocrine	Cyclophosphamide Ifosfamide Radiation	Sexual dysfunction Growth abnormalities Sterilization Menstrual cycle changes	Routine laboratory values: follicle-stimulating hormone, luteinizing hormone, sperm analysis, triiodothyronine, thyroxine, and thyroid-stimulating hormone Sperm donation (men) (before chemotherapy and radiation if area is included in field) Education during treatment Hormonal support Referral to endocrinologist or fertility specialist
Hematopoietic	Anthracyclines Epipodophyllotoxins (etoposide) Radiation to marrow-containing bones	Acute myeloid leukemia	Routine physical exam Routine complete blood count with differential
Central nervous system	Radiation to spine Surgical manipulation near spine Vincristine Cisplatin Carboplatin	Paresthesias Chronic pain Seizures Neuropathy Ototoxicity	Computed tomography and magnetic resonance imaging Referral to neurology Audiological evaluation, speech and language therapy
Gastrointestinal	Radiation to abdomen Concomitant use of actinomycin and doxorubicin Irinotecan Methotrexate	Fibrosis and strictures Malabsorption Anorexia, nausea, vomiting Change in bowel habits Food intolerance Jaundice	Growth charts Routing laboratory values (chemistries and complete blood count) Referral to gastroenterologist
Musculoskeletal	Radiation to long bones, spine, any growing bone/muscle area Amputation or limb salvage Methotrexate	Muscle or bone asymmetry Muscle or bone hypoplasia Limb length discrepancy Alterations in growth Gait changes Functional deficits Chronic pain Reduced bone mineral density	Bone age films Standing and sitting heights Encourage physical activity Encourage weight control Referral to orthopedist Referral to physical and occupational therapy Bone density evaluation

References

Baggott CR, Association of Pediatric Oncology Nurses (U.S.) (2002) Nursing care of children and adolescents with cancer. Saunders, Philadelphia

Black KL, Caufield C (2007) Standardization of telephone triage in pediatric oncology. J Pediatr Oncol Nurs 24:190–199

Brown CG, Cantril C, Mcmullen L, Barkley DL, Dietz M, Murphy CM, Fabrey LJ (2012) Oncology nurse navigator role delineation study: an oncology nursing society report. Clin J Oncol Nurs 16:581–585

Cherven B, Mertens A, Meacham LR, Williamson R, Boring C, Wasilewski-Masker K (2014) Knowledge and risk perception of late effects among childhood cancer survivors and parents before and after visiting a childhood cancer survivor clinic. J Pediatr Oncol Nurs 31:339–349

Eilers J, Million R (2007) Prevention and management of oral mucositis in patients with cancer. Semin Oncol Nurs 23:201–212

Francz S (2014) Who is the nurse navigator [Online]. Available: http://nconn.membershipsoftware. org/content.asp?contentid=51. Accessed 16 Oct 2014

Garcia S (2014) The effects of education on anxiety levels in patients receiving chemotherapy for the first time: an integrative review. Clin J Oncol Nurs 18: 516–521

Griffie J, Godfroy J (2014) Improving cancer-related fatigue outcomes. Clin J Oncol Nurs 18:21–24

Heiney SP, Wells LM (1995) Developing, implementing, and evaluating a handbook for parents of pediatric hematology/oncology patients. J Pediatr Oncol Nurs 12:129–134

Hewitt ME, Ganz PA, Institute of Medicine (U.S.), American Society of Clinical Oncology (U.S.) (2006) From cancer patient to cancer survivor : lost in transition : an American Society of Clinical Oncology and Institute of Medicine Symposium. National Academies Press, Washington, DC

Horowitz ME, Fordis M, Krause S, Mckellar J, Poplack DG (2009) Passport for care: implementing the survivorship care plan. J Oncol Pract 5:110–112

Howitt MJ (2011) The family care coordinator: paving the way to seamless care. J Pediatr Oncol Nurs 28: 107–113

Hudson MM, Hester A (2013) Reducing the risk of second cancers [Online]. Children's Oncology Group. Available: http://www.survivorshipguidelines.org/pdf/ healthlinks/English/reducing_the_risk_of_second_ cancers_Eng.pdf. Accessed 13 Oct 2014

Kelly KP, Porock D (2005) A survey of pediatric oncology nurses' perceptions of parent educational needs. J Pediatr Oncol Nurs 22:58–66

Lahl M, Fisher VL, Laschinger K (2008) Ewing's sarcoma family of tumors: an overview from diagnosis to survivorship. Clin J Oncol Nurs 12:89–97

Latour K (2014) The Nurse's Guide to Cancer Survivorship Care Plans. CURE Media Group, Dallas

Mcclellan W, Klemp JR, Krebill H, Ryan R, Nelson EL, Panicker J, Sharma M, Stegenga K (2013) Understanding the functional late effects and informational needs of adult survivors of childhood cancer. Oncol Nurs Forum 40:254–262

Mize L, Harris N, Stokhuyzen A, Avery T, Cash J, Kasse M, Sanborn C, Leonardelli A, Rodgers C, Hockenberry M (2014) Neutropenia precautions for children receiving chemotherapy or stem cell transplantation for cancer. J Pediatr Oncol Nurs 31:200–210

Murphy K (2011) The Children's Oncology Group Family Handbook for Children with Cancer. [Online]. Children's Oncology Group. Available: https://www. childrensoncologygroup.org/index.php/cog-family-handbook. Accessed 13 Oct 2014

New Nurse Navigator Program simplifies the complicated health care journey for pediatric cancer patients and their parents [Online]. Available: http://www.miller-childrenshospitallb.org/about-us/featured-articles/new-nurse-navigator-program-simplifies-the-complicated-health-care-journey. Accessed 21 Aug 2014

Pearson M (2009) Caring for children and adolescents with osteosarcoma: a nursing perspective. Cancer Treat Res 152:385–394

Pedersen A, Hack TF (2010) Pilots of oncology health care: a concept analysis of the patient navigator role. Oncol Nurs Forum 37:55–60

Rheingans JI (2008) Pediatric oncology nurses' management of patients' symptoms. J Pediatr Oncol Nurs 25:303–311

Society ON (2013) Oncology nursing society oncology nurse navigator core competencies [Online]. Available: https://www.ons.org/sites/default/files/ ONNCompetencies_rev.pdf. Accessed Oct 21 2014

Wilcox B, Bruce SD (2010) Patient navigation: a "win-win" for all involved. Oncol Nurs Forum 37:21–25

Wohlschlaeger A (2004) Prevention and treatment of mucositis: a guide for nurses. J Pediatr Oncol Nurs 21:281–287

Cynthia A. Gerhardt, Amii C. Steele, Amanda L. Thompson, and Tammi K. Young-Saleme

Contents

12.1 Introduction 202

12.2 Theoretical Perspectives 202

12.3 Psychosocial Functioning of Children with Cancer 203

12.4 Psychosocial Functioning in Survivors of Bone Tumors 204

12.5 Psychosocial Functioning of Families 205

12.6 Recommendations for Supportive Care 206

12.7 Directions for Future Research 207

12.8 Summary 207

References 208

C.A. Gerhardt, PhD (✉)
Center for Biobehavioral Health, The Research Institute at Nationwide Children's Hospital,
700 Children's Drive, Columbus, OH 43205, USA
e-mail: Cynthia.gerhardt@nationwidechildrens.org

A.C. Steele, PhD
Division of Hematology/Oncology and Blood Marrow Transplant, Levine Children's Hospital,
1001 Blythe Boulevard, Suite 601,
Charlotte, NC 28203, USA
e-mail: Amii.steele@carolinashealthcare.org

A.L. Thompson, PhD
Center for Cancer and Blood Disorders,
Children's National Medical Center,
111 Michigan Avenue, NW,
Washington, DC 20010, USA
e-mail: althomps@childrensnational.org

T.K. Young-Saleme, PhD
Department of Psychology/Neuropsychology,
Nationwide Children's Hospital,
700 Children's Drive, Columbus, OH 43205, USA
e-mail: Tammi.youngsaleme@nationwidechildrens.org

Abstract

The diagnosis of a bone tumor in childhood is a significant stressor that has implications for the psychosocial well-being of the entire family from diagnosis to survivorship and/or end of life. In general, many children with cancer adjust well over the first year, but there is greater risk for parent distress, particularly among mothers. Risk for psychosocial difficulties is also elevated for parents and siblings who are bereaved. Supportive care should be interdisciplinary and evidence-based to address information needs, decision making, adjustment, and long-term challenges. Consideration of the family system and developmental context of the diagnosis and treatment is important. Because the vast majority of research to date has not focused on outcomes for families of children with bone tumors specifically, implications for future research are also described.

© Springer International Publishing Switzerland 2015
T.P. Cripe, N.D. Yeager (eds.), *Malignant Pediatric Bone Tumors - Treatment & Management*,
Pediatric Oncology, DOI 10.1007/978-3-319-18099-1_12

12.1 Introduction

Even under the best circumstances when the chance of cure is good, children and families may experience considerable stress when their child is diagnosed with a bone tumor. In addition to adjusting to the diagnosis and making difficult treatment decisions, families must cope with the side effects of therapy, disruptions in family routines, financial costs, challenging conversations with healthcare providers and other family members, and the lingering possibility of relapse or death (Rodriguez et al. 2012). Disruption of normative activities, such as school and extracurricular activities, is common for children during treatment (Katz and Madan-Swain 2006). In survivorship, a significant proportion of families must also deal with the child's late effects as discussed in Chap. 16. Thus, the diagnosis of a bone tumor in childhood has significant and enduring implications for the psychosocial well-being of the entire family.

We begin this chapter by highlighting theoretical models that guide our research and supportive care of families of children with cancer. Research on the psychosocial outcomes of children with cancer, parents, and siblings is summarized across the continuum during diagnosis and treatment, survivorship, and/or end of life. Although limited research has examined psychosocial outcomes specific to children with bone tumors, we highlight this work when possible. Attention is paid to implications for the psychosocial assessment and ongoing care of the family. Finally, directions for future research are summarized.

12.2 Theoretical Perspectives

Disability, stress, and coping theories recognize that stressors, such as cancer, can pose a significant threat to child and family adjustment (Wallander and Varni 1992; Compas et al. 2012). The degree of perceived threat and controllability may influence an individual's choice of coping strategies to manage the stressor. Research suggests that coping strategies focused on disengaging from the stressor (e.g., denial, wishful thinking) increase risk for difficulties, while active engagement strategies that aim to change the situation or adapt to it (e.g., problem solving, acceptance) tend to be associated with resilience (Compas et al. 2012; Connor-Smith et al. 2000). Thus, stressors, such as a cancer diagnosis, have important implications for coping and the emergence of psychopathology or successful adaptation in children and families.

Family systems and socio-ecological models emphasize that the stress of childhood cancer affects all members of the family, as individuals make adjustments to accommodate the illness and treatment in the family system (Alderfer and Kazak 2006). A child's diagnosis occurs within the context of a family that has preexisting patterns of relationships and interactions. This climate, or the common values, rules, and beliefs within the family, provides a framework for how parents and children respond to one another about the challenges presented throughout treatment and thereafter. For example, family environment influences how openly the family speaks about the diagnosis, shares emotion and affect, as well as collaborates in decision making. Family members are interdependent, such that a person's adjustment is influenced not only by intrinsic characteristics, but also by the significant others in his or her life. In other words, family functioning may set the stage for how the family will manage cancer-related stress as a system.

Consideration of child development is also important in the context of cancer. As a growing number of childhood cancer survivors mature into adults, we have gained a better understanding of the evolving and lasting impact of cancer on the developing child. Because the needs of children with cancer are ongoing and complex, research and care are optimized when considered within a life-span developmental perspective. This approach requires sensitivity to the dynamic context of the child and family's illness experience over time (Holmbeck et al. 2010; Kazak 2001). Transitions between developmental periods are also important, as major changes in social roles and contexts can alter the course of physical and psychosocial well-being. For example, the child's age or the timing of diagnosis and treatment are important with respect to risk for psychosocial effects and provision of appropriate supportive care. The developmental context of cancer has particular relevance for the child's concept of illness and death, medical knowledge, and involvement in self-care and decision making into survivorship or at the end of life. Finally, there is evidence that childhood cancer can affect the transition between developmental periods after diagnosis, including the attainment of socially valued milestones (e.g., graduation, employment).

As many children with bone tumors are diagnosed in the second decade of life, it is helpful to acknowledge the primary developmental tasks of adolescence and emerging adulthood (i.e., ages 18–25). These years are characterized by numerous biological, psychological, and social changes (Feldman and Elliott 1993). A greater capacity for abstract thought, higher-order reasoning, perspective taking, and emotion regulation evolves. Socially, adolescents develop greater autonomy from parents and gravitate toward the peer group. Psychosexual development includes dating, sexual exploration, and more intimate emotional connections with romantic partners. At the same time, youth are also at higher risk for psychopathology, risky health behaviors, and nonadherence to medical regimens (Shaw 2001; Gibbons et al. 2012; Cicchetti and Rogosch 2002). Many health behaviors (e.g., nutrition, exercise) decline markedly in adolescence (Dumith et al. 2011; Lytle and Kubik 2003), and experimentation in risk-taking behaviors (e.g., alcohol use, unprotected sex) is common, further blurring the distinction between normative and abnormal functioning during this time (Cicchetti and Rogosch 2002).

During emerging adulthood, one gains increasing independence, acquires more responsibility, and forms an identity that will likely endure throughout adulthood (Arnett 2000). The decisions and actions that occur during this time can affect education levels, occupational attainment, and social status across the life span (Chisholm and Hurrelmann 1995). Typically, parent–child relationships improve in early adulthood as children become more independent, geographically distant (e.g., away at college), and similar to their parents with regard to roles and responsibilities (e.g., adult work or spousal roles) (Buhl 2007). Hallmark characteristics of this period are exploration and multiple life changes, such as dating different partners, moving frequently, seeking temporary or part-time employment, and pursuing various educational alternatives. Therefore, it is valuable to understand the challenges families face in balancing the demands of cancer with the normal developmental tasks of adolescence and emerging adulthood.

12.3 Psychosocial Functioning of Children with Cancer

In general, children with cancer may have an increased risk for internalizing problems (e.g., depressed mood, anxiety) near diagnosis, but these symptoms tend to dissipate over the first year (Sawyer et al. 2000). Although most survivors are not at risk for severe psychopathology over the long-term, there is some risk for internalizing and for social problems, particularly among children with brain tumors or those who received central nervous system (CNS) directed therapies (Vannatta and Gerhardt 2003; Eiser et al. 2000). As evidence of enhanced functioning or lower rates of psychopathology has been found among children with cancer (Phipps et al. 2001; Noll et al. 1999), there has also been a growing emphasis on positive outcomes, such as benefit finding, posttraumatic growth, and the emergence of other competencies in response to stress (Barakat et al. 2006; Phipps et al. 2007).

Because survivors appear to have limited psychopathology, research has focused on more subtle indicators of functioning, such as the attainment of socially valued outcomes or developmental milestones (e.g., graduation rates, employment, parenthood). Survivors of childhood cancer may not reach certain developmental milestones, or they may have delays in achieving life goals, such as completing their education and finding employment (Stam et al. 2006; Gurney et al. 2009; Lund et al. 2010). A recent meta-analysis (de Boer et al. 2006) reported that adult survivors of childhood cancer were disproportionately likely to be unemployed relative to controls. There is some evidence that survivors of childhood cancer may experience early social difficulties, as well as delays in marriage and parenthood relative to peers (Stam et al. 2006; Gurney et al. 2009; Lund et al. 2010). However, this risk is primarily accounted for by deficits among brain tumor survivors.

With respect to health behaviors, children with cancer demonstrate reduced physical activity and a lower capacity for exercise both during treatment and long-term (Tillmann et al. 2002; Warner et al. 1998). Adherence to sun protection has been noted as the least-frequent health behavior practiced by survivors (Tercyak et al. 2006). Furthermore, screening behaviors, such as breast or testicular self-examination, have been suboptimal among survivors (Yeazel et al. 2004). Experimenting in high-risk or health-compromising behaviors (e.g., sexual activity, substance use) is especially problematic for survivors of childhood cancer and may increase vulnerability to further health problems or secondary malignancies. Although children and adolescents with cancer may be protected from some high-risk behaviors, especially during treatment, participation in these activities at rates similar to peers is still of concern (Hollen and Hobbie 1996; Thompson et al. 2009; Klosky et al. 2012).

12.4 Psychosocial Functioning in Survivors of Bone Tumors

Research specific to children with bone tumors is sparse, with reports primarily focused on long-term functional or quality of life outcomes, as well as developmental milestones. Often, this work comes from the Childhood Cancer Survivor Study (CCSS) (Robison et al. 2009). Comparison samples vary across studies, including normative samples, sibling controls, other malignancies, or within-group comparisons based on amputation and limb salvage procedures. One review suggests that survivors of childhood bone tumors

enjoy a favorable quality of life and have psychosocial outcomes similar to the general population (Mosher and McCarthy 1998). Another found no differences in outcomes between amputee and limb salvage survivors, but a third review concluded that there is some evidence that bone tumor survivors may fare less well relative to other cancer survivors (Langeveld et al. 2002).

Self-reported global functioning and psychological adjustment are generally good compared to normative samples or epidemiological controls (Felder-Puig et al. 1998; Teall et al. 2013; Nagarajan et al. 2009). However, Felder-Puig (1998) found that bone tumor survivors had lower rates of marriage, living independently, and parenthood. Survivors diagnosed in adolescence also had more social problems compared to those diagnosed in childhood or early adulthood. In other reports that compared bone tumor survivors to siblings, survivors were more likely to have some functional difficulty and employment disability (Nicholson et al. 1992). Those with amputations had greater deficits in education, employment, and health insurance coverage (Nagarajan et al. 2003). Although Zeltzer et al. (2008) found more psychosocial difficulties and poorer quality of life among bone tumor survivors than siblings, mean scores fell in the normal range.

Relative to survivors of other malignancies, survivors of bone tumors may have a higher likelihood of reporting adverse health status in at least one domain (e.g., activity limitations) (Nagarajan et al. 2011; Hudson et al. 2003). Interest has also focused on the relative superiority of limb salvage vs. amputation. This research tends to support some physical complications from limb salvage but generally similar quality of life and psychosocial functioning across groups (Postma et al. 1992; Nagarajan et al. 2002, 2004). However, quality of life may be lower for survivors who are female, have less education, and are older (Nagarajan et al. 2004). A final study found similar psychological functioning between groups, but survivors with amputations were more likely to have negative effects on marriage and work (Christ et al. 1996).

12.5 Psychosocial Functioning of Families

While many individual and family factors can contribute to the development of psychopathology more generally, often proximal factors (e.g., parental depression, family conflict) are the most common contributors to a child's risk in the context of cancer (Robinson et al. 2007; Drotar 1997). This finding mirrors the developmental literature indicating the two primary factors that buffer the impact of stress on children are often intelligence and having a warm and consistent caregiver (Masten 2001). For example, both parental depression and anxiety have been positively associated with distress in children (Brennan et al. 2002; Langrock et al. 2002; Whaley et al. 1999).

Transmission of distress between family members may be accounted for or modified by family environment. In general, children in families high in conflict are more prone to difficulties (Hammen et al. 2004; Holmes et al. 1999), while children in a positive family environment are more likely to adjust better to stress (Drotar 1997; Ivanova and Israel 2006; Varni et al. 1996). Varni and colleagues (1996) found that in families of children with newly diagnosed with cancer, cohesion and expressiveness were associated with fewer child internalizing problems. Thus, a positive family environment may be protective for children with cancer.

Interestingly, parents of children treated for cancer may be at greater risk for adverse psychological outcomes than children themselves. A meta-analysis found that parents of children receiving treatment for cancer, particularly mothers, have greater distress than comparison samples (Pai et al. 2007). While many parents do not report clinical levels of distress, a subgroup of parents may be at risk for difficulties, particularly internalizing symptoms. Single mothers, and those with fewer socioeconomic resources, may be at the highest risk for internalizing symptoms and benefit the most from clinical assistance (Dolgin et al. 2007). Distress tends to be higher near diagnosis and during treatment but usually declines over the first couple of years. However, elevations in posttraumatic stress symptoms have been reported for parents both during and after their child's cancer treatment (Kazak et al. 2005).

Little research has focused on the experience of parents near the end of their child's life. Caring for a seriously ill child can have deleterious effects on parental quality of life, mood, sleep, and fatigue, with fear of the child's death and physical symptoms as frequent concerns (Klassen et al. 2008; Carter 2003; Gedaly-Duff et al. 2006; Theunissen et al. 2007). About half of parents of children with advanced cancer have been found to have high rates of distress (Rosenberg et al. 2013). These outcomes may be worse for parents of children with poorer health status, more intense treatment, less time since diagnosis, and more economic hardship (Klassen et al. 2008; Rosenberg et al. 2013). In fact, parents whose children have a "difficult death" or unrelieved pain, anxiety, and sleep disruption may have a higher risk for internalizing symptoms and poorer quality of life 4–9 years after the death (Kreicbergs et al. 2005; Jalmsell et al. 2010). Not surprisingly, bereaved parents are at risk for depression, anxiety, guilt, posttraumatic stress symptoms, and anger (Rosenberg et al. 2012). They routinely score worse on most scales of adjustment, especially internalizing problems, relative to norms and controls (Rosenberg et al. 2012). Although parental grief is more prolonged than in other types of loss, over time, some parents can also recognize personal growth and positive outcomes in response to a child's illness and death (Hogan and Schmidt 2002; Helgeson et al. 2006).

Siblings are often overlooked in research, and most work is qualitative in nature (Sharpe and Rossiter 2002). In many cases, there are several years of treatment during which much of the family's attention and resources are directed toward the ill child (Wilkins and Woodgate 2005). Older siblings are often caregivers for their brother or sister with cancer and can assume other adult roles in the home (Martinson and Campos 1991; Gaab et al. 2014). This stress, coupled with parents who are less available or impaired by the child's illness and/or death, poses significant risk for siblings.

A meta-analysis found siblings of children with chronic illness are at risk for multiple difficulties (Sharpe and Rossiter 2002), but a recent review suggests only a subset of siblings of children with cancer experience symptoms of posttraumatic stress, emotional distress, or reduced quality of life (Alderfer et al. 2010). When a child dies, bereaved siblings have been noted to have lower social competence and more internalizing and externalizing problems relative to norms or controls within 2 years of the death (Birenbaum et al. 1989; Hutton and Bradley 1994; McCown and Davies 1995). Grief symptoms can resurface years later as children mature and reflect on the loss from a different perspective. However, there is also evidence of positive growth, such as having a better outlook on life, being kinder, and more tolerant of others (Hogan and Greenfield 1991; Hogan and DeSantis 1996).

12.6 Recommendations for Supportive Care

Providing supportive care that is sensitive to the context of child development and the family system is important throughout cancer treatment, survivorship, and/or end of life. Currently, comprehensive standards for psychosocial care in pediatric psycho-oncology are under development. Interdisciplinary psychosocial services that include access to chaplains, child life, creative arts therapies (e.g., art and music therapy), school intervention, social work, psychologists, and psychiatrists are ideal. However, resources are limited, and the availability of clinical services varies both between and within centers. Recommendations for interdisciplinary care of children with cancer include assistance with the practical and financial burdens of treatment and rehabilitation; communication about diagnosis and treatment decisions between the family and healthcare providers; routine screening for risk and protective factors that may contribute to overall adjustment; cognitive behavioral strategies for coping with symptoms, procedural distress, adherence, and emotional and behavioral adjustment; and school reintegration services to sustain normal academic and social functioning (Noll and Kazak 2004).

Support for adjustment among parents and siblings is also important, but often challenging with respect to visitor restrictions or access in the case of siblings.

Recent models of care acknowledge that some families may not require extensive services to do well during treatment, recommending instead that psychosocial services be available depending upon individual risk profile (Kazak et al. 2007). Regular screening for psychosocial challenges and the assessment of strengths and available resources can more accurately inform the allocation of services. Referrals should be made for evidence-based treatments to reduce psychological problems when warranted (Pai et al. 2006; Kazak 2005). A focus on pain management and adherence to physical therapy should be priorities to help children regain optimal functioning during rehabilitation. The ability to provide ongoing support, such as educational accommodations, physical accessibility, or vocational rehabilitation, during treatment and later survivorship may help optimize the survivor's success at achieving developmental milestones in adulthood. Interdisciplinary clinics that include psychosocial providers and other specialists are key to long-term care and surveillance in survivorship.

Supportive care is vitally important at end of life, particularly with respect to facilitating communication between the family and healthcare providers. Unfortunately, referrals to palliative or end-of-life care are often late or abrupt in pediatrics (Field and Behrman 2003), and children with cancer experience significant symptom burden at the end of life (Wolfe et al. 2000; Jalmsell et al. 2006). Attention should focus on symptom communication and management, assessing family beliefs about death and previous losses, helping parents talk about death with the ill child and siblings, giving the child a chance to ask questions and express themselves through developmentally appropriate means (e.g., journal, artwork), supporting the child in creating a legacy, allowing the family to share feelings for one another, and preparing them to say goodbye. Some children may wish to give gifts or will belongings to loved ones, participate in funeral planning, and make special requests for after their death (Foster et al. 2009). These discussions, while difficult, have the potential to promote healing, provide closure, and minimize guilt and regrets after the death.

Advance care planning should take place when possible and consider the cultural, spiritual, and moral values of the child and family (Kirkwood 2005; Matlins and Magida 2003), as well as ethical and legal guidelines. Consensus building and assessing family preferences for end of life, such as life-sustaining treatment, mechanical support, DNR status, and place of death is important. For patients over age 18, advance directives (e.g., living will, durable power of attorney) should be addressed. Advance care plans should include the family and medical team and should be documented in writing. Evidence-based clinical tools such a "Five Wishes" and "Voicing my Choices" can facilitate these conversations and elicit preferences of children at different developmental stages (Wiener et al. 2012). They may also require periodic revision depending on changes in the child's status and reevaluation of family needs and preferences. Systematic follow-up or postbereavement care for parents and siblings should also be a priority.

12.7 Directions for Future Research

While we are gaining more knowledge about the impact of cancer and its treatment on children, there is more to learn. A growing body of research has focused on outcomes of children with cancer more generally or diagnostic groups (e.g., leukemia, brain tumors) at higher risk for psychosocial difficulties in survivorship. However, little research has focused specifically on children with bone tumors or during the end-of-life phase. Much of our knowledge of psychosocial outcomes among survivors comes from seminal work through the Childhood Cancer Survivor Study (Robison et al. 2009). Such epidemiological studies allow for screening of large cohorts, but many participants received treatments that are quite different from what are offered today. No studies have followed a large cohort of children with bone tumors prospectively from diagnosis into adulthood to gain an in-depth

assessment of predictors and processes related to psychosocial outcomes. Researchers must understand the explanatory factors that account for variation in outcomes over time, as well as how development differs from typical peers who have not experienced cancer.

Other methodological points for research include the need for multiple informants and mixed method approaches that move beyond paper and pencil measures. Assessments such as lab-based tasks, "real world" observation, qualitative interviews, biological measures (e.g., actigraphy, psychoneuroimmunology), and functional imaging will enhance the quality of our science. Most importantly, research that can inform the development and evaluation of interventions to prevent difficulties and promote psychosocial resilience is paramount. These interventions will be most effective if they can capitalize on innovative technologies or approaches that allow for wider dissemination and easy access to underserved populations.

Arnett (2007) has argued success in adulthood is not measured simply by the attainment of developmental milestones, but also by a subjective sense of having reached adulthood or feeling satisfied in life. In western countries, emerging adults now desire not just a mate, but a soul mate, and not just a job, but a career or dream job. These are lofty goals for many as evidenced by current divorce and unemployment rates, but it remains unknown whether these idealistic goals are more difficult to achieve for cancer survivors relative to their peers. While research has examined subjective sense of well-being and life satisfaction among adults with cancer, we know less about these concepts in pediatric cancer survivors. Do they have a sense of reaching adulthood at different ages than peers? Are they more or less happy in life? Are they more or less fulfilled, or do they just have different priorities after facing cancer?

12.8 Summary

We now expect that most children diagnosed with cancer will live long and hopefully full and happy lives. Thus, considering the long-term implications of their experience within a family and life span developmental context will help ensure the provision of appropriate supportive care and optimize outcomes. Ongoing research that is methodologically rigorous will advance our understanding of issues relevant to families of children with bone tumors and inform evidence-based care. With these goals in mind, we can ensure that more children with cancer are not only surviving, but thriving.

References

Alderfer MA, Kazak AE (2006) Family issues when a child is on treatment for cancer. In: Brown RT (ed) Comprehensive handbook of childhood cancer and sickle cell disease: a biopsychosocial approach. Oxford University Press, New York

Alderfer MA, Long KA, Lown EA et al (2010) Psychosocial adjustment of siblings of children with cancer: a systematic review. Psychooncology 19:789–805

Arnett JJ (2000) Emerging adulthood: a theory of development from the late teens through the twenties. Am Psychol 55:469–480

Arnett JJ (2007) Emerging adulthood: what is it good for? Child Dev Perspect 1:68–73

Barakat LP, Alderfer MA, Kazak AE (2006) Posttraumatic growth in adolescent survivors of cancer and their mothers and fathers. Special issue: posttraumatic stress related to pediatric illness and injury. J Pediatr Psychol 31:413–419

Birenbaum LK, Robinson MA, Phillips DS et al (1989) The response of children to the dying and death of a sibling. Omega 20:213–228

Brennan, PA, Hammen, C, Katz, AR et al. (2002) Maternal depression, paternal psychopathology, and adolescent diagnostic outcomes. Journal of Consulting and Clinical Psychology 70:1075–1085

Buhl HM (2007) Well-being and the child-parent relationship at the transition from university to work life. J Adolesc Res 22:550–571

Carter PA (2003) Family caregivers' sleep loss and depression over time. Cancer Nurs 26:253–259

Chisholm L, Hurrelmann K (1995) Adolescence in modern Europe: pluralized transition patterns and their implications for personal and social risk. J Adolesc 18:129–158

Christ GH, Lane JM, Marcove R (1996) Psychosocial adaptation of long-term survivors of bone sarcoma. J Psychosoc Oncol 13:1–22

Cicchetti D, Rogosch FA (2002) A developmental psychopathology perspective on adolescence. J Counsulting Clin Psychol 70:6–20

Compas BE, Jaser SS, Dunn MJ et al (2012) Coping with chronic illness in childhood and adolescence. Annu Rev Clin Psychol 8:15.1–15.26

Connor-Smith JK, Compas BE, Wadsworth ME et al (2000) Responses to stress in adolescence: measurement of coping and involuntary stress responses. J Consult Clin Psychol 68:976–992

De Boer AG, Verbeek JH, Van Dijk FJ (2006) Adult survivors of childhood cancer and unemployment: a meta-analysis. Cancer 107:1–11

Dolgin MJ, Phipps S, Fairclough DL et al (2007) Trajectories of adjustment in mothers of children with newly diagnosed cancer: a natural history investigation. J Pediatr Psychol 32:771–782

Drotar D (1997) Relating parent and family functioning to the psychological adjustment of children with chronic health conditions: what have we learned? What do we need to know? J Pediatr Psychol 22:149–165

Dumith SC, Gigante DP, Domingues MR et al (2011) Physical activity change during adolescence: a systematic review and a pooled analysis. Int J Epidemiol 40:685–698

Eiser C, Hill JJ, Vance YH (2000) Examining the psychological consequences of surviving childhood cancer: systematic review as a research method in pediatric psychology. J Pediatr Psychol 25:449–460

Felder-Puig R, Formann AK, Mildner A et al (1998) Quality of life and psychosocial adjustment of young patients after treatment of bone cancer. Cancer 83: 69–75

Feldman SS, Elliott GR (1993) At the threshold: the developing adolescent. Harvard University Press, Cambridge

Field MJ, Behrman RE (eds) (2003) When children die: improving palliative and end-of-life care for children and their families. Institute of Medicine, National Academies Press, Washington, DC

Foster TL, Gilmer MJ, Davies B et al (2009) Bereaved parents' and siblings' reports of legacies created by children with cancer. J Pediatr Oncol Nurs 26:369–376

Gaab EM, Owens GR, Macleod RD (2014) Siblings caring for and about pediatric palliative care patients. J Palliat Med 17:62–67

Gedaly-Duff V, Lee KA, Nail LM et al (2006) Pain, sleep disturbance, and fatigue in children with leukemia and their parents: a pilot study. Oncol Nurs Forum 33:614–646

Gibbons FX, Kingsbury JH, Gerrard M (2012) Social-psychological theories and adolescent health risk behavior. Soc Personal Psychol Compass 6:170–183

Gurney JG, Krull KR, Kadan-Lottick NS et al (2009) Social outcomes in the childhood cancer survivor study cohort. J Clin Oncol 27:2390–2395

Hammen, C, Brennan, PA & Shih, JH (2004) Family discord and stress predictors of depression and other disorders in adolescent children of depressed and nondepressed women. Journal of the American Academy of Child & Adolescent Psychiatry 43:994–1002

Helgeson VS, Reynolds KA, Tomich PL (2006) Meta-analytic review of benefit finding and growth. J Consult Clin Psychol 74:797–816

Hogan NS, Desantis L (1996) Adolescent sibling bereavement: toward a new theory. In: CORR CA, BALK DE (eds) Handbook of adolescent death and bereavement. Springer, New York

Hogan NS, Greenfield DB (1991) Adolescent sibling bereavement: symptomatology in a large community sample. J Adolesc Res 6:97–112

Hogan NS, Schmidt LA (2002) Testing the grief to personal growth model using structural equation modeling. Death Stud 26:615–634

Hollen PJ, Hobbie WL (1996) Decision making and risk behaviors of cancer-surviving adolescents and their peers. J Pediatr Oncol Nurs 13:121–134

Holmbeck GN, Bauman LJ, Essner BS et al (2010) Developmental context: the transition from adolescence to emerging adulthood for youth with disabilities and chronic health conditions. In: Lollar D (ed) Launching into adulthood: an integrated response to suport transition of youth with chronic health conditions and disabilities. Paul H. Brooks Publishing Company, Baltimore

Holmes, CS, Yu, Z & Frentz, J (1999) Chronic and discrete stress as predictors of children's adjustment. Journal of Consulting and Clinical Psychology 67:411–419

Hudson MM, Mertens AC, Yasui Y et al (2003) Health status of adult long-term survivors of childhood cancer: a report from the Childhood Cancer Survivor Study. JAMA 290:1583–1592

Hutton CJ, Bradley BS (1994) Effects of sudden infant death on bereaved siblings: a comparative study. J Child Psychol Psychiatry 35:723–732

Ivanova, MY & Israel, AC (2006) Family stability as a protective factor against psychopathology for urban children receiving psychological services. Journal of Clinical Child & Adolescent Psychology 35:564–570

Jalmsell L, Kreicbergs U, Onelov E et al (2006) Symptoms affecting children with malignancies during the last month of life: a nationwide follow-up. Pediatrics 117:1314–1320

Jalmsell L, Kreicbergs U, Onelov E et al (2010) Anxiety is contagious – symptoms of anxiety in the terminally ill child affect long-term psychological well-being in bereaved parents. Pediatr Blood Cancer 54:751–757

Katz ER, Madan-Swain A (2006) Maximizing school, academic, and social outcomes in children and adolescents with cancer. In: Brown RT (ed) Comprehensive handbook of childhood cancer and sickle cell disease: a biopsychosocial approach

Kazak AE (2001) Comprehensive care for children with cancer and their families: a social ecological framework guiding research, practice, and policy. Child Serv Soc Policy Res Pract 4:217–233

Kazak AE (2005) Evidence-based interventions for survivors of childhood cancer and their families. J Pediatr Psychol 30:29–39

Kazak AE, Simms S, Alderfer MA et al (2005) Feasibility and preliminary outcomes from a pilot study of a brief psychological intervention for families of children newly diagnosed with cancer. J Pediatr Psychol 30:644–655

Kazak AE, Rourke MT, Alderfer MA et al (2007) Evidence-based assessment, intervention and psychosocial care in pediatric oncology: a blueprint for comprehensive services across treatment. J Pediatr Psychol 32:1099–1110

Kirkwood NA (2005) A hospital handbook on multiculturalism and religion. Morehouse Publishing, Harrisburg

Klassen AF, Klassen R, Dix D et al (2008) Impact of caring for a child with cancer on parents' health-related quality of life. J Clin Oncol 26:1–6

Klosky JL, Howell CR, Li Z et al (2012) Health behavior among adolescents in the childhood cancer study cohort. J Pediatr Psychol 37:634–646

Kreicbergs U, Valdimarsdottir U, Onelov E et al (2005) Care-related distress: a nationwide study of parents who lost their child to cancer. J Clin Oncol 23:9162–9171

Langeveld N, Stam H, Grootenhuis M et al (2002) Quality of life in young adult survivors of childhood cancer. Support Care Cancer 10:579–600

Lund LW, Schmiegelow K, Rechnitzer C et al (2010) A systematic review of studies on psychosocial late effects of childhood cancer: structures of society and methodological pitfalls may challenge the conclusions. Pediatr Blood Cancer 56:532–543

Lytle LA, Kubik MY (2003) Nutritional issues for adolescents. Best Pract Res Clin Endocrinol Metab 17: 177–189

Martinson IM, Campos RG (1991) Adolescent bereavement: long-term responses to a sibling's death from cancer. J Adolesc Res 6:54–69

Masten AS (2001) Ordinary magic. Resilience processes in development. Am Psychol 56:227–238

Matlins SM, Magida AJ (2003) How to be a perfect stranger, 3rd edition: the essential religious etiquette handbook. SkyLight Paths Publishing, Woodstock

Mccown DE, Davies B (1995) Patterns of grief in young children following the death of a sibling. Death Stud 19:41–53

Mosher RB, Mccarthy BJ (1998) Late effects in survivors of bone tumors. J Pediatr Oncol Nurs 15:72–84

Nagarajan R, Neglia JP, Clohisy DR et al (2002) Limb salvage and amputation in survivors of pediatric lower-extremity bone tumors: what are the long-term implications? J Clin Oncol 20:4493–4501

Nagarajan R, Neglia JP, Clohisy DR et al (2003) Education, employment, insurance, and marital status among 694 survivors of pediatric lower extremity bone tumors. Cancer 97:2554–2564

Nagarajan R, Clohisy DR, Neglia JP et al (2004) Function and quality-of-life of survivors of pelvic and lower extremity osteosarcoma and Ewing's sarcoma: the Childhood Cancer Survivor Study. Br J Cancer 91:1858–1865

Nagarajan R, Mogil R, Neglia JP et al (2009) Self-reported global function among adult survivors of childhood lower-extremity bone tumors: a report from the Childhood Cancer Survivor Study (CCSS). J Cancer Surviv 3:59–65

Nagarajan R, Kamruzzaman A, Ness KK et al (2011) Twenty years of follow-up of survivors of childhood osteosarcoma. Cancer 117:625–634

Nicholson HS, Mulvihill JJ, Byrne J (1992) Late effects of therapy in adult survivors of osteosarcoma and Ewing's sarcoma. Med Pediatr Oncol 20:6–12

Noll RB, Kazak AE (2004) Psychosocial care. In: Altman A (ed) Supportive care of children with cancer: current therapy and guidelines from the Children's Oncology Group. Johns Hopkins University Press, Baltimore

Noll RB, Gartstein MA, Vannatta K et al (1999) Social, emotional, and behavioral functioning of children with cancer. Pediatrics 103:71–78

Pai ALH, Drotar D, Zebracki K et al (2006) A meta-analysis of the effects of psychological interventions in pediatric oncology on outcomes of psychological distress and adjustment. J Pediatr Psychol 31:978–988

Pai ALH, Lewandowski A, Youngstrom E et al (2007) A meta-analytic review of the influence of pediatric cancer on parent and family functioning. J Fam Psychol 21:407–415

Phipps S, Steele RG, Hall K et al (2001) Repressive adaptation in children with cancer: a replication and extension. Health Psychol 20:445–451

Phipps S, Long AM, Ogden J (2007) Benefit finding scale for children: preliminary findings from a childhood cancer population. J Pediatr Psychol 32:1264–1271

Postma A, Kingma A, De Ruiter JH et al (1992) Quality of life in bone tumor patients comparing limb salvage and amputation of the lower extremity. J Surg Oncol 51:47–51

Robinson KE, Gerhardt CA, Vannatta K et al (2007) Parent and family factors associated with child adjustment to pediatric cancer. J Pediatr Psychol 32:400–410

Robison LL, Armstrong GT, Boice JD et al (2009)The Childhood Cancer Survivor Study: A National Cancer Institute–Supported Resource for Outcome and Intervention Research. J Clin Oncol 27:2308–2318

Rodriguez EM, Dunn MJ, Zuckerman T et al (2012) Cancer-related sources of stress for children with cancer and their parents. J Pediatr Psychol 37:185–197

Rosenberg AR, Baker KS, Syrjala K et al (2012) Systematic review of psychosocial morbidities among bereaved parents of children with cancer. Pediatr Blood Cancer 58:503–512

Rosenberg AR, Dussel V, Kang T et al (2013) Psychological distress in parents of children with advanced cancer. JAMA Pediatr 167:537–543

Sawyer M, Antoniou G, Toogood I et al (2000) Childhood cancer: a 4-year prospective study of the psychological adjustment of children and parents. J Pediatr Hematol Oncol 22:214–220

Sharpe D, Rossiter L (2002) Siblings of children with a chronic illness: a meta-analysis. J Pediatr Psychol 27:699–710

Shaw RJ (2001) Treatment adherence in adolescents: development and psychopathology. Clin Child Psychol Psychiatry 6:137–150

Stam H, Hartman EE, Deurloo JA et al (2006) Young adult patients with a history of pediatric disease: impact on course of life and transition into adulthood. J Adolesc Health 39:4–13

Teall T, Barrera M, Barr R et al (2013) Psychological resilience in adolescent and young adult survivors of lower extremity bone tumors. Pediatr Blood Cancer 60:1223–1230

Tercyak KP, Donze JR, Prahlad S et al (2006) Multiple behavioral risk factors among adolescent survivors of childhood cancer in the survivor health and resilience education (SHARE) program. Pediatr Blood Cancer 47:825–830

Theunissen JM, Hoogerbrugge PM, Van Achterberg T et al (2007) Symptoms in the palliative phase of children with cancer. Pediatr Blood Cancer 49:160–165

Thompson AL, Gerhardt CA, Miller KS et al (2009) Survivors of childhood cancer and comparison peers: the influence of early peer factors on externalizing behavior in emerging adulthood. J Pediatr Psychol 34:1119–1128

Tillmann V, Darlington AS, Eiser C et al (2002) Male sex and low physical activity are associated with reduced spine bone mineral density in survivors of childhood acute lymphoblastic leukemia. J Bone Miner Res 17:1073–1080

Vannatta K, Gerhardt CA (2003) Pediatric oncology: psychosocial outcomes for children and families. In: Roberts MC (ed) Handbook of pediatric psychology, 4th edn. Guilford Press, New York

Wallander J, Varni JW (1992) Adjustment in children with chronic physical disorders: programmatic research on a disability-stress-coping model. In: Lagreca A, Siegel L, Wallander J, Walker C (eds) Stress and coping in child health. Guilford Press, New York

Warner JT, Bell W, Webb DK et al (1998) Daily energy expenditure and physical activity in survivors of childhood malignancy. Pediatr Res 43:607–613

Whaley, SE, Pinto, A & Sigman, M (1999) Characterizing interactions between anxious mothers and their children. Journal of Consulting and Clinical Psychology 67:826–836

Wiener L, Zadeh S, Battles H et al (2012) Allowing adolescents and young adults to plan their end-of-life care. Pediatrics 130:897–905

Wilkins KL, Woodgate RL (2005) A review of qualitative research on the childhood cancer experience from the perspective of siblings: the need to give them a voice. J Pediatr Oncol Nurs 22:305–319

Wolfe J, Grier HE, Klar N et al (2000) Symptoms and suffering at the end of life in children with cancer. N Engl J Med 342:326–333

Varni, JW, Katz, ER, Colegrove, R et al. (1996) Family functioning predictors of adjustment in children with newly diagnosed cancer: A prospective analysis. Journal of Child Psychology & Psychiatry & Allied Disciplines 37:321–328

Yeazel MW, Oeffinger KC, Gurney JG et al (2004) The cancer screening practices of adult survivors of childhood cancer. Cancer 100:631–640

Zeltzer LK, Lu Q, Leisenring W et al (2008) Psychosocial outcomes and health-related quality of life in adult childhood cancer survivors: a report from the childhood cancer survivor study. Cancer Epidemiol Biomarkers Prev 17:435–446

Bhuvana A. Setty

Contents

13.1 **Introduction**. 211

13.2 **Objective Response to Treatment
of Bone Tumors**. 212
13.2.1 World Health Organization
(WHO) Definitions. 212
13.2.2 RECIST Criteria. 212

13.3 **Role of Blood Work in Surveillance** 213
13.3.1 CBC for MDS. 213
13.3.2 LDH/Alk Phos 214

13.4 **Surveillance During Chemotherapy** 214
13.4.1 Rationale, Modalities,
and Frequency of Imaging 214

13.5 **Surveillance Post Chemotherapy** 215
13.5.1 Modalities of Imaging 215

Conclusion 217

References. 217

Abstract

Survival of patients with pediatric bone tumors have slowly improved, with more than half with localized disease staying alive 5 years after primary diagnosis. Post chemotherapy surveillance detects disease that can be managed by therapeutic options. The WHO and RECIST criteria utilize tumor response criteria as an endpoint for many clinical trials. International cooperative groups such as the Children's Oncology Group Bone tumor committee have put forth consensus guidelines for surveillance. This chapter aims to discuss the rationale, utility and standard recommendations for surveillance post chemotherapy for those with pediatric bone tumors.

13.1 Introduction

With the advent of newer therapies to treat pediatric bone tumors, rates of survival have slowly improved. More than half of patients with localized bone tumors are alive 5 years after primary diagnosis. It is now possible to sustain stable disease in relapsed patients with the use of newer cytotoxic chemotherapy and targeted agents. The primary reason for surveillance post chemotherapy is to detect disease that can be managed by therapeutic options. Oncologists utilize comparable regimens of imaging modalities for diagnosis at presentation, with continued

B.A. Setty, MD
Division of Hematology/Oncology/BMT,
Nationwide Children's Hospital,
700 Children's Drive, Columbus, OH 43205, USA
e-mail: Bhuvana.setty@nationwidechildrens.org

© Springer International Publishing Switzerland 2015
T.P. Cripe, N.D. Yeager (eds.), *Malignant Pediatric Bone Tumors - Treatment & Management*,
Pediatric Oncology, DOI 10.1007/978-3-319-18099-1_13

monitoring while on therapy and for surveillance following completion of therapy. Imaging is desirable at frequent intervals to determine the status of primary and metastatic disease and is recommended for a minimum of 10 years after the completion of chemotherapy. Various consensus guidelines have been put forth by international cooperative groups, including the Children's Oncology Group (COG) Bone Tumor Committee that is comprised of oncologists and members of the surgical, radiation oncology, imaging, and nursing committees, and are discussed below (Meyer et al. 2008).

13.2 Objective Response to Treatment of Bone Tumors

The efficacy of anticancer therapies is important for medical decision-making and outcomes of clinical trials (Therasse 2002). Oncologists routinely monitor efficacy of treatments for bone tumors by serial radiographic evaluation. Shrinkage of tumor lesions with standard cytotoxic chemotherapy is a method of determining tumor response. Anatomic and functional imaging is utilized to assist with treatment response. However, with the availability of newer agents that target immunological, antiangiogenic, antihormonal, and antimetabolic pathways, methods of assessing efficacy of treatments are being reevaluated (Ganten et al. 2014). A summary of differences between WHO and RECIST criteria is described below (Table 13.1).

13.2.1 World Health Organization (WHO) Definitions

Recommendations were put together by the WHO in the 1980s to standardize the response assessment of anticancer therapy (Miller et al. 1981). In the 1980s, members of the WHO met to put forth recommendations that investigators would use to report patient data and outcomes following a standardized pattern. This methodology helped various researchers to compare their results. These recommendations introduced the concept of utilizing tumor response criteria as an endpoint for many clinical trials. Assessment of tumor burden was determined by bidimensional lesion measurements. The WHO recommendations utilized any change from baseline evaluation as response to therapeutic interventions (Miller et al. 1981). A high rate of interobserver variability and imprecise definitions for practical implementation led to the development of the RECIST criteria.

13.2.2 RECIST Criteria (1.1)

Important endpoints of early phase clinical trials are evaluated by tumor shrinkage and time to development of disease progression (Eisenhauer et al. 2009). Some issues with the WHO criteria included methods of incorporating change in size of measurable disease, minimum number of lesions to be recorded, and definition of progressive disease (Therasse et al. 2000). The lack of clearly stated criteria led to modifications by the coopera-

Table 13.1 Summary of changes between WHO criteria and RECIST 1.1

Criterion	WHO	RECIST 1.1
Definition of measurable disease	Bidimensional, no minimum lesion size	Minimum size of 10 mm on anatomic imaging
Method of measurement	Sum of the product of diameter (SPD)	Largest diameter (other than lymph nodes)
Lymph nodes	Unspecified	Short axis, target lesions ≥15 mm, nontarget lesions 10–15 mm, nonpathological lesions <10 mm
Definition of progressive disease	≥25 % increase in SPD	≥20 % increase in size
Number of lesions measured	N/A	Five lesions (≤2 in one organ)
New lesions	N/A	Provides guidance to determine if lesion is considered new
Guidance for imaging studies	N/A	CT, MRI, FDG-PET

tive groups and pharmaceutical companies. Valid comparisons were unable to be performed to adequately interpret the results of clinical trials (Tonkin et al. 1985). Due to these circumstances and introduction of newer radiographic technologies, the International Working Group was created in the 1990s to help clarify and revisit standard definitions of response criteria. These criteria were called RECIST, Response Evaluation Criteria in Solid Tumors, and were published in 2000. These guidelines were widely accepted by the EORTC, US NCI, NCI Canada Clinical Trials Group, and other cooperative groups and play a large role in current early phase clinical trials to determine overall evaluation of tumor burden and response to therapy. Several of the recommendations put forth in this version were based on retrospective clinical data. Because of this, large-scale validation studies were performed to monitor the implementation of these guidelines in prospective studies (Therasse et al. 2006). The International Cancer Imaging Society (ICIS) and radiology groups reported concerns regarding lesion measurements, especially in patients with bone or nodal metastases, methods of measuring maximum diameter, and the need for standardizing reporting techniques in relation to measurements, contrast enhancement of lesions, and adequate comparisons to prior imaging studies (Bellomi and Preda 2004; Husband et al. 2004).

RECIST criteria are now used to define response rate and time to progression irrespective of the stage of development of new cancer therapeutics. Overall tumor burden is defined at baseline and then used as comparison for subsequent measurements. Measurable disease is defined by the presence of one measurable lesion. This is measured in at least one dimension in the longest diameter, with a minimum of 10 mm by CT scan or 20 mm by chest X-ray. Lymph nodes must be $\geq$15 mm in short axis by CT scan. Other lesions <10 mm or pathological lymph nodes $\geq$10 mm and <15 mm are considered non-measurable. Other non-measurable lesions include leptomeningeal disease, ascites, pleural or pericardial effusion, abdominal masses, or abdominal organomegaly that is identified by physical exam that is not seen on reproducible imaging techniques (Eisenhauer et al. 2009).

Complete response (CR) is defined as disappearance of all target lesions and reduction of any patho-

logical lymph nodes to <10 mm. Partial response (PR) is defined as at least 30 % decrease in the sum of the diameters of the target lesions from baseline measurements. Progressive disease (PD) is defined as at least 20 % increase in the sum of the diameters of the target lesions. In addition to this increase, the sum must also demonstrate an absolute increase of at least 5 mm. The appearance of one or more new lesions is also considered progression. Stable disease (SD) is defined as neither sufficient shrinkage that qualifies for PR nor sufficient increase that qualifies for PD with reference to the smallest sum diameter of the baseline lesions. Best overall response is the best response recorded from the start of the study treatment until the end of the treatment.

Despite all these recommendations, there are multiple biases when reporting size criteria. More recently, RECIST has been modified to take functional biological information into consideration (Ganten et al. 2014). The PERCIST (PET Response Criteria in Solid Tumors) was proposed in 2009 and takes into account biological information from PET imaging, especially in those patients treated with newer therapies, during response evaluation. Most new cancer therapies are more cytostatic than cytocidal. Tumor response may be associated with a decrease in metabolism rather than a major decrease in tumor size (Tirkes et al. 2013). This concept has been put forth in practice for response categories for patients with lymphomas (Wahl et al. 2009; Cheson et al. 2007). Response is evaluated as a percentage change in SUV_{max} or SUL (lean body mass-normalized SUV) for the most active lesion at each time of evaluation. Adherence to standardized PET/CT scanning protocol that includes consistency in injected dose, postinjection delay, and SUV normalization technique is crucial (Tirkes et al. 2013). These criteria continue to be modified to adapt to advancing technology and drug development.

13.3 Role of Blood Work in Surveillance

13.3.1 CBC for MDS

Exposure to DNA-damaging cytotoxic drugs results in approximately 20 % of cases of therapy-related acute myeloid leukemia (t-AML) and myelodysplastic syndrome (MDS) (Morton et al. 2013). Commonly used chemotherapeutic agents for bone tumors include alkylating agents such as cyclophosphamide and anthracyclines such as doxorubicin alone and in combination with the use of radiation therapy are thought to contribute to the development of MDS or t-AML (Gale et al. 2014). However, the exact incidence after treatment of bone tumors is not known. Laboratory testing of complete blood count (CBC) is recommended at diagnosis, during therapy, and at each post-therapy follow-up visit.

13.3.2 LDH/Alk Phos

Other specific laboratory tests for bone tumors have been identified, but their clinical utility is still largely unknown. Serum alkaline phosphatase (ALP) and serum lactate dehydrogenase (LDH) have been studied but have not shown strong direct correlation. Markedly elevated levels have shown to be associated with adverse outcomes. In adults with osteosarcoma, a high ALP level is considered valuable. However, due to the variable serum levels in children based on age, gender, and Tanner stage, these have not proven their value in the pediatric population. Serum acid phosphatase (ACP) has been recently studied due to similar patterns of expression as ALP in children and adolescents. When obtained at diagnosis, the ratio of ALP/ACP was found to be more predictive of a diagnosis of osteosarcoma than serum ALP levels alone. There does not appear to be much value in monitoring serial levels after initiation and completion of therapy for bone tumors (Bielack et al. 2009; Shimose et al. 2014).

The utility of LDH has been studied for application in bone tumors. A recent meta-analysis of ten studies shows that elevated levels of serum LDH is associated with a lower overall survival rate in patients with osteosarcoma and can be used as an effective prognostic marker (Chen et al. 2014). High serum LDH levels are considered a poor prognostic factor in Ewing sarcoma; however, it has not proven to have value in post-therapy surveillance (Paulussen et al. 2009). Another retrospective multicenter analysis evaluating prognostic factors and treatment outcomes of children and teenagers with osteosarcoma

revealed that high serum LDH and high serum ALP level at baseline are concurrent with poorer overall outcomes (Durnali et al. 2013). We now know that these values have prognostic value but have not been deemed useful to determine recurrent disease.

13.4 Surveillance During Chemotherapy

13.4.1 Rationale, Modalities, and Frequency of Imaging

The role of imaging during chemotherapy is to intermittently assess primary and metastatic sites of disease. This is generally accomplished by various modalities that include radiographs, computed tomography (CT), magnetic resonance imaging (MRI), and functional imaging with ^{18}F-FDG-PET imaging studies. The results of these studies determine whether ongoing regimen will be continued, in case of stable or improving disease burden, or whether a change in treatment is necessary due to progression of disease. The frequency of imaging is arbitrary but based on each patient's treatment regimen. As a general rule of thumb, it is recommended to perform imaging of bone disease by bone radiographs and MRI or CT of the primary site and CT evaluation of the lungs for assessment of metastatic disease. If abnormal findings are seen, then more extensive imaging is performed with MRI or CT and bone scintigraphy or FDG-PET studies to guide therapeutic decision-making. Functional imaging has been recommended at the end of chemotherapy as a baseline for future clinical trials. Patients with Ewing sarcoma do not require FDG-PET imaging unless bone scintigraphy was negative and FDG-PET positive on prior imaging. For those with osteosarcoma, bone scintigraphy is recommended. However, due to technological advances, and subsequent clinical trials utilizing FDG-PET results for therapeutic decision-making, these studies are being obtained at diagnosis, prior to local control, and at the completion of therapy (Meyer et al. 2008).

MRI is utilized for preoperative planning and for surveillance imaging while on chemotherapy

Table 13.2 Current guidelines for post-therapy surveillance in osteosarcoma

| Site | Imaging | | Frequency of imaging |
	Anatomic imaging	Functional imaging	
Primary and metastatic bone lesions	AP and lateral radiographs		q 3 months × 8, then q 6 months × 6, then q 12 months × 5
Primary and metastatic bone lesions	CT imaging MRI with contrast		PRN symptoms or abnormal imaging
Chest	CT		q 3 months × 8, then q 6 months × 2
Chest	AP and lateral radiographs		q 12 months × 7. To begin after the last scheduled CT
Whole body		MDP bone scintigraphy	PRN for symptoms or abnormal imaging
Whole body		FDG-PET	PRN for symptoms or abnormal imaging

Adapted from Children's Oncology Group Protocol AOST06P1

and after completion of therapy. Interpretation post chemotherapy may be complicated due to an osteoblastic reaction (Iwasawa et al. 1997). Up until recently, the ultimate criterion to determine response to preoperative chemotherapy has been analysis of histopathology, specifically degree of necrosis. Pathological analysis does not always seem to correlate with reduction in tumor volume on imaging studies, though a decrease in the T2-weighted signal in the extraosseous component is associated with a favorable response (Shin et al. 2000; Holscher et al. 1995). Delineation of the margin of tumor or changes in the extent of the joint effusion do not predict a favorable histologic response (Holscher et al. 1992). PET imaging for patients with osteosarcoma and Ewing sarcoma has gained popularity. It has been reported that a SUVmax of ≥5 g/ml after chemotherapy is associated with a poor histologic response and a SUVmax of 2 to ≤2.5 g/ml correlates with a good histologic response (Cheon et al. 2009).

13.5 Surveillance Post Chemotherapy

Follow-up of bone tumors is to detect local recurrences or development of metastatic disease when early treatment is still possible and may show effectiveness. Imaging of the primary lesion and lung imaging with chest X-ray or CT chest

are the recommended norm. There are no randomized data that describe the frequency and extent of follow-up in patients with bone sarcomas. Overall, the majority of those with osteosarcoma recur with lung metastasis, and those with the Ewing family of tumors have a higher incidence of skeletal metastasis (Ferrari et al. 2013). Various guidelines have been put together by the COG and the European Working Groups. Recommended intervals by the ESMO/EuroBoNet working group suggests every 6 weeks to 3 months for the first 2 years after completion of chemotherapy, every 2–4 months during years 3–4, every 6 months for years 5–10, and then approximately every year (Hogendoorn et al. 2010). Similar recommendations have been put forth by the COG and are described below for osteosarcoma and Ewing sarcoma (Tables 13.2 and 13.3).

13.5.1 Modalities of Imaging

13.5.1.1 Chest X-Ray vs. Chest CT for Lung Nodules

There continues to be an ongoing debate about the utilization of chest radiographs for adequate surveillance of metastatic lesions from bone tumors. Higher sensitivity is seen with the use of chest CT when compared to radiographs; however, multinational groups still recommend chest X-rays during the first few years after completion

Table 13.3 Current guidelines for post-therapy surveillance in Ewing sarcoma

Site	Imaging		Frequency of imaging
	Anatomic imaging	Functional imaging	
Primary site	AP and lateral radiographs		Recommended for bone tumors of extremity and pelvic sites: q 3 months × 8, then q 6 months × 6, then q 12 months × 5
Primary site	CT imaging MRI with contrast		PRN symptoms or abnormal imaging
Chest	AP and lateral radiographs		q 3 months × 8, then q 6 months × 6, then q 12 months × 5
Chest	CT imaging		If abnormal chest radiographs
Whole body		MDP bone scintigraphy	PRN for symptoms or abnormal imaging
Whole body		FDG-PET	PRN for symptoms or abnormal imaging

Adapted from Children's Oncology Group Protocol AEWS1031

of therapy. The American College of Radiology published guidelines for follow-up of malignant musculoskeletal tumors (Vanel et al. 1984). These state that CT is more precise in determining lung parenchymal metastatic lesions. In a retrospective study it was determined that the use of CT of the lungs for staging and follow-up was found to be cost-effective only in large, high-grade malignancies (Ferrari et al. 2013). Lung metastases in patients with Ewing sarcoma are thought to be adequately screened by chest radiographs. Patients with osteosarcoma are recommended to obtain intermittent chest CT imaging to identify lung nodules. Multinational collaborative corporations continue to discuss the best method of identification and surveillance of lung nodules due to metastatic disease. Currently, CT scans are indicated for early surveillance, but frequency remains controversial (Meyer et al. 2008).

13.5.1.2 MRI/PET vs. CT/PET

MRI continues to be one of the preferred imaging modalities for diagnosis and T-staging of malignant bone tumors (Hogendoorn et al. 2010). It has been shown that the utility of MRI for diagnosis is approximately 94 %. This study also determined that with the utilization of ^{18}F-FDG PET/CT for T-staging, the accuracy increases to approximately 96 %. These data were interesting, considering the inferior soft tissue contrast of CT when compared to MRI (Buchbender et al. 2012; Tateishi et al. 2007). There are little published data about PET/MRI for staging and surveillance of pediatric bone tumors. There is some expected benefit of a whole-body PET/MRI to increase accuracy of TNM staging (Buchbender et al. 2012). Detecting lymph node metastases from primary bone tumors is expected to have similar accuracy with PET/MRI and PET/CT imaging. Integrated PET/MRI also helps with pairing high-resolution local staging with a sensitive metabolic whole-body staging examination.

No guidelines have been established that incorporate metabolic imaging for routine surveillance. ^{18}F-FDG PET/CT has shown to have a high accuracy for restaging, with a sensitivity and specificity of 87 % and 97 %, respectively (Gerth et al. 2007). Responders and nonresponders can be differentiated by ^{18}F-FDG-PET, but CT and MRI assess tumor volume that does not accurately differentiate one from the other (Denecke et al. 2010). Currently PET/CT still maintains popularity for end-of-therapy imaging and is recommended during surveillance only if abnormal findings are visible on anatomic imaging.

13.5.1.3 Risk of Radiation Exposure

Frequent incidences of imaging studies are postulated to be associated with risk of radiation exposure. The recommendations for interval and duration of CT scans post therapy remain controversial. Since the early 2000s, there has been ongoing discussion about balancing the risk-benefit with exposure to radiation. Certain groups have reported that increased use of CT imaging modalities will lead to radiation-induced malignancies in children. Approximately 600,000 abdominal and head CT examinations are performed annually in children younger than 15 years of age. It is estimated that 500 of these individuals may develop CT radiation-induced cancer (Brenner et al. 2001). These reported data were based on the computer models that estimate cancer risk from atomic bomb survivors and CT radiation doses that are higher than used by most pediatric radiologists (Rice et al. 2007). The best available data for radiation-induced malignancies are the Japanese survival data; however, that population was directly exposed to alpha and gamma radiation from contaminated food and water and gamma and beta radiation from the bombs, whereas computed tomography modalities utilize only gamma radiation (Herzog and Rieger 2004). Despite the knowledge of this association, the reported overall risk is quite low. A retrospective study revealed that patients who received a cumulative dose of about 50 mGy may triple the risk of leukemia and those who received a dose of 60 mGy may triple the risk of brain tumors. However, only one incidence of leukemia and one incidence of brain tumor were reported in this very large adult cohort. Due to the rarity of pediatric malignancies, this overall risk is relatively very low (Pearce et al. 2012). As a rule, pediatric protocols utilize more specific, low-dose modalities in concordance with manufacturer standards. Automatic adjustment control technique performs automatic adjustments based on the size and body region imaged to obtain high-quality images with lower radiation doses. This method is widely utilized in pediatric practice (Kalra et al. 2005). Despite this ongoing debate, it is imperative to presume that low-level radiation may have a small risk of causing cancer and should be considered while determining the type of imaging for post-therapy surveillance (Brody et al. 2007). There is no reported information about the risk of serial subsequent CT scans after an initial CT scan. Pediatric patients treated with cytotoxic chemotherapy are at a slight elevated risk of secondary malignancies later in life, and it is unclear whether repeated CT scans add further to this risk. The risk of recurrence of bone tumors is high during the first 5 years from beginning of treatment. Local recurrences and risk of lung metastases also decrease at 5 years after completion of therapy (Bacci et al. 2006; Papagelopoulos et al. 2000) Thus, the Children's Oncology Group recommends decreasing frequency of CT imaging for surveillance imaging during the first 5 years of therapy.

> **Conclusion**
>
> One of the cornerstones of staging and surveillance monitoring includes imaging studies. Various modalities are used, but anatomic imaging remains popular with functional studies done at diagnosis or to confirm abnormal findings seen on MRI or CT scans. RECIST criteria have undergone many modifications since inception and most recently include the use of functional imaging studies in determining response to treatment. Laboratory studies, although easy to obtain and monitor, have not shown to have value in determining recurrent disease. Frequent surveillance is a necessity to help determine early metastases to allow for intervention with chemotherapy and surgical treatment that may positively influence post-relapse survival.

References

Bacci G, Longhi A, Versari M et al (2006) Prognostic factors for osteosarcoma of the extremity treated with neoadjuvant chemotherapy: 15-year experience in 789 patients treated at a single institution. Cancer 106:1154–1161

Bellomi M, Preda L (2004) Evaluation of the response to therapy of neoplastic lesions. Radiol Med 107:450–458

Bielack S, Carrle D, Casali PG (2009) Osteosarcoma: ESMO clinical recommendations for diagnosis, treatment and follow-up. Ann Oncol 20(Suppl 4):137–139

Brenner D, Elliston C, Hall E et al (2001) Estimated risks of radiation-induced fatal cancer from pediatric CT. AJR Am J Roentgenol 176:289–296

Brody AS, Frush DP, Huda W et al (2007) Radiation risk to children from computed tomography. Pediatrics 120:677–682

Buchbender C, Heusner TA, Lauenstein TC et al (2012) Oncologic PET/MRI, part 2: bone tumors, soft-tissue tumors, melanoma, and lymphoma. J Nucl Med 53:1244–1252

Chen J, Sun MX, Hua YQ et al (2014) Prognostic significance of serum lactate dehydrogenase level in osteosarcoma: a meta-analysis. J Cancer Res Clin Oncol 140:1205–1210

Cheon GJ, Kim MS, Lee JA et al (2009) Prediction model of chemotherapy response in osteosarcoma by 18F-FDG PET and MRI. J Nucl Med 50:1435–1440

Cheson BD, Pfistner B, Juweid ME et al (2007) Revised response criteria for malignant lymphoma. J Clin Oncol 25:579–586

Denecke T, Hundsdorfer P, Misch D et al (2010) Assessment of histological response of paediatric bone sarcomas using FDG PET in comparison to morphological volume measurement and standardized MRI parameters. Eur J Nucl Med Mol Imaging 37:1842–1853

Durnali A, Alkis N, Cangur S et al (2013) Prognostic factors for teenage and adult patients with high-grade osteosarcoma: an analysis of 240 patients. Med Oncol 30:624

Eisenhauer EA, Therasse P, Bogaerts J et al (2009) New response evaluation criteria in solid tumours: revised RECIST guideline (version 1.1). Eur J Cancer 45:228–247

Ferrari S, Balladelli A, Palmerini E et al (2013) Imaging in bone sarcomas. The chemotherapist's point of view. Eur J Radiol 82:2076–2082

Gale RP, Hlatky L, Sachs RK et al (2014) Why is there so much therapy-related AML and MDS and so little therapy-related CML? Leuk Res 38(10):1162–1164. doi:10.1016/j.leukres.2014.08.002. Epub 2014 Aug 11

Ganten MK, Ganten TM, Schlemmer HP (2014) Radiological monitoring of the treatment of solid tumors in practice. Röfo 186:466–473

Gerth HU, Juergens KU, Dirksen U et al (2007) Significant benefit of multimodal imaging: PET/CT compared with PEt alone in staging and follow-up of patients with Ewing tumors. J Nucl Med 48:1932–1939

Herzog P, Rieger CT (2004) Risk of cancer from diagnostic X-rays. Lancet 363:340–341

Hogendoorn PC, Athanasou N, Bielack S et al (2010) Bone sarcomas: ESMO clinical practice guidelines for diagnosis, treatment and follow-up. Ann Oncol 21(Suppl 5):v204–v213

Holscher HC, Bloem JL, Vanel D et al (1992) Osteosarcoma: chemotherapy-induced changes at MR imaging. Radiology 182:839–844

Holscher HC, Bloem JL, Van Der Woude HJ et al (1995) Can MRI predict the histopathological response in patients with osteosarcoma after the first cycle of chemotherapy? Clin Radiol 50:384–390

Husband JE, Schwartz LH, Spencer J et al (2004) Evaluation of the response to treatment of solid tumours – a consensus statement of the International Cancer Imaging Society. Br J Cancer 90:2256–2260

Iwasawa T, Tanaka Y, Aida N et al (1997) Microscopic intraosseous extension of osteosarcoma: assessment on dynamic contrast-enhanced MRI. Skelet Radiol 26:214–221

Kalra MK, Naz N, Rizzo SM et al (2005) Computed tomography radiation dose optimization: scanning protocols and clinical applications of automatic exposure control. Curr Probl Diagn Radiol 34:171–181

Meyer JS, Nadel HR, Marina N et al (2008) Imaging guidelines for children with Ewing sarcoma and osteosarcoma: a report from the Children's Oncology Group Bone Tumor Committee. Pediatr Blood Cancer 51:163–170

Miller AB, Hoogstraten B, Staquet M et al (1981) Reporting results of cancer treatment. Cancer 47:207–214

Morton LM, Dores GM, Tucker MA et al (2013) Evolving risk of therapy-related acute myeloid leukemia following cancer chemotherapy among adults in the United States, 1975–2008. Blood 121:2996–3004

Papagelopoulos PJ, Galanis EC, Vlastou C et al (2000) Current concepts in the evaluation and treatment of osteosarcoma. Orthopedics 23:858–867; quiz 868–869

Paulussen M, Bielack S, Jurgens H et al (2009) Ewing's sarcoma of the bone: ESMO clinical recommendations for diagnosis, treatment and follow-up. Ann Oncol 20(Suppl 4):140–142

Pearce MS, Salotti JA, Little MP et al (2012) Radiation exposure from CT scans in childhood and subsequent risk of leukaemia and brain tumours: a retrospective cohort study. Lancet 380:499–505

Rice HE, Frush DP, Farmer D et al (2007) Review of radiation risks from computed tomography: essentials for the pediatric surgeon. J Pediatr Surg 42:603–607

Shimose S, Kubo T, Fujimori J et al (2014) A novel assessment method of serum alkaline phosphatase for the diagnosis of osteosarcoma in children and adolescents. J Orthop Sci 19:997–1003

Shin KH, Moon SH, Suh JS et al (2000) Tumor volume change as a predictor of chemotherapeutic response in osteosarcoma. Clin Orthop Relat Res (376):200–208

Tateishi U, Yamaguchi U, Seki K et al (2007) Bone and soft-tissue sarcoma: preoperative staging with fluorine 18 fluorodeoxyglucose PET/CT and conventional imaging. Radiology 245:839–847

Therasse P (2002) Evaluation of response: new and standard criteria. Ann Oncol 13(Suppl 4):127–129

Therasse P, Arbuck SG, Eisenhauer EA et al (2000) New guidelines to evaluate the response to treatment in solid tumors. European Organization for Research and Treatment of Cancer, National Cancer Institute of the

United States, National Cancer Institute of Canada. J Natl Cancer Inst 92:205–216

Therasse P, Eisenhauer EA, Verweij J (2006) RECIST revisited: a review of validation studies on tumour assessment. Eur J Cancer 42:1031–1039

Tirkes T, Hollar MA, Tann M et al (2013) Response criteria in oncologic imaging: review of traditional and new criteria. Radiographics 33:1323–1341

Tonkin K, Tritchler D, Tannock I (1985) Criteria of tumor response used in clinical trials of chemotherapy. J Clin Oncol 3:870–875

Vanel D, Henry-Amar M, Lumbroso J et al (1984) Pulmonary evaluation of patients with osteosarcoma: roles of standard radiography, tomography, CT, scintigraphy, and tomoscintigraphy. AJR Am J Roentgenol 143:519–523

Wahl RL, Jacene H, Kasamon Y et al (2009) From RECIST to PERCIST: evolving considerations for PET response criteria in solid tumors. J Nucl Med 50(Suppl 1):122S–150S

Recurrent Bone Tumors

Joanne Lagmay and Nicholas D. Yeager

Contents

14.1   **Recurrent Osteosarcoma**   222
14.1.1   Incidence of Recurrence   222
14.1.2   Risk Factors for Relapse   222
14.1.3   Prognostic Factors After Relapse   223
14.1.4   Outcome After Relapse   225
14.1.5   Therapeutic Approach   225
14.1.6   Emerging Targets and Therapies   232
14.1.7   The Future for Osteosarcoma   237

14.2   **Recurrent Ewing Sarcoma**   237
14.2.1   Incidence of Recurrence   237
14.2.2   Outcomes at Recurrence   238
14.2.3   Risk Factors for Recurrence   239
14.2.4   Prognostic Factors at Recurrence   240
14.2.5   Therapeutic Approach   244
14.2.6   Emerging Targets   249
14.2.7   Future of Ewing Sarcoma   251

References   252

J. Lagmay, MD (✉)
Division of Pediatric Hematology/Oncology, Shands
Hospital for Children, University of Florida, 1515
SW Archer Road, Gainesville, FL 32608, USA
e-mail: jplagmay@ufl.edu

N.D. Yeager, MD
Division of Hematology/Oncology/BMT, Nationwide
Children's Hospital, 700 Children's Drive, Columbus,
OH 43205, USA
e-mail: Nicholas.yeager@nationwidechildrens.org

Abstract

Multimodal approach to treatment has led to
the dramatically improved outcome of patients
with osteosarcoma and Ewing sarcoma.
However, despite intensive therapies and
incorporation of novel agents in trials, the
therapeutic plateau in recurrent osteosarcoma
and Ewing sarcoma has not yet been overcome. Cure for these patients remain a daunting challenge with dismal survival rate after
relapse despite best efforts. Certain clinical
factors help prognosticate quality of relapse of
these tumors. Because patient characteristics
are different upon disease recurrence, therapeutic approach to these patients vary widely.

Further improvements in outcome for
patients with recurrent disease will depend on
refinement of therapy using agents with clinical
activity based on understanding of tumor biology, and within a trial design that optimally
detects drug activity. There is a growing list of
targets for osteosarcoma and Ewings sarcoma.
A significant biology effort has been established by cooperative groups, as well as preclinical drug evaluation systems created
towards more rapid identification and validation of compounds active in osteosarcoma and
Ewing sarcoma. High throughput screens of
novel agents should accelerate clinical trial
development. Finally, there are now various
national and international cooperative groups to
efficiently test new agents in these rare tumors.

© Springer International Publishing Switzerland 2015
T.P. Cripe, N.D. Yeager (eds.), *Malignant Pediatric Bone Tumors - Treatment & Management*,
Pediatric Oncology, DOI 10.1007/978-3-319-18099-1_14

14.1 Recurrent Osteosarcoma

In the last three decades, introduction of chemotherapy has greatly improved the prognosis of patients with osteosarcoma (Fuchs et al. 1998; Giuliano et al. 1984; Goorin et al. 1991; Jaffe et al. 1983; Longhi et al. 2006; Saeter et al. 1995). Currently however, despite multimodal intensive treatment, a plateau in the survival and cure rates of osteosarcoma has been reached (Chou and Gorlick 2006). About three fourths of patients with metastases at diagnosis will relapse (Marina et al. 1993; Meyers et al. 1993; Ward et al. 1994). For patients with localized disease at initial presentation, 30–40 % will develop recurrence (Fuchs et al. 1998; Goorin et al. 1991; Jaffe et al. 1983; Kempf-Bielack et al. 2005; Longhi et al. 2006; Saeter et al. 1995). Survival rates continue to be unsatisfactory for patients with metastatic and recurrent disease, with a 10-year overall survival (OS) of 23–29 % (Carrle and Bielack 2009; Kager et al. 2003) and less than 20 % (Kempf-Bielack et al. 2005), respectively. Subjects enrolled on INT-0133 who experienced recurrence had an overall survival of 20 % at 10 years, similar to outcomes reported by other groups. Bielack et al. (2009) reported 5 year OS and event-free survival (EFS) estimates with second and subsequent osteosarcoma recurrences: 16 % and 9 % for the second, 14 % and 0 % for the third, 13 % and 6 % for the fourth, and 18 % and 0 % for the fifth recurrences, respectively. In this study, the median interval from the first to second recurrence was about 9 months, and the median interval between subsequent recurrences remained at approximately 6 months.

14.1.1 Incidence of Recurrence

14.1.1.1 Timing of Recurrence

Most patients developed disease recurrence within 2 years of initial diagnosis (Bacci et al. 2001, 2008; Chou et al. 2005; Duffaud et al. 2003; Ferrari et al. 2003; Hawkins and Arndt 2003; Kempf-Bielack et al. 2005). In the Cooperative Osteosarcoma Study Group (COSS) report of 576 patients who had achieved first complete remission (CR) then developed recurrent disease, the median time from diagnosis to first relapse was 1.6 years (Kempf-Bielack et al. 2005). This was identical to what was described in Chi et al. (2004), Duffaud et al. (2003), and Hawkins and Arndt (2003), but approximately half a year shorter than the median time of 23 months from the first complete remission reported by the Rizzolli Institute ($n = 162$) (Ferrari et al. 2003).

14.1.1.2 Sites of Recurrence

The lungs were involved in more than 80 % of all patients with recurrent disease and as the only site in nearly two thirds of all patients (Briccoli et al. 2010; Chi et al. 2004; Chou et al. 2005; Duffaud et al. 2003; Ferrari et al. 2003; Goorin et al. 1984, 1991; Hawkins and Arndt 2003; Huth and Eilber 1989; Kempf-Bielack et al. 2005; Meyers and Gorlick 1997; Saeter et al. 1995). Local recurrence occurs in approximately 10 % of patients treated with limb-sparing surgery (Meyers and Gorlick 1997; Saeter et al. 1995; Weeden et al. 2001). In the COSS study, about 10 % relapsed in the bone other than the primary site and 10 % with multifocal recurrence (Kempf-Bielack et al. 2005). As also observed in other reports (Saeter et al. 1995), solitary relapses were more likely to occur in patients without primary metastases ($p = 0.01$) and more likely to be late relapses ($p = 0.001$).

14.1.2 Risk Factors for Relapse

Several independent risk factors are associated with the probability to develop osteosarcoma recurrence. Surgically inaccessible primary sites such as the axial skeleton as well as the pelvis, the large size of a primary tumor, and the presence of metastases at diagnosis make it very challenging to secure surgical local control, hence having higher propensity for relapse (Bielack et al. 2002).

Of the factors associated with initial disease presentation and treatment, response to first-line chemotherapy has been shown to be a predictive factor for relapse and correlates significantly with survival (Bielack et al. 2002; Martini et al.

1971; Spanos et al. 1976). Contrary to this, however, there is evidence that response to first-line chemotherapy is not an independent prognostic value for outcome after recurrence (Hawkins and Arndt 2003; Kempf-Bielack et al. 2005), as it seems like the benefit for relapsing good responders may have been mediated by longer times to recurrence. In addition, dose intensification of conventional cytotoxic agents, although leading to greater necrosis after preoperative chemotherapy, does not seem alter the poor outcome of patients with metastatic osteosarcoma (Gorlick and Meyers 2003; Meyers et al. 1998).

14.1.3 Prognostic Factors After Relapse

Outcome after osteosarcoma relapse is largely dictated by onset and location of recurrence, as well as ability to secure surgical local control. However, the reported overall survival rate in patients with relapsed osteosarcoma had a wide range of 13–58 % (Ferrari et al. 1997, 2003; Goorin et al. 1984, 1991; Martini et al. 1971; Rosenburg et al. 1979; Saeter et al. 1995; Schaller et al. 1982; Spanos et al. 1976; Ward et al. 1994). The discrepancies in outcome published by different studies could be from differences in the selection criteria for the type of relapse (i.e., lung relapse only versus all relapses). In addition, variability among prognostic factors in several series could be from studies with small study populations and differences in the treatment approach to recurrence.

14.1.3.1 Timing of Recurrence

While some studies failed to detect association with time to relapse and post-relapse survival (Carter et al. 1991; Goorin et al. 1984, 1991; McCarville et al. 2001; Meyer et al. 1987; Saeter et al. 1995; Tabone et al. 1994), there are numerous reports that confirm that patients with late relapses fared better. Improved survival has been associated by prolonged recurrence-free interval (RFI) (Ferrari et al. 2003; Hawkins and Arndt 2003; Korholz et al. 1998; Putnam et al. 1983; Thompson Jr. et al. 2002), variably defined as longer than 6 months (Putnam et al. 1983), 8 months (Ward et al. 1994), and 24 months

(Briccoli et al. 2010; Chou et al. 2005; Ferrari et al. 1997, 2003; Hawkins and Arndt 2003). In a study by Chou et al. (2005), patients who developed disease recurrence before 24 months after primary diagnosis did significantly worse than those who recurred after 24 months. In a separate study, significantly higher disease-free survival (DFS) and OS were associated with RFI of >24 months (Hawkins and Arndt 2003). Bricolli et al. (2010) demonstrated that the EFS was significantly correlated with relapse interval, greatest in patients with >24 months RFI, followed by RFI 12–24 months, and the least in patients with RFI <12 months. This is in accordance to outcome data reported by Duffaud et al. (2003) ($n = 24$) and Harting et al. (2006) ($n = 137$). Unfortunately, even in patients who develop late relapse, the survival curve does not reach a plateau, and the ultimate course of disease tends to be relentless in most cases (Kempf-Bielack et al. 2005). Surgery and second CR were more likely to have been reported in patients with late or solitary relapses than in others ($p < 0.001$) (Chou et al. 2005).

14.1.3.2 Location of Recurrence

Lung

Solitary Versus Multiple Recurrence
In the COSS series of 576 patients (Kempf-Bielack et al. 2005), 39 % had solitary versus 36 % bilateral lung recurrence. Several earlier studies indicate that the number of pulmonary nodules detected at first relapse did not correlate with survival (Carter et al. 1991; Chou et al. 2005; Goorin et al. 1984, 1991; Tabone et al. 1994). However, there is significant evidence that suggests patients with multiple lesions fared worse than those with solitary relapses (Chou et al. 2005; Duffaud et al. 2003; Ferrari et al. 2003; Hawkins and Arndt 2003; Meyer et al. 1987; Putnam et al. 1983; Saeter et al. 1995; Thompson et al. 2002; Ward et al. 1994). Solitary pulmonary recurrence was associated with improved DFS and survival rates compared to multiple pulmonary nodules, likely because isolated pulmonary recurrence achieved a second complete remission

(CR2) rate of 83 % (Hawkins and Arndt 2003), similar to other reported rates (Carter et al. 1991; Ferrari et al. 2003; Goorin et al. 1984; Pastorino et al. 1991; Putnam et al. 1983; Rosenburg et al. 1979; Saeter et al. 1995; Tabone et al. 1994).

Unilateral Versus Bilateral Recurrence

In the COSS study (Kempf-Bielack et al. 2005), about 50 % had unilateral and 50 % had bilateral disease. In some studies (Carter et al. 1991; Chou et al. 2005; Goorin et al. 1984, 1991; Pastorino et al. 1991; Tabone et al. 1994), bilateral lung recurrence did not significantly correlate with survival (22 % versus 54 % $p=0.14$). In contrast, presence of metastatic nodules in both lungs significantly correlated with poor survival (Hawkins and Arndt 2003; Kempf-Bielack et al. 2005; Saeter et al. 1995; Ward et al. 1994). Again, this is likely due to amenability to surgical local control in unilateral disease versus bilateral recurrence.

Pleural Involvement

Pleural metastases in patients with osteosarcoma may occur via two mechanisms, direct contact of pleura with metastatic lesions in the lungs and/or hematogenous spread of osteosarcoma. In general, pleural involvement of underlying cancer confers worse prognosis. This may be due to the relative difficulty of addressing surgical local control of pleural metastases and possible decreased distribution of chemotherapeutic agents to the pleura. Of note, early relapses to the lungs tend to disrupt the pleura (Kempf-Bielack et al. 2005; Saeter et al. 1995). In a study by Kempf-Bielack et al. (2005), the incidence of pleural disruption was noted at 11 %, and patients with pleural disruption by lung metastases fared worse than those without ($p<0.0001$).

Other Prognostic Factors After Lung Relapse

In a large study of patients with extremity osteosarcoma with pulmonary involvement, either with recurrent disease or at initial presentation (Briccoli et al. 2010), it was found that outcome significantly correlated with tumor stage at presentation. The 5 year EFS for patients with localized disease who later relapsed in the lungs was 36 % versus those with resectable lung metastases at presentation 9 % ($p<0.0001$). Outcome also significantly correlated with the presence of local recurrence in addition to lung metastases ($p=0.019$). The number of thoracotomies performed in a single patient also correlated with outcome, with 5 year EFS of 38 % for patients who had only one thoracotomy versus 8.5 % in patients who had two or more thoracotomies ($p<0.0001$). Of note there was no difference between two or three thoracotomies versus four or five ($p=0.29$). Interestingly in this study, second-line salvage chemotherapy after relapse did not have an impact on outcome.

Other Metastatic Sites

Extrapulmonary recurrence is often believed to carry a grave prognosis, particularly distant bone recurrence of osteosarcoma (Tabone et al. 1994; Ward et al. 1994). Ferrari et al. (1997) reported no surviving patients among four patients with bone recurrence. In a subsequent study by Ferrari (Ferrari et al. 2003), the 5-year post-recurrence survival was 11 % in 37 patients with extrapulmonary recurrence, most of whom had distant bone recurrence.

In contrast, the COSS series (Kempf-Bielack et al. 2005) results imply that it is not the extrapulmonary site, but rather the high likelihood that extrapulmonary metastases are part of a disseminated disease process that leads to this impression. Recent reports have demonstrated that metachronous osteosarcoma limited to distant bone is not associated with a bleak prognosis (Aung et al. 2003; Jaffe et al. 2003; San-Julian et al. 2003). Multimodal therapy may have contributed to the survival of patients with extrapulmonary recurrences, as was noted by Hawkins et al. (Hawkins and Arndt 2003) where 20 % of patients with distant bone recurrence, either initial or subsequent recurrence, survived without active disease. The location and number of lesions cannot be viewed independently from resectability. There are long-term survivors exclusively among patients who achieved a second surgical remission (Carter et al. 1991; Duffaud et al. 2003; Ferrari et al. 2003; Goorin et al. 1984, 1991; Hawkins and Arndt 2003; Huth and Eilber 1989; Putnam et al. 1983; Saeter et al. 1995; Tabone et al. 1994; Ward et al. 1994).

14.1.3.3 Ability to Achieve Surgical Remission

Ability to achieve complete surgical control of disease is required for cure. The most important factor associated with prolonged survival was the achievement of second remission (CR2) via complete surgical excision. In the COSS series (Kempf-Bielack et al. 2005), failure to do surgery was the strongest negative prognostic factor for the entire cohort (any surgery $p < 0.0001$, macroscopically complete surgery $p < 0.0001$). The 4-year survival rate was 33 % for patients who achieved CR2 with a median survival period of 31 months versus 0 % survival rate and median survival period of 7.4 months in patients without CR2 ($p < 0.001$) (Hawkins and Arndt 2003). In a separate study, complete resection of all disease sites is correlated with survival (26 % versus 17 %, $p = 0.05$) (Chou et al. 2005). Inability to achieve surgical CR2 was associated with exceptionally poor outcome in other studies, with OS rates from 0 % to 8 % (Carter et al. 1991; Ferrari et al. 2003; Pastorino et al. 1991; Putnam et al. 1983; Saeter et al. 1995; Strauss et al. 2004).

14.1.4 Outcome After Relapse

Overall survival after osteosarcoma recurrence is <30 % (Bacci et al. 2001; Chi et al. 2004; Ferrari et al. 1997; Meyers et al. 1998; Strauss et al. 2004). Chou et al. (2005) reported in a cohort of 43 patients, the OS at 36 months was 35 %, relapse-free survival (RFS) 14 %, and average survival for patients treated with both chemotherapy and surgery was 29.6 months. In the COSS series (Kempf-Bielack et al. 2005), post-relapse actuarial OS at 5 and 10 years was 0.23 and 0.18, respectively. The median time to second relapse in 249 of 339 patients that were surgically disease-free was 0.8 year, shorter than the first relapse-free interval. The median survival was 1.2 years for all patients and 4.2 years for 148 survivors, whereby 82 patients were in CR2 with EFS 0.13 and 0.11 at 5 years and 10 years, respectively. In this cohort of patients, eventually only 37 were alive at the conclusion of the study, with 24 in CR3, 7 in CR4, 4 in CR5 4, 1 in CR7, and 1 in CR8.

Hawkins and Arndt (2003) reported, in a study with 59 patients, that the overall 4y OS was 23 % and 4-year disease-free survival (DFS) was 6 %. The discrepancy between DFS and survival rates for the entire study (6 % versus 23 %) and for patients with isolated pulmonary recurrence who achieved CR2 (7 % versus 28 %) showed the high probability of second disease recurrence. Despite the ability to achieve CR2, most patients with recurrent OS developed other disease recurrence. DFS analysis also demonstrated that the time to second disease recurrence was rapid at a median of 8.8 months after achieving CR2 in patients with isolated pulmonary recurrence.

In the Bricolli et al. study (Briccoli et al. 2010) of 323 extremity osteosarcoma patients with either resectable lung metastases at diagnosis or localized disease who relapsed with resectable lung metastases, 29 % were alive and disease-free, 4 % were alive with controlled disease, and 67 % died from progressive disease. The 5 year OS was 37 %. Other studies confirm poor overall prognosis of recurrent osteosarcoma, with an OS rate after recurrence ranging from 13 to 57 % (Bacci et al. 2001; Carter et al. 1991; Ferrari et al. 1997; Goorin et al. 1984, 1991; Kempf-Bielack et al. 2005; Martini et al. 1971; Pastorino et al. 1991; Putnam et al. 1983; Rosenburg et al. 1979; Saeter et al. 1995; Spanos et al. 1976; Tabone et al. 1994; Ward et al. 1994).

The most common cause of death in patients with relapsed osteosarcoma is progressive disease (Briccoli et al. 2010; Chou et al. 2005; Hawkins and Arndt 2003; Kempf-Bielack et al. 2005). In minority of cases, other causes implicated were sepsis/multiorgan failure, ARDS, perioperative complications, thromboembolic events, cardiomyopathy, pulmonary fibrosis, and treatment-associated AML/MDS (Chou et al. 2005; Kempf-Bielack et al. 2005).

14.1.5 Therapeutic Approach

14.1.5.1 General Approach

More than 90 % of patients with osteosarcoma had already been exposed to at least three of the agents considered most active against the disease: high-dose methotrexate, doxorubicin, cisplatin and ifosfamide. Majority of patients receive multi-agent chemotherapy in combination with aggressive surgery for treatment at relapse. The treatment for isolated pulmonary recurrence varied, most frequently involving surgery alone, or in combination with chemotherapy. The treatment of second disease recurrence was highly variable: surgery alone, surgery in combination with chemotherapy or a novel agent via enrollment in a trial, surgery plus radiation therapy or palliative therapy (Briccoli et al. 2010; Chou et al. 2005; Hawkins and Arndt 2003; Kempf-Bielack et al. 2005). For repeated relapses, use of second-line salvage chemotherapy with drugs not used in previous treatments or with the same drugs used at higher doses (methotrexate, ifosfamide), particularly when metastatic pattern suggests a particularly aggressive tumor behavior (i.e., patients with metastases at diagnosis, less than 2 years disease-free interval from the beginning of any treatment and first relapse, multiple lung metastases, or when complete surgical removal of all tumor was not feasible) (Briccoli et al. 2010).

14.1.5.2 Surgical Approach

Importance of Surgical Local Control

Ability to achieve complete surgical control of disease is required for cure (Briccoli et al. 2010; Chou et al. 2005; Ferrari et al. 2003; Goorin et al. 1991; Hawkins and Arndt 2003; Kempf-Bielack et al. 2005; Saeter et al. 1995). The general approach for late recurrence and presence of a solitary metastatic lung nodule is to do surgery alone (Chou et al. 2005). Hawkins and Arndt (2003) showed that for patients with solitary pulmonary recurrence, surgical resection alone provided a better 4-year survival compared with chemotherapy in addition to surgery (47 % versus 13 %, $p=0.005$), and DFS rate was similar for patients treated with either surgery alone or surgery with chemotherapy. A subgroup analysis of patients with completely excised isolated pulmonary recurrence showed a superior 5-year survival with surgery alone, compared with surgery and second-line chemotherapy. For patients with short RFI, 5-year survival rate was 30 % with surgery alone versus 6 % with surgery and second-line chemotherapy ($p=0.0001$).

For patients with one or two pulmonary nodules, 5-year survival rate of 65 % was noted with surgery alone versus 30 % with surgery and second-line chemotherapy ($p=0.02$). This may be due to selection of patients with recurrence amenable to surgical local control only salvage strategies versus patients who have disseminated disease at relapse who were deemed to require systemic chemotherapy for disease control.

Among treatment-related variables, surgery and a second surgical CR were correlated with improved OS ($p<0.0001$), and failure to achieve second surgical remission was the strongest negative prognostic factor for the entire cohort (Kempf-Bielack et al. 2005). About 25 % of patients who relapsed with lung-only metastases could become long-term survivors and perhaps also be definitely cured by thoracic surgery alone or in combination with chemotherapy.

Durable remissions have been achieved in patients who experience two or more lung relapses. Bricolli et al. (2010) reported that among 323 patients with relapsed osteosarcoma, complete remission rate was 26 % for patients who had one relapse only and 18 % for patients who had four relapses ($p=0.79$). Of the five patients who had five relapses, one is alive and disease-free 5 years from last relapse. In another study, 30 % (10 out of 33) remained in complete remission at a median follow-up of 34 months from surgery of metastatic lung nodules (Duffaud et al. 2003). In addition, Tabone et al. (1994) showed that 31 % (13 out of 42) were in complete remission after repeated surgeries at a median follow-up of 39 months. These studies showed that all patients in complete remission at the last follow-up had a complete surgical resection of all metastatic tumor tissue, but those who were not operated or only had a trial removal of disease did not survive (Briccoli et al. 2010; Duffaud et al. 2003; Tabone et al. 1994). Several series including Hawkins and Arndt (2003) and Bricolli et al. (2010) have shown the curative potential of pulmonary metastasectomy, with or without further adjuvant therapy.

Variable Reported Outcomes After Surgery

There are different possible reasons for variable reported outcomes after surgery in patients with recurrent osteosarcoma. First, the definition of complete resection varies, and often a loose criteria for complete remission (CR) in different studies is used. In a study by Goorin et al. (1984), a much more stringent criteria for CR was used: complete removal of macroscopic disease, negative margins, and no histologic evidence of pleural disruption by tumor. The use of such rigid criteria narrows down considerably the number of patients assumed to have achieved a second CR, possibly allowing a better definition of the subgroup from which survivors will originate (Kempf-Bielack et al. 2005). Second, threshold for resectability varies per institution and surgeon's experience. In a large study (Briccoli et al. 2010), criteria for resectability of metastatic lung lesions included primary tumor under control, no pleural or pericardial effusions, no metastasis in other organs besides the lungs, and complete resectability leaving adequate residual pulmonary functions. These variables likely contribute to the variability of outcome in relapsed patients following surgery.

14.1.5.3 Chemotherapy

Unclear Role of Chemotherapy in Relapse Setting

Unlike in the treatment for primary disease, the role of chemotherapy in the setting of disease recurrence has been less clear as that of surgery. Although the benefit of multi-agent chemotherapy in addition to complete resection of all areas of tumor involvement has been proven in the initial therapy of OS in a randomized trial (Link et al. 1986), there has been no randomized study evaluating the benefit of chemotherapy after osteosarcoma recurrence.

Many investigators consider patients who relapse after completing modern chemotherapy resistant to further systemic treatment (Goorin et al. 1984; Pratt et al. 1987). Several studies (Ferrari et al. 2003; Pastorino et al. 1991; Tabone et al. 1994), have shown there was no benefit or observed difference in survival after second-line chemotherapy in the setting of relapse. In a large study (Briccoli et al. 2010), second-line salvage chemotherapy did not influence outcome, with EFS of 23 % for those who received chemotherapy ($n=111$) versus 27 % for those who were treated with surgery alone ($n=212$) ($p=0.42$).

There are factors that complicate the analysis of the published literature regarding DFS and survival after osteosarcoma recurrence which make interpretation of impact of chemotherapy not well defined. First, in the past, chemotherapy given to patients who received neoadjuvant or adjuvant treatments often differed significantly from regimens used currently, including relatively inactive or non-intensive agents (Goorin et al. 1984; Gorlick and Meyers 2003; Pastorino et al. 1991; Putnam et al. 1983; Rosenburg et al. 1979; Schaller et al. 1982; Tabone et al. 1994; Ward et al. 1994). Second, most series only reported survival rates, and very few reported DFS or EFS after disease recurrence (Ferrari et al. 2003; Goorin et al. 1991; Tabone et al. 1994) making it difficult to evaluate impact of chemotherapy. Third, in many series, the number of patients treated with second-line chemotherapy was too small to draw conclusions regarding its impact on survival (Ellis et al. 1997; Rosenburg et al. 1979). More importantly, some series (Schaller et al. 1982; Spanos et al. 1976; Temeck et al. 1995) included selected cohorts of patients amenable to surgical excision, thereby excluding patients with unresectable, and therefore unfavorable, recurrent tumors. The superior surgical survival rates observed for patients treated with surgery alone were likely due to biased use of chemotherapy in patients with marginally excised or difficult to resect tumors, early or multiple recurrences, or short relapse-free interval (<1 year) (Chou et al. 2005; Hawkins and Arndt 2003). Because of these limitations, an unambiguous conclusion regarding the role of second-line chemotherapy could not be drawn.

Evidence to Support Chemotherapy

When primary mode of treatment for osteosarcoma involved surgery alone, most patients recurred in the lungs within 12 months (Friedman and Carter 1972). Introduction of chemotherapy has greatly improved prognosis for these patients (Fuchs et al. 1998; Goorin et al. 1991; Jaffe et al. 1983; Link et al. 1986; Longhi et al. 2006; Saeter et al. 1995). Moreover, the incorporation of chemotherapy to treatment of osteosarcoma has made DFS significantly longer and the number of lung metastases significantly lower compared to patients treated with surgery alone (Fuchs et al. 1998; Longhi et al. 2006; Saeter et al. 1995). This relapse pattern change seems to indicate a partial effect of combined chemotherapy, which may also benefit patients who relapsed (Briccoli et al. 2010). The adjuvant effect of chemotherapy is much less obvious than that of first-line treatment and may be easily missed when analyzing small cohorts. There might be some selection bias, as chemotherapy efficacy may have been underestimated as the patients who received chemotherapy were more likely to have presented with more extensive recurrences.

Several studies have demonstrated the possible benefit of second-line chemotherapy in the relapse setting. In a study by Saeter et al. (1995), survival improved in those patients ($n=60$) with recurrent disease who received "adequate" chemotherapy, defined as receiving at least one agent to which the patient had not been previously exposed or a dose escalation of methotrexate, in addition to surgery.

It seems that impact of chemotherapy is a bit more obvious in patients who have not achieved second surgical remission. In the Cooperative Osteosarcoma Study Group (COSS) study (Kempf-Bielack et al. 2005), the use of chemotherapy is correlated with overall survival for patients who did not achieve a second complete remission ($p=0.0001$). It was also noted in this study that chemotherapy use also was found to correlate with event-free survival for patients who were able to achieve a CR2 ($p=0.016$). When multidrug chemotherapy was compared with no chemotherapy or single-agent chemotherapy, multidrug chemotherapy is correlated with overall survival in the total cohort ($p=0.012$). The use of second-line chemotherapy is correlated with good response to first-line chemotherapy ($p=0.022$), multiple lesions at relapse ($p=0.001$), and bilateral pulmonary involvement ($p=0.001$), but not the time to relapse ($p=0.953$). Most patients treated without chemotherapy for a first relapse will undoubtedly receive chemotherapy for subsequent recurrences, and analysis of overall survival compare immediate with delayed chemotherapy rather than chemotherapy with observation. This bias does not apply to analyses of event-free survival, which stop at second recurrence. By performing such analysis, in this study Kempf-Bielack et al. (2005) were able to expand previous observations of a positive correlation between second-line chemotherapy and outcome to patients achieving a second surgical remission, suggesting an adjuvant effect, albeit limited, even in these heavily pretreated patients.

Ferrari et al. (2003) showed that in 162 patients with relapsed osteosarcoma, chemotherapy was given when surgical remission was not achievable or when pattern of disease recurrence suggested a particularly aggressive tumor. This study concluded that for the majority of patients in whom surgical remission was achieved, the use of second-line chemotherapy did not affect survival. However, for those patients who were not able to achieve surgical remission, the use of chemotherapy was found to increase survival.

Systemic Agents

Ifosfamide ± Etoposide

Ifosfamide is an oxazaphosphorine nitrogen mustard that has proven activity as a single agent against a variety of neoplasms, including bone (Carli et al. 2003). In adults, it is clinically active in advanced soft tissue sarcoma, with higher response rates achieved using higher doses. Interestingly, high-dose ifosfamide has also been proven effective in patients previously treated with conventional dose ifosfamide (Elias et al. 1990; Le Cesne et al. 1995; Palumbo et al. 1997; Patel et al. 1997). In a phase I and II combination studies with other agents, ifosfamide has significant activity in recurrent or metastatic osteosarcoma (Goorin et al. 2002; Miser et al. 1987), with objective responses reported in 30–50 % (Miser et al. 1987).

Since high-dose ifosfamide was found to have increased response rate in patients with osteosarcoma (Goorin et al. 2002), the 2.8 $g/m^2/$ day $\times 5$ days with mesna has become widely used by pediatric oncologists. Often, etoposide is added at a dose of 100 mg/m²/day×5 days (Chou et al. 2005). The response rate to ifosfamide and etoposide regimen is 38 % (Miser et al. 1987).

Ifosfamide can also be given as a prolonged 14-day infusion which was found to be well tolerated in pediatric patients with favorable toxicity profile, not requiring hospitalization for administration and thereby promoting patient's QOL as well as decreasing cost. A response rate of 35 % in heavily pretreated patients is a promising finding, even in patients who were already previously treated with ifosfamide (Meazza et al. 2010). This study reported very low incidence of nausea, no encephalopathy or renal toxicity, low incidence of bladder toxicity, and reduction in cytopenias.

MTP-PE

Muramyl tripeptide phosphatidylethanolamine (MTP) is a nonspecific immunomodulator that is a synthetic analogue of a component of bacterial cell walls. Incorporation of MTP into liposomes has allowed targeted delivery of this agent to monocytes and macrophages in areas such as the lungs, activating these cells to be tumoricidal (Chou et al. 2009). Preclinical models in mice and canine osteosarcoma have confirmed antitumor effects of MTP (Anderson 2006; Asano and Kleinerman 1993; Kleinerman et al. 1993; MacEwen et al. 1989; Nardin et al. 2006). Moreover, concurrent administration of chemotherapy does not interfere with antitumor effects of MTP (Kleinerman et al. 1995; Meyers et al. 2005).

In a study by Meyers et al. (2005), patients with newly diagnosed metastatic osteosarcoma ($n=677$) were randomly assigned to receive or not to receive ifosfamide and/or MTP in a 2×2 factorial design, in addition to standard chemotherapy (methotrexate, doxorubicin, and cisplatin). The 3y EFS for patients treated with standard arm of therapy, addition of MTP to standard therapy, addition of ifosfamide to standard therapy, and addition of both ifosfamide and MTP were 71 %, 68 %, 61 %, and 78 %, respectively. There was an observed interaction between the addition of ifosfamide and addition of MTP. From this study, it was concluded that the addition of MTP to chemotherapy might improve EFS. A follow-up analysis (Meyers et al. 2008) showed

no evidence of interaction of ifosfamide and MTP, and both chemotherapy regimens resulted in similar EFS and OS. The addition of MTP to chemotherapy resulted in a statistically significant improvement in OS (6y OS increased from 70 to 78 %, $p=0.03$) and a trend toward better EFS ($p=0.08$).

An access study (MTP-OS-403, NCT00631631) (Anderson et al. 2014a) for MTP in patients with relapsed and/or recurrent osteosarcoma was done after initial approval by the European Medical Agency and at the request of the US Food and Drug Administration. This study also helped better define pharmacodynamics, pharmacokinetics, and safety profile of this drug in osteosarcoma. Resection of recurrence or metastases was encouraged but was not required for study entry. Concurrent chemotherapy was also allowed. Greater than or equal to grade 3 toxicity attributed to MTP was far less common than those attributed to chemotherapy. Among 50 patients whose disease was completely resected, >50 % remained alive more than 2 years from study entry. Many of these patients had already received ≥2 lines of therapy. MTP is currently available in Europe, Mexico, South Korea, Switzerland, and Israel for nonmetastatic osteosarcoma.

Gemcitabine/Docetaxel

Gemcitabine is a difluorinated deoxycytidine analogue, which is taken up by cells and depletes deoxynucleotide stores and interferes with DNA elongation and ultimately DNA synthesis. Docetaxel is a semisynthetic analogue of paclitaxel, a taxane, which stabilizes microtubules against depolymerization resulting in cell cycle arrest and apoptosis.

In phase 1 and 2 trials with gemcitabine alone (Reid et al. 2004; Wagner-Bohn et al. 2006), disease stabilization was reported in 4 of 13 patients with osteosarcoma. Modest responses in patients with Ewing sarcoma, rhabdomyosarcoma, and osteosarcoma have been observed with docetaxel as a single agent (Blaney et al. 1997; Seibel et al. 1999; Zwerdling et al. 2006). In a phase 2 trial of docetaxel (125 mg/m² every 21 days) in 55 patients with recurrent bone and soft tissue sarcomas, there were 6 objective responses, 2 of which have underlying osteosarcoma (Zwerdling et al. 2006).

Combination of gemcitabine and docetaxel was proven to be synergistic in terms of antitumor activity against different cell lines, including osteosarcoma cells (Leu et al. 2004; Ricotti et al. 2003). In a retrospective case review, 22 patients with recurrent or refractory bone or soft tissue sarcoma were given gemcitabine (675 mg/m^2 IV on days 1 and 8) and docetaxel (75–100 mg/m^2 IV on day 8) (Navid et al. 2008a). Osteosarcoma was the most common diagnosis in this cohort ($n = 18$). Of the 14 patients evaluable for response, 3 patients with osteosarcoma achieved a partial response and 1 had stable disease. The overall objective response rate (CR+PR) was 29 %. Median duration of response was 4.8 months (1.6–13 months). Toxicity was manageable, primarily thrombocytopenia and neutropenia. The authors concluded that this combination demonstrated antitumor activity, especially against recurrent or refractory osteosarcoma. Response Evaluation Criteria in Solid Tumors (RECIST) showed shrinkage or stabilization of tumor in heavily pretreated patients with osteosarcoma and compared favorably with ifosfamide and cyclophosphamide/etoposide regimens (Miser et al. 1987; Rodriguez-Galindo et al. 2002b; Van Winkle et al. 2005).

In a phase II trial through Sarcoma Alliance for Research Collaboration (SARC), gemcitabine (675 mg/m^2 IV on days 1 and 8) and docetaxel (75–100 mg/m^2 IV on day 8) were given every 21 days in children and adults with recurrent ES, osteosarcoma, or unresectable or recurrent chondrosarcoma (Fox et al. 2012). Out of 53 evaluable patients, there were no complete responses observed, and partial responses included 1 (out of 14) osteosarcoma, 2 (out of 14) ES, and 2 (out of 25) chondrosarcoma patients. For this study, gemcitabine and docetaxel combination was associated with the probability of reaching the target of 35 % response rate <5 % in osteosarcoma and 5.6 % in EWS.

14.1.5.4 Other Local Control Measures

Radiation Therapy (RT)

Traditionally, osteosarcoma has been considered a relatively radioresistant neoplasm. Viable tumor cells have been observed in surgical specimen after a dose of 60–70 Gy or more (Cade 1955; de Moor 1975). In contrast, there is evidence of a direct relationship between radiation dose and percent tumor necrosis (DeLaney et al. 2005; Gaitan-Yanguas 1981).

Delaney et al. (2005) reviewed 41 patients who received RT for osteosarcoma that was unresected or resected with positive margins. Local control was achieved in 78.4 % for patients with gross total resection, 77.8 % who had subtotal resection, and 40 % for those who had biopsy only. Control is also correlated with radiation dose, and a dose of >55 Gy achieved 71 % local control versus in <55 Gy only 53.6 % local control rate. This study concluded that RT can help provide local control of osteosarcoma for patients in whom surgical resection with widely negative margins is not possible. RT was specifically noted to be effective in situations in which microscopic or minimal residual disease is being treated.

Machak et al. (2003) determined the effectiveness of radiation therapy for local control of nonmetastatic osteosarcoma of the extremities after induction chemotherapy. Thirty-one patients refusing surgical local control were treated with neoadjuvant chemotherapy followed by standard fractionated external beam radiotherapy with median dose 60 Gy. The 5 year OS was 61 %, local progression-free survival 56 %, and metastases-free survival 62 %. Local treatment failure occurred median time of 18 months. As with DeLaney et al. (2005), the incidence of local relapse was higher when the dose was <50 Gy than those with >50 Gy. No definite correlation was found between the rate of local failure and regimen of fractionation. The outcome is correlated significantly with imaging and biochemical surrogate markers (alkaline phosphatase). Of note, survival probability was largely determined by whether a patient's tumor responded to the induction of systemic therapy. In the COSS series (Kempf-Bielack et al. 2005), RT was almost exclusively administered to patients failing to achieve a second CR. RT was associated with prolonged survival only in the subgroup without a second CR ($p = 0.0001$).

Nowadays, there are multiple and advanced ways of delivering RT. Intensity-modulated RT

(IMRT) has the potential to deliver higher doses to the tumor bed while sparing adjacent organs. This can be used for primaries in the pelvis, vertebrae, and chest wall. Another mode of delivering RT is with protons. Ciernik et al. (2011) demonstrated that high dose proton therapy allowed locally curative treatment for some patients with unresectable or incompletely resected osteosarcoma. After a median dose of 68.4 Gy, local control after 3 years and 5 years was 82 % and 72 %, respectively, with distant failure rate of 26 % after 5 years. In this study, the 5-year DFS was 65 % and OS 67 %. The extent of surgical resection did not correlate with the outcome. Risk factors for local failure were ≥ 2 grade disease ($p<0.0001$) and total treatment length ($p=0.0008$).

The effectiveness of the conventional, fractionated radiotherapeutic approach is probably limited by tumor cell repair of sublethal radiation injury and a relatively high fraction of hypoxic tumor cells (van Putten 1968; Weichselbaum et al. 1977). To overcome these causes, radiation is combined with various radiosensitizers (Kinsella and Glatstein 1987; Martinez et al. 1985). Radiotherapy combined with chemotherapy has been used in animal and human osteosarcoma to enhance local control over that achieved with radiation therapy alone (Caceres et al. 1984; Withrow et al. 1993). Concurrent use of ifosfamide during RT has been the standard of care for patients with Ewing sarcoma. Caceres (Caceres et al. 1984) was able to show complete tumor devitalization on 80 % of patients with osteosarcoma treated with high-dose methotrexate, doxorubicin, and 60 Gy of RT. Chemotherapy agents that combine systemic osteosarcoma control and also increase radiation effectiveness include ifosfamide, cisplatin, high-dose methotrexate, and gemcitabine (Leu et al. 2004). Gemcitabine, an active drug against a variety of sarcomas, is a potent radiosensitizer. Concentrations of 1,000-fold lower than typical plasma levels can be effective (Joschko et al. 1997; Lawrence et al. 1997), when given at least 2 hours prior to radiation with an effect lasting up to 48–60 hours after a dose (Wilson et al. 2006). Severe radiation recall is rare with gemcitabine

compared to anthracyclines and taxanes, and might involve proinflammatory cytokine production (Friedlander et al. 2004).

There is evidence that chemotherapy markedly improves the effectiveness of local control using RT (Anderson 2003; Machak et al. 2003). In addition, there is also data that radiation dose required for adequate osteosarcoma control is less when combined with chemotherapy. In canine osteosarcoma, the radiation dose predicted to cause 90 % tumor necrosis when radiation was given with cisplatin was 36 Gy, but needed 50 Gy when radiation was given alone (Withrow et al. 1993). Mahajan et al. (2008) analyzed the exposure of 39 high-risk metastatic and/or recurrent osteosarcoma during consecutive 20 months. The median radiation dose was 30 Gy in 10 fractions. Chemotherapy was used in 80 % of radiotherapy courses. Their results confirmed that external beam radiotherapy with systemic treatment may provide a successful multimodality approach to local control and symptom relief.

In summary, RT can reduce the likelihood of positive margins and can be given after surgery if there are close or positive margins. RT is an option for patients with unresectable or incompletely resected tumors, for patients who refuse surgery, and for palliation of symptomatic metastases (DeLaney et al. 2005; Schwarz et al. 2009).

Thermal Ablation

The term "tumor ablation" refers to the destruction of tumor tissues in situ. The use of thermal extremes to ablate the tumor has been used widely in specific clinical scenarios. Lesions must be detectable using CT or ultrasound (>1 cm) and not so large (<5 cm) that heating and freezing uniformaly within lesion become difficult.

Radiofrequency ablation (RFA) is used to coagulate and destroy tumor tissue by direct application of radiofrequency (RF)-generated heat. An RF probe is placed into the tumor, and an RF generator is used to deliver high-frequency (375–480 Hz) alternating current to generate heat within the tumor to temperatures above 60 °C. After access is obtained, percutaneous delivery of thermal energy is used to destroy the tumor. The necrotic tissue is then resorbed and eliminated by the body. RFA requires anesthesia, but with short recovery time of 1–2 days (Rybak 2009).

Traditionally, symptomatic bone metastases have been addressed with chemotherapy and/or radiation with surgery reserved in cases of impending pathologic fracture. Not all lesions however are amenable to these first-line therapies. Lack of tumor sensitivity or an unacceptable risk of damage to adjacent organs may obviate the use of these treatment methods. For many patients, escalating use of opioids to treat pain may be too debilitating. In these cases, RFA may offer a minimally invasive alternative for local control of disease and pain palliation. The main goal of RF treatment of metastases for palliation is the complete ablation of the tumor interface with nearby tumor bone, as this is correlated directly with level of pain relief (Goetz et al. 2004; Simon and Dupuy 2006). In one study (Petsas et al. 2007), 95 % experienced decreased pain that was considered clinically significant.

RFA has been demonstrated to be an effective method, especially in lesions <3 cm in several adult malignancies. In a pilot study of 16 patients with recurrent pediatric solid tumors including 8 refractory osteosarcomas with lung metastases, Hoffer et al. (2009) was able to demonstrate feasibility and safety of RFA. In a later study (Saumet et al. 2014), 10 patients enrolled with osteosarcoma in French Society of Childhood Cancer centers had 22 treatment to lung metastases <3 cm and >1 cm from the large bronchi, trachea, and esophagus. Seven had complete remission at last follow-up (median 24 months after RFA), and none had recurrence at RFA sites. Eight sessions were done for bone lesions, and of three that were curative intent, all were in remission for >3 years. There are various other studies that showed RFA to be beneficial in alleviating pain from symptomatic metastases (Callstrom et al. 2006; Goetz et al. 2004; Rybak 2009; Santiago et al. 2009).

Side effects associated with RFA include immediate post-procedural hemoptysis and pneumothorax, as well as a paradoxic increase in pain up to the first week after RFA. Patients may have post-ablation syndrome, characterized by general malaise and fatigue believed to result from systemic release of cytokines caused by tumor cell death. Patients with lesions in the spine or in weight-bearing areas such as the acetabulum may be at risk for fracture.

On the other extreme, cryoablation involves freezing the tumor to below −20 °C. Cell death is induced by direct cellular injury involving formation of extracellular ice resulting in a relative imbalance of solutes between the intra- and extracellular environment, resulting in cellular dehydration and damage to cell membrane and enzymatic machinery (Baust and Gage 2005; Robinson et al. 2001). Primary use of cryoablation is in palliation of bone metastases (Corby et al. 2008) and primary bone tumors. Cryotherapy has also been used where definitive surgery would result in significant morbidity (i.e., hemipelvectomy for a large pelvic lesion) or may be used as a preliminary debulking measure thus allowing more limited surgical resection.

14.1.6 Emerging Targets and Therapies

14.1.6.1 Radionuclides

Samarium

Samarium-153 ethylenediamine tetramethylene phosphonic acid (^{153}Sm-EDTMP) is a bone-seeking radiopharmaceutical designed to selectively deliver radiation to osteoblastic skeletal metastases (Anderson and Nunez 2007; Anderson et al. 2002). The radioisotope ^{153}Sm emits an electron (beta particle) which induces targeted cytotoxicity. Its photon emissions help with scintigraphic imaging, thereby allowing both confirmation of agent localization and quantification of the absorbed dose delivered to target lesions.

^{153}Sm-EDTMP has been used in the treatment of patients with high-risk recurrent or unresectable osteosarcoma. A phase I study found that up to 30 mCi/kg could be administered with autologous stem cell support; the only significant toxicity was myelosuppression (Anderson et al. 2002, 2005). In an effort to improve efficacy, Anderson et al. (2005) combined samarium with gemcitabine, a radiosensitizer. Although some patients achieved partial responses, none of these were durable. In a dose-finding study (Loeb et al. 2009) to see how much [153]Sm-EDTMP can be given that would allow hematopoietic recovery within 6 weeks without use of stem cell support in patients with osteosarcoma bone metastases, the maximally tolerated dose of [153]Sm-EDTMP was 1.21 mCi/kg with dose-limiting toxicity (DLT) confined to hematologic toxicity, mainly platelet recovery.

A phase 2 study reported safety and response of high-risk osteosarcoma to tandem doses of [153]Sm-EDTMP (37–51.8 MBq/kg followed by 222 MBq/kg) and autologous stem cell rescue in a cohort of heavily pretreated patients (Loeb et al. 2010). Nine patients were enrolled and six had disease stabilization; however, this was not considered a response, so the study was terminated early. There was no correlation between positron emission tomography tumor uptake possibly from tumor inflammation and absorbed dose or time to progression. The median time to progression for the entire group was 79 days. Interestingly, one patient with disseminated lung and lymph node disease had a prolonged period of progression-free survival, and pulmonary nodules had >95 % necrosis of his pulmonary nodules. Another patient with pulmonary parenchymal disease also had disease stabilization. These cases support the idea that [153]Sm-EDTMP is cytotoxic to extraosseous disease.

Aside from nonselective toxicity to the bone marrow, another limitation of [153]Sm-EDTMP is the significant variability of tumor absorbed dose (Anderson et al. 2002, 2005; Loeb et al. 2009). To circumvent this problem, it would be ideal to administer an individually targeted tumoricidal absorbed dose of the pharmaceutical. Another option is to combine [153]Sm-EDTMP with a vascular disrupting agent or a radiosensitizer. In addition, this may have limited efficacy for large tumors since a beta particle such as [153]Sm-EDTMP has short path length, meaning that large areas of the tumor are inadequately treated. To augment the effect may need delivery of external beam radiation. Further investigation of this novel form for biophysically targeted therapy is warranted.

Radium

Another investigational bone-seeking radiopharmaceutical is radium ([223]Ra). Compared to [226]Ra which was initially evaluated for internal radiotherapy, [223]Ra has favorable decay characteristics, and radon daughter decay is rapid (4 s) providing much less of a chance of "off target" radon diffusion (Anderson et al. 2014b). Experience with [223]Ra in phase I (Nilsson et al. 2005) and phase II trials in patients with metastatic prostate cancer confirmed excellent activity against bone metastases and a low toxicity profile (Nilsson et al. 2007). In a phase III prostate cancer trial with 809 patients, [223]Ra significantly improved overall survival ($p = 0.002$) (Parker et al. 2013). It was also associated with low myelosuppression rates and fewer adverse events.

Radium should be suitable for use in combination with chemotherapy because of its higher therapeutic index (low bone marrow toxicity, higher effect on malignant forming cells) than 153Sm-EDTMP. There is currently an ongoing phase I dose escalation of monthly intravenous [223]Ra dichloride in osteosarcoma (NCT01833520, clinicaltrials.gov).

14.1.6.2 Novel Delivery Systems

Inhaled Cisplatin (SLIT™ Cisplatin)

Inhalation therapy has potential advantages in the treatment of patients with pulmonary metastatic disease. Inhaled liposomal cisplatin has pharmacokinetic properties that maximize lung tissue delivery of cisplatin with minimal systemic exposure. Cisplatin is one of the most active agents in osteosarcoma and when encapsulated in liposomes limits its undesired side effects like nephrotoxicity, myelosuppression, ototoxicity, and nausea/vomiting (Wittgen et al. 2007). A study using inhaled lipid cisplatin (ILC) in 19 patients, administered via nebulizer every 2 weeks, and whenever possible metastasectomy was undertaken after 2 treatments (Chou et al. 2013). Eleven patients had bulky disease, and all progressed prior to cycle 7, while three of eight patients who had less bulky disease (<2 cm) had sustained benefit. This was well tolerated with only one patient experiencing ≥grade 3 respiratory toxicity.

Liposomal Doxorubicin

Liposomal delivery of doxorubicin allows for selective delivery of therapeutic agent to target tissues such as the lungs. The pegylated formulation of liposomal doxorubicin (Doxil) is a unique form of liposomal doxorubicin in which the liposomes are coated with ethylene glycol, resulting in a diminished uptake by the reticuloendothelial system, leading to a longer half-life in the blood and a different toxicity profile than nonpegylated liposomes (Ta et al. 2009). In a study of methylene diphosphonate (MDP)-conjugated adriamycin liposomes (MDP-LADMs), tumor growth and animal survival rates were evaluated after UMR106 osteosarcomas were established in Sprague–Dawley rats, and SOSP-M pulmonary metastatic osteosarcoma models were established in nude mice, respectively (Wu and Wan 2012). The toxicity assay revealed a significantly higher median lethal dose for MDP-LADMs than for free Adriamycin and LADMs ($p < 0.05$), and animal survival in the MDP-LADMs group was significantly higher ($p < 0.05$). These findings indicate that MDP-LADMs have higher therapeutic efficacy against osteosarcomas, demonstrate lower toxicity, and targeted osteosarcomas more clearly than the stand-alone systems.

In a phase II study of Doxil in previously heavily treated sarcoma patients ($n = 47$, 6 with osteosarcoma) considered unresponsive to chemotherapy (Skubitz 2003), a dose of 55 mg/m^2 every 4 weeks was used which was well tolerated without documented cardiac toxicity. Three of the 47 patients received a CR or PR, although 15 of the 47 patients were felt to have derived clinical benefit from the treatment. These data suggest that pegylated liposomal doxorubicin has activity in this population of poor prognosis sarcoma and that this treatment is associated with modest toxicity. In a dose-finding study of temsirolimus 20 mg/m^2 weekly and liposomal doxorubicin (30 mg/m^2 monthly) for patients with recurrent and refractory bone and soft tissue sarcoma, this combination was shown to be safe for heavily pretreated sarcoma patients (Thornton et al. 2013). The phase II expansion portion of this study is ongoing.

14.1.6.3 Inhibition of Signaling Receptors and Transduction

Mammalian Target of Rapamycin (mTOR) Inhibitors

mTOR regulates protein synthesis and cell proliferation, survival, and angiogenesis. Ezrin is a protein with a role in cell–cell interactions and signal transduction and when upregulated drives metastasis (Hunter 2004). It appears to mediate its metastatic actions through the MAPK signaling pathway. Increased ezrin expression in pediatric osteosarcoma patients is associated with reduced disease-free intervals, and downregulation of ezrin expression in a mouse model of human osteosarcoma is associated with inhibition of pulmonary metastasis (Khanna et al. 2004). Rapamycin, an mTOR inhibitor, has been found to inhibit ezrin-mediated pathways leading to reduced lung metastases in a mouse model in osteosarcoma (Wan et al. 2005).

Response activity to rapamycin was high in one osteosarcoma xenograft (CR) and intermediate in five tumors (Houghton et al. 2008). Combination with cyclophosphamide or vincristine resulted in increased activity in osteosarcoma models (Houghton et al. 2010b). A randomized phase II trial of ridaforolimus as single-agent therapy met primary end point of improved PFS in two osteosarcoma patients (Chawla et al. 2012). Use of mTOR inhibitors in the treatment of osteosarcoma patients is under investigation as single-dose therapy (everolimus, NCT01216826; sirolimus, NCT01331135) and multi-agent therapy (sirolimus and cyclophosphamide, NCT00743509).

Multi-tyrosine Kinase Inhibitors (TKIs)

Tyrosine kinases (TKs) regulate cellular proliferation, survival, differentiation, function, and motility. Osteosarcoma has shown overexpression of several TKs (Rettew et al. 2012).

Src Kinase Pathway

Src is found to be overexpressed in osteosarcoma and mediates PI3K/Akt anoikis resistance (Diaz-

Montero et al. 2006). Inhibition of Src prevents cell invasion and induces apoptosis in vitro and reduces tumor growth in vivo (Akiyama et al. 2008). Dasatinib was tested against osteosarcoma xenograft panels and was found to have intermediate activity (Kolb et al. 2008). Hingorani et al. (2009) demonstrated dasatinib to be active in primary osteosarcoma tumor, but not against pulmonary metastasis suggesting that this process may be independent of Src activation. There is a phase I/II study (NCT00788125) of dasatinib in combination with ifosfamide, carboplatin, and etoposide in young patients with metastatic or recurrent solid tumors including osteosarcoma. SARC has a randomized trial using Src inhibitor saracatinib in patients with recurrent osteosarcoma localized to the lung (NCT00752206).

Sorafenib

Sorafenib is an oral multi-TKI that targets Raf kinases and other RTKs involved in tumor progression (FLT-3, KIT, fibroblast growth factor receptor, RET) and angiogenesis (VEGFR and PDGFR-β). Several of these molecular targets are involved in the pathogenesis of osteosarcoma: Raf (Ikeda et al. 1989), PDGF (Sulzbacher et al. 2003), VEGF (Yang et al. 2007), and KIT (Smithey et al. 2002). Sorafenib has been shown to inhibit ERK1/2, MCL-1, and phospho-ezrin/radixin/moesin (P-ERM) pathways which are activated in osteosarcoma cell lines (Pignochino et al. 2009).

Insulinlike Growth Factor-1 Receptor (IGF-1R) Inhibition

IGF-1R has been implicated in the development of sarcomas, and inhibition of IGF-1R function has been demonstrated to reduce growth in osteosarcoma, ES, and rhabdomyosarcoma (Scotlandi 2006; Toretsky et al. 1997b). More than 25 antibodies and small molecules that specifically inhibit IGF-1R have undergone preclinical and clinical testing in both adults and children. Two humanized monoclonal antibodies (mAb) have been evaluated by the Pediatric Preclinical Testing Program (PPTP). Preliminary evidence of antitumor activity was reported in a phase II study of SCH717454 in subjects with relapsed osteosarcoma and Ewing sarcoma (NCT00617890). The mAb cixutumumab (IMC-A12) has been shown to induce intermediate responses in three of five osteosarcoma xenografts (Houghton et al. 2010a). In a phase II COG trial, cixutumumab was well tolerated as a single agent in patients with solid tumors (Malempati et al. 2012). In the phase II study which included patients with osteosarcoma, the combination of cixutumumab and temsirolimus showed clinical activity in patients, but did not have an effect on median progression-free survival (Schwartz et al. 2013). Despite evidence of benefits in some pediatric patients, several drug companies have curtailed or stopped anti-IGF-1R programs because observed clinical benefits did not meet primary end points in many adult trials.

14.1.6.4 Altering Tumor Microenvironment

Receptor Activator of Nuclear Factor-Kappa B Ligand (RANKL) Inhibitors

Zoledronic acid (ZA) is a potent third-generation bisphosphonate which targets the microenvironment of the bone, improves bone strength, and reduces tumor-related pain and skeletal-related events in several adult cancers through inhibition of osteoclast activity and bone resorption. It is approved by the US FDA in adults with solid tumors and bone metastases (Lipton et al. 2003; Rosen et al. 2003).

Preclinical studies suggest that ZA has direct antitumor activity in a variety of tumors, including osteosarcoma. ZA has been shown to inhibit primary tumor growth, reduce lung metastases, and prolong survival in animal models of osteosarcoma (Dass and Choong 2007; Labrinidis et al. 2009; Ory et al. 2005). The COG has completed a feasibility and dose discovery analysis of ZA with concurrent chemotherapy in the treatment of newly diagnosed metastatic osteosarcoma (Goldsby et al. 2013).

Denosumab is a fully human monoclonal antibody targeting receptor activator of the nuclear factor-kappa B ligand (RANKL) which interacts with its receptor RANK to regulate bone turnover. It is approved by the FDA for the prevention of fracture in postmenopausal women with osteoporosis, for prevention of skeletal-related events in adults with solid tumor bone metastases, and for giant cell tumor of the bone (Ellis et al. 2008; McClung et al. 2006). RANKL and its receptor RANK have the physiologic function of regulating bone turnover. In response to RANKL–RANK binding, osteoclast precursors differentiate and become activated resulting in bone resorption. RANK is expressed in 57 % of human osteosarcomas, most human osteosarcoma cell lines and 70 % of canine osteosarcomas (Barger et al. 2007; Mori et al. 2007). In osteosarcoma, RANKL activates downstream signaling and modulates gene expression (Akiyama et al. 2010). A phase II single-arm study using denosumab in recurrent osteosarcoma is currently being developed by COG.

Inhibition of Angiogenesis

Angiogenesis is closely related to tumor development and metastasis, as is seen in osteosarcoma. Endostatin is a broad-spectrum angiogenesis inhibitor. Endostar, a human recombinant endostatin, enhances the antineoplastic effects of combretastatin, a vascular disrupting agent in an osteosarcoma xenograft (Fu et al. 2011). In a trial to evaluate the clinical efficacy of Endostar (Xu et al. 2013), a human recombinant endostatin is combined with chemotherapy in the treatment of 116 newly diagnosed osteosarcoma patients. Immunohistochemistry was used to measure VEGF and CD31 expression. Chemotherapy was noted to increase VEGF expression and the presence of microvessels in osteosarcoma tissues compared with pre-chemotherapy. Although no significant difference was observed in the OS rate between the Endostar treatment and nontreatment groups, Endostar treatment significantly inhibited the chemotherapy-induced VEGF expression and the presence of microvessels. The Endostar group had a higher increase in the event-free survival rate and decreased the occurrence of metastases.

14.1.6.5 Other Targets

Anti-mitotic Activity

Eribulin is a fully synthetic analogue of halichondrin B, which is capable of inducing irreversible mitotic blockade and apoptosis by inhibiting microtubule dynamic instability, which differs from the mode of action of both vinca alkaloids and taxanes (Jordan and Wilson 2004). In an initial testing by the Pediatric Preclinical Testing Program (PPTP), eribulin induced significant differences in EFS distribution compared to control in 29 of 35 (83 %) of the solid tumors. Objective responses were observed in 18 of 35 (51 %) solid tumor xenografts, including complete responses (CR) or maintained CR that were observed in osteosarcoma xenografts (Kolb et al. 2013). A single-arm phase II study using eribulin for recurrent osteosarcoma is currently open to accrual (COG AOST1322).

Targeting Disialoganglioside (GD2)

Disialoganglioside GD2 is a sialic acid containing glycosphingolipid expressed in many tumor surfaces. Targeting of disialoganglioside GD2 with immunotherapy has resulted in improved outcomes for patients with neuroblastoma. It is highly expressed by osteosarcoma cells (>90 %) and thought to play an important role in the attachment of tumor cells to extracellular matrix proteins (Shibuya et al. 2012; Yu et al. 1998). Expression of GD2 may confer worse prognosis. In a report by Roth et al. (2014), osteosarcoma tissue obtained at the time of disease recurrence demonstrated a higher intensity of staining compared with samples obtained at initial biopsy and definitive surgery ($p=0.016$). In another study, results suggested that expression of GD2/GD3 is responsible for the enhancement of the malignant features of osteosarcomas (Shibuya et al. 2012). These findings support GD2 as a great candidate for molecular-targeted therapy in osteosarcoma. Currently, there are ongoing trials targeting GD2 in patients with osteosarcoma (anti-GD2 CAR NCT02107963, humanized anti-GD2 antibody NCT00743496).

Targeting Glycoprotein Nonmetastatic Melanoma Protein B (GPNMB)

GPNMB is a transmembrane glycoprotein highly expressed in various types of cancer. It promotes the migration, invasion, and metastasis of tumor cells. Glembatumumab is an antibody–drug conjugate targeting GPNMB which has entered clinical evaluation for adult cancers that express GPNMB, including melanoma and breast cancer (Zhou et al. 2012). PPTP found that, among all xenografts, GPNMB was primarily expressed on osteosarcoma xenografts, all of which expressed GPNMB at the RNA level (Kolb et al. 2014). Glembatumumab induced statistically significant differences ($p<0.05$) in EFS distribution compared to control in each of the six osteosarcoma models studied. Glembatumumab yielded high-level activity against three of the six osteosarcoma xenografts, two of which showed the highest GPNMB expression at the RNA level, an evidence for response being related to GPNMB expression levels.

14.1.7 The Future for Osteosarcoma

Osteosarcoma demonstrates high genetic instability, tumor heterogeneity, local aggressiveness, and early metastatic potential, all of which contribute to the aggressiveness of this disease. Hence, understanding the biology of osteosarcoma is of paramount importance in the design of therapeutic trials that will hopefully impact the survival of patients, especially the ones with metastatic and recurrent disease. In the past, hypothesis failure of several early phase trials was due to lack of clinical activity of tested novel agents against osteosarcoma. Metastasis is a consistent feature of osteosarcoma biology that is responsible for patient mortality, and shortcomings in our understanding of the biology of osteosarcoma metastatic process preclude any judgments on the value of agents that target metastatic process.

It is clear that there is a need for changes in the trial design which should be specifically curtailed to the underlying biology of osteosarcoma. The traditional phase II study design assesses radiographic response in patients with measurable disease. This end point as a means to evaluate efficacy of treatment is difficult in patients with recurrent osteosarcoma as pathologically responding lesions may not change in size radiographically owing to mineralization of tumors with treatment, leading to a conclusion that investigational treatment is ineffective in error. In addition, many patients with recurrent osteosarcoma may not be considered for phase II agents if all sites of disease recurrence are amenable to surgical resection. Hence, these patients frequently have complete resection without a trial of second-line chemotherapy, excluding them from a phase II trial and limiting the number of patients available to investigate novel treatment strategies. Novel biologic therapies may not be effective in patients with gross residual disease, but might improve outcome in patients with minimal residual disease after surgical excision.

Ongoing biology efforts through pediatric consortium studies are underway, and tumor specimens from this bank have been used as part of the NCI Therapeutically Applicable Research to Generate Effective Treatments (TARGET) initiative and NCI-led genome-wide association study. Preclinical drug evaluation systems created toward more rapid identification and validation of compounds active in osteosarcoma have been established such as the Pediatric Preclinical Testing Program in the United States and Innovative Therapies for Children with Cancer in Europe. High-throughput screens of novel agents should accelerate clinical trial development. Finally, the clinical infrastructure is primed, and there are now various national and international cooperative groups to efficiently test new agents.

14.2 Recurrent Ewing Sarcoma

14.2.1 Incidence of Recurrence

Ewing sarcoma (ES) is an aggressive tumor whose prognosis is critically determined by the adequacy of local control of primary lesion through surgery, radiation, or both and by the efficacy of the systemic chemotherapy aimed at the control of micrometastatic disease. Multimodal approach to the treatment has led to the dramatically improved outcome of patients with localized ES. However, recurrences remain a daunting challenge with dismal survival rate after relapse despite best efforts. Approximately 30–40 % of patients with initially localized disease at diagnosis still died of their disease (Burgert et al. 1990; Craft et al. 1998; Nesbit et al. 1990; Nilbert et al. 1998; Oberlin et al. 1985, 2001; Paulussen et al. 2001). About 60–80 % of patients with metastatic disease at initial diagnosis will relapse (Leavey and Collier 2008).

Most patients recur within 2 years from initial diagnosis (Bacci et al. 2006; Barker et al. 2005; Leavey et al. 2008; McTiernan et al. 2006; Shankar et al. 2003; Stahl et al. 2011). Patients diagnosed initially with metastatic disease relapsed significantly earlier compared to those who relapsed with initially localized disease at diagnosis (median time to recurrence 434 days versus 563 days, respectively, $p<0.001$). The overall median survival after first relapse was 9–14 months (Bacci et al. 2006; Barker et al. 2005; Leavey et al. 2008; McTiernan et al. 2006; Shankar et al. 2003; Stahl et al. 2011). It was noted that in subsequent relapses, there was a higher rate of patients who relapsed with disseminated disease at multiple sites versus local recurrences ($p<0.0001$) (Bacci et al. 2006). In 714 patients with first recurrence treated by Cooperative Ewing Sarcoma Studies (CESS) and European Intergroup CESS (EICESS 92), the patterns of relapse were as follows: 15 % local, 12 % combined systemic and local, and 73 % systemic. Pattern of relapse seems to change according to the stage of disease at presentation. In this series, among patients who were initially diagnosed with localized disease, 20 % relapsed locally, 73 % had systemic relapse, and 12 % had combined local and systemic relapse. When primary disease was disseminated at initial diagnosis, systemic relapse was seen in 82 %, 13 % combined, and 5 % localized relapse (Stahl et al. 2011). Barker et al. (2005) reported that among

71 % metastatic relapse without associated local relapse, the most common sites were the distant bone (35 %) and lung (18 %), with isolated recurrences occurring in 11 % of patients.

14.2.2 Outcomes at Recurrence

Whereas current intensive multimodal treatment enables patients with localized disease to be cured, in those with metastatic spread or recurrent disease, its benefit is more often limited to extending progression-free survival (Esiashvili et al. 2008; Leavey and Collier 2008). The outcome for patients with initially metastatic disease remains poor with 5 year EFS 28 % (Miser et al. 2007). The outlook for patients with recurrent EWS is even worse at less than 20 % in most series (Bacci et al. 2003, 2006; Barker et al. 2005; Cotterill et al. 2000; McTiernan et al. 2006; Robinson et al. 2013; Rodriguez-Galindo et al. 2002a Shankar et al. 2003; Stahl et al. 2011) despite aggressive multimodal treatment. Patients with recurrent disease have a reported 5-year post-relapse survival (PRS) of 7–23 % (Bacci et al. 2003, 2006; Barker et al. 2005; Leavey et al. 2008; Shankar et al. 2003) and 5-year post-relapse EFS (PREFS) of 7.9–13.8 % (Bacci et al. 2003, 2006). In a single-center case series of 114 patients, only 12.3 % remained alive at a median follow-up of 61 months (Whelan et al. 2012). In a retrospective study by Bacci et al. (2003), of 195 patients with relapsed ES, a second complete remission was achieved in only 26 patients (13.3 %). Of the 169 patients who never achieved disease-free status, 164 died of disease. Among patients who entered remission ($n=26$), 12 relapsed once again with none of these patients achieving CR3, and all died of the disease. In the end, 14 patients were alive and free of disease. With a mean follow-up of 9.5 years, the 5-year PR EFS and OS were 9.7 % and 13.8 %, respectively. This study's outcome was worse than reported in St. Jude's cohort (Rodriguez-Galindo et al. 2002a) which included patients with metastatic disease at initial diagnosis, with a 5 year PRS of 23.7 % ($n=71$) and similar to the UKCCSG ET-2 study ($n=64$) with localized ES who had relapsed (Craft et al. 1998). Another study by Bacci et al. (2006) with 290 relapsed ES patients, the 5-year PREFS and PRS 5.1 % and 7.9 %, respectively. The median follow-up was 16.8 years from the start of primary treatment and 13.6 years from first recurrence. This is similar to ones reported by Craft et al. (1998), Oberlin et al. (1992), and Sauer et al. (1987). In a separate series with 114 patients with relapsed or progressive ES, the 2- and 5-year PRS were 23.5 % and 15.2 %, respectively (McTiernan et al. 2006). For all patients with recurrent ES, the 5-year PFS rate was estimated to be 20 % and 5 year PRS 23 % (Barker et al. 2005).

14.2.3 Risk Factors for Recurrence

The Children's Oncology Group (COG) phase III multi-institutional study (INT0091) showed that older age, tumor size, primary site, advanced tumor stage, and serum LDH were all associated with decreased EFS and risk of recurrence (Grier et al. 2003). This was similar to those in previous studies of Ewing sarcoma (Cotterill et al. 2000; Oberlin et al. 1992; Meyer et al. 1992). Specifically, patients with large tumors (maximal diameter of at least 8 cm) had a poorer outcome than those with smaller tumors (5 year EFS 55 % versus 75 % percent, $p<0.001$). The site of the tumor was also correlated with the outcome with the 5 year EFS 68 % among patients with tumors of the distal extremity, 61 % among patients with tumors of the proximal extremity, and 50 % among those with primary tumors of the pelvis ($p=0.003$).

Grier et al. (2003) reported that younger patients had a better outcome than older patients. The 5 year EFS was 70 % for patients under 10 years, 60 % for those 10 years to 17 years, and 44 % for those 18 years or older (relative risk as compared with those under 10 years was 2.5; $p=0.001$). Interestingly in this study, even though ifosfamide and etoposide benefited patients with localized ES, older age remained an adverse prognostic factor despite this addition. Other studies also supported older age (>14 years) being associated with poor outcome (Cotterill et al. 2000; Kolb et al. 2003; Siegel et al. 1988;

Picci et al. 1997). The explanation of this is unclear. Some series suggest no differences between age-groups in terms of metastasis at diagnosis, tumor location, or histological response to neoadjuvant chemotherapy (Verrill et al. 1997; Bacci et al. 2007). However, there is a higher incidence of increased tumor size and extraskeletal primaries among patients >40 years (Pieper et al. 2008; Maki 2008). Older patients (>18 years) were also noted to have not benefited from compressed cycles of vincristine, Adriamycin, and cyclophosphamide alternating with ifosfamide and etoposide (VAD/IE) every 2 weeks instead of 3 weeks (Womer et al. 2012). In the study by Bacci et al. (2000), it is interesting to note that some of the factors that influenced initial EFS also impacted the pattern of relapse and the length of survival. For instance, in this series, in patients less than <12 years who relapsed, time to relapse and time to death were significantly longer than patients who are older than 12 years when their disease recurred.

Overt metastatic disease at diagnosis is established as one of the strongest indicators of poor outcome (Cotterill et al. 2000; Grier et al. 2003; Bacci et al. 2000). Initial pretreatment serum LDH correlates with tumor burden and has also been shown to be an adverse prognostic factor for outcome in ES (Bacci et al. 2000, 2003). Pathologic assessment of response to therapy involves evaluation of the treated tumor for degree of necrosis similar to what is done for osteosarcoma. There is general agreement that a complete response (inability to detect viable tumor cells with extensive sampling) is associated with better outcome than residual gross disease in the resection specimen (Picci et al. 1993, 1997; Bacci et al. 2000). Five-year EFS was 77.2 % and was noted for patients with good histologic response versus only 28 % for poor responders ($p<0.001$) (Bacci et al. 2000). Moreover, patients who had good histologic response who relapsed and died of their cancer had significantly longer survival time versus poor responders ($p=0.03$). However, histologic response to chemotherapy is hard to be properly defined as a prognostic factor because it is not assessable for patients who did not undergo surgery for local treatment. Other studies show conflicting data with regard to impact of tumor necrosis with post-relapse survival (Bacci et al. 2003, 2006).

14.2.4 Prognostic Factors at Recurrence

14.2.4.1 Time to Recurrence

Several studies have documented that outcome is significantly correlated with time to relapse, with patients who relapsed early (within 2 years of initial diagnosis) having worse prognosis compared to those who experienced late recurrence (≥ 2 years after initial diagnosis) (Shankar et al. 2003; Leavey et al. 2008; Bacci et al. 2006; McTiernan et al. 2006; Stahl et al. 2011; Barker et al. 2005; Robinson et al. 2013). There was an observed significantly better outcome in patients who had late versus early relapse, with 5 year PRS 14 % versus 7 % ($p<0.001$), respectively, and PREFS was 5 % versus 19 % ($p<0.003$) for early versus late relapse, respectively (Bacci et al. 2003). In a separate study, 5-year PREFS is significantly correlated with time to first relapse ($p<0.0009$) (Bacci et al. 2006). In a study by Leavey et al. (2008), the disease-free interval (DFI) was shown to be significantly associated to the risk for post-recurrence death, with 5 year EFS of those who recurred >2 years from initial diagnosis 30 % versus 7 % for those whose disease recurred <2 years ($p<0.0001$). The DFI for those who relapsed >2 years is 23 months, 1–2 years is 10 months, and <1 year is 5 months. Robinson et al. (2013) reported that time to relapse was a significant predictor of 5 year PRS, with early relapse (<2 year) at 12 % versus late relapse (>2 year) at 50 % ($p=0.003$). In this study, those who had late relapses also had a greater PREFS than those who relapsed early (16 % versus 0 %).

Disease-free interval in between relapses is noted to be shorter with every relapse. Bacci et al. (2006) reported that the mean time to relapse was 27 months since the start of primary treatment, 17.6 months for second relapse, 13.7 months to third relapse, and 4 months for those who experienced fourth relapse. Moreover, the time to first relapse was significantly longer for patients who achieved second remission after treatment than for those who were never free of

disease (52 months versus 23.5 months, $p<0.0001$) (Bacci et al. 2003). This association in terms of time of recurrence is similar to findings in other studies (Nesbit et al. 1990; Oberlin et al. 1985; Paulussen et al. 2001; Rodriguez-Galindo et al. 2002a; Schuck et al. 2003).

14.2.4.2 Location of Recurrence

Local Versus Distant Relapse

Shankar et al. (2003) reported no difference in OS between local and systemic relapse and site relapse. In a study by Robinson et al. (2013), the 5 year PRS (35 %) was similar in all patients with distant relapse (lung-only metastases and other patterns of failure). In this study, however, the 5yearear PRS for those with localized relapse was significantly better than distant relapse (55 % versus 22 %, $p=0.045$). Patients with combined relapse (local and distant) fared worse with a 5 year PRS for combined recurrence that was 12.5 % ± 8.3 % versus 21.7 % ± 7.8 % for those with localized relapse (Rodriguez-Galindo et al. 2002a). This is similar to a report by Stahl et al. (2011).

Isolated Lung Recurrence: Unilateral Versus Bilateral

Leavey et al. (2008) reported that 30 % of relapsed patients recurred in the lungs, but only 17 % had isolated pulmonary recurrence. In this cohort of patients, pulmonary recurrence was not predictive of post-recurrence survival (PRS), with isolated pulmonary recurrence not shown to be a statistically significant advantage compared with combined pulmonary recurrence (17 months versus 9 months, $p=0.08$). This is in contrast to findings by Bacci et al. (2003) and McTiernan et al. (2006) who reported that for those with lung-only recurrence, those with bilateral disease has a significantly worse outcome compared to those with unilateral lung recurrence.

Recurrence in the Lungs Versus Other Sites

Some studies did not show a difference in the outcome of patients who had lung recurrence compared to other distant sites (Shankar et al. 2003; Robinson et al. 2013), although this can be due to smaller sample size of these studies. On the contrary, several studies have reported improved survival in patients who had lung-only relapses versus those with combination of distant recurrences (Bacci et al. 2003, 2006; McTiernan et al. 2006; Stahl et al. 2011). Specifically, Bacci et al. (2003) reported a significantly better outcome in patients who had lung-only metastases versus the ones with combined lung and outside lung metastases with a 5 year PREFS 14 % versus 0.9 % ($p<0.0001$). In McTiernan's study (McTiernan et al. 2006), patients with local relapse or lung-only relapse fared better compared to those with extrapulmonary recurrence. Moreover, patients with disease confined locally or to the lungs at both diagnosis and relapse had superior survival to those with extrapulmonary disease at any time.

14.2.4.3 Treatment for Recurrence

Treatment for relapsed ES varies because of the many different types of recurrences that occur (localized, systemic, or combined), the site of distant relapse (lung, bone, lung and bone, other sites), the number of pulmonary metastases, and the type of first-line local and systemic treatment performed. The treatment is consequently tailored on an individual basis. Depending on what patients received at diagnosis, those who have local recurrence typically have local treatment with surgery or radiation therapy (RT) with our without systemic therapy.

Local Control

Shankar et al. (2003) reported that patients who received multimodal treatment had significantly higher response rate, but outcome was no different to those who only received single modality treatment. In another study, outcome significantly correlated with treatment performed after relapse, with all patients free of disease treated with surgery alone or combined with radiation therapy or a second-line chemotherapy (Bacci et al. 2003). In this study, there was a significantly better outcome in patients who had definitive local control (surgery and/or radiotherapy) alone, or in combination with chemotherapy, versus the ones who had chemotherapy alone (15.4 % versus 0.9 % $p<0.0001$). In a separate study, the rate of the first remission was significantly higher for patients treated with surgery alone (93.6 %) or combined

with chemotherapy (91.6 %) than those treated with conventional (2.2 %) or high-dose chemotherapy (11 %) or by radiotherapy (22 %) (Bacci et al. 2006). This however needs to be interpreted with caution since patients treated with surgery alone likely had isolated local or lung recurrences, and the ones who were treated with chemotherapy alone were highly selected and restricted to patients with unresectable disease and not amenable for curative intent radiotherapy.

Comparing local control strategies, second remission was achieved with complete surgical resection (45 %) compared to radiotherapy (13 %) ($p<0.001$) (Robinson et al. 2013). However, McTiernan et al. (2006) reported that among 114 patients, definitive local treatment was a strong predictor of outcome, whether the local control modality was surgery or radiotherapy. Radical surgery for those with local recurrence had significantly higher 5 year PRS of 31.4 % ± 11.6 % versus other strategies 9.1 % ± 6.1 % ($p=0.023$). Use of RT alone for local control (especially doses <35 Gy) was observed to contribute to high local failure rate (Rodriguez-Galindo et al. 2002a).

Data supporting resection of lung metastases in ES is conflicting. Some reports demonstrate improved survival (Lanza et al. 1987; Briccoli et al. 2004); however, others did not (Paulussen et al. 2001). In the St. Jude cohort (Rodriguez-Galindo et al. 2002a), lung RT in patients with isolated pulmonary relapse had significantly prolonged survival (5 year PRS 30.3 % ± 12.5 % versus 16.7 % ± 10.8 %, $p=0.018$). In a separate study (Robinson et al. 2013), patients who underwent complete surgical resection of recurrence or definitive RT had three times higher likelihood of 5 year PRS and significantly improved 5 year PREFS. On the contrary, there is evidence that indicates only a small effect from the use of lung irradiation (Hawkins et al. 2000), especially when second-line treatment for ES fails.

Chemotherapy

Analysis of patients who received vincristine, doxorubicin, and cyclophosphamide, alternating with ifosfamide and etoposide (VDC/IE) for initial diagnosis versus the ones who did not, the 5 year PRS was different (16 % versus 31 %, respectively) although difference was not statistically significant (Robinson et al. 2013). However, patients who received VDC/IE had significantly later first relapse ($p=0.004$). In this study, the use of chemotherapy at first recurrence did not significantly improve outcome. In a separate study, the type of first-line chemotherapy did not matter to rate of achieving remission after relapse since no patient who did not undergo surgery after relapse was alive and free of disease (Bacci et al. 2006).

Use of second-line chemotherapy was highly variable among different studies in patients with relapsed ES. A significant number of patients also received multimodal therapy (chemotherapy and local control), making it hard to evaluate specific benefit from systemic therapy. In general, chemotherapy seems to be employed when relapse is deemed not amenable to local control strategies (surgery and/or radiation). In one study Nesbit et al. (1990), 17 % received chemotherapy alone, and all of these patients subsequently died due to disease progression. In another study Oberlin et al. (1985), 65 % received chemotherapy at first relapse. There was a trend for benefit of systemic therapy but did not achieve statistical difference in 5 year PRS ($p=0.67$).

Bacci et al. (2003) reported that among 195 patients with relapsed ES, about 50 % received chemotherapy mostly in the setting of multimodal therapy and up to a third of these patients in the context of high-dose chemotherapy with stem cell transplant. None of the patients who received chemotherapy alone were long-term survivors. In another study by Bacci et al. (2006) with 378 recurrent ES, only 6 % received adjuvant chemotherapy after surgery, 13 % chemotherapy alone, and 5 % high-dose chemotherapy with stem cell transplant. None of the patients who did not get surgical local control survived, irrespective of whether they received concurrent chemotherapy or not. Their conclusion is that multimodal therapy seems to be beneficial for relapsed patients; nonetheless, surgical local control still has the leading role in relapsed ES.

The relationship between second remission and type of salvage treatment should be considered with caution mainly due to selection bias. Patients who have more isolated and localized recurrences are amenable to surgical resection, and therefore better outcome, compared to patients who have disseminated relapse who receive chemotherapy and are not candidates for local control.

14.2.4.4 Second Complete Remission (CR2)

Rate of CR2 is influenced by the type of relapse and treatment. In one report, the rate of patients who achieved second remission was 83.3 % for those who had local recurrence, 48 % who relapsed with isolated lung metastases ($p<0.0004$), 20 % who relapsed with isolated bone metastases ($p<0.0002$), and 2.4 % who relapsed with combined bone and lung mets ($p<0.004$) (Bacci et al. 2003). This pattern was similar to reports by Shakar et al. (2003), Bacci et al. (2006), and Stahl et al. (2011). This is likely due to the fact that the ones who had local or isolated relapses tend to be more amenable to complete surgical resection. The type of treatment influenced the rate of remission. Bacci et al. (2003) reported 86.6 % CR2 rate for those treated with surgery and chemotherapy, 66.7 % for surgery alone, 33.3 % for radiotherapy plus chemotherapy, 6 % for radiotherapy alone, and 0.9 % for chemotherapy alone. These differences are highly significant ($p<0.0001$).

Relapse-free interval was significantly longer for patients who achieved CR2 (39 months) versus those who did not (21 month) ($p<0.0001$) (Bacci et al. 2006). Improved 5 year PFS (40 % versus 0 %) and 5 year PRS (46 % versus 0 %) were both associated with response to second-line therapy ($p<0.0001$), with the median survival time for patients who responded to second-line treatment of 36 months versus 4 months for those who did not respond to second-line treatment (Barker et al. 2005). This was similar in other reports (Bacci et al. 2003; Hayes et al. 1987). PR EFS was significantly higher in patients who had second surgical remission versus those whose disease was not completely resected at relapse or had disease not amenable to definitive RT (16 % versus 0 %) (Robinson et al. 2013).

14.2.4.5 Metastatic Disease at Diagnosis

The presence of metastasis at diagnosis seems to be the worst prognostic factor for patients with ES, and unfortunately, systemic chemotherapy trials have not been able to improve durable remission rates for patients with metastatic ES (Cotterill et al. 2000; Navid et al. 2008a). Metastatic disease at initial diagnosis was correlated with significantly poorer PRS compared to localized disease ($p<0.0001$) (McTiernan et al. 2006), similar to findings in other studies (Leavey et al. 2008; Barker et al. 2005). However, when controlling for response to second-line therapy in this study, metastatic disease at initial diagnosis was not associated with worse outcome. Surprisingly, in initial intergroup ewings sarcoma study (IESS), patients with metastatic disease achieved a 30 % 5-year OS with standard chemotherapy (Paulussen et al. 2001; Hayes et al. 1987; Cangir et al. 1990) or TBI followed by auto-BMT (Miser et al. 2004; Burdach et al. 2003; Horowitz et al. 1993). Here it seems like patients with metastatic EWS at presentation have a more favorable outcome than nonmetastatic disease who relapsed after combined treatment (Sauer et al. 1987). This may be because patients with metastases at presentation who had never received chemotherapy before diagnosis might be more sensitive to systemic treatment in comparison to patients who have relapsed after initial aggressive chemotherapy.

14.2.4.6 Impact of Initial Prognostic Factors on Outcome

Patient age has been associated with outcome. In a report by Robinson et al. (Robinson et al. 2013), patients 18 years and older with initially localized disease had a 5 year PRS that was 30 %. In this study, adult patients with ES who have disease relapse after primary treatment of localized disease will continue to have recurrences regardless of modality of salvage therapy. Worse prognosis remains for adult patients who have had distant relapse and recurrence less than 2 years after initial diagnosis. On the contrary, reports from other studies (Leavey et al. 2008; Bacci et al. 2003, 2006; McTiernan et al. 2006) indicated that age did not influence outcome.

Several prognostic indicators at initial diagnosis did not continue to have prognostic significance in multivariate analysis with post-recurrence survival, such as gender, primary tumor site (extremity versus pelvic versus other sites), tumor volume, and histologic response to chemotherapy, and did not affect survival after relapse (Shankar et al. 2003; Leavey et al. 2008; Bacci et al. 2003, 2006; McTiernan et al. 2006; Rodriguez-Galindo et al. 2002a). Serum LDH was significantly associated with outcome after recurrence (Leavey et al. 2008), but this was not found to be true in several studies (Shankar et al. 2003; Bacci et al. 2003, 2006; McTiernan et al. 2006; Rodriguez-Galindo et al. 2002a).

Prognostic factors evaluated in these studies need to be interpreted with caution. The major limitation of most studies is that majority are done retrospectively and cannot control for selection bias. In addition, incomplete or ambiguous data, patient, disease, or treatment-related factors taint analysis. There is also lack of standard values in reporting measurable variables such as age, tumor size, necrosis, and the small numbers of patients in most series.

It seems that relapsed patients can be divided into two groups, the ones that can be cured with traditional treatments (late relapse, relapse to lungs only, and patients whose recurrences can be surgically treated with or without chemotherapy or RT) versus those who have early relapse with combined metastases to lungs and other sites who seem to gain no benefit from traditional therapies (Bacci et al. 2003, 2006). In multivariate analyses (McTiernan et al. 2006; Stahl et al. 2011; Barker et al. 2005), the most significant factors associated with improved survival were disease confined locally or to the lungs, time to relapse (early <2 years versus late ≥2 years from initial diagnosis), and response to second-line treatment. Most studies suggest the importance of local control, specifically surgery, and an aggressive approach to local failure. The benefit of chemotherapy in the relapse setting is hard to tease out given that most patients receive multimodal treatment, as well as selection bias for use of systemic treatment in patients who have disseminated disease and therefore are not candidates for adequate local control.

14.2.5 Therapeutic Approach

14.2.5.1 Chemotherapy

Chemotherapy has been used in relapsed ES mainly to control disease, address micro-/macrometastatic disease, and facilitate local control or primary tumor. Unfortunately, new combinations of traditional drugs and use of novel agents have yet to significantly affect the outcome of patients with high-risk disease (DuBois ct al. 2009; Mora et al. 2009; Jacobs et al. 2010; Fox et al. 2010; Chao et al. 2010; Hunold et al. 2006; Langevin et al. 2008; Van Winkle et al. 2005). Several different regimens are employed reflecting patient factors such as organ function, duration of remission, need for mobilization and collection of stem cells, and evolving practice.

Ifosfamide- or Carboplatin-Based Regimen

Historically, majority of patients were treated with second-line regimens, principally carboplatin- or ifosfamide-based chemotherapy: ifosfamide and etoposide (IE) or ifosfamide, carboplatin, and etoposide (ICE) (Barker et al. 2005; Rodriguez-Galindo et al. 2002a). When short durations of response with carboplatin regimens were observed, high-dose ifosfamide, at a median dose of 15 g/m2 (range 12–18 g/m2), was employed (Ladenstein et al. 1995a).

Irinotecan/Temozolomide

The combination of irinotecan and temozolomide has been used with encouraging results for various relapsed adult and pediatric solid tumors in recent years (Reardon et al. 2005; Jones et al. 2003; Wagner et al. 2004; Kushner et al. 2006). Irinotecan is a camptothecin prodrug that is metabolized by carboxylesterase enzymes to a topoisomerase I inhibitor, SN-38, which is approximately 1,000 times more potent than the prodrug (Thompson et al. 2008). It offers the advantages of cytotoxicity at relatively nonmyelosuppressive doses and manageable non-hematological toxicity, the most common of which is diarrhea. Temozolomide is a second-generation imidazotetrazine prodrug that is metabolized to the active metabolite monomethyl triazenoimidazole carboxamide. This agent promotes cytotoxicity, leading to base pair mismatch and eventual inhibition of DNA replication, resulting in cell cycle arrest (Wagner et al. 2004; Newlands et al. 1997). It has the advantages of excellent oral bioavailability, ability to cross the blood–brain barrier, and a favorable toxicity profile.

Although each agent alone has minimal activity against ES, preclinical and clinical studies demonstrate the combination of irinotecan and temozolomide to have schedule-dependent synergy and antineoplastic activity in relapsed solid tumors, including ES (Wagner et al. 2004, 2007; Houghton et al. 2000). A pediatric phase I trial of temozolomide combined with protracted irinotecan for refractory solid tumors demonstrated the MTD to be temozolomide 100 mg/m^2/day × 5 and irinotecan 10 mg/m^2/day (daily × 5 × 2) every 28 days (Wagner et al. 2004). For patients with advanced ES treated with this regimen, overall response rates of up to 60 % have been reported (Wagner et al. 2007; Anderson et al. 2008). Experience at Memorial Sloan Kettering Cancer Center (MSKCC) (Casey et al. 2009) with 19 recurrent/progressive ES using this regimen yielded 5 complete and 7 partial responses (a 63 % overall objective response), with a median time to progression (TTP) for all patients at 8.3 months and for the subset of 14 patients with recurrent ES at 16.2 months. Median TTP was better for patients who sustained a 2-year first remission than for those who relapsed <2 years from diagnosis and for patients with primary localized versus metastatic disease. In a study by Mascarenhas et al. (2010), two treatment schedules of irinotecan with vincristine were evaluated for relapsed rhabdomyosarcoma patients and showed that there was no difference in response and toxicity in maximizing the dose of irinotecan 50 mg/m^2/day intravenously for 5 days every 21-day cycle (instead of 20 mg/m2/day intravenously for 10 days). Because this regimen is shorter and more convenient, this is the more commonly used drug dose and schedule in the outpatient setting.

Topotecan/Cyclophosphamide

Cyclophosphamide is well studied in ES with proven efficacy (Hunold et al. 2006; Sutow and

Sullivan 1962; Bernstein et al. 2006). Its combination with topotecan, a derivative of camptothecin that inhibits topoisomerase I, has proved to be synergistic with proven efficacy in EWS (Anderson et al. 2008; Hunold et al. 2006). In a phase II study of patients with recurrent solid tumors using cyclophosphamide (250 mg/m²/dose) and topotecan (0.75 mg/m²/dose) given for 5 days every 21-day cycle, which included 17 patients with Ewing sarcoma, 2 achieved complete response (CR), 4 partial response (PR), and 6 had stable disease (SD), with an overall objective response of 35 % (Saylors et al. 2001). In a therapeutic window study conducted by the Children's Oncology Group (COG), treatment of patients with Ewing sarcoma with cyclophosphamide/topotecan resulted in PR in 21 of 37 patients, accounting for a response rate of 56 %, and 15 more patients had SD (Bernstein et al. 2006). A review of the German experience with this regimen, in patients with Ewing sarcoma who received cyclophosphamide/topotecan at either first or second relapse, showed a response rate of 32.6 % (Hunold et al. 2006). In this study, one third of the patients were alive at a median follow-up of 14.5 months (range, 2.1–59.8 months), of whom a proportion had subsequently received other therapies.

In a separate study in relapsed ES using cyclophosphamide/topotecan (Farhat et al. 2013), response was assessable in 13 patients and showed progressive disease in 6 (46 %), stable disease in 4 (31 %), and partial response in 3 (23 %). Nine patients had local control (radical surgery in two, radiation in three, and a combination in four patients). Response, when it occurred, was maintained for a median of 8 months (range 4–28 months). Four patients (29 %) are alive at 3, 7, 9, and 10 months after relapse. COG opened a phase II study (AEWS0521) combining bevacizumab with vincristine, topotecan, and cyclophosphamide for patients with first recurrent Ewing sarcoma. This combination was found to be feasible, but further study of bevacizumab in combination with cytotoxic therapy for patients with recurrent EWS is still warranted.

Gemcitabine and Docetaxel

In a phase 2 study from the COG using docetaxel alone in pediatric patients with refractory solid tumors, Zwerdling et al. (2006) showed 3 PR and no CR among 21 ES patients. A retrospective case review of 22 patients with recurrent/refractory bone sarcoma treated with gemcitabine (675 mg/m2 IV on day 1 and day 8) and docetaxel (75–100 mg/m2 IV on day 8) was conducted (Navid et al. 2008b). In this cohort, two patients had relapsed ES, with one patient with SD and no CR/PR. The overall objective response for this study was 29 %, with a median duration of response of 4.8 months and manageable ambulatory toxicity.

In another series (Mora et al. 2009), ten patients with relapsed/refractory pediatric sarcoma, including six Ewing sarcomas, two synovial sarcomas, one osteosarcoma, and one undifferentiated sarcoma, were treated prospectively with gemcitabine (1,000 mg/m² over 90 min on day 1 and 8) and docetaxel (100 mg/m² over 2–4 h on day 8 of a 21-day cycle). By Response Evaluation Criteria in Solid Tumors (RECIST), four (40 %) patients had CR, one (10 %) had PR, three (30 %) had SD, and two (20 %) had progressive disease (PD), which provides an objective response rate of 50 %, with a median duration of response of 10 months (range: 6–32+ months). Five out of the ten patients (50 %) were alive, with a median follow-up of 48 months from diagnosis. Mild toxicities (no grades 3–4) were encountered and managed in the ambulatory setting. The study concluded that the gemcitabine and docetaxel regimen demonstrated antitumor activity against advanced pediatrics, mainly Ewing sarcoma, allowing for good quality of life.

A SARC phase 2 trial (SARC) was conducted using gemcitabine (675 mg/m2 IV on days 1 and 8) and docetaxel (75–100 mg/m2 IV on day 8) given every 21 days in children and adults with recurrent ES, osteosarcoma, or unresectable or recurrent chondrosarcoma (Fox et al. 2012). Primary objective response rate was based on RECIST, and out of 53 evaluable patients, there was no complete response observed, and partial responses included 2 out of 14 enrolled relapsed ES. In this study, gemcitabine and docetaxel combination was associated with 5.6 % probability of reaching the target of 35 % response rate in ES.

14.2.5.2 High-Dose Chemotherapy with Stem Cell Transplant (HDT-SCT)

Evidence That HDT-SCT Is Beneficial

Benefit of HDT-SCT in Ewing sarcoma has been controversial. Over the years, there have been numerous attempts in trying to answer this question, but the answer is still elusive. Several studies have alluded to its benefit, especially in the setting of high-risk ES. McTiernan et al. (2006) reported the use of HDT-SCT after second-line chemotherapy with curative intent among 29 (of 77) patients with progressed or relapsed Ewing sarcoma. HDT-SCT conditioning regimens included the following: busulfan–melphalan (BuMel) in 19 patients, melphalan only 2, melphalan/TBI 1, melphalan/etoposide 7, melphalan/etoposide/TBI 3, and busulfan/cyclophosphamide 3. The median time from diagnosis to relapse was 23 months for those who proceeded to HDT-SCT after relapse. After HDT-SCT, there were 13 CR, 8 PR, 7 responding disease, and 1 progressive disease. Out of three patients who died from the entire cohort due to treatment-related causes, two underwent HDT-SCT. Findings indicate that HDT-SCT was the strongest predictor of survival in univariate analysis, with a 5-year PRS of 50.6 % (±9.5 %) for those who received HDT-SCT compared to 3.5 % (±2.0 %) for those who did not ($p < 0.001$).

In a series of 33 patients who received HDT-SCT using BuMel as conditioning regimen, univariate analysis showed improved 5 year EFS (21 %) associated with treatment with HDT-SCT compared to patients who received standard dose chemotherapy (0 %) (Bacci et al. 2003). Of note, however, multivariate analysis was not done to control for other prognostic factors.

The European Intergroup Cooperative Ewing Sarcoma Study (EICESS) reported that a subgroup of patients especially those with early relapses showed benefit from HDT-SCT (Burdach et al. 1993; Ladenstein et al. 1992). It must be noted that patients who underwent HDT-SCT were a selected cohort primarily by being responsive to salvage therapy, achieved either CR or VGPR, and remained in remission long enough for HDT-SCT.

Barker et al. (2005) reported 13 patients with relapsed ES who received HDT-SCT. Only patients who responded to second-line therapy received HDT-SCT. Most of these patients (10 of 13) achieved complete surgical excision of all recurrent disease, while 3 of 13 had partial excision of recurrent disease. Median time between relapse and HDT-SCT was 5 months. All patients received busulfan, melphalan, and thiotepa (BuMelTT) as preparative regimen, and 12 of 13 received autologous stem cell transplant. Five-year PFS (61 % versus 7 %, $p < 0.0001$) and OS (77 % versus 7 %, $p < 0.0001$) were superior in this group compared with patients who did not receive HDT-SCT for relapse. No patient died of HDT-SCT-related complications. There were five patients who developed second recurrence after HDT-SCT, with median time between the first and second recurrence of 20 months. Six out of nine patients who received tandem HDT-SCT are alive without recurrence. Two out of four patients who received BuMel only are alive without recurrence. Optimal conditioning regimen for Ewing sarcoma remains unclear, and most regimens use BuMel and often with TBI.

Review of the European Bone Marrow Transplantation Solid Tumor Registry (EBMTR) showed advantage of BuMel versus TBI (Ladenstein et al. 1992). A report from Perentesis et al. (1999) have used identical BuMelTT regimen for high-risk Ewing sarcoma (initially metastatic or recurrent) with encouraging early survival data.

Al-Faris et al. (2007) evaluated the role of HDT-SCT as consolidation therapy for children with high-risk Ewing sarcoma. High-risk Ewing sarcoma was defined as metastatic at diagnosis or relapsed disease. Forty-five children were identified, and 20 patients received autologous SCT after induction with VDC/IE. All patients had adequate local control: patients with resectable tumor or lung metastases underwent surgery, and those with non-resectable tumors were treated with radiation. At relapse, patients were treated with topotecan and cyclophosphamide, followed by ICE and local control with surgery and/or irradiation. Ten of the 20 patients treated with HDT-SCT are alive (median follow-up 6 years), with 8 out of 10 being in remission more than 5 years from diagnosis. The 3 year OS for HDT-SCT was 59 %, compared to 34 % ($p=0.06$) for patients treated with conventional chemotherapy (CC). The 3 year EFS for the ASCT was 39 % compared to 32 % in the CC group ($p=0.08$). Authors concluded that HDT-SCT appears to add some benefit to conventional multimodality therapy for children with high-risk ES.

No Benefit from HDT-SCT

On the contrary, there have also been numerous reports about the lack of evidence that HDT-SCT provides additional benefit in the treatment of patients with high-risk Ewing sarcoma. There are some plausible explanations why HDT-SCT may not necessarily work for patients with high-risk Ewing sarcoma. Patients having aggressive disease that do not respond to initial treatment particularly chemotherapy likely have chemoresistant disease and may have residual disease even after HDT-SCT. There have also been some reports of stem cell or marrow product contaminated with tumor cells (Hayes et al. 1987; Miser et al. 2004; Leung et al. 1998; Fischmeister et al. 1999). Overall survival remains unchanged despite a significant risk of death approaching 8 % from treatment-related complications such as secondary leukemia and myelodysplasia.

Several earlier studies suggest that HDT-SCT failed to improve survival when compared to historical controls (Kolb et al. 2003; Burdach et al. 2000, 2003; Ladenstein et al. 1995b; Paulussen et al. 1998; Meyers et al. 2001). Although patient number was small, HDT-SCT did not significantly make a difference in outcome of patients with relapsed EWS (Shankar et al. 2003). Four out of seven had recurrence after HDT-SCT, two alive with one disease-free for 42 months after distant skeletal relapse, and the other with recurrent disease 15 months after relapse. Progression-free interval after HDT-SCT is 16 months. Bacci et al. (2003) reported that none of the 15 patients who underwent HDT-SCT reached remission.

Meyers et al. (2001) conducted a study to determine whether consolidation therapy with high-dose melphalan, etoposide, and total body irradiation (TBI) with autologous stem cell support would improve the prognosis of 32 patients with newly diagnosed ES metastatic to bone and/or bone marrow. All patients received VDC/IE and local control. Twenty-three patients who had a good response to initial therapy proceeded to consolidation therapy with HDT-SCT. Three patients died from toxicity during HDT-SCT. The majority of the patients who underwent high-dose consolidation therapy experienced relapse and died with progressive disease. The 2 year EFS for all eligible patients was 20 %, compared to the 2-year post-stem cell reconstitution EFS for 23 patients who received HDT-SCT of 24 %. This study concluded that high-dose melphalan, etoposide, and TBI with autologous stem cell support failed to improve the probability of EFS in this cohort of patients with newly diagnosed metastatic ES.

In another study by Kushner and Meyers (2001), 21 patients with newly diagnosed ES metastatic to bone/bone marrow received VDC/IE for induction. Patients in complete or very good partial remission (CR/VGPR) after VDC/IE received myeloablative therapy with either total body irradiation TBI/melphalan or thiotepa/carboplatin. Only one patient became a long-term event-free survivor; all but one relapse was in a distant site. In eight patients treated with TBI/melphalan, four relapsed 2–7 months after transplantation, two died early of toxicity, one died of pulmonary failure 17 months after transplantation without evidence of ES, and one remains in CR at more than 7 years. The three patients treated with thiotepa/carboplatin relapsed 3–4 months after transplantation. All reports on large series of unselected patients with ES/PNET metastatic to bone/BM showed similarly unsatisfactory results and no improvements in event-free survival rates (Meyer et al. 1992; Cangir et al. 1990; Horowitz et al. 1993; Paulussen et al. 1998; Wexler et al. 1996; Sandoval et al. 1996). Secondary leukemia emerged as a major risk with dose-intensive regimens.

Poor outcome of recurrent Ewing sarcoma has led several investigators to use high-dose chemotherapy in the attempt to overcome chemotherapy resistance (Burdach et al. 1993, 2003; Hawkins et al. 2000; Ladenstein et al. 1992). However, the role of HDT-SCT in Ewing sarcoma remains unproven due to variations in approach. Different types of myeloablative regimens and sources of stem cells have been used. Also, selection criteria for eligible patients are varied among different studies. Patients who have had response to second-line therapy and/or had good performance status were candidates for HDT-SCT (Burdach et al. 1993, 2003; Ladenstein et al. 1992). This creates a selection bias for patients able to go through HDT-SCT by excluding patients who have especially aggressive or therapy-resistant disease. Also, a lot of studies were retrospective in nature and had small sample size with short follow-up. In addition, different patient-related factors, such as presence of metastatic disease at initial diagnosis, induction and treatment at relapse, and extent and timing of relapse from initial diagnosis, may have influenced outcome after HDT-SCT.

Clearly, there is a need for a prospective randomized controlled trial to answer the controversies of the role of HDT-SCT in Ewing sarcoma. Short of this trial format, statistical analyses may minimize the biases, but unlikely to eliminate it. In addition, defining a specific group of patients that will likely benefit from this approach is necessary. Barker et al. (2005), adjusting for selection bias in patients deemed eligible for HDT-SCT by performing multivariate analysis that controls for RFI and response to therapy, reported that patients with prolonged RFI and have response to therapy have an improved PFS and PRS with HDT-SCT. EBMTR (Ladenstein et al. 1995b) reported that favorable outcome was limited to relapsed patients with localized disease at initial diagnosis. In a separate study (Oberlin et al. 2006), 97 patients with newly diagnosed metastatic Ewing sarcoma who had CR or VGPR after induction chemotherapy received HDT-SCT with BuMel. Local therapy (surgery and/or radiation therapy) was performed before or after HDT-SCT. The 5 year EFS for all 97 patients was

37 %, and the overall survival (OS) rate was 38 %, whereas EFS after HDT-SCT was 47 %, 52 % for the 44 patients with lung-only metastases, and 36 % for patients with bone metastases without bone marrow involvement. From this study, it seemed that HDT-SCT benefited patients who responded well to systemic therapy and had lung- or bone-only metastases. In a report by Burke et al. (2007), HDT-SCT was offered to eight patients with high-risk Ewing sarcoma (defined as pelvic primary and/or metastatic disease). This study yielded four CR with mean follow-up of 6.25 years, and all had tandem HDT-SCT. Two other survivors constituted truly high-risk patients with bone metastases who have not had local control (surgery of radiation) of metastatic sites and had no evidence of disease. This study endorses HDT-SCT for high-risk patients, especially the ones with bone metastases and for whom local control measures cannot be adequately administered.

EURO-E.W.I.N.G. 99

The EURO-E.W.I.N.G. 99 trial is the first international randomized evaluation of the role of HDT-SCT for patients with metastatic ES at initial diagnosis. In this study, all patients received an intensive induction chemotherapy consisting of vincristine, ifosfamide, doxorubicin, and etoposide (VIDE) for six courses. Following local control, patients with localized tumors and a good response to induction were randomized to either ifosfamide-containing (VAI) or cyclophosphamide-containing (VAC) consolidation chemotherapy. Patients with isolated pulmonary/pleural metastases or with localized tumors and poor response to induction therapy were randomized to either VAI conventional consolidation chemotherapy or HDT-SCT using BuMel for consolidation. This study had lower than anticipated accrual to the R2 randomization because of the higher than predicted rate of good responding patients with localized tumors.

In a study by Ladenstein et al. (2010), 281 patients with primary disseminated multifocal ES were enrolled onto the EURO-E.W.I.N.G.99 (R3) study. Median age was 16.2 years (range, 0.4–49 years). Recommended treatment consisted of six cycles of VIDE, one cycle of VAI, local treatment (surgery and/or radiotherapy), and high-dose busulfan–melphalan followed by autologous stem cell transplantation (HDT-SCT). After a median follow-up of 3.8 years, 3 year EFS and OS for all 281 patients were 27 %±3 % and 34 %±4 %, respectively. Six VIDE cycles were completed by 250 patients (89 %); 169 patients (60 %) received HDT-SCT. The estimated 3 year EFS from the start of HDT-SCT was 45 % for 46 children younger than 14 years. Cox regression analyses demonstrated increased risk at diagnosis for patients older than 14 years (hazard ratio (HR) 1.6), a primary tumor volume more than 200 mL (HR = 1.8), more than one bone metastatic site (HR = 2.0), bone marrow metastases (HR = 1.6), and additional lung metastases (HR = 1.5). An up-front risk score based on these HR factors identified three groups with EFS rates of 50 % for score ≤3 (82 patients), 25 % for score more than 3 to less than 5 (102 patients), and 10 % for score ≥5 (70 patients) ($p = 0.0001$). This study concludes that patients with high-risk ES may survive with intensive multimodal therapy, and risk-adapted treatment approach may help tailor management.

14.2.5.3 Local Therapies (Surgery and Radiation)

Robinson et al. (2013) reported that patients who received multimodal treatment had significantly higher response rate, but outcome was no different to those who only received single modality treatment. In another study, outcome is significantly correlated with treatment performed after relapse, with all patients free of disease treated with surgery alone or combined with radiation therapy or a second-line chemotherapy (Bacci et al. 2003). In this study, there was a significantly better outcome in patients who had definitive local control (surgery and/or radiotherapy) alone, or in combination with chemotherapy, versus the ones who had chemotherapy alone (15.4 % versus 0.9 % $p < 0.0001$). In a separate study, the rate of first remission was significantly higher for patients treated with surgery alone (93.6 %) or combined with chemotherapy (91.6 %) than those treated with conventional

(2.2 %) or high-dose chemotherapy (11 %) or by radiotherapy (22 %) (Bacci et al. 2006). This however needs to be interpreted with caution since patients treated with surgery alone had isolated local or lung recurrences, and the ones who were treated with chemotherapy alone were highly selected and restricted to patients with unresectable disease and not amenable for curative intent radiotherapy.

Comparing local control strategies, second remission was achieved with complete surgical resection (45 %) compared to radiotherapy (13 %) ($p < 0.001$) (Robinson et al. 2013). However, McTiernan et al. (2006) reported that among 114 patients, definitive local treatment was a strong predictor of outcome, whether the local control modality was surgery or radiotherapy. Radical surgery for those with local recurrence had significantly higher 5 year PRS of 31.4 %±11.6 % versus other strategies 9.1 %±6.1 % ($p = 0.023$). Use of RT alone for local control (especially dose <35 Gy) was hypothesized to contribute to high local failure rate (Rodriguez-Galindo et al. 2002a).

14.2.6 Emerging Targets

Targeting EWS-FLI1
EWS-FLI1 is critical for Ewing cell survival. Direct targeting of this transcription factor has been for a long time felt to be "undruggable." There is therapeutic promise in disrupting interactions between EWS–FLI1 and other protein complexes thought to be required for oncogenesis such as RNA helicase and lysine-specific demethylase 1 (Erkizan et al. 2009; Sankar et al. 2013). In vitro downregulation of the EWS-FLI1 translocation via antisense oligonucleotides, dominant negative transcripts, and RNAi has been shown to limit the malignant transformation and reduce cell growth (Kovar et al. 1996; Toretsky et al. 1997a; Lambert et al. 2000).

Toretsky's group reported their work on a small molecule YK-4-279 which blocks EWS-FLI1 from interacting with RNA helicase A (RHA) (Barber-Rotenberg et al. 2012). In vivo studies confirm prior in vitro experiments showing the enantiomer (S)-YK-4-279 as the EWS-FLI1-specific enantiomer demonstrating both induction of apoptosis and reduction of EWS-FLI1-regulated caveolin-1 protein. Rat xenograft model of ES treated with (S)-YK-4-279 led to a sustained complete response in two of six ES tumors (Hong et al. 2014).

Mithramycin, an older antibiotic, is a drug that binds GC-rich regions of the genome and regulates the expression of specific genes including SRC, MYC, and MDR1 often by inhibiting the SP1 family of transcription factors. This agent was identified in a high-throughput drug screen to inhibit expression of EWS-FLI1 downstream targets and decrease the growth of ES cells in mouse xenografts (Grohar et al. 2011).

PARP Inhibitors

Great interest emerged with poly (ADP-ribose) polymerase (PARP) inhibitors which are small molecules that have been studied in a variety of malignancies (Fong et al. 2009; Foulkes et al. 2010). PARP messenger RNA and proteins are amassed in very high levels in ES cell lines (Soldatenkov et al. 1999). ES cells, primary tumor xenografts, and tumor metastases were shown to be all highly sensitive to PARP1 inhibition (Soldatenkov et al. 1999; Garnett et al. 2012). Mechanistic investigations revealed that DNA damage induced by expression of EWS-FLI1 or EWS-ERG fusion genes was potentiated by PARP1 inhibition in ESFT cell lines. Notably, EWS-FLI1 fusion genes acted in a positive feedback loop to maintain the expression of PARP1, which was required for EWS-FLI-mediated transcription, thereby enforcing oncogene-dependent sensitivity to PARP1 inhibition. This response was specific to ESFT, as this did not have an effect on osteosarcoma and rhabdomyosarcoma cell lines. These findings offer a strong preclinical rationale to target the EWS-FLI1–PARP1 intersection as a therapeutic strategy to improve the treatment of ESFTs. Addition of a PARP1 inhibitor to the second-line chemotherapeutic agent temozolomide resulted in complete responses of all treated tumors in an EWS-FLI1-driven mouse xenograft model of ESFT (Brenner et al. 2012). Although a single-agent study did not show clinical activity, combination studies with temozolomide are being pursued (NCT01858168, NCT02044120).

IGF-1R Inhibition

Over the past 5 years, significant work has been focused on insulinlike growth factor 1 receptor (IGF-1R), which is a receptor tyrosine kinase that is overexpressed in ES cells. Activation of this receptor has been found to be essential for EWS-FLI1-induced malignant transformation of murine fibroblasts (Toretsky et al. 1997b; Manara et al. 2007). For a small subset of refractory ES patients, dramatic responses were seen with monoclonal antibodies to IGF-1R (Juergens et al. 2011; Malempati and Hawkins 2012; Pappo et al. 2011). Anti-IGF-1R antibodies have been used with mammalian target of rapamycin (mTOR) inhibitors in refractory pediatric patients (O'Reilly et al. 2006), with a few complete responses and sustained stable disease (Naing et al. 2012; Schwartz et al. 2013).

A phase I expansion cohort study of figitumumab in 29 patients, 16 of whom had ES, had objective responses (one complete response, one partial response). Eight patients had disease stabilization for 4–16 months, of whom six had ES (Olmos et al. 2010). A phase I study of R1507 was conducted on 37 patients with advanced solid tumors. Of nine patients who had ES, two had durable partial responses of 11.5 and >26 months, and two had stable disease (Kurzrock et al. 2010). In a multicenter phase II trial of R1507 in 133 patients with recurrent or refractory Ewing sarcoma/PNET, overall complete/partial response rate was 10 % with a median duration of response of 29 weeks and median survival of 7.6 months (Pappo et al. 2011). Finally there also is the theoretical potential for combining IGF-1R inhibitors with other drugs such as mTOR inhibitors with the prospect of enhanced treatment efficacy.

Mammalian Target of Rapamycin (mTOR) Inhibition

Different types of EWS-FLI1 express differing levels of total and phosphorylated mTOR protein. The use of rapamycin as a cytostatic treatment has been evaluated in Ewing sarcoma/PNET cell lines with heterogeneous EWS-FLI1 fusion genes. ES has been shown to have upregulated p-Akt and p-mTOR (Subbiah et al. 2013). Rapamycin was found to inhibit cell line proliferation by causing G1 phase arrest with concurrent downregulation of EWS-FLI1 protein and restoration of expression of TGF-b type 2 receptor. TGF-b type 2 receptor is transcriptionally repressed in Ewing sarcoma cells, and exposure to rapamycin resulted in a marked increase in TGF-b receptor 2 mRNA in the cell lines tested with concomitant-increased susceptibility to TGF-b inhibition of growth (Mateo-Lozano et al. 2003). COG conducted a phase 1 trial of temsirolimus in combination with irinotecan and temozolomide in patients with recurrent/refractory solid tumors. Of 71 eligible patients, 7 had ES. Six patients had objective responses confirmed by central review including patient with ES, with three sustained responses through ≥14 cycles of therapy (Bagatell et al. 2014).

Epigenetic Targeting

Agents that target chromatin structure would be expected to have activity in ES since this is a disease driven by a transcription factor. There has been note of dysregulation of protein complexes involved in the regulation of chromatin structure. The resulting changes in the epigenome play a major role in the biology of ES and have been linked to alterations in gene expression, malignant transformation, and even drug resistance (Lawlor and Thiele 2012). Studies have investigated the role of HDAC inhibitors in particular signaling pathways mediated by EWS–FLI1 (Li et al. 2012; Matsumoto et al. 2001). In the clinic, the HDAC inhibitor vorinostat has been evaluated in children in the relapsed refractory setting. Unfortunately, single-agent activity in Ewing sarcoma has not been observed, although only two patients with Ewing sarcoma received the drug (Fouladi et al. 2010). EWS-FLI1 drives the expression of genes that in turn suppress a large percentage of the genome by modifying the availability of chromatin to the transcriptional machinery, allowing ES cells to evade senescence and apoptosis in the setting of genetic damage. Further investigation of these agents in ES is warranted.

VEGF Inhibition

Angiogenesis plays an important role in the biology of ES oncogenesis and tumor growth and development (Stewart and Kleinerman 2011; Yu et al. 2010). Also, the EWS-FLI1 chimeric fusion gene is known to upregulate VEGF-A in preclinical models (Nagano et al. 2009). Clinical experience with bevacizumab as monotherapy demonstrated stable disease at best for at least 4 months in three out of five patients with Ewing sarcoma enrolled in a COG phase I clinical study (Glade Bender et al. 2008). COG evaluated the use of bevacizumab with VTC (AEWS0521) with recurrent EWS, and addition of bevacizumab was feasible but did not improve outcome.

14.2.7 Future of Ewing Sarcoma

Recent novel therapies produced dramatic responses thought to have overcome the therapeutic plateau in patients with ES. Unfortunately, these therapies benefited only a minority of patients, and even those patients who had favorable responses initially inevitably developed resistance. It is clear that further understanding of the complex biology of ES is warranted. Various prognostic molecular markers have been recently identified for ES, as well as prognostic gene expression signatures. Since most ES express EWS-FLI1 and EWS-ERG transcription factors, there is a realistic chance for targeted therapeutics that may impact those with newly diagnosed as well as recurrent disease. Continued systematic clinical investigation that integrates active agents into ES therapy will hopefully lead to improved outcomes. A significant biology effort has been established in ES through COG AEWS02B1 and AEWS07B1 studies. This endeavor allows for molecular profiling as well as development of tissue resources such as microarrays containing tumor samples that are linked to therapeutic studies and can be used for evaluation of prognostic factors.

The rarity of this tumor is a significant obstacle for drug development. However, with optimism and global collaboration, significant number of patients can be accrued in short time frames. Considering the demographics, high lethality, and defined molecular pathogenesis, targeted therapeutics of ES is an area of importance for collaborative international clinical trials.

References

Akiyama T, Dass CR, Choong PF (2008) Novel therapeutic strategy for osteosarcoma targeting osteoclast differentiation, bone-resorbing activity, and apoptosis pathway. Mol Cancer Ther 7(11):3461–3469. doi:10.1158/1535-7163.MCT-08-0530

Akiyama T, Choong PF, Dass CR (2010) RANK-Fc inhibits malignancy via inhibiting ERK activation and evoking caspase-3-mediated anoikis in human osteosarcoma cells. Clin Exp Metastasis 27(4):207–215. doi:10.1007/s10585-010-9319-y

Al-Faris N, Al Harbi T, Goia C, Pappo A, Doyle J, Gassas A (2007) Does consolidation with autologous stem cell transplantation improve the outcome of children with metastatic or relapsed Ewing sarcoma? Pediatr Blood Cancer 49(2):190–195. doi:10.1002/pbc.21140

Anderson PM (2003) Effectiveness of radiotherapy for osteosarcoma that responds to chemotherapy. Mayo Clin Proc 78(2):145–146. doi:10.4065/78.2.145

Anderson P (2006) Liposomal muramyl tripeptide phosphatidyl ethanolamine: ifosfamide-containing chemotherapy in osteosarcoma. Future Oncol 2(3):333–343. doi:10.2217/14796694.2.3.333

Anderson P, Nunez R (2007) Samarium lexidronam (153Sm-EDTMP): skeletal radiation for osteoblastic bone metastases and osteosarcoma. Expert Rev Anticancer Ther 7(11):1517–1527. doi:10.1586/14737140.7.11.1517

Anderson PM, Wiseman GA, Dispenzieri A, Arndt CA, Hartmann LC, Smithson WA, Bruland OS (2002) High-dose samarium-153 ethylene diamine tetramethylene phosphonate: low toxicity of skeletal irradiation in patients with osteosarcoma and bone metastases. J Clin Oncol 20(1):189–196

Anderson PM, Wiseman GA, Erlandson L, Rodriguez V, Trotz B, Dubansky SA, Albritton K (2005) Gemcitabine radiosensitization after high-dose samarium for osteoblastic osteosarcoma. Clin Cancer Res 11(19 Pt 1):6895–6900. doi:10.1158/1078-0432.CCR-05-0628

Anderson P, Kopp L, Anderson N, Cornelius K, Herzog C, Hughes D, Huh W (2008) Novel bone cancer drugs: investigational agents and control paradigms for primary bone sarcomas (Ewing's sarcoma and osteosarcoma). Expert Opin Investig Drugs 17(11):1703–1715. doi:10.1517/13543784.17.11.1703

Anderson PM, Meyers P, Kleinerman E, Venkatakrishnan K, Hughes DP, Herzog C, Chou A (2014a) Mifamurtide in metastatic and recurrent osteosarcoma: a patient access study with pharmacokinetic, pharmacodynamic, and safety assessments. Pediatr Blood Cancer 61(2):238–244. doi:10.1002/pbc.24686

Anderson PM, Subbiah V, Rohren E (2014b) Bone-seeking radiopharmaceuticals as targeted agents of osteosarcoma:

samarium-153-EDTMP and radium-223. Adv Exp Med Biol 804:291–304. doi:10.1007/978-3-319-04843-7_16

Asano T, Kleinerman ES (1993) Liposome-encapsulated MTP-PE: a novel biologic agent for cancer therapy. J Immunother Emphasis Tumor Immunol 14(4):286–292

Aung L, Gorlick R, Healey JH, Shi W, Thaler HT, Shorter NA, Meyers PA (2003) Metachronous skeletal osteosarcoma in patients treated with adjuvant and neoadjuvant chemotherapy for nonmetastatic osteosarcoma. J Clin Oncol 21(2):342–348

Bacci G, Ferrari S, Bertoni F, Rimondini S, Longhi A, Bacchini P, Picci P (2000) Prognostic factors in nonmetastatic Ewing's sarcoma of bone treated with adjuvant chemotherapy: analysis of 359 patients at the Istituto Ortopedico Rizzoli. J Clin Oncol 18(1):4–11

Bacci G, Ferrari S, Longhi A, Perin S, Forni C, Fabbri N, Smith KV (2001) Pattern of relapse in patients with osteosarcoma of the extremities treated with neoadjuvant chemotherapy. Eur J Cancer 37(1):32–38

Bacci G, Ferrari S, Longhi A, Donati D, De Paolis M, Forni C, Barbieri E (2003) Therapy and survival after recurrence of Ewing's tumors: the Rizzoli experience in 195 patients treated with adjuvant and neoadjuvant chemotherapy from 1979 to 1997. Ann Oncol 14(11):1654–1659

Bacci G, Longhi A, Ferrari S, Mercuri M, Barbieri E, Bertoni F, Picci P (2006) Pattern of relapse in 290 patients with nonmetastatic Ewing's sarcoma family tumors treated at a single institution with adjuvant and neoadjuvant chemotherapy between 1972 and 1999. Eur J Surg Oncol 32(9):974–979. doi:10.1016/j.ejso.2006.01.023

Bacci G, Balladelli A, Forni C, Ferrari S, Longhi A, Benassi MS, Picci P (2007) Adjuvant and neoadjuvant chemotherapy for Ewing's sarcoma family tumors and osteosarcoma of the extremity: further outcome for patients event-free survivors 5 years from the beginning of treatment. Ann Oncol 18(12):2037–2040. doi:10.1093/annonc/mdm382

Bacci G, Rocca M, Salone M, Balladelli A, Ferrari S, Palmerini E, Briccoli A (2008) High grade osteosarcoma of the extremities with lung metastases at presentation: treatment with neoadjuvant chemotherapy and simultaneous resection of primary and metastatic lesions. J Surg Oncol 98(6):415–420. doi:10.1002/jso.21140

Bagatell R, Norris R, Ingle AM, Ahern C, Voss S, Fox E, Blaney S (2014) Phase 1 trial of temsirolimus in combination with irinotecan and temozolomide in children, adolescents and young adults with relapsed or refractory solid tumors: a Children's Oncology Group Study. Pediatr Blood Cancer 61(5):833–839. doi:10.1002/pbc.24874

Barber-Rotenberg JS, Selvanathan SP, Kong Y, Erkizan HV, Snyder TM, Hong SP, Toretsky JA (2012) Single enantiomer of YK-4-279 demonstrates specificity in targeting the oncogene EWS-FLI1. Oncotarget 3(2):172–182

Barger AM, Fan TM, de Lorimier LP, Sprandel IT, O'Dell-Anderson K (2007) Expression of receptor activator of nuclear factor kappa-B ligand (RANKL) in neoplasms of dogs and cats. J Vet Intern Med 21(1):133–140

Barker LM, Pendergrass TW, Sanders JE, Hawkins DS (2005) Survival after recurrence of Ewing's sarcoma family of tumors. J Clin Oncol 23(19):4354–4362. doi:10.1200/JCO.2005.05.105

Baust JG, Gage AA (2005) The molecular basis of cryosurgery. BJU Int 95(9):1187–1191. doi:10.1111/j.1464-410X.2005.05502.x

Bernstein ML, Devidas M, Lafreniere D, Souid AK, Meyers PA, Gebhardt M, Children's Oncology G. (2006) Intensive therapy with growth factor support for patients with Ewing tumor metastatic at diagnosis: Pediatric Oncology Group/Children's Cancer Group Phase II Study 9457–a report from the Children's Oncology Group. J Clin Oncol 24(1):152–159. doi:10.1200/JCO.2005.02.1717

Bielack SS, Kempf-Bielack B, Delling G, Exner GU, Flege S, Helmke K, Winkler K (2002) Prognostic factors in high-grade osteosarcoma of the extremities or trunk: an analysis of 1,702 patients treated on neoadjuvant cooperative osteosarcoma study group protocols. J Clin Oncol 20(3):776–790

Bielack SS, Kempf-Bielack B, Branscheid D, Carrle D, Friedel G, Helmke K, Jurgens H (2009) Second and subsequent recurrences of osteosarcoma: presentation, treatment, and outcomes of 249 consecutive cooperative osteosarcoma study group patients. J Clin Oncol27(4):557–565.doi:10.1200/JCO.2008.16.2305

Blaney SM, Seibel NL, O'Brien M, Reaman GH, Berg SL, Adamson PC, Balis FM (1997) Phase I trial of docetaxel administered as a 1-h infusion in children with refractory solid tumors: a collaborative pediatric branch, National Cancer Institute and Children's Cancer Group trial. J Clin Oncol 15(4):1538–1543

Brenner JC, Feng FY, Han S, Patel S, Goyal SV, Bou-Maroun LM, Chinnaiyan AM (2012) PARP-1 inhibition as a targeted strategy to treat Ewing's sarcoma. Cancer Res 72(7):1608–1613. doi:10.1158/0008-5472.CAN-11-3648

Briccoli A, Rocca M, Ferrari S, Mercuri M, Ferrari C, Bacci G (2004) Surgery for lung metastases in Ewing's sarcoma of bone. Eur J Surg Oncol 30(1):63–67

Briccoli A, Rocca M, Salone M, Guzzardella GA, Balladelli A, Bacci G (2010) High grade osteosarcoma of the extremities metastatic to the lung: long-term results in 323 patients treated combining surgery and chemotherapy, 1985–2005. Surg Oncol 19(4):193–199. doi:10.1016/j.suronc.2009.05.002

Burdach S, Jurgens H, Peters C, Nurnberger W, Mauz-Korholz C, Korholz D et al (1993) Myeloablative radiochemotherapy and hematopoietic stem-cell rescue in poor-prognosis Ewing's sarcoma. J Clin Oncol 11(8):1482–1488

Burdach S, van Kaick B, Laws HJ, Ahrens S, Haase R, Korholz D, el Go U (2000) Allogeneic and autologous stem-cell transplantation in advanced Ewing tumors. An update after long-term follow-up from two centers of the European Intergroup study EICESS. Stem-Cell Transplant Programs at Dusseldorf University Medical Center, Germany and St. Anna Kinderspital, Vienna, Austria. Ann Oncol 11(11):1451–1462

Burdach S, Meyer-Bahlburg A, Laws HJ, Haase R, van Kaik B, Metzner B, Juergens H (2003) High-dose therapy for patients with primary multifocal and early relapsed Ewing's tumors: results of two consecutive regimens assessing the role of total-body irradiation. J Clin Oncol 21(16):3072–3078. doi:10.1200/JCO.2003.12.039

Burgert EO Jr, Nesbit ME, Garnsey LA, Gehan EA, Herrmann J, Vietti TJ et al (1990) Multimodal therapy for the management of nonpelvic, localized Ewing's sarcoma of bone: intergroup study IESS-II. J Clin Oncol 8(9):1514–1524

Burke MJ, Walterhouse DO, Jacobsohn DA, Duerst RE, Kletzel M (2007) Tandem high-dose chemotherapy with autologous peripheral hematopoietic progenitor cell rescue as consolidation therapy for patients with high-risk Ewing family tumors. Pediatr Blood Cancer 49(2):196–198. doi:10.1002/pbc.21182

Caceres E, Zaharia M, Valdivia S, Misad O, de la Flor J, Tejada F, Zubrod G (1984) Local control of osteogenic sarcoma by radiation and chemotherapy. Int J Radiat Oncol Biol Phys 10(1):35–39

Cade S (1955) Osteogenic sarcoma; a study based on 133 patients. J R Coll Surg Edinb 1(2):79–111

Callstrom MR, Charboneau JW, Goetz MP, Rubin J, Atwell TD, Farrell MA, Maus TP (2006) Image-guided ablation of painful metastatic bone tumors: a new and effective approach to a difficult problem. Skeletal Radiol 35(1):1–15. doi:10.1007/s00256-005-0003-2

Cangir A, Vietti TJ, Gehan EA, Burgert EO Jr, Thomas P, Tefft M, Pritchard D (1990) Ewing's sarcoma metastatic at diagnosis. Results and comparisons of two intergroup Ewing's sarcoma studies. Cancer 66(5):887–893

Carli M, Passone E, Perilongo G, Bisogno G (2003) Ifosfamide in pediatric solid tumors. Oncology 65(Suppl 2):99–104. doi: 73369

Carrle D, Bielack S (2009) Osteosarcoma lung metastases detection and principles of multimodal therapy. Cancer Treat Res 152:165–184. doi:10.1007/978-1-4419-0284-9_8

Carter SR, Grimer RJ, Sneath RS, Matthews HR (1991) Results of thoracotomy in osteogenic sarcoma with pulmonary metastases. Thorax 46(10):727–731

Casey DA, Wexler LH, Merchant MS, Chou AJ, Merola PR, Price AP, Meyers PA (2009) Irinotecan and temozolomide for Ewing sarcoma: the Memorial Sloan-Kettering experience. Pediatr Blood Cancer 53(6):1029–1034. doi:10.1002/pbc.22206

Chao J, Budd GT, Chu P, Frankel P, Garcia D, Junqueira M, Chow WA (2010) Phase II clinical trial of imatinib mesylate in therapy of KIT and/or PDGFRalpha-expressing Ewing sarcoma family of tumors and desmoplastic small round cell tumors. Anticancer Res 30(2):547–552

Chawla SP, Staddon AP, Baker LH, Schuetze SM, Tolcher AW, D'Amato GZ, Demetri GD (2012) Phase II study of the mammalian target of rapamycin inhibitor ridaforolimus in patients with advanced bone and soft tissue sarcomas. J Clin Oncol 30(1):78–84. doi:10.1200/JCO.2011.35.6329

Chi SN, Conklin LS, Qin J, Meyers PA, Huvos AG, Healey JH, Gorlick R (2004) The patterns of relapse in osteosarcoma: the Memorial Sloan-Kettering experience. Pediatr Blood Cancer 42(1):46–51. doi:10.1002/pbc.10420

Chou AJ, Gorlick R (2006) Chemotherapy resistance in osteosarcoma: current challenges and future directions. Expert Rev Anticancer Ther 6(7):1075–1085. doi:10.1586/14737140.6.7.1075

Chou AJ, Merola PR, Wexler LH, Gorlick RG, Vyas YM, Healey JH, Meyers PA (2005) Treatment of osteosarcoma at first recurrence after contemporary therapy: the Memorial Sloan-Kettering Cancer Center experience. Cancer 104(10):2214–2221. doi:10.1002/cncr.21417

Chou AJ, Kleinerman ES, Krailo MD, Chen Z, Betcher DL, Healey JH, Children's Oncology G (2009) Addition of muramyl tripeptide to chemotherapy for patients with newly diagnosed metastatic osteosarcoma: a report from the Children's Oncology Group. Cancer 115(22):5339–5348. doi:10.1002/cncr.24566

Chou AJ, Gupta R, Bell MD, Riewe KO, Meyers PA, Gorlick R (2013) Inhaled lipid cisplatin (ILC) in the treatment of patients with relapsed/progressive osteosarcoma metastatic to the lung. Pediatr Blood Cancer 60(4):580–586. doi:10.1002/pbc.24438

Ciernik IF, Niemierko A, Harmon DC, Kobayashi W, Chen YL, Yock TI, Delaney TF (2011) Proton-based radiotherapy for unresectable or incompletely resected osteosarcoma. Cancer 117(19):4522–4530. doi:10.1002/cncr.26037

Corby RR, Stacy GS, Peabody TD, Dixon LB (2008) Radiofrequency ablation of solitary eosinophilic granuloma of bone. AJR Am J Roentgenol 190(6):1492–1494. doi:10.2214/AJR.07.3415

Cotterill SJ, Ahrens S, Paulussen M, Jurgens HF, Voute PA, Gadner H, Craft AW (2000) Prognostic factors in Ewing's tumor of bone: analysis of 975 patients from the European Intergroup Cooperative Ewing's Sarcoma Study Group. J Clin Oncol 18(17):3108–3114

Craft A, Cotterill S, Malcolm A, Spooner D, Grimer R, Souhami R, Lewis I (1998) Ifosfamide-containing chemotherapy in Ewing's sarcoma: the Second United Kingdom Children's Cancer Study Group and the Medical Research Council Ewing's Tumor study. J Clin Oncol 16(11):3628–3633

Dass CR, Choong PF (2007) Zoledronic acid inhibits osteosarcoma growth in an orthotopic model. Mol Cancer Ther 6(12 Pt 1):3263–3270. doi:10.1158/1535-7163.MCT-07-0546

de Moor NG (1975) Osteosarcoma a review of 72 cases treated by megavoltage radiation therapy, with or without surgery. S Afr J Surg 13(3):137–146

DeLaney TF, Park L, Goldberg SI, Hug EB, Liebsch NJ, Munzenrider JE, Suit HD (2005) Radiotherapy for local control of osteosarcoma. Int J Radiat Oncol Biol Phys 61(2):492–498. doi:10.1016/j.ijrobp.2004.05.051

Diaz-Montero CM, Wygant JN, McIntyre BW (2006) PI3-K/Akt-mediated anoikis resistance of human osteosarcoma cells requires Src activation. Eur J Cancer 42(10):1491–1500. doi:10.1016/j.ejca.2006.03.007

DuBois SG, Krailo MD, Lessnick SL, Smith R, Chen Z, Marina N, Children's Oncology G. (2009) Phase II study of intermediate-dose cytarabine in patients with relapsed or refractory Ewing sarcoma: a report from the Children's Oncology Group. Pediatr Blood Cancer 52(3):324–327. doi:10.1002/pbc.21822

Duffaud F, Digue L, Mercier C, Dales JP, Baciuchka-Palmaro M, Volot F, Favre R (2003) Recurrences following primary osteosarcoma in adolescents and adults previously treated with chemotherapy. Eur J Cancer 39(14):2050–2057

Elias AD, Eder JP, Shea T, Begg CB, Frei E 3rd, Antman KH (1990) High-dose ifosfamide with mesna uroprotection: a phase I study. J Clin Oncol 8(1):170–178

Ellis PM, Tattersall MH, McCaughan B, Stalley P (1997) Osteosarcoma and pulmonary metastases: 15-year experience from a single institution. Aust N Z J Surg 67(9):625–629

Ellis GK, Bone HG, Chlebowski R, Paul D, Spadafora S, Smith J, Jun S (2008) Randomized trial of denosumab in patients receiving adjuvant aromatase inhibitors for nonmetastatic breast cancer. J Clin Oncol 26(30):4875–4882. doi:10.1200/JCO.2008.16.3832

Erkizan HV, Kong Y, Merchant M, Schlottmann S, Barber-Rotenberg JS, Yuan L, Toretsky JA (2009) A small molecule blocking oncogenic protein EWS-FLI1 interaction with RNA helicase A inhibits growth of Ewing's sarcoma. Nat Med 15(7):750–756. doi:10.1038/nm.1983

Esiashvili N, Goodman M, Marcus RB Jr (2008) Changes in incidence and survival of Ewing sarcoma patients over the past 3 decades: surveillance epidemiology and end results data. J Pediatr Hematol Oncol 30(6):425–430. doi:10.1097/MPH.0b013e31816e22f3

Farhat R, Raad R, Khoury NJ, Feghaly J, Eid T, Muwakkit S, Saab R (2013) Cyclophosphamide and topotecan as first-line salvage therapy in patients with relapsed Ewing sarcoma at a single institution. J Pediatr Hematol Oncol 35(5):356–360. doi:10.1097/MPH.0b013e318270a343

Ferrari S, Bacci G, Picci P, Mercuri M, Briccoli A, Pinto D, Brach del Prever A (1997) Long-term follow-up and post-relapse survival in patients with non-metastatic osteosarcoma of the extremity treated with neoadjuvant chemotherapy. Ann Oncol 8(8):765–771

Ferrari S, Briccoli A, Mercuri M, Bertoni F, Picci P, Tienghi A, Bacci G (2003) Postrelapse survival in osteosarcoma of the extremities: prognostic factors for long-term survival. J Clin Oncol 21(4):710–715

Fischmeister G, Zoubek A, Jugovic D, Witt V, Ladenstein R, Fritsch G, Kovar H (1999) Low incidence of molecular evidence for tumour in PBPC harvests from patients with high risk Ewing tumours. Bone Marrow Transplant 24(4):405–409. doi:10.1038/sj.bmt.1701924

Fong PC, Boss DS, Yap TA, Tutt A, Wu P, Mergui-Roelvink M, de Bono JS (2009) Inhibition of poly(ADP-ribose) polymerase in tumors from BRCA mutation carriers. N Engl J Med 361(2):123–134. doi:10.1056/NEJMoa0900212

Fouladi M, Park JR, Stewart CF, Gilbertson RJ, Schaiquevich P, Sun J, Adamson PC (2010) Pediatric phase I trial and pharmacokinetic study of vorinostat: a Children's Oncology Group phase I consortium report. J Clin Oncol 28(22):3623–3629. doi:10.1200/JCO.2009.25.9119

Foulkes WD, Smith IE, Reis-Filho JS (2010) Triple-negative breast cancer. N Engl J Med 363(20):1938–1948. doi:10.1056/NEJMra1001389

Fox E, Aplenc R, Bagatell R, Chuk MK, Dombi E, Goodspeed W, Balis FM (2010) A phase 1 trial and pharmacokinetic study of cediranib, an orally bio-available pan-vascular endothelial growth factor receptor inhibitor, in children and adolescents with refractory solid tumors. J Clin Oncol 28(35):5174–5181. doi:10.1200/JCO.2010.30.9674

Fox E, Patel S, Wathen JK, Schuetze S, Chawla S, Harmon D, Helman LJ (2012) Phase II study of sequential gemcitabine followed by docetaxel for recurrent Ewing sarcoma, osteosarcoma, or unresectable or locally recurrent chondrosarcoma: results of Sarcoma Alliance for Research Through Collaboration Study 003. Oncologist 17(3):321. doi:10.1634/theoncologist.2010-0265

Friedlander PA, Bansal R, Schwartz L, Wagman R, Posner J, Kemeny N (2004) Gemcitabine-related radiation recall preferentially involves internal tissue and organs. Cancer 100(9):1793–1799. doi:10.1002/cncr.20229

Friedman MA, Carter SK (1972) The therapy of osteogenic sarcoma: current status and thoughts for the future. J Surg Oncol 4(5):482–510

Fu XH, Li J, Zou Y, Hong YR, Fu ZX, Huang JJ, Zheng S (2011) Endostar enhances the antineoplastic effects of combretastatin A4 phosphate in an osteosarcoma xenograft. Cancer Lett 312(1):109–116. doi:10.1016/j.canlet.2011.08.008

Fuchs N, Bielack SS, Epler D, Bieling P, Delling G, Korholz D, Winkler K (1998) Long-term results of the co-operative German-Austrian-Swiss osteosarcoma study group's protocol COSS-86 of intensive multi-drug chemotherapy and surgery for osteosarcoma of the limbs. Ann Oncol 9(8):893–899

Gaitan-Yanguas M (1981) A study of the response of osteogenic sarcoma and adjacent normal tissues to radiation. Int J Radiat Oncol Biol Phys 7(5):593–595

Garnett MJ, Edelman EJ, Heidorn SJ, Greenman CD, Dastur A, Lau KW, Benes CH (2012) Systematic identification of genomic markers of drug sensitivity in cancer cells. Nature 483(7391):570–575. doi:10.1038/nature11005

Giuliano AE, Feig S, Eilber FR (1984) Changing metastatic patterns of osteosarcoma. Cancer 54(10):2160–2164

Glade Bender JL, Adamson PC, Reid JM, Xu L, Baruchel S, Shaked Y, Children's Oncology Group, S (2008) Phase I trial and pharmacokinetic study of bevacizumab in pediatric patients with refractory solid tumors: a Children's Oncology Group Study. J Clin Oncol 26(3):399–405. doi:10.1200/JCO.2007.11.9230

Goetz MP, Callstrom MR, Charboneau JW, Farrell MA, Maus TP, Welch TJ, Rubin J (2004) Percutaneous image-guided radiofrequency ablation of painful metastases involving bone: a multicenter study. J Clin Oncol 22(2):300–306. doi:10.1200/JCO.2004.03.097

Goldsby RE, Fan TM, Villaluna D, Wagner LM, Isakoff MS, Meyer J, Marina N (2013) Feasibility and dose discovery analysis of zoledronic acid with concurrent chemotherapy in the treatment of newly diagnosed metastatic osteosarcoma: a report from the Children's Oncology Group. Eur J Cancer 49(10):2384–2391. doi:10.1016/j.ejca.2013.03.018

Goorin AM, Delorey MJ, Lack EE, Gelber RD, Price K, Cassady JR et al (1984) Prognostic significance of complete surgical resection of pulmonary metastases in patients with osteogenic sarcoma: analysis of 32 patients. J Clin Oncol 2(5):425–431

Goorin AM, Shuster JJ, Baker A, Horowitz ME, Meyer WH, Link MP (1991) Changing pattern of pulmonary metastases with adjuvant chemotherapy in patients with osteosarcoma: results from the multiinstitutional osteosarcoma study. J Clin Oncol 9(4):600–605

Goorin AM, Harris MB, Bernstein M, Ferguson W, Devidas M, Siegal GP, Grier HE (2002) Phase II/III trial of etoposide and high-dose ifosfamide in newly diagnosed metastatic osteosarcoma: a pediatric oncology group trial. J Clin Oncol 20(2):426–433

Gorlick R, Meyers PA (2003) Osteosarcoma necrosis following chemotherapy: innate biology versus treatment-specific. J Pediatr Hematol Oncol 25(11):840–841

Grier HE, Krailo MD, Tarbell NJ, Link MP, Fryer CJ, Pritchard DJ, Miser JS (2003) Addition of ifosfamide and etoposide to standard chemotherapy for Ewing's sarcoma and primitive neuroectodermal tumor of bone. N Engl J Med 348(8):694–701. doi:10.1056/NEJMoa020890

Grohar PJ, Woldemichael GM, Griffin LB, Mendoza A, Chen QR, Yeung C, Helman LJ (2011) Identification of an inhibitor of the EWS-FLI1 oncogenic transcription factor by high-throughput screening. J Natl Cancer Inst 103(12):962–978. doi:10.1093/jnci/djr156

Harting MT, Blakely ML, Jaffe N, Cox CS Jr, Hayes-Jordan A, Benjamin RS, Lally KP (2006) Long-term survival after aggressive resection of pulmonary metastases among children and adolescents with osteosarcoma. J Pediatr Surg 41(1):194–199. doi:10.1016/j.jpedsurg.2005.10.089

Hawkins DS, Arndt CA (2003) Pattern of disease recurrence and prognostic factors in patients with osteosarcoma treated with contemporary chemotherapy. Cancer 98(11):2447–2456. doi:10.1002/cncr.11799

Hawkins D, Barnett T, Bensinger W, Gooley T, Sanders J (2000) Busulfan, melphalan, and thiotepa with or without total marrow irradiation with hematopoietic stem cell rescue for poor-risk Ewing-Sarcoma-Family tumors. Med Pediatr Oncol 34(5):328–337

Hayes FA, Thompson EI, Kumar M, Hustu HO (1987) Long-term survival in patients with Ewing's sarcoma relapsing after completing therapy. Med Pediatr Oncol 15(5):254–256

Hingorani P, Zhang W, Gorlick R, Kolb EA (2009) Inhibition of Src phosphorylation alters metastatic potential of osteosarcoma in vitro but not in vivo. Clin Cancer Res 15(10):3416–3422. doi:10.1158/1078-0432.CCR-08-1657

Hoffer FA, Daw NC, Xiong X, Anghelescu D, Krasin M, Yan X, Spunt SL (2009) A phase 1/pilot study of radiofrequency ablation for the treatment of recurrent pediatric solid tumors. Cancer 115(6):1328–1337. doi:10.1002/cncr.24158

Hong SH, Youbi SE, Hong SP, Kallakury B, Monroe P, Erkizan HV, Toretsky JA (2014) Pharmacokinetic modeling optimizes inhibition of the 'undruggable' EWS-FLI1 transcription factor in Ewing sarcoma. Oncotarget 5(2):338–350

Horowitz ME, Kinsella TJ, Wexler LH, Belasco J, Triche T, Tsokos M et al (1993) Total-body irradiation and autologous bone marrow transplant in the treatment of high-risk Ewing's sarcoma and rhabdomyosarcoma. J Clin Oncol 11(10):1911–1918

Houghton PJ, Stewart CF, Cheshire PJ, Richmond LB, Kirstein MN, Poquette CA, Brent TP (2000) Antitumor activity of temozolomide combined with irinotecan is partly independent of O6-methylguanine-DNA methyltransferase and mismatch repair phenotypes in xenograft models. Clin Cancer Res 6(10):4110–4118

Houghton PJ, Morton CL, Kolb EA, Gorlick R, Lock R, Carol H, Smith MA (2008) Initial testing (stage 1) of the mTOR inhibitor rapamycin by the pediatric preclinical testing program. Pediatr Blood Cancer 50(4):799–805. doi:10.1002/pbc.21296

Houghton PJ, Morton CL, Gorlick R, Kolb EA, Keir ST, Reynolds CP, Smith MA (2010a) Initial testing of a monoclonal antibody (IMC-A12) against IGF-1R by the Pediatric Preclinical Testing Program. Pediatr Blood Cancer 54(7):921–926. doi:10.1002/pbc.22367

Houghton PJ, Morton CL, Gorlick R, Lock RB, Carol H, Reynolds CP, Smith MA (2010b) Stage 2 combination testing of rapamycin with cytotoxic agents by the Pediatric Preclinical Testing Program. Mol Cancer Ther 9(1):101–112. doi:10.1158/1535-7163.MCT-09-0952

Hunold A, Weddeling N, Paulussen M, Ranft A, Liebscher C, Jurgens H (2006) Topotecan and cyclophosphamide in patients with refractory or relapsed Ewing tumors. Pediatr Blood Cancer 47(6):795–800. doi:10.1002/pbc.20719

Hunter KW (2004) Ezrin, a key component in tumor metastasis. Trends Mol Med 10(5):201–204. doi:10.1016/j.molmed.2004.03.001

Huth JF, Eilber FR (1989) Patterns of recurrence after resection of osteosarcoma of the extremity. Strategies for treatment of metastases. Arch Surg 124(1):122–126

Ikeda S, Sumii H, Akiyama K, Watanabe S, Ito S, Inoue H, Oda T (1989) Amplification of both c-myc and c-raf-1 oncogenes in a human osteosarcoma. Jpn J Cancer Res 80(1):6–9

Jacobs S, Fox E, Krailo M, Hartley G, Navid F, Wexler L, Widemann BC (2010) Phase II trial of ixabepilone administered daily for five days in children and young adults with refractory solid tumors: a report from the children's oncology group. Clin Cancer Res 16(2):750–754. doi:10.1158/1078-0432.CCR-09-1906

Jaffe N, Smith E, Abelson HT, Frei E 3rd (1983) Osteogenic sarcoma: alterations in the pattern of pulmonary metastases with adjuvant chemotherapy. J Clin Oncol 1(4):251–254

Jaffe N, Pearson P, Yasko AW, Lin P, Herzog C, Raymond K (2003) Single and multiple metachronous osteosarcoma tumors after therapy. Cancer 98(11):2457–2466. doi:10.1002/cncr.11800

Jones SF, Gian VG, Greco FA, Miranda FT, Shipley DL, Thompson DS, Burris HA 3rd (2003) Phase I. Trial of irinotecan and temozolomide in patients with solid tumors. Oncology (Williston Park) 17(5 Suppl 5):41–45

Jordan MA, Wilson L (2004) Microtubules as a target for anticancer drugs. Nat Rev Cancer 4(4):253–265. doi:10.1038/nrc1317

Joschko MA, Webster LK, Groves J, Yuen K, Palatsides M, Ball DL, Millward MJ (1997) Enhancement of radiation induced regrowth delay by gemcitabine in a human tumor xenograft model. Radiat Oncol Investig 5(2):62–71. doi:10.1002/(SICI)1520-6823(1997)5:2<62::AID-ROI4>3.0.CO;2-H

Juergens H, Daw NC, Geoerger B, Ferrari S, Villarroel M, Aerts I, Gualberto A (2011) Preliminary efficacy of the anti-insulin-like growth factor type 1 receptor antibody figitumumab in patients with refractory Ewing sarcoma. J Clin Oncol 29(34):4534–4540. doi:10.1200/JCO.2010.33.0670

Kager L, Zoubek A, Potschger U, Kastner U, Flege S, Kempf-Bielack B, Cooperative German-Austrian-Swiss Osteosarcoma Study, G. (2003) Primary metastatic osteosarcoma: presentation and outcome of patients treated on neoadjuvant Cooperative Osteosarcoma Study Group protocols. J Clin Oncol 21(10):2011–2018. doi:10.1200/JCO.2003.08.132

Kempf-Bielack B, Bielack SS, Jurgens H, Branscheid D, Berdel WE, Exner GU, Winkler K (2005) Osteosarcoma relapse after combined modality therapy: an analysis of unselected patients in the Cooperative Osteosarcoma Study Group (COSS). J Clin Oncol 23(3):559–568. doi:10.1200/JCO.2005.04.063

Khanna C, Wan X, Bose S, Cassaday R, Olomu O, Mendoza A, Helman LJ (2004) The membrane-cytoskeleton linker ezrin is necessary for osteosarcoma metastasis. Nat Med 10(2):182–186. doi:10.1038/nm982

Kinsella TJ, Glatstein E (1987) Clinical experience with intravenous radiosensitizers in unresectable sarcomas. Cancer 59(5):908–915

Kleinerman ES, Maeda M, Jaffe N (1993) Liposome-encapsulated muramyl tripeptide: a new biologic response modifier for the treatment of osteosarcoma. Cancer Treat Res 62:101–107

Kleinerman ES, Gano JB, Johnston DA, Benjamin RS, Jaffe N (1995) Efficacy of liposomal muramyl tripeptide (CGP 19835A) in the treatment of relapsed osteosarcoma. Am J Clin Oncol 18(2):93–99

Kolb EA, Kushner BH, Gorlick R, Laverdiere C, Healey JH, LaQuaglia MP, Meyers PA (2003) Long-term event-free survival after intensive chemotherapy for Ewing's family of tumors in children and young adults. J Clin Oncol 21(18):3423–3430. doi:10.1200/JCO.2003.10.033

Kolb EA, Gorlick R, Houghton PJ, Morton CL, Lock RB, Tajbakhsh M, Smith MA (2008) Initial testing of dasatinib by the pediatric preclinical testing program. Pediatr Blood Cancer 50(6):1198–1206. doi:10.1002/pbc.21368

Kolb EA, Gorlick R, Reynolds CP, Kang MH, Carol H, Lock R, Smith MA (2013) Initial testing (stage 1) of eribulin, a novel tubulin binding agent, by the pediatric preclinical testing program. Pediatr Blood Cancer 60(8):1325–1332. doi:10.1002/pbc.24517

Kolb EA, Gorlick R, Billups CA, Hawthorne T, Kurmasheva RT, Houghton PJ, Smith MA (2014) Initial testing (stage 1) of glembatumumab vedotin (CDX-011) by the pediatric preclinical testing program. Pediatr Blood Cancer 61(10):1816–1821. doi:10.1002/pbc.25099

Korholz D, Verheyen J, Kemperdick HF, Gobel U (1998) Evaluation of follow-up investigations in osteosarcoma patients: suggestions for an effective follow-up program. Med Pediatr Oncol 30(1):52–58

Kovar H, Aryee DN, Jug G, Henockl C, Schemper M, Delattre O, Gadner H (1996) EWS/FLI-1 antagonists induce growth inhibition of Ewing tumor cells in vitro. Cell Growth Differ 7(4):429–437

Kurzrock R, Patnaik A, Aisner J, Warren T, Leong S, Benjamin R, Gore L (2010) A phase I study of weekly R1507, a human monoclonal antibody insulin-like growth factor-I receptor antagonist, in patients with advanced solid tumors. Clin Cancer Res 16(8):2458–2465. doi:10.1158/1078-0432.CCR-09-3220

Kushner BH, Meyers PA (2001) How effective is dose-intensive/myeloablative therapy against Ewing's sarcoma/primitive neuroectodermal tumor metastatic to bone or bone marrow? The Memorial Sloan-Kettering experience and a literature review. J Clin Oncol 19(3):870–880

Kushner BH, Kramer K, Modak S, Cheung NK (2006) Irinotecan plus temozolomide for relapsed or refractory neuroblastoma. J Clin Oncol 24(33):5271–5276. doi:10.1200/JCO.2006.06.7272

Labrinidis A, Hay S, Liapis V, Ponomarev V, Findlay DM, Evdokiou A (2009) Zoledronic acid inhibits both the osteolytic and osteoblastic components of osteosarcoma lesions in a mouse model. Clin Cancer Res 15(10):3451–3461. doi:10.1158/1078-0432.CCR-08-1616

Ladenstein R, Lasset C, Philip T (1992) Treatment duration before bone marrow transplantation in stage IV neuroblastoma. European Bone Marrow Transplant Group Solid Tumour Registry. Lancet 340(8824):916–917

Ladenstein R, Gadner H, Hartmann O, Pico J, Biron P, Thierry P (1995a) The European experience with megadose therapy and autologous bone marrow transplantation in solid tumors with poor prognosis Ewing sarcoma, germ cell tumors and brain tumors). Wien Med Wochenschr 145(2-3):55–57

Ladenstein R, Lasset C, Pinkerton R, Zucker JM, Peters C, Burdach S, Coze C (1995b) Impact of megatherapy in children with high-risk Ewing's tumours in complete remission: a report from the EBMT Solid Tumour Registry. Bone Marrow Transplant 15(5):697–705

Ladenstein R, Potschger U, Le Deley MC, Whelan J, Paulussen M, Oberlin O, Jurgens H (2010) Primary disseminated multifocal Ewing sarcoma: results of the Euro-EWING 99 trial. J Clin Oncol 28(20):3284–3291. doi:10.1200/JCO.2009.22.9864

Lambert G, Bertrand JR, Fattal E, Subra F, Pinto-Alphandary H, Malvy C, Couvreur P (2000) EWS fli-1 antisense nanocapsules inhibits ewing sarcoma-related tumor in mice. Biochem Biophys Res Commun 279(2):401–406. doi:10.1006/bbrc.2000.3963

Langevin AM, Bernstein M, Kuhn JG, Blaney SM, Ivy P, Sun J, Children's Oncology G. (2008) A phase II trial of rebeccamycin analogue (NSC #655649) in children with solid tumors: a Children's Oncology Group study. Pediatr Blood Cancer 50(3):577–580. doi:10.1002/pbc.21274

Lanza LA, Miser JS, Pass HI, Roth JA (1987) The role of resection in the treatment of pulmonary metastases from Ewing's sarcoma. J Thorac Cardiovasc Surg 94(2):181–187

Lawlor ER, Thiele CJ (2012) Epigenetic changes in pediatric solid tumors: promising new targets. Clin Cancer Res 18(10):2768–2779. doi:10.1158/1078-0432.CCR-11-1921

Lawrence TS, Chang EY, Hahn TM, Shewach DS (1997) Delayed radiosensitization of human colon carcinoma cells after a brief exposure to 2′,2′-difluoro-2′-deoxycytidine (Gemcitabine). Clin Cancer Res 3(5):777–782

Le Cesne A, Antoine E, Spielmann M, Le Chevalier T, Brain E, Toussaint C et al (1995) High-dose ifosfamide: circumvention of resistance to standard-dose ifosfamide in advanced soft tissue sarcomas. J Clin Oncol 13(7):1600–1608

Leavey PJ, Collier AB (2008) Ewing sarcoma: prognostic criteria, outcomes and future treatment. Expert Rev Anticancer Ther 8(4):617–624. doi:10.1586/14737140.8.4.617

Leavey PJ, Mascarenhas L, Marina N, Chen Z, Krailo M, Miser J, Children's Oncology G. (2008) Prognostic factors for patients with Ewing sarcoma (EWS) at first recurrence following multi-modality therapy: a report from the Children's Oncology Group. Pediatr Blood Cancer 51(3):334–338. doi:10.1002/pbc.21618

Leu KM, Ostruszka LJ, Shewach D, Zalupski M, Sondak V, Biermann JS, Baker LH (2004) Laboratory and clinical evidence of synergistic cytotoxicity of sequential treatment with gemcitabine followed by docetaxel in the treatment of sarcoma. J Clin Oncol 22(9):1706–1712. doi:10.1200/JCO.2004.08.043

Leung W, Chen AR, Klann RC, Moss TJ, Davis JM, Noga SJ, Civin CI (1998) Frequent detection of tumor cells in hematopoietic grafts in neuroblastoma and Ewing's sarcoma. Bone Marrow Transplant 22(10):971–979. doi:10.1038/sj.bmt.1701471

Li Y, Li X, Fan G, Fukushi J, Matsumoto Y, Iwamoto Y, Zhu Y (2012) Impairment of p53 acetylation by EWS-Fli1 chimeric protein in Ewing family tumors. Cancer Lett 320(1):14–22. doi:10.1016/j.canlet.2012.01.018

Link MP, Goorin AM, Miser AW, Green AA, Pratt CB, Belasco JB et al (1986) The effect of adjuvant chemotherapy on relapse-free survival in patients with osteosarcoma of the extremity. N Engl J Med 314(25):1600–1606. doi:10.1056/NEJM198606193142502

Lipton A, Zheng M, Seaman J (2003) Zoledronic acid delays the onset of skeletal-related events and progression of skeletal disease in patients with advanced renal cell carcinoma. Cancer 98(5):962–969. doi:10.1002/cncr.11571

Loeb DM, Garrett-Mayer E, Hobbs RF, Prideaux AR, Sgouros G, Shokek O, Schwartz CL (2009) Dose-finding study of 153Sm-EDTMP in patients with poor-prognosis osteosarcoma. Cancer 115(11):2514–2522. doi:10.1002/cncr.24286

Loeb DM, Hobbs RF, Okoli A, Chen AR, Cho S, Srinivasan S, Schwartz CL (2010) Tandem dosing of samarium-153 ethylenediamine tetramethylene phosphoric acid with stem cell support for patients with high-risk osteosarcoma. Cancer 116(23):5470–5478. doi:10.1002/cncr.25518

Longhi A, Errani C, De Paolis M, Mercuri M, Bacci G (2006) Primary bone osteosarcoma in the pediatric age: state of the art. Cancer Treat Rev 32(6):423–436. doi:10.1016/j.ctrv.2006.05.005

MacEwen EG, Kurzman ID, Rosenthal RC, Smith BW, Manley PA, Roush JK, Howard PE (1989) Therapy for osteosarcoma in dogs with intravenous injection of liposome-encapsulated muramyl tripeptide. J Natl Cancer Inst 81(12):935–938

Machak GN, Tkachev SI, Solovyev YN, Sinyukov PA, Ivanov SM, Kochergina NV, Glebovskaya VV (2003) Neoadjuvant chemotherapy and local radiotherapy for high-grade osteosarcoma of the extremities. Mayo Clin Proc 78(2):147–155. doi:10.4065/78.2.147

Mahajan A, Woo SY, Kornguth DG, Hughes D, Huh W, Chang EL, Anderson P (2008) Multimodality treatment of osteosarcoma: radiation in a high-risk cohort. Pediatr Blood Cancer 50(5):976–982. doi:10.1002/pbc.21451

Maki RG (2008) Pediatric sarcomas occurring in adults. J Surg Oncol 97(4):360–368. doi:10.1002/jso.20969

Malempati S, Hawkins DS (2012) Rhabdomyosarcoma: review of the Children's Oncology Group (COG) Soft-Tissue Sarcoma Committee experience and rationale for current COG studies. Pediatr Blood Cancer 59(1):5–10. doi:10.1002/pbc.24118

Malempati S, Weigel B, Ingle AM, Ahern CH, Carroll JM, Roberts CT, Blaney SM (2012) Phase I/II trial and pharmacokinetic study of cixutumumab in pediatric patients with refractory solid tumors and Ewing sarcoma: a report from the Children's Oncology Group. J Clin Oncol 30(3):256–262. doi:10.1200/JCO.2011.37.4355

Manara MC, Landuzzi L, Nanni P, Nicoletti G, Zambelli D, Lollini PL, Scotlandi K (2007) Preclinical in vivo study of new insulin-like growth factor-I receptor–specific inhibitor in Ewing's sarcoma. Clin Cancer Res 13(4):1322–1330. doi:10.1158/1078-0432.CCR-06-1518

Marina NM, Pratt CB, Shema SJ, Brooks T, Rao B, Meyer WH (1993) Brain metastases in osteosarcoma. Report of a long-term survivor and review of the St Jude Children's Research Hospital experience. Cancer 71(11):3656–3660

Martinez A, Goffinet DR, Donaldson SS, Bagshaw MA, Kaplan HS (1985) Intra-arterial infusion of radiosensitizer (BUdR) combined with hypofractionated irradiation and chemotherapy for primary treatment of osteogenic sarcoma. Int J Radiat Oncol Biol Phys 11(1):123–128

Martini N, Huvos AG, Mike V, Marcove RC, Beattie EJ Jr (1971) Multiple pulmonary resections in the treatment of osteogenic sarcoma. Ann Thorac Surg 12(3):271–280

Mascarenhas L, Lyden ER, Breitfeld PP, Walterhouse DO, Donaldson SS, Paidas CN, Hawkins DS (2010) Randomized phase II window trial of two schedules of irinotecan with vincristine in patients with first relapse or progression of rhabdomyosarcoma: a report from the Children's Oncology Group. J Clin Oncol 28(30):4658–4663. doi:10.1200/JCO.2010.29.7390

Mateo-Lozano S, Tirado OM, Notario V (2003) Rapamycin induces the fusion-type independent downregulation of the EWS/FLI-1 proteins and inhibits Ewing's sarcoma cell proliferation. Oncogene 22(58):9282–9287. doi:10.1038/sj.onc.1207081

Matsumoto Y, Tanaka K, Nakatani F, Matsunobu T, Matsuda S, Iwamoto Y (2001) Downregulation and forced expression of EWS-Fli1 fusion gene results in changes in the expression of G(1)regulatory genes. Br J Cancer 84(6):768–775. doi:10.1054/bjoc.2000.1652

McCarville MB, Kaste SC, Cain AM, Goloubeva O, Rao BN, Pratt CB (2001) Prognostic factors and imaging patterns of recurrent pulmonary nodules after thoracotomy in children with osteosarcoma. Cancer 91(6):1170–1176

McClung MR, Lewiecki EM, Cohen SB, Bolognese MA, Woodson GC, Moffett AH, Group, A. M. G. B. L. S (2006) Denosumab in postmenopausal women with low bone mineral density. N Engl J Med 354:821–831. doi:10.1056/NEJMoa044459

McTiernan A, Driver D, Michelagnoli MP, Kilby AM, Whelan JS (2006) High dose chemotherapy with bone marrow or peripheral stem cell rescue is an effective treatment option for patients with relapsed or progressive Ewing's sarcoma family of tumours. Ann Oncol 17(8):1301–1305. doi:10.1093/annonc/mdl108

Meazza C, Casanova M, Luksch R, Podda M, Favini F, Cefalo G, Ferrari A (2010) Prolonged 14-day continuous infusion of high-dose ifosfamide with an external portable pump: feasibility and efficacy in refractory pediatric sarcoma. Pediatr Blood Cancer 55(4):617–620. doi:10.1002/pbc.22596

Meyer WH, Schell MJ, Kumar AP, Rao BN, Green AA, Champion J, Pratt CB (1987) Thoracotomy for pulmonary metastatic osteosarcoma. An analysis of prognostic indicators of survival. Cancer 59(2):374–379

Meyer WH, Kun L, Marina N, Roberson P, Parham D, Rao B, Pratt CB (1992) Ifosfamide plus etoposide in newly diagnosed Ewing's sarcoma of bone. J Clin Oncol 10(11):1737–1742

Meyers PA, Gorlick R (1997) Osteosarcoma. Pediatr Clin North Am 44(4):973–989

Meyers PA, Heller G, Vlamis V (1993) Osteosarcoma of the extremities: chemotherapy experience at Memorial Sloan-Kettering. Cancer Treat Res 62:309–322

Meyers PA, Gorlick R, Heller G, Casper E, Lane J, Huvos AG, Healey JH (1998) Intensification of preoperative chemotherapy for osteogenic sarcoma: results of the Memorial Sloan-Kettering (T12) protocol. J Clin Oncol 16(7):2452–2458

Meyers PA, Krailo MD, Ladanyi M, Chan KW, Sailer SL, Dickman PS, Gorlick RG (2001) High-dose melphalan, etoposide, total-body irradiation, and autologous stem-cell reconstitution as consolidation therapy for high-risk Ewing's sarcoma does not improve prognosis. J Clin Oncol 19(11):2812–2820

Meyers PA, Schwartz CL, Krailo M, Kleinerman ES, Betcher D, Bernstein ML, Grier H (2005) Osteosarcoma: a randomized, prospective trial of the addition of ifosfamide and/or muramyl tripeptide to cisplatin, doxorubicin, and high-dose methotrexate. J Clin Oncol 23(9):2004–2011. doi:10.1200/JCO.2005.06.031

Meyers PA, Schwartz CL, Krailo MD, Healey JH, Bernstein ML, Betcher D, Children's Oncology G. (2008) Osteosarcoma: the addition of muramyl tripeptide to chemotherapy improves overall survival–a report from the Children's Oncology Group. J Clin Oncol 26(4):633–638. doi:10.1200/JCO.2008.14.0095

Miser JS, Kinsella TJ, Triche TJ, Tsokos M, Jarosinski P, Forquer R, Magrath I (1987) Ifosfamide with mesna uroprotection and etoposide: an effective regimen in the treatment of recurrent sarcomas and other tumors of children and young adults. J Clin Oncol 5(8):1191–1198

Miser JS, Krailo MD, Tarbell NJ, Link MP, Fryer CJ, Pritchard DJ, Grier HE (2004) Treatment of metastatic Ewing's sarcoma or primitive neuroectodermal tumor of bone: evaluation of combination ifosfamide and etoposide–a Children's Cancer Group and Pediatric Oncology Group study. J Clin Oncol 22(14):2873–2876. doi:10.1200/JCO.2004.01.041

Miser JS, Goldsby RE, Chen Z, Krailo MD, Tarbell NJ, Link MP, Grier HE (2007) Treatment of metastatic Ewing sarcoma/primitive neuroectodermal tumor of bone: evaluation of increasing the dose intensity of chemotherapy–a report from the Children's Oncology Group. Pediatr Blood Cancer 49(7):894–900. doi:10.1002/pbc.21233

Mora J, Cruz CO, Parareda A, de Torres C (2009) Treatment of relapsed/refractory pediatric sarcomas with gemcitabine and docetaxel. J Pediatr Hematol Oncol 31(10):723–729. doi:10.1097/MPH.0b013e3181b2598c

Mori K, Le Goff B, Berreur M, Riet A, Moreau A, Blanchard F, Heymann D (2007) Human osteosarcoma cells express functional receptor activator of nuclear factor-kappa B. J Pathol 211(5):555–562. doi:10.1002/path.2140

Nagano A, Miyamoto K, Nishimoto H, Hosoe H, Suzuki N, Shimizu K (2009) Transforaminal lumbar interbody fusion for failed Graf ligamentoplasty: a report of two cases. J Orthop Surg (Hong Kong) 17(2):220–222

Naing A, LoRusso P, Fu S, Hong DS, Anderson P, Benjamin RS, Kurzrock R (2012) Insulin growth factor-receptor (IGF-1R) antibody cixutumumab combined with the mTOR inhibitor temsirolimus in patients with refractory Ewing's sarcoma family tumors. Clin Cancer Res 18(9):2625–2631. doi:10.1158/1078-0432.CCR-12-0061

Nardin A, Lefebvre ML, Labroquere K, Faure O, Abastado JP (2006) Liposomal muramyl tripeptide phosphatidylethanolamine: targeting and activating macrophages for adjuvant treatment of osteosarcoma. Curr Cancer Drug Targets 6(2):123–133

Navid F, Billups C, Liu T, Krasin MJ, Rodriguez-Galindo C (2008a) Second cancers in patients with the Ewing sarcoma family of tumours. Eur J Cancer 44(7):983–991. doi:10.1016/j.ejca.2008.02.027

Navid F, Willert JR, McCarville MB, Furman W, Watkins A, Roberts W, Daw NC (2008b) Combination of gemcitabine and docetaxel in the treatment of children and young adults with refractory bone sarcoma. Cancer 113(2):419–425. doi:10.1002/cncr.23586

Nesbit ME Jr, Gehan EA, Burgert EO Jr, Vietti TJ, Cangir A, Tefft M et al (1990) Multimodal therapy for the management of primary, nonmetastatic Ewing's sarcoma of bone: a long-term follow-up of the First Intergroup study. J Clin Oncol 8(10):1664–1674

Newlands ES, Stevens MF, Wedge SR, Wheelhouse RT, Brock C (1997) Temozolomide: a review of its discovery, chemical properties, pre-clinical development and clinical trials. Cancer Treat Rev 23(1):35–61

Nilbert M, Saeter G, Elomaa I, Monge OR, Wiebe T, Alvegard TA (1998) Ewing's sarcoma treatment in Scandinavia 1984–1990–ten-year results of the Scandinavian Sarcoma Group Protocol SSGIV. Acta Oncol 37(4):375–378

Nilsson S, Larsen RH, Fossa SD, Balteskard L, Borch KW, Westlin JE, Bruland OS (2005) First clinical experience with alpha-emitting radium-223 in the treatment of skeletal metastases. Clin Cancer Res 11(12):4451–4459. doi:10.1158/1078-0432.CCR-04-2244

Nilsson S, Franzen L, Parker C, Tyrrell C, Blom R, Tennvall J, Bruland OS (2007) Bone-targeted radium-223 in symptomatic, hormone-refractory prostate cancer: a randomised, multicentre, placebo-controlled phase II study. Lancet Oncol 8(7):587–594. doi:10.1016/S1470-2045(07)70147-X

Oberlin O, Patte C, Demeocq F, Lacombe MJ, Brunat-Mentigny M, Demaille MC, Lemerle J (1985) The response to initial chemotherapy as a prognostic factor in localized Ewing's sarcoma. Eur J Cancer Clin Oncol 21(4):463–467

Oberlin O, Habrand JL, Zucker JM, Brunat-Mentigny M, Terrier-Lacombe MJ, Dubousset J et al (1992) No benefit of ifosfamide in Ewing's sarcoma: a nonrandomized study of the French Society of Pediatric Oncology. J Clin Oncol 10(9):1407–1412

Oberlin O, Deley MC, Bui BN, Gentet JC, Philip T, Terrier P, French Society of Paediatric, O (2001) Prognostic factors in localized Ewing's tumours and peripheral neuroectodermal tumours: the third study of the French Society of Paediatric Oncology (EW88 study). Br J Cancer 85(11):1646–1654. doi:10.1054/bjoc.2001.2150

Oberlin O, Rey A, Desfachelles AS, Philip T, Plantaz D, Schmitt C, Societe Francaise des Cancers de, l. E. (2006) Impact of high-dose busulfan plus melphalan as consolidation in metastatic Ewing tumors: a study by the Societe Francaise des Cancers de l'Enfant. J Clin Oncol 24(24):3997–4002. doi:10.1200/JCO.2006.05.7059

Olmos D, Postel-Vinay S, Molife LR, Okuno SH, Schuetze SM, Paccagnella ML, Haluska P (2010)

Safety, pharmacokinetics, and preliminary activity of the anti-IGF-1R antibody figitumumab (CP-751,871) in patients with sarcoma and Ewing's sarcoma: a phase 1 expansion cohort study. Lancet Oncol 11(2):129–135. doi:10.1016/S1470-2045(09)70354-7

O'Reilly KE, Rojo F, She QB, Solit D, Mills GB, Smith D, Rosen N (2006) mTOR inhibition induces upstream receptor tyrosine kinase signaling and activates Akt. Cancer Res 66(3):1500–1508. doi:10.1158/0008-5472.CAN-05-2925

Ory B, Heymann MF, Kamijo A, Gouin F, Heymann D, Redini F (2005) Zoledronic acid suppresses lung metastases and prolongs overall survival of osteosarcoma-bearing mice. Cancer 104(11):2522–2529. doi:10.1002/cncr.21530

Palumbo R, Palmeri S, Antimi M, Gatti C, Raffo P, Villani G, Toma S (1997) Phase II study of continuous-infusion high-dose ifosfamide in advanced and/or metastatic pretreated soft tissue sarcomas. Ann Oncol 8(11):1159–1162

Pappo AS, Patel SR, Crowley J, Reinke DK, Kuenkele KP, Chawla SP, Baker LH (2011) R1507, a monoclonal antibody to the insulin-like growth factor 1 receptor, in patients with recurrent or refractory Ewing sarcoma family of tumors: results of a phase II Sarcoma Alliance for Research through Collaboration study. J Clin Oncol 29(34):4541–4547. doi:10.1200/JCO.2010.34.0000

Parker C, Nilsson S, Heinrich D, Helle SI, O'Sullivan JM, Fossa SD, Investigators A (2013) Alpha emitter radium-223 and survival in metastatic prostate cancer. N Engl J Med 369(3):213–223. doi:10.1056/NEJMoa1213755

Pastorino U, Gasparini M, Tavecchio L, Azzarelli A, Mapelli S, Zucchi V, Ravasi G (1991) The contribution of salvage surgery to the management of childhood osteosarcoma. J Clin Oncol 9(8):1357–1362

Patel SR, Vadhan-Raj S, Papadopolous N, Plager C, Burgess MA, Hays C, Benjamin RS (1997) High-dose ifosfamide in bone and soft tissue sarcomas: results of phase II and pilot studies–dose-response and schedule dependence. J Clin Oncol 15(6):2378–2384

Paulussen M, Ahrens S, Burdach S, Craft A, Dockhorn-Dworniczak B, Dunst J, Jurgens H (1998) Primary metastatic (stage IV) Ewing tumor: survival analysis of 171 patients from the EICESS studies. European Intergroup Cooperative Ewing Sarcoma Studies. Ann Oncol 9(3):275–281

Paulussen M, Ahrens S, Dunst J, Winkelmann W, Exner GU, Kotz R, Jurgens H (2001) Localized Ewing tumor of bone: final results of the cooperative Ewing's Sarcoma Study CESS 86. J Clin Oncol 19(6):1818–1829

Perentesis J, Katsanis E, DeFor T, Neglia J, Ramsay N (1999) Autologous stem cell transplantation for high-risk pediatric solid tumors. Bone Marrow Transplant 24(6):609–615. doi:10.1038/sj.bmt.1701950

Petsas T, Megas P, Papathanassiou Z (2007) Radiofrequency ablation of two femoral head chondroblastomas. Eur J Radiol 63(1):63–67. doi:10.1016/j.ejrad.2007.03.024

Picci P, Rougraff BT, Bacci G, Neff JR, Sangiorgi L, Cazzola A et al (1993) Prognostic significance of histopathologic response to chemotherapy in nonmetastatic Ewing's sarcoma of the extremities. J Clin Oncol 11(9):1763–1769

Picci P, Bohling T, Bacci G, Ferrari S, Sangiorgi L, Mercuri M, Bertoni F (1997) Chemotherapy-induced tumor necrosis as a prognostic factor in localized Ewing's sarcoma of the extremities. J Clin Oncol 15(4):1553–1559

Pieper S, Ranft A, Braun-Munzinger G, Jurgens H, Paulussen M, Dirksen U (2008) Ewing's tumors over the age of 40: a retrospective analysis of 47 patients treated according to the International Clinical Trials EICESS 92 and EURO-E.W.I.N.G. 99. Onkologie 31(12):657–663. doi:10.1159/000165361

Pignochino Y, Grignani G, Cavalloni G, Motta M, Tapparo M, Bruno S, Aglietta M (2009) Sorafenib blocks tumour growth, angiogenesis and metastatic potential in preclinical models of osteosarcoma through a mechanism potentially involving the inhibition of ERK1/2, MCL-1 and ezrin pathways. Mol Cancer 8:118. doi:10.1186/1476-4598-8-118

Pratt CB, Epelman S, Jaffe N (1987) Bleomycin, cyclophosphamide, and dactinomycin in metastatic osteosarcoma: lack of tumor regression in previously treated patients. Cancer Treat Rep 71(4):421–423

Putnam JB Jr, Roth JA, Wesley MN, Johnston MR, Rosenberg SA (1983) Survival following aggressive resection of pulmonary metastases from osteogenic sarcoma: analysis of prognostic factors. Ann Thorac Surg 36(5):516–523

Reardon DA, Quinn JA, Rich JN, Desjardins A, Vredenburgh J, Gururangan S, Friedman HS (2005) Phase I trial of irinotecan plus temozolomide in adults with recurrent malignant glioma. Cancer 104(7):1478–1486. doi:10.1002/cncr.21316

Reid JM, Qu W, Safgren SL, Ames MM, Krailo MD, Seibel NL, Holcenberg J (2004) Phase I trial and pharmacokinetics of gemcitabine in children with advanced solid tumors. J Clin Oncol 22(12):2445–2451. doi:10.1200/JCO.2004.10.142

Rettew AN, Young ED, Lev DC, Kleinerman ES, Abdul-Karim FW, Getty PJ, Greenfield EM (2012) Multiple receptor tyrosine kinases promote the in vitro phenotype of metastatic human osteosarcoma cell lines. Oncogenesis 1, e34. doi:10.1038/oncsis.2012.34

Ricotti L, Tesei A, De Paola F, Ulivi P, Frassineti GL, Milandri C, Zoli W (2003) In vitro schedule-dependent interaction between docetaxel and gemcitabine in human gastric cancer cell lines. Clin Cancer Res 9(2):900–905

Robinson D, Halperin N, Nevo Z (2001) Two freezing cycles ensure interface sterilization by cryosurgery during bone tumor resection. Cryobiology 43(1):4–10. doi:10.1006/cryo.2001.2312

Robinson SI, Ahmed SK, Okuno SH, Arndt CA, Rose PS, Laack NN (2013) Clinical outcomes of adult patients with relapsed Ewing sarcoma: a 30-year single-institution experience. Am J Clin Oncol. doi:10.1097/COC.0b013e318281d6ab

Rodriguez-Galindo C, Billups CA, Kun LE, Rao BN, Pratt CB, Merchant TE, Pappo AS (2002a) Survival after recurrence of Ewing tumors: the St Jude Children's Research Hospital experience, 1979–1999. Cancer 94(2):561–569. doi:10.1002/cncr.10192

Rodriguez-Galindo C, Daw NC, Kaste SC, Meyer WH, Dome JS, Pappo AS, Pratt CB (2002b) Treatment of refractory osteosarcoma with fractionated cyclophosphamide and etoposide. J Pediatr Hematol Oncol 24(4):250–255

Rosen LS, Gordon D, Kaminski M, Howell A, Belch A, Mackey J, Seaman JJ (2003) Long-term efficacy and safety of zoledronic acid compared with pamidronate disodium in the treatment of skeletal complications in patients with advanced multiple myeloma or breast carcinoma: a randomized, double-blind, multicenter, comparative trial. Cancer 98(8):1735–1744. doi:10.1002/cncr.11701

Rosenburg SA, Flye MW, Conkle D, Seipp CA, Levine AS, Simon RM (1979) Treatment of osteogenic sarcoma. II. Aggressive resection of pulmonary metastases. Cancer Treat Rep 63(5):753–756

Roth M, Linkowski M, Tarim J, Piperdi S, Sowers R, Geller D, Gorlick R (2014) Ganglioside GD2 as a therapeutic target for antibody-mediated therapy in patients with osteosarcoma. Cancer 120(4):548–554. doi:10.1002/cncr.28461

Rybak LD (2009) Fire and ice: thermal ablation of musculoskeletal tumors. Radiol Clin North Am 47(3):455–469. doi:10.1016/j.rcl.2008.12.006

Saeter G, Hoie J, Stenwig AE, Johansson AK, Hannisdal E, Solheim OP (1995) Systemic relapse of patients with osteogenic sarcoma. Prognostic factors for long term survival. Cancer 75(5):1084–1093

Sandoval C, Meyer WH, Parham DM, Kun LE, Hustu HO, Luo X, Pratt CB (1996) Outcome in 43 children presenting with metastatic Ewing sarcoma: the St. Jude Children's Research Hospital experience, 1962 to 1992. Med Pediatr Oncol 26(3):180–185. doi:10.1002/(SICI)1096-911X(199603)26:3<180::AID-MPO6>3.0.CO;2-G

San-Julian M, Diaz-de-Rada P, Noain E, Sierrasesumaga L (2003) Bone metastases from osteosarcoma. Int Orthop 27(2):117–120. doi:10.1007/s00264-002-0407-8

Sankar S, Bell R, Stephens B, Zhuo R, Sharma S, Bearss DJ, Lessnick SL (2013) Mechanism and relevance of EWS/FLI-mediated transcriptional repression in Ewing sarcoma. Oncogene 32(42):5089–5100. doi:10.1038/onc.2012.525

Santiago FR, Del Mar Castellano Garcia M, Montes JL, Garcia MR, Fernandez JM (2009) Treatment of bone tumours by radiofrequency thermal ablation. Curr Rev Musculoskelet Med 2(1):43–50. doi:10.1007/s12178-008-9042-3

Sauer R, Jurgens H, Burgers JM, Dunst J, Hawlicek R, Michaelis J (1987) Prognostic factors in the treatment of Ewing's sarcoma. The Ewing's Sarcoma Study Group of the German Society of Paediatric Oncology CESS 81. Radiother Oncol 10(2):101–110

Saumet L, Deschamps F, Marec-Berard P, Gaspar N, Corradini N, Petit P, Brugieres L (2014) Radiofrequency ablation of metastases from osteosarcoma in patients under 25 years: the SCFE experience. Pediatr Hematol Oncol. doi:10.3109/08880018.2014.926469

Saylors RL 3rd, Stine KC, Sullivan J, Kepner JL, Wall DA, Bernstein ML, Pediatric Oncology G (2001) Cyclophosphamide plus topotecan in children with recurrent or refractory solid tumors: a Pediatric Oncology Group phase II study. J Clin Oncol 19(15):3463–3469

Schaller RT Jr, Haas J, Schaller J, Morgan A, Bleyer A (1982) Improved survival in children with osteosarcoma following resection of pulmonary metastases. J Pediatr Surg 17(5):546–550

Schuck A, Ahrens S, Paulussen M, Kuhlen M, Konemann S, Rube C, Jurgens H (2003) Local therapy in localized Ewing tumors: results of 1058 patients treated in the CESS 81, CESS 86, and EICESS 92 trials. Int J Radiat Oncol Biol Phys 55(1):168–177

Schwartz GK, Tap WD, Qin LX, Livingston MB, Undevia SD, Chmielowski B, Maki RG (2013) Cixutumumab and temsirolimus for patients with bone and soft-tissue sarcoma: a multicentre, open-label, phase 2 trial. Lancet Oncol 14(4):371–382. doi:10.1016/S1470-2045(13)70049-4

Schwarz R, Bruland O, Cassoni A, Schomberg P, Bielack S (2009) The role of radiotherapy in osteosarcoma. Cancer Treat Res 152:147–164. doi:10.1007/978-1-4419-0284-9_7

Scotlandi K (2006) Targeted therapies in Ewing's sarcoma. Adv Exp Med Biol 587:13–22

Seibel NL, Blaney SM, O'Brien M, Krailo M, Hutchinson R, Mosher RB, Reaman GH (1999) Phase I trial of docetaxel with filgrastim support in pediatric patients with refractory solid tumors: a collaborative Pediatric Oncology Branch, National Cancer Institute and Children's Cancer Group trial. Clin Cancer Res 5(4):733–737

Shankar AG, Ashley S, Craft AW, Pinkerton CR (2003) Outcome after relapse in an unselected cohort of children and adolescents with Ewing sarcoma. Med Pediatr Oncol 40(3):141–147. doi:10.1002/mpo.10248

Shibuya H, Hamamura K, Hotta H, Matsumoto Y, Nishida Y, Hattori H, Furukawa K (2012) Enhancement of malignant properties of human osteosarcoma cells with disialyl gangliosides GD2/GD3. Cancer Sci 103(9):1656–1664. doi:10.1111/j.1349-7006.2012.02344.x

Siegel RD, Ryan LM, Antman KH (1988) Adults with Ewing's sarcoma. An analysis of 16 patients at the Dana-Farber Cancer Institute. Am J Clin Oncol 11(6):614–617

Simon CJ, Dupuy DE (2006) Percutaneous minimally invasive therapies in the treatment of bone tumors: thermal ablation. Semin Musculoskelet Radiol 10(2):137–144. doi:10.1055/s-2006-939031

Skubitz KM (2003) Phase II trial of pegylated-liposomal doxorubicin (Doxil) in sarcoma. Cancer Invest 21(2):167–176

Smithey BE, Pappo AS, Hill DA (2002) C-kit expression in pediatric solid tumors: a comparative immunohistochemical study. Am J Surg Pathol 26(4):486–492

Soldatenkov VA, Albor A, Patel BK, Dreszer R, Dritschilo A, Notario V (1999) Regulation of the human poly(ADP-ribose) polymerase promoter by the ETS transcription factor. Oncogene 18(27):3954–3962. doi:10.1038/sj.onc.1202778

Spanos PK, Payne WS, Ivins JC, Pritchard DJ (1976) Pulmonary resection for metastatic osteogenic sarcoma. J Bone Joint Surg Am 58(5):624–628

Stahl M, Ranft A, Paulussen M, Bolling T, Vieth V, Bielack S, Dirksen U (2011) Risk of recurrence and survival after relapse in patients with Ewing sarcoma. Pediatr Blood Cancer 57(4):549–553. doi:10.1002/pbc.23040

Stewart KS, Kleinerman ES (2011) Tumor vessel development and expansion in Ewing's sarcoma: a review of the vasculogenesis process and clinical trials with vascular-targeting agents. Sarcoma 2011:165837. doi:10.1155/2011/165837

Strauss SJ, McTiernan A, Whelan JS (2004) Late relapse of osteosarcoma: implications for follow-up and screening. Pediatr Blood Cancer 43(6):692–697. doi:10.1002/pbc.20154

Subbiah V, Brown RE, Jiang Y, Buryanek J, Hayes-Jordan A, Kurzrock R, Anderson PM (2013) Morphoproteomic profiling of the mammalian target of rapamycin (mTOR) signaling pathway in desmoplastic small round cell tumor (EWS/WT1), Ewing's sarcoma (EWS/FLI1) and Wilms' tumor(WT1). PLoS One 8(7):e68985. doi:10.1371/journal.pone.0068985

Sulzbacher I, Birner P, Trieb K, Traxler M, Lang S, Chott A (2003) Expression of platelet-derived growth factor-AA is associated with tumor progression in osteosarcoma. Mod Pathol 16(1):66–71. doi:10.1097/01.MP.0000043522.76788.0A

Sutow WW, Sullivan MP (1962) Cyclophosphamide therapy in children with Ewing's sarcoma. Cancer Chemother Rep 23:55–60

Ta HT, Dass CR, Larson I, Choong PF, Dunstan DE (2009) A chitosan-dipotassium orthophosphate hydrogel for the delivery of Doxorubicin in the treatment of osteosarcoma. Biomaterials 30(21):3605–3613. doi:10.1016/j.biomaterials.2009.03.022

Tabone MD, Kalifa C, Rodary C, Raquin M, Valteau-Couanet D, Lemerle J (1994) Osteosarcoma recurrences in pediatric patients previously treated with intensive chemotherapy. J Clin Oncol 12(12):2614–2620

Temeck BK, Wexler LH, Steinberg SM, McClure LL, Horowitz M, Pass HI (1995) Metastasectomy for sarcomatous pediatric histologies: results and prognostic factors. Ann Thorac Surg 59(6):1385–1389; discussion 1390

Thompson RC Jr, Cheng EY, Clohisy DR, Perentesis J, Manivel C, Le CT (2002) Results of treatment for metastatic osteosarcoma with neoadjuvant chemotherapy and surgery. Clin Orthop Relat Res (397):240–247

Thompson PA, Gupta M, Rosner GL, Yu A, Barrett J, Bomgaars L, Mondick J (2008) Pharmacokinetics of irinotecan and its metabolites in pediatric cancer patients: a report from the children's oncology group. Cancer Chemother Pharmacol 62(6):1027–1037. doi:10.1007/s00280-008-0692-z

Thornton KA, Chen AR, Trucco MM, Shah P, Wilky BA, Gul N, Loeb DM (2013) A dose-finding study of temsirolimus and liposomal doxorubicin for patients with recurrent and refractory bone and soft tissue sarcoma. Int J Cancer 133(4):997–1005. doi:10.1002/ijc.28083

Toretsky JA, Connell Y, Neckers L, Bhat NK (1997a) Inhibition of EWS-FLI-1 fusion protein with antisense oligodeoxynucleotides. J Neurooncol 31(1–2):9–16

Toretsky JA, Kalebic T, Blakesley V, LeRoith D, Helman LJ (1997b) The insulin-like growth factor-I receptor is required for EWS/FLI-1 transformation of fibroblasts. J Biol Chem 272(49):30822–30827

van Putten LM (1968) Tumour reoxygenation during fractionated radiotherapy; studies with a transplantable mouse osteosarcoma. Eur J Cancer 4(2):172–182

Van Winkle P, Angiolillo A, Krailo M, Cheung YK, Anderson B, Davenport V, Cairo MS (2005) Ifosfamide, carboplatin, and etoposide (ICE) reinduction chemotherapy in a large cohort of children and adolescents with recurrent/refractory sarcoma: the Children's Cancer Group (CCG) experience. Pediatr Blood Cancer 44(4):338–347. doi:10.1002/pbc.20227

Verrill MW, Judson IR, Harmer CL, Fisher C, Thomas JM, Wiltshaw E (1997) Ewing's sarcoma and primitive neuroectodermal tumor in adults: are they different from Ewing's sarcoma and primitive neuroectodermal tumor in children? J Clin Oncol 15(7):2611–2621

Wagner LM, Crews KR, Iacono LC, Houghton PJ, Fuller CE, McCarville MB, Santana VM (2004) Phase I trial of temozolomide and protracted irinotecan in pediatric patients with refractory solid tumors. Clin Cancer Res 10(3):840–848

Wagner LM, McAllister N, Goldsby RE, Rausen AR, McNall-Knapp RY, McCarville MB, Albritton K (2007) Temozolomide and intravenous irinotecan for treatment of advanced Ewing sarcoma. Pediatr Blood Cancer 48(2):132–139. doi:10.1002/pbc.20697

Wagner-Bohn A, Henze G, von Stackelberg A, Boos J (2006) Phase II study of gemcitabine in children with relapsed leukemia. Pediatr Blood Cancer 46(2):262. doi:10.1002/pbc.20632

Wan X, Mendoza A, Khanna C, Helman LJ (2005) Rapamycin inhibits ezrin-mediated metastatic behavior in a murine model of osteosarcoma. Cancer Res 65(6):2406–2411. doi:10.1158/0008-5472.CAN-04-3135

Ward WG, Mikaelian K, Dorey F, Mirra JM, Sassoon A, Holmes EC, Eckardt JJ (1994) Pulmonary metastases of stage IIB extremity osteosarcoma and subsequent pulmonary metastases. J Clin Oncol 12(9):1849–1858

Weeden S, Grimer RJ, Cannon SR, Taminiau AH, Uscinska BM, European Osteosarcoma I (2001) The effect of local recurrence on survival in resected osteosarcoma. Eur J Cancer 37(1):39–46

Weichselbaum R, Little JB, Nove J (1977) Response of human osteosarcoma in vitro to irradiation: evidence for unusual cellular repair activity. Int J Radiat Biol Relat Stud Phys Chem Med 31(3):295–299

Wexler LH, DeLaney TF, Tsokos M, Avila N, Steinberg SM, Weaver-McClure L, Horowitz ME (1996) Ifosfamide and etoposide plus vincristine, doxorubicin, and cyclophosphamide for newly diagnosed Ewing's sarcoma family of tumors. Cancer 78(4):901–911. doi:10.1002/(SICI)1097-0142(19960815)78:4<901::AID-CNCR30>3.0.CO;2-X

Whelan J, McTiernan A, Cooper N, Wong YK, Francis M, Vernon S, Strauss SJ (2012) Incidence and survival of malignant bone sarcomas in England 1979–2007. Int J Cancer 131(4):E508–E517. doi:10.1002/ijc.26426

Wilson GD, Bentzen SM, Harari PM (2006) Biologic basis for combining drugs with radiation. Semin Radiat Oncol 16(1):2–9. doi:10.1016/j.semradonc.2005.08.001

Withrow SJ, Thrall DE, Straw RC, Powers BE, Wrigley RH, Larue SM et al (1993) Intra-arterial cisplatin with or without radiation in limb-sparing for canine osteosarcoma. Cancer 71(8):2484–2490

Wittgen BP, Kunst PW, van der Born K, van Wijk AW, Perkins W, Pilkiewicz FG, Postmus PE (2007) Phase I study of aerosolized SLIT cisplatin in the treatment of patients with carcinoma of the lung. Clin Cancer Res 13(8):2414–2421. doi:10.1158/1078-0432.CCR-06-1480

Womer RB, West DC, Krailo MD, Dickman PS, Pawel BR, Grier HE, Weiss AR (2012) Randomized controlled trial of interval-compressed chemotherapy for the treatment of localized Ewing sarcoma: a report from the Children's Oncology Group. J Clin Oncol 30(33):4148–4154. doi:10.1200/JCO.2011.41.5703

Wu D, Wan M (2012) Methylene diphosphonate-conjugated adriamycin liposomes: preparation, characteristics, and targeted therapy for osteosarcomas in vitro and in vivo. Biomed Microdevices 14(3):497–510. doi:10.1007/s10544-011-9626-3

Xu M, Xu CX, Bi WZ, Song ZG, Jia JP, Chai W, Wang Y (2013) Effects of endostar combined multidrug chemotherapy in osteosarcoma. Bone 57(1):111–115. doi:10.1016/j.bone.2013.07.035

Yang SY, Yu H, Krygier JE, Wooley PH, Mott MP (2007) High VEGF with rapid growth and early metastasis in a mouse osteosarcoma model. Sarcoma 2007:95628. doi:10.1155/2007/95628

Yu AL, Uttenreuther-Fischer MM, Huang CS, Tsui CC, Gillies SD, Reisfeld RA, Kung FH (1998) Phase I trial of a human-mouse chimeric anti-disialoganglioside monoclonal antibody ch14.18 in patients with refractory neuroblastoma and osteosarcoma. J Clin Oncol 16(6):2169–2180

Yu L, Su B, Hollomon M, Deng Y, Facchinetti V, Kleinerman ES (2010) Vasculogenesis driven by bone marrow-derived cells is essential for growth of Ewing's sarcomas. Cancer Res 70(4):1334–1343. doi:10.1158/0008-5472.CAN-09-2795

Zhou LT, Liu FY, Li Y, Peng YM, Liu YH, Li J (2012) Gpnmb/osteoactivin, an attractive target in cancer immunotherapy. Neoplasma 59(1):1–5. doi:10.4149/neo_2012_001

Zwerdling T, Krailo M, Monteleone P, Byrd R, Sato J, Dunaway R, Children's Oncology G. (2006) Phase II investigation of docetaxel in pediatric patients with recurrent solid tumors: a report from the Children's Oncology Group. Cancer 106(8):1821–1828. doi:10.1002/cncr.21779

Novel Therapies on the Horizon

15

Timothy P. Cripe, Kellie B. Haworth, and Peter J. Houghton

Contents

15.1 **Introduction** 265

15.2 **Antimitotic Agents** 266
15.2.1 Eribulin............................. 266
15.2.2 Glembatumumab Vedotin............... 267

15.3 **Targeted Inhibitors**.................. 268
15.3.1 IGF-1 Receptor Inhibitors 268
15.3.2 mTOR Inhibitors 269
15.3.3 Agents That Target EWS-FLI 271

15.4 **Immunotherapy** 274
15.4.1 Cytokines 276
15.4.2 Adoptive Transfer of Immunologically
Active Cells 277
15.4.3 Vaccines 278
15.4.4 Checkpoint Inhibitors.................. 279
15.4.5 Antibodies and CAR T Cells 280

15.5 **Virotherapy**........................ 281
15.5.1 Reolysin............................. 282
15.5.2 Seneca Valley Virus 282
15.5.3 HSV1716 282

15.5.4 JX-594 282
15.5.5 Other Vectors 283

15.6 **Summary**.......................... 283

References............................. 283

T.P. Cripe, MD, PhD • K.B. Haworth, MD
Division of Hematology/Oncology/BMT,
Nationwide Children's Hospital,
700 Children's Drive, Columbus, OH 43205, USA
e-mail: Timothy.cripe@nationwidechildrens.org;
Kellie.haworth@nationwidechildrens.org

P.J. Houghton, PhD (✉)
Center for Childhood Cancer and Blood Diseases,
The Research Institute at Nationwide Children's
Hospital, 700 Children's Drive, Columbus,
OH 43205, USA
e-mail: Peter.houghton@nationwidechildrens.org

Abstract

As many of the prior chapters illustrate, we have had many successes in the treatment of children with malignant bone tumors. Nevertheless, there is a substantial fraction of patients who are not cured by current therapies. In addition, even those who are long term survivors often suffer chronic side effects of treatment. Thus, we need to continue to explore novel therapies both to increase the cure rates and decrease complications. In this chapter we review available data for a variety of new therapies including novel small molecules, immunotherapies, and virotherapy, with an emphasis on findings in preclinical models or early phase clinical trials in patients with bone cancers.

15.1 Introduction

An overview of experimental therapeutics for pediatric bone tumors is difficult to include in a book as it is a rapidly evolving topic and much of what is written may be out of date at the time

© Springer International Publishing Switzerland 2015
T.P. Cripe, N.D. Yeager (eds.), *Malignant Pediatric Bone Tumors - Treatment & Management*,
Pediatric Oncology, DOI 10.1007/978-3-319-18099-1_15

of publication. New drugs and approaches often become fashionable or show promise in preclinical or early phase clinical studies and then fade into obscurity because of failure to meet primary objectives in adult studies. Nevertheless, we felt compelled to include a chapter on novel therapies as some of them are likely to gain a foothold: if not the particular agents, then at least perhaps the general class of agents or the strategy. Here we discuss several compounds or drugs that show promise for pediatric bone tumors. Many of the small molecules and biologics have been tested as part of the National Cancer Institute's Pediatric Preclinical Testing Program (PPTP, http://pptp.nchresearch.org), which includes a cadre of osteosarcoma and Ewing sarcoma models.

15.2 Antimitotic Agents

Microtubules function by rapidly polymerizing and depolymerizing tubulin monomeric subunits and are critical for cell division and migration. Drugs that inhibit microtubule function include the *vinca* alkaloids, *taxanes*, and *epothilones*, which play a major role in treatment of human malignant diseases. The taxanes and epothilones stabilize microtubules, reducing the dynamics necessary for cell movement and division. *Vinca* alkaloids inhibit microtubule function by causing depolymerization leading to mitotic arrest and possibly interphase death of cells. Halichondrin B analogs are a relatively new class of microtubule-targeted agents with a novel mechanism of action. Eribulin is a fully synthetic macrocyclic ketone analog of halichondrin B, a natural product derived from the marine sponge *Halichondria okadai* (Bai et al. 1991; Towle et al. 2001). Eribulin induces irreversible mitotic blockade and apoptosis by inhibiting microtubule "dynamic instability" (Jordan and Wilson 2004), the growth and shortening of microtubules required for mitosis. Microtubule growth is inhibited by eribulin binding with high affinity at the plus ends (Smith et al. 2010a). Eribulin is distinctive from that of other tubulin-binding antimitotic agents in that eribulin suppresses the growth parameters at microtubule plus ends with-

out affecting microtubule shortening parameters (Jordan et al. 2005; Smith et al. 2010a). With a novel mechanism of inhibition of microtubule dynamic instability coupled with prolonged cellular retention (Towle et al. 2011), eribulin has promise as an antineoplastic for multiple cancer histologies (Jain and Vahdat 2011).

Somewhat related to antitubulin agents are anti-tropomyosin drugs. The actin cytoskeleton has been long sought as a potential cancer target because of its importance in cell integrity and growth. Because it is so universal to cells, however, safely targeting actin in cancer cells without harming normal cells has proven challenging. Recently, it was reported that one of actin's partner proteins, tropomyosin, exists in multiple isoforms, some of which are selectively upregulated in cancer, and anti-tropomyosin drugs are currently under development (Stehn et al. 2013). These agents have not yet been tested in bone tumors but may be another avenue for impairing the cancer cytoskeleton.

15.2.1 Eribulin

Eribulin demonstrated a remarkably high level of activity against the Pediatric Preclinical Testing Program (PPTP) solid tumor and ALL in vivo models (Kolb et al. 2013). The obvious comparison for the eribulin in vivo results are to those previously obtained for vincristine, an agent used in standard of care regimens for soft tissue sarcomas and ALL. Vincristine is also used in upfront regimens for patients with Ewing sarcoma, with the current COG standard therapy for newly diagnosed nonmetastatic Ewing sarcoma prescribing 18 doses of vincristine over an approximately 9-month treatment course. The PPTP results showed a number of similarities between the activity pattern for the two agents, with both showing activity for Wilms' tumor, rhabdomyosarcoma, glioblastoma, and osteosarcoma xenograft models. The most noticeable difference between the two agents is the high level of activity observed for eribulin for the Ewing sarcoma xenografts (four of five models with complete regressions) compared to vincristine (zero of five models with CR or maintained complete response).

For osteosarcoma, vincristine is not used in standard upfront therapy regimens and in commonly employed retrieval regimens. Vincristine was highly active against one osteosarcoma xenograft, while eribulin showed high activity against three osteosarcoma xenografts. While vincristine has been used in the past to treat osteosarcoma (Rosen et al. 1981), it is a drug not normally considered active in this disease. There are, however, only limited single-agent data for vincristine for patients with osteosarcoma, most of which are from patients treated in the 1960s (Sutow 1968; Sutow et al. 1971). Pharmacokinetic data for eribulin suggest that the systemic exposure in mice per treatment course at the 1 mg/kg dose that is highly active in the mouse models is similar to that observed in humans at the 1.4 mg/m^2 recommended phase II dose (Goel et al. 2009; Taur et al. 2011). A phase I trial of eribulin is currently recruiting (NCT02082626), and a trial for refractory or recurrent osteosarcoma is planned (NCT02097238).

15.2.2 Glembatumumab Vedotin

Glembatumumab vedotin is an antibody-auristatin conjugate that targets cells expressing the transmembrane glycoprotein NMB (GPNMB, also known as osteoactivin). GPNMB is a transmembrane glycoprotein primarily expressed in intracellular compartments (e.g., lysosomes and melanosomes) in nonmalignant cells such as melanocytes, osteoclasts, and osteoblasts (Bachner et al. 2002; Ripoll et al. 2007; Tomihari et al. 2009). In hepatocellular carcinoma (Onaga et al. 2003), breast cancer (Rose et al. 2010; Rose and Siegel 2007), glioblastoma (Kuan et al. 2006), and melanoma (Tomihari et al. 2009; Tse et al. 2006), membrane GPNMP is overexpressed, making it a reasonable candidate for targeted therapeutics. GPNMB may also play a role in the inhibition of T cell activation by antigen-presenting cells (Chung et al. 2007a, b; Schwarzbich et al. 2012). Six of seven osteosarcoma xenografts also express GPNMB at the RNA level and by immunohistochemistry, whereas none of the rhabdomyosarcoma xenografts in the PPTP panel expressed GPNMB.

Glembatumumab vedotin is an antibody-drug conjugate (ADC) that combines an anti-GPNMB antibody with the antimitotic agent monomethyl auristatin E (vedotin) (Tse et al. 2006). When internalized, vedotin is released and results in cell cycle arrest and cell death (Carter and Senter 2008). In vitro glembatumumab vedotin showed cytotoxicity that was related to the level of GPNMB expression, and it induced complete regressions in GPNMB-expressing melanoma and breast cancer xenografts (Pollack et al. 2007; Rose et al. 2010; Tse et al. 2006). In the PPTP screen, glembatumumab vedotin induced statistically significant differences in event-free survival (EFS) distribution compared to control in each of the six osteosarcoma models studied. Three of six osteosarcoma xenografts demonstrated a maintained complete response. Two other xenografts showed progressive disease with growth delay, while the final xenograft showed progressive disease with no growth delay. Two of the osteosarcoma xenografts with maintained complete responses showed the highest GPNMB expression at the RNA level. Conversely, the xenograft with the lowest GPNMB mRNA expression had the poorest response to glembatumumab vedotin. Neither GPNMB-negative rhabdomyosarcomas examined responded to glembatumumab vedotin.

Historically, microtubule inhibitors have not been incorporated into standard neoadjuvant therapy regimens or in retrieval regimens for osteosarcoma. Limited single-agent data on vincristine in osteosarcoma is available from early studies (Sutow 1968; Sutow et al. 1971). Several subsequent single-arm and randomized trials combining vincristine with other conventional agents failed to clearly demonstrate a role for vincristine in neoadjuvant chemotherapy (Edmonson et al. 1984; Eilber et al. 1987; Krailo et al. 1987; Pratt et al. 1990; Rosen et al. 1981; Souhami et al. 1997). There have been few recent clinical trials of microtubule-targeted therapy although a response to vinorelbine was observed in one of five patients with osteosarcomas (Casanova et al. 2002). Currently, there are no planned clinical trials to evaluate this agent against osteosarcoma.

15.3 Targeted Inhibitors

15.3.1 IGF-1 Receptor Inhibitors

IGF-1 receptor has become a major focus for adult cancer therapeutics development with at least eight fully human or humanized antibodies in adult phase I or II clinical trials (Braczkowski et al. 2002; Cohen et al. 2005; Guerreiro et al. 2006; Kurmasheva and Houghton 2006; Sachdev and Yee 2006, 2007; Wang et al. 2005). These agents show specificity for the IGF-1R, blocking ligand binding, although they may also inhibit chimeric receptors formed through heterodimerization with the insulin receptor (IR). In preclinical cancer models, antibody-mediated downregulation of IGF-1R significantly retards proliferation of many tumors (Sachdev et al. 2003) and induces regressions when combined with cytotoxic agents (Cohen et al. 2005; Goetsch et al. 2005). These results are consistent with the significant literature that implicates IGF-1 signaling in survival of cells exposed to different cellular stresses (Kurmasheva and Houghton 2006). Several classes of small-molecule inhibitors of IGF-1R have been described, including tyrphostins, pyrrolopyrimidines (Mitsiades et al. 2004; Scotlandi et al. 2005), substituted benzimidazole derivatives (Haluska et al. 2006), and diarylureas (Gable et al. 2006). In contrast to the antibodies, small-molecule ATP-competitive IGF-1R inhibitors do not induce downregulation of the receptor (Sachdev et al. 2006), an effect that may be important for the activity of anti-IGF-1R directed antibody treatments (Jackson-Booth et al. 2003). In addition, in most cases these small-molecule inhibitors do not discriminate between the insulin receptor (IR) and the IGF-1R (Haluska et al. 2006; Wittman et al. 2007). As a consequence they may have pronounced effects on glucose homeostasis (hyperglycemia and hyperinsulinemia).

Deregulated insulin-like growth factor signaling through the type 1 receptor (IGF-1R) appears to be common to many childhood solid tumors and offers an important molecular target for pediatric therapeutics development. IGF-1R is a potent mediator of autocrine growth in Ewing sarcoma (Scotlandi et al. 1996, 1998). Cases of Ewing sarcoma with the type 1 EWS-FLI1 chimeric transcription factor are associated with an improved prognosis and with lower IGF-1R expression compared to cases with non-type 1 translocations (de Alava et al. 2000). EWS-FLI1 silencing leads to increased levels of insulin-like growth factor binding protein 3 gene (IGFBP-3), a major regulator of IGF-1 (Prieur et al. 2004). Additionally, IGF-1 is a mitogen for osteosarcoma cells (Bostedt et al. 2001; MacEwen et al. 2004; Pollak and Richard 1990).

The murine monoclonal antibody αIR-3 has demonstrated in vivo activity against rhabdomyosarcoma (Kalebic et al. 1994), and antisera to IGF-1 or IGF-2 significantly inhibited proliferation of Ewing sarcoma cells in vitro (Braczkowski et al. 2002). For SCH 717454 (robatumumab), in vivo testing has revealed marked growth inhibition against A2780, an aggressive ovarian carcinoma cell line (Wang et al. 2005). For CP-751,871 (figitumumab), another fully human anti-IGF-1R monoclonal antibody, in vivo growth inhibition was observed against several xenografts, including MCF7 (breast cancer), Colo-205 (colon cancer), and H460 lung cancer (Cohen et al. 2005). Two antibodies (SCH717545 and IMC-A12) were tested in the PPTP screen. Cumulative results indicate modest activity although complete regressions were observed in one of five Ewing sarcoma, one of six rhabdomyosarcoma, and two of six osteosarcoma models (overall response rate 4 of 32 tests [12.5 %]). Similarly, IGF-1R inhibition by R1507 induced tumor growth delays and improvement in event-free survival in four of six osteosarcoma xenograft tumor lines (Kolb et al. 2010). Of interest, R1507 induced a complete response in one model, whereas it had no efficacy against the model that responded to SCH717545, suggesting that each of the anti-IGF-1R antibodies may have individual characteristics.

Clinical studies also indicate some activity of IGF-1R-targeted antibodies in bone tumors as well as soft tissue sarcoma (Olmos et al. 2010; Pappo et al. 2011, 2014; Tolcher et al. 2009; Toretsky and Gorlick 2010). In Ewing sarcoma the response rate was ~10 % for each of the antibodies tested, similar to the predicted response rate from the PPTP xenograft models. However, in several studies there was a cohort of patients that had disease stabilization for several months. Because the IGF-1R-targeted antibodies showed relatively poor activity in adult malignancies, most have been withdrawn from clinical development. At least two antibodies (IMC-A12 [Imclone] and MK0646 [Merck]) are still in development, although the future of these antibodies, like those already abandoned, is uncertain (Yee 2012). Although the objective response rate is quite low, clear activity in both osteosarcoma and Ewing sarcoma has been demonstrated. Several preclinical studies have suggested that IGF-1R-targeted antibodies may have additive activity when combined with rapamycin (Kolb et al. 2012; Kurmasheva et al. 2009; Wan et al. 2007). Clinical studies combining cixutumumab and temsirolimus showed 12-week progression-free rates of 31 % and 35 % for IGF-1R-positive soft tissue sarcoma and bone sarcoma, respectively, although the progression-free rate was similar for patients with IGF-1R-negative tumor (39 %) (Schwartz et al. 2013). Similarly, regression of tumor >20 % was documented in 29 % of Ewing sarcoma patients, with prolonged stabilization of disease for 8–27 months (Naing et al. 2012). Signaling through the IGF-1R is also required for VEGF-driven proliferation and differentiation of human umbilical cord vascular endothelial cells (HUVECs) in vitro, and IGF-1R-targeting antibodies block angiogenesis in mouse models (Bid et al. 2012). Thus, in part, disease stabilization may be a result from the antiangiogenic activities of IGF-1R-targeted antibodies. The mechanisms for intrinsic or acquired resistance to IGF-1R-targeted antibodies are not well understood. Downregulation of IGF binding protein 2 (IGFBP2) has been reported to be associated with acquired resistance both in vitro and in vivo (Kang et al. 2013). Similarly, IGFBP ratios have been associated with sensitivity, where the IGFBP-5/IGFBP-4 expression ratio may serve as a surrogate biomarker of IGF pathway activation and predict sensitivity to anti-IGF-1R targeting (Becker et al. 2012). AXL expression was highly elevated in a subline of Rh41 rhabdomyosarcoma selected for resistance to the anti-IGF-1R antibody MAB391

(Huang et al. 2010). While MEDI-573, a ligand binding antibody with high affinity for binding IGF-2, had no single-agent activity, a combination of an IGF-1R-targeted antibody had some additive effects in several sarcoma xenograft models supporting the conjecture that tumor-secreted IGF-2 was responsible for circumventing the block on IGF-1R, signaling through the IR to maintain proliferation and angiogenesis (Bid et al. 2012, 2013). Thus, there appear to be multiple mechanisms associated with resistance to this class of agents.

There is less information on the activity of small-molecule inhibitors in models of bone tumors. The PPTP screen demonstrated some growth inhibition for Ewing sarcoma and osteosarcoma models treated with BMS-754807, but no regressions were reported (Kolb et al. 2011). Acquired resistance to BMS-754807 was attributed to amplification and overexpression of platelet-derived growth factor receptor α (PDGFRα), and knockdown of PDGFRα by small interfering RNA in Rh41-807R resensitized the cells to BMS-754807 (Huang et al. 2010). Huang et al. recently demonstrated that IGF-1R, IGF-1, and IGF-2 are highly expressed in cell lines sensitive to another IGF-1R inhibitor (BMS-536924), while IGF binding proteins (IGFBP-3 and IGFBP-6) are highly expressed in resistant cell lines. Overexpression of EGFR and downstream components of EGFR signaling was also noted in BMS-536924-resistant tumor lines (Huang et al. 2009). In hepatocellular carcinoma cell lines, HER3 activation by EGFR in response to IGR-1R inhibition seems to be one potential mechanism of resistance (Desbois-Mouthon et al. 2009). There are no available data on the activity of OSI-906 or LDK-378 (also an inhibitor of ALK) in bone tumor models.

15.3.2 mTOR Inhibitors

In mammalian cells, the serine/threonine kinase mTOR (target of rapamycin), a member of the PI3 kinase like kinase (PIKK) superfamily, exists in two complexes: mTORC1, comprising mTOR, raptor, PRAS40, and mLst8 (GβL), and mTORC2 (mTOR, rictor, Sin1, mLst8, mAvo3) (Guertin and Sabatini 2009; Wullschleger et al. 2006). Increasing evidence has implicated mTORC1 as a sensor that integrates extracellular and intracellular events, coordinating cell size (growth), proliferation, and survival. mTORC1 may directly or indirectly regulate cap-dependent translation initiation, membrane trafficking, protein degradation, ribosome biogenesis and tRNA synthesis, as well as transcription (Bjornsti and Houghton 2004; Wullschleger et al. 2006). mTORC1 signaling is negatively regulated by amino acid deficiency, hypoxia, DNA damage, and increased AMP levels, suppressing cap-dependent protein synthesis. Thus, mTORC1 in concert with the tuberous sclerosis complex (TSC) and Rheb appears to sense nutrient and growth factor status, as well as energy charge, and regulates progression from G1 to S phase. The mTORC2 complex phosphorylates Akt(Ser473) leading to its full activation and regulates F-actin and the cytoskeleton. Over the past few years, the role of mTOR complexes in tumorigenesis and survival has become apparent (Bjornsti and Houghton 2004; Wullschleger et al. 2006). Hence, inhibition of mTOR has become a focus for drug development (Guertin and Sabatini 2009). In epithelial cancers, such as breast and prostate, there is clear evidence that the PI3K/TOR pathway is activated through mutations (PI3K), loss of suppressors (PTEN), as well as amplification of growth factor receptors (Her2) that increase signaling flux through the pathway. Although signaling via IGF-1R activates the PI3K/TOR pathway, there is less compelling evidence that bone cancers are dependent or "addicted" to this pathway.

Rapamycin, a macrocyclic lactone antibiotic, is the prototypic allosteric inhibitor of mTOR. Rapamycin is a selective inhibitor of mTORC1 signaling, inhibits the proliferation of many tumor cell lines in vitro including cell lines derived from childhood cancers (Dilling et al. 1994; Houghton et al. 2008), and showed significant antitumor activity against syngeneic tumor models in the NCI in vivo screening program (Houchens et al. 1983). In the PPTP screen rapamycin induced significant differences in event-free survival (EFS) distribution in 28 of 36 solid tumor xenografts and in 5 of 8 ALL xeno-grafts with objective responses being observed in several panels including one complete response in an osteosarcoma model with undetectable IGF-1R (Houghton et al. 2008). Blockade of the mTOR pathway with rapamycin or its analog, temsirolimus, led to significant inhibition of experimental osteosarcoma lung metastasis in vivo, suggesting that blocking the mTOR/S6K1/4E-BP1 pathway may be an appropriate target for strategies to reduce tumor cell metastasis (Wan et al. 2005). A phosphorus-containing rapalog also inhibited growth and angiogenesis in two osteosarcoma models (Liu et al. 2013).

Rapalogs in general have shown only modest single-agent preclinical activity, predominantly in sarcoma and acute lymphoblastic leukemia models; thus, combinations have been explored, as described above for combination with IGF-1R-targeted antibodies. A combination of temsirolimus with zoledronic acid augmented the inhibition of cancer cell proliferation and led to a decrease in PI3K/mTOR signaling compared with either treatment alone and reduced tumor development in two murine models of osteoblastic or osteolytic osteosarcoma. Furthermore, zoledronic acid reversed temsirolimus resistance in osteosarcoma, limiting osteosarcoma cell growth when combined with everolimus (Ferrari and Palmerini 2007; Moriceau et al. 2010). Rapamycin potentiated the antitumor activity of both cyclophosphamide and vincristine in studies reported by the PPTP (Houghton et al. 2010a). For two Ewing sarcoma and one osteosarcoma models, a combination of rapamycin with vincristine, cisplatin, or cyclophosphamide was either additive or supra-additive in activity (Houghton et al. 2010a). Rapalogs also potentiate the effects of ionizing radiation in glioblastoma (Eshleman et al. 2002) and prostate cancer cells (Schiewer et al. 2012). Both rapamycin and AZD8055, a TOR kinase inhibitor, downregulate FANCD2, a protein involved in homologous recombination repair of DNA damage, and AZD8055 potentiates the effect of ionizing radiation in vitro and in xenograft models of rhabdomyosarcoma (Shen et al. 2013). The effect of TOR inhibitors on bone tumor response to ionizing radiation has not been reported, but the observation that inhibition of TOR downregulates FANCD2 in diverse cell lines and enhances tumor responses to ionizing radiation therapy suggests that this approach would be of some use for treatment of bone tumors.

Selective TOR kinase inhibitors have recently been developed. AZD8055 and MLN-0128, both ATP-competitive highly potent TOR kinase inhibitors, have been evaluated in the PPTP screen using daily dosing schedules (Kang et al. 2014; Lock et al. 2012). Both agents demonstrated very modest activity with some growth inhibition in several osteosarcoma and Ewing sarcoma models. Despite clear evidence of TOR kinase inhibition, as determined by the absence of detectable phospho-4E-BP1 and phospho-S6, there were no tumor regressions in any of the models where the drugs were tested. No combination studies have been reported for these drugs. Other agents that inhibit PI3K and Akt also had modest single-agent activity against the models in the PPTP screen (Gorlick et al. 2012; Houghton et al. 2010a; Reynolds et al. 2013), suggesting a lack of dependence on this pathway for bone tumors.

The rapamycin analogs (rapalogs) temsirolimus (CCI-779) and everolimus (RAD001) have been approved for treatment of refractory renal cell carcinoma (Hudes et al. 2007; Motzer et al. 2008), and temsirolimus demonstrates a high response rate against mantle cell lymphoma at relapse (Witzig et al. 2005). Both temsirolimus (Spunt et al. 2011) and everolimus (Fouladi et al. 2007) have completed phase I trials in pediatric patients. Both agents showed evidence of antitumor activity, although not in patients with bone sarcomas. Ridaforolimus did show activity with confirmed PR in two osteosarcoma patients, although the overall response rate in sarcoma was low (1.9 %) (Chawla et al. 2012). Phase I trials combining rapalogs with standard chemotherapy are ongoing. The combination of irinotecan, temozolomide, and temsirolimus demonstrated activity in patients with refractory Ewing sarcoma (Bagatell et al. 2014), and a combination of rapamycin (sirolimus) with vinblastine (Morgenstern et al. 2014) or bevacizumab (Piha-Paul et al. 2014) has shown activity but not in bone cancers. Temsirolimus has been combined with liposomal doxorubicin to treat adult patients with recurrent or refractory bone and soft tissue sarcoma (Thornton et al. 2013), based on the observation that at high concentrations rapamycin could sensitize TC-71 Ewing sarcoma ALDH^{High} "stem cells" to doxorubicin. Temsirolimus has also been combined with vinorelbine and cyclophosphamide for treatment of soft tissue sarcoma (NCT01222715). There are currently no trials with TOR kinase inhibitors being planned, although preclinical studies indicate that these agents may enhance radiation sensitivity.

15.3.3 Agents That Target EWS-FLI

Ewing sarcoma is characterized by the t(11;22) (q24;q12) chromosomal translocation, which joins the *EWS* gene located on chromosome 22 with the *FLI1* gene located on chromosome 11. The translocation fuses the 5′ portion of the EWSR1 gene on chromosome 22 to the 3′ portion of the FLI1 (friend leukemia integration locus-1) gene on chromosome 11 (Delattre et al. 1992; Zucman et al. 1992). FLI1 encodes the FLI protein, a member of the ETS family of transcription factors, and is involved in the control of cellular proliferation, development, and tumorigenesis (Hromas and Klemsz 1994). EWS-FLI binds DNA via its FLI-derived ETS domain and regulates gene expression through the EWS portion of the fusion. The validity of targeting EWS-FLI1 directly is demonstrated by the finding that RNAi-mediated downregulation of EWS-FLI1 increased apoptosis (Prieur et al. 2004). In addition, expression of EWS-FLI1 or EWS-ERG in NIH3T3 cells inhibits stress-induced apoptosis (Yi et al. 1997), while antisense inhibition of EWS-FLI increases susceptibility to chemotherapy-induced apoptosis in Ewing sarcoma cell lines.

15.3.3.1 Cytosine Arabinoside

Because EWS-FLI1 is a validated target, a screen was undertaken to identify drugs that would alter the expression profile of Ewing sarcoma cells in a manner similar to that found after RNAi-mediated suppression of EWS-FLI1. Screening a small-molecule library enriched for FDA-approved drugs identified the antileukemic drug cytosine arabinoside (Ara-C) as a modulator of EWS-FLI. Ara-C reduced EWS/FLI protein abundance and accordingly diminished cell viability and transformation. The Ewing sarcoma cell line used, A549, was more sensitive to Ara-C than several epithelial cancer lines derived from colon or breast carcinomas. In vivo, using the A673 xenograft, five daily treatments with Ara-C caused tumor regression. In contrast, none of six Ewing sarcoma xenograft models were sensitive to Ara-C in the PPTP evaluation, and Ewing sarcoma cells were greater than 20-fold less sensitive to Ara-C than a panel of acute lymphoblastic leukemia cell lines in vitro (Houghton et al. 2010b). Similar to the PPTP result, Ara-C given at the dose and schedule utilized in the phase II trial had minimal activity in the treatment of patients with relapsed or refractory Ewing sarcoma (DuBois et al. 2009). Although several reasons for the failure of Ara-C in treatment of Ewing sarcoma have been postulated, the observation that a panel of Ewing sarcoma cells are significantly less sensitive to Ara-C than ALL suggests that appropriate comparator cell lines to identify differential drug sensitivity are essential to accurately translating preclinical results to the clinic.

15.3.3.2 Mithramycin

Mithramycin is a cytotoxic agent that intercalates DNA possibly causing cross-linking in GC-rich promoter sequences and suppressing Src transcription after incubation of cells for 18 h at 50–100 nM (Remsing et al. 2003). In an early study, mithramycin was reported to have activity against Ewing sarcoma (Kofman et al. 1973). Mithramycin was identified in a high-throughput screen of more than 50,000 compounds for inhibition of EWS-FLI1 activity in TC32 Ewing sarcoma cells. The screen used a TC32 cell-based luciferase reporter screen using the EWS-FLI1-regulated NR0B1 promoter and a gene signature secondary screen to sort and prioritize "active" compounds. The lead compound, mithramycin, was characterized based on its ability to inhibit EWS-FLI1 activity in vitro using microarray

expression profiling, quantitative reverse transcription-polymerase chain reaction, and immunoblot analysis and in vivo using immunohistochemistry. Six-hour exposure to mithramycin (10–200 nM) inhibited NR0B1 promoter activity and at 100 nM inhibited expression of EWS-FLI1 downstream targets at the mRNA and protein levels. Mithramycin decreased the growth of Ewing sarcoma cells at half maximal inhibitory concentrations between 10 and 15 nM. Mithramycin suppressed the growth of two different Ewing xenograft tumors TC-32 and to a lesser extent TC-71 and prolonged the event-free survival of Ewing sarcoma xenograft-bearing mice by causing a decrease in mean tumor volume. In contrast, while mithramycin treatment suppressed the growth of the MNNG-HOS osteosarcoma model (no EWS-FLI1) similarly to TC-71, strangely, it did not increase event-free survival (Grohar et al. 2011). Differential cell sensitivity to mithramycin and several analogs was not determined in limited in vitro screening by the PPTP (Houghton, 2014). As mithramycin is a very potent cytotoxin, and drug concentrations that cause meaningful changes in transcription are far in excess of the IC_{50} concentrations, it is difficult to determine whether the antiproliferative or cytotoxic effects of mithramycin are indeed the consequence of altered EWS-FLI1 activity.

15.3.3.3 YK-4-279

Transcription factors, such as EWS-FLI1, lack enzymatic activity and because of their intrinsically disordered domains (Darnell 2002) have been considered "undruggable." However, a small molecule, YK-4-279, was identified that blocks the interaction of EWS-FLI1 with RNA helicase A (RHA), thought to be important for EWS-FLI1 transcriptional activity (Erkizan et al. 2009; Toretsky et al. 2006). EWS-FLI1 binds RHA in a unique region that is not occupied by other transcriptional or RNA metabolism proteins (Toretsky et al. 2006); hence, potentially disrupting the interaction between EWS-FLI1 and RHA could suppress EWS-FLI1 activity. YK-4-279 was identified by screening an NCI small-molecule library using surface plasmon resonance binding to an EWS-FLI1 peptide. This agent reduced growth of CHP-100 Ewing sarcoma xenografts but had no activity against a prostate cancer model that does not express EWS-FLI1. Further studies showed that it is the *S* enantiomer that is the active component (Barber-Rotenberg et al. 2012) and that administration using continuous infusions of YK-4-279 in Ewing sarcoma xenografts in an athymic nude rat model optimized antitumor activity (Hong et al. 2014). Thus, this agent is continuing to be developed as an Ewing sarcoma-specific therapeutic.

15.3.3.4 Poly(ADP-Ribose) Polymerase (PARP) Inhibitors

The observation that cells defective in homologous recombination as a consequence of mutation in *BRCA1* or *BRCA2* are hypersensitive to inhibitors of poly(ADP-ribose) polymerase (PARP) has spurred the development of PARP inhibitors. Early clinical trials, largely focused on breast cancer, have demonstrated a high frequency of tumor responses in BRCA-mutant patients (Fong et al. 2010; Tutt et al. 2010). In the absence of functional homologous recombination, cells become dependent upon base excision repair (BER) for repair of DNA single-strand breaks and repair of apurinic sites within DNA. PARP-1 and PARP-2 play an essential role in BER, and enhanced cytotoxicity associated with PARP inhibition correlates closely with PARP-1 binding to the 5′-deoxyribose phosphate group-containing BER intermediate (Horton and Wilson 2013). Even in the presence of an inhibitor, PARP binds damaged DNA, and it is considered that the inactive-DNA-bound PARP-1 is persistent, inhibiting the BER process. Inhibition of PARP-1 catalytic activity may result in trapping of the enzyme on DNA, as catalytic inhibitors prevent dissociation of PARP from DNA. Dissociation of the enzyme from DNA is required for completion of DNA repair (Murai et al. 2012). The cytotoxicity of inhibited PARP bound to DNA is linked to formation of replication-dependent DNA double-strand breaks and induction of both p53-dependent and p53-independent cell deaths (Nguyen et al. 2011). PARP-1 and PARP-2 knockout mice have

severe deficiencies in DNA repair and increased sensitivity to alkylating agents or ionizing radiation (Masutani et al. 2000).

Recently, a systematic screen to identify biomarkers of drug sensitivity identified Ewing sarcoma cells as being hypersensitive to inhibitors of PARP (Garnett et al. 2012). Simultaneously, another report (Brenner et al. 2012) proposed that Ewing sarcoma cells were hypersensitive to PARP inhibitors as a consequence of EWS-FLI1 or EWS-ERG binding PARP1, mediated by the ETS DNA-binding domain (Brenner et al. 2011). PARP1 may also be positively regulated by EWS-FLI1, as the ETS transcription factor regulates this gene (Soldatenkov et al. 1999), and maintain the expression of PARP1 that is required for EWS-FLI1-mediated transcription. Thus, hypothetically, inhibition of PARP1, in the context of EWS-FLI1, would reduce EWS-FLI1-mediated transcription and induce apoptosis. In addition to its role in BER, PARP1 is also involved in transcription through remodeling of chromatin by PARylating histones and relaxing chromatin structure, thus allowing transcription complexes to access genes. Of note, while cells with EWS-FLI1 expression were more sensitive to the PARP inhibitor olaparib, the single-agent activity against the RD-ES Ewing sarcoma xenograft was quite modest (53 % inhibition of tumor growth). Similar results were obtained with talazoparib (BMN-673), a potent stereoselective PARP1/2 inhibitor when tested across the in vitro and in vivo panels of solid tumors and acute leukemia models in the PPTP (Smith et al. 2015). In vitro, Ewing sarcoma cell lines were significantly more sensitive to talazoparib than other cell lines. The in vitro results showing hypersensitivity of Ewing sarcoma cells compared to other cell types extend previous observations regarding the relationship between *SLFN11* expression and the in vitro activity of PARP inhibitors like talazoparib to childhood cancer cell lines (Murai et al. 2014b). The PPTP results suggest that the primary effect of *SLFN11* expression is in promoting a cytotoxic rather than a cytostatic response to PARP inhibition. Among the PPTP cell lines, *SLFN11* expression was significantly higher for the Ewing cell lines providing one mechanism that may contribute to the preferential response of Ewing cell lines to PARP inhibitors. The single-agent in vivo BMN673 antitumor activity against 43 solid tumor and ALL xenograft models was modest activity with progressive disease in all five Ewing sarcoma xenografts. Expanded testing demonstrated no meaningful tumor inhibition in ten Ewing sarcoma xenografts.

As discussed above, it was thought that PARP1 inhibitors potentiate the activity of chemotherapy agents through their inhibition of the catalytic activity PARP1, leading to accumulation of DNA single-strand breaks (Plummer 2010). However, recent studies have indicated that some PARP1 inhibitors have a second mechanism of action related to their ability to tightly trap PARP1 to DNA at sites of DNA single-strand breaks (Kedar et al. 2012; Murai et al. 2012). The PARP-DNA complexes are more cytotoxic than unrepaired DNA single-stand breaks caused by inhibition of PARP enzymatic activity (Murai et al. 2012). The ability of PARP inhibitors to trap PARP is unrelated to their potency in inhibiting PARP1 enzymatic activity, and the inhibitors differ in their potency at PARP trapping with talazoparib being the most potent and veliparib being the least potent (Murai et al. 2012, 2014a). Chemotherapy agents likewise differ in their ability to induce PARP1 trapping, with methylating agents such as methyl methanesulfonate (MMS) and temozolomide being highly effective and with agents like camptothecins, cisplatin, or etoposide being ineffective (Murai et al. 2012, 2014a, c). This variability is consistent with a failure to demonstrate synergy when olaparib was combined with cyclophosphamide and topotecan in xenograft models (Norris et al. 2014).

Despite the relatively modest activity of PARP inhibitors as single agents, there is marked synergy when combined with temozolomide (Brenner et al. 2012). Talazoparib dramatically increased the cytotoxic potency of temozolomide up to 70-fold, with marked potentiation in three of four Ewing sarcoma lines (30–50-fold), as well as some leukemia cell lines. In vivo, talazoparib potentiated the toxicity of temozolomide, and maximum tolerated doses of temozolomide, when combined with low-dose or high-dose BMN-673, demonstrated significant synergism

against five of ten Ewing sarcoma xenografts. Of interest is that four Ewing sarcoma xenograft models had poor responses to the combinations, yet all express the type 1 EWS-FLI1 fusion. In contrast to the results with Ewing sarcoma xenografts, there was little antitumor activity against four osteosarcoma xenografts when high-dose BMN-673 was combined with lower dose temozolomide, further emphasizing the distinctive sensitivity of Ewing sarcoma to this combination. PARP1 inhibition by RNAi or olaparib treatment also uniquely sensitized Ewing sarcoma cell lines to ionizing radiation, and this effect was abrogated when EWS-FLI1 was silenced (Lee et al. 2013). A combination of olaparib with 4 Gy radiation effectively halted growth of the SK-N-MC Ewing sarcoma xenograft in mice.

At least seven PARP inhibitors are in clinical development. Multiple PARP inhibitors have shown single-agent activity against cancers arising in patients with *BRCA1* or *BRCA2* mutations (De Bono et al. 2013; Kaufman et al. 2013; Sandhu et al. 2013), and phase III clinical trials are ongoing for ovarian cancer (olaparib, NCT01874353; olaparib, NCT01844986; niraparib, NCT01847274; rucaparib, NCT01968213) and breast cancer (olaparib, NCT02000622; olaparib, NCT02032823; niraparib, NCT01905592; talazoparib, NCT01945775). However, a recent study failed to demonstrate single-agent activity for olaparib in adult patients with recurrent or metastatic Ewing sarcoma (Choy et al. 2013). Two combination trials with temozolomide are currently accruing patients: niraparib with temozolomide in previously treated, incurable Ewing Sarcoma (NCT02044120) for patients 13 years and older and talazoparib with temozolomide in patients 13 months to 30 years of age (NCT02116777).

15.4 Immunotherapy

Improvements in traditional pediatric cancer treatments such as chemotherapy and radiation have been made over the past several decades through the use of clinical trials, with resultant increases in survival rates for select cancer subtypes. Advancement using traditional cytotoxic chemotherapies for pediatric bone cancers, however, has plateaued, and toxicities remain substantially problematic (Smith et al. 2010b). Therefore, research for pediatric malignancies has shifted its focus to not only increase survival rates but to tailor therapies to specifically target cancer cells, thus sparing healthy cells from toxicity. Advances in the knowledge of the molecular biology and genetics of tumors have led to the development of drugs targeted at particular pathways involved in tumorigenesis, growth, and metastasis. Further understanding of tumor immunology has also resulted in the discovery of several promising candidates for therapeutic targeting. Finally, after decades of unfulfilled promise, cancer immunotherapies have come to culmination, with numerous FDA-approved products now available and several more exhibiting potential therapeutic aptitude in clinical trials for both adult and pediatric cancers. In fact, immune-based therapies are gaining traction with increasing reports of antitumor efficacy in adult cancers and have shown promise in liquid tumors such as leukemia in the pediatric realm. Presently utilized immunotherapeutic approaches include the infusion of cytokines, adoptive transfer of immunologic effector cells, vaccines, and T cells engineered to express chimeric receptors and bispecific antibodies. A plethora of current research is aimed at the immunologic microenvironment of solid tumors, with the expectation that these targeted therapies will ultimately provide the answer to the stalled success burdening the pediatric bone tumor world.

Suspicion that the immune system's response may play an important role in the eventual rejection of tumors is not novel. In the late nineteenth century, surgical oncologist William Coley introduced intratumoral injections of "Coley's toxin" in sarcoma patients. This potent infectious-based toxin induced a significant systemic immune response, sometimes leading to the eventual death of the patient. However, it was found that for those patients capable of overcoming the infection, the responses to their cancers were improved (Coley 1933). This may have been the first notion that the immune system may play a role in the fight against cancer, and inducing an immune response in cancer patients may be beneficial. Another, more recent immunologic-based

treatment for sarcoma patients is muramyl tripeptide (MTP), derived from bacterial cell wall and thought to induce macrophage activity. Inhaled MTP was used in an effort to eradicate micrometastatic lung disease via provoking an inflammatory response to the substance, the resultant recruitment of immune cells, and therefore the death of tumor cells (Meyers and Chou 2014). Studied in the COG 7921/INT-0133 (POG-9351) protocol, it was found that patients who received MTP had an increased 6-year OS (78 %) compared to patients who did not receive MTP (70 %) ($p = 0.03$) (Meyers et al. 2005). In a more recent study, NCT00631631 in high-risk osteosarcoma patients was completed in October of 2012, with results currently pending at the time of this writing.

Discoveries of potential immunologic targets on pediatric bone tumors are being reported frequently. Cancer testis antigens (CTAs) are relatively recently detected proteins expressed on several malignancies. Some of these are highly immunogenic and represent possible immunotherapy targets (Akers et al. 2010; Hofmann et al. 2008; Orentas et al. 2012b). Genes encoding cancer testis antigens are expressed in germ cells of the testis and ovary and/or the placenta and also in tumors, with two or less non-germline normal tissues exhibiting expression (Akers et al. 2010). Although highly expressed in testis, CTA genes display heterogeneous expression and are therefore categorized as testis restricted, testis/brain restricted, or testis selective (Hofmann et al. 2008). Over 265 CTA genes have been described to date (Dobrynin et al. 2013). There exist non-CTA antigens in pediatric cancers as well, including differentiation antigens and oncogenes, some of which are already incorporated as targets in immunotherapeutic trials (Orentas et al. 2012a).

Some studies have focused on the integration of immunotherapies into a multimodal regimen for the treatment of pediatric high-risk sarcomas. It was demonstrated that this approach using consolidative immunotherapy results in significantly improved 5-year overall survival (43 %) versus that for patients who did not receive consolidative immunotherapy (15 %) (Mackall et al. 2008). Patients who received immunotherapy were noted to experience minimal toxicity as well.

15.4.1 Cytokines

Cell signaling molecules, the cytokines, include chemokines, interferons (IFNs), interleukins (ILs), and tumor necrosis factor. These molecules serve to regulate the immune system through activation, suppression, proliferation, and apoptotic signaling. Cytokine-based immunotherapies have also been reported to enhance the antigen-nonspecific effects of memory T cells (Tietze et al. 2012). Cytokines including GM-CSF, IL-2, IL-7, IL-12, IL-15, IL-18, and IL-21 have been utilized for recent immunotherapy clinical trials in patients with advanced cancers (Lee and Margolin 2011). Unfortunately, systemic administration of these agents can yield nonspecific immune activation and potentially significant toxicities, including autoimmunity (Lechner et al. 2011).

15.4.1.1 Interferons (IFNs)

The IFNs are characterized by their binding abilities to either type I, II, or III receptors. Type I IFNs, consisting of IFNα and IFNβ, are secreted by most somatic cells and are chiefly involved in antiviral cellular immune responses via activation of the JAK-STAT signaling pathway (Lee and Margolin 2011). As a result, they activate cytotoxic T lymphocytes (CTLs), natural killer (NK) cells, and macrophages and, in addition, induce the maturation of dendritic cells and upregulate major histocompatibility complex (MHC) class I expression, resulting in increased tumoral antigen presentation (Lee and Margolin 2011). Type I IFNs also can induce antiangiogenic and apoptotic effects.

IFNα is the only approved adjuvant therapy for patients with high-risk stage II or III melanomas, based upon clinical trials with evidence of improved disease-free survival. It is also approved for the treatment of some hematologic malignancies and AIDS-related Kaposi's sarcoma and used in combinations for other cancers. It has shown efficacy against hairy cell leukemia and chronic myelogenous leukemia as well, though relapses after therapy were common (Lee and Margolin 2011). Toxicities of IFNα are dose related and seem to be mostly self-limiting.

Constitutional symptoms of fatigue, fever, headache, GI upset, and myalgias are reported to occur in >80 % of patients. Hepatic transaminitis, marrow suppression including thrombocytopenia, leukopenia, and neutropenia are relatively common. Psychiatric manifestations including depression, often serious, confusion, and mania are possible. Autoimmune disease development has been reported (Lee and Margolin 2011).

IFNβ demonstrates more potent antiproliferative effects than IFNα in preclinical cancer models. However, its low bioavailability and persistent side effects limit its therapeutic usefulness (Lee and Margolin 2011).

IFNγ, the only type II IFN, also works through the JAK-STAT pathway (Lee and Margolin 2011). It activates macrophages and induces increased antigen presentation by a variety of ways. Firstly, it upregulates MHC class I, MHC class II, and costimulatory molecule expression on antigen-presenting cells (APCs). Secondly, it causes changes within the proteasome. In addition to improved antigenic epitope presentation, IFNγ also promotes CD4+ T cellular differentiation toward a Th1 phenotype. Its clinical usefulness is limited, however, due to its narrow therapeutic index (Lee and Margolin 2011).

The recently described type III interferons, consisting of IFN-y1, IFN-y2, and IFN-y3, have not yet been established as therapeutically relevant. Notably, their receptor expression is limited to only cells of epithelial origin (Lee and Margolin 2011).

15.4.1.2 IL-2 and Family

IL-2 and its family members (IL-4, IL-7, IL-9, IL-15, and IL-21) are potent T cell signaling molecules that result in the proliferation and activation of CD4+ and CD8+ T cells and NK cells. IL-2 has been shown to suppress T cells through the competitive activation of Tregs, thereby characterizing it as a regulatory cytokine and mediator of the overall T cell immune response. Currently, IL-2 is utilized clinically in the treatment of patients with metastatic melanoma and metastatic clear cell renal carcinoma (Lechner et al. 2011; Lee and Margolin 2011) and in pediatric tumors as an adjunctive therapy against neuroblastoma. Systemic IL-2 therapy invariably leads to untargeted immune stimulation. Side effects include severe inflammatory responses, with capillary leak syndrome (hypotension, tachycardia, peripheral edema, pulmonary edema) being the most prominent. Other symptoms include fever, chills, fatigue, GI upset, and hepatic transaminitis.

In the treatment of pediatric bone tumor patients, NCT00001564, a pilot study of tumor-specific peptide vaccination and IL-2 with or without autologous T cell transplantation in recurrent pediatric sarcomas, IL-2 is used as an adjunct to other immunotherapeutic approaches. This trial conducted by the NCI was opened in December of 1996 and closed in October of 2007. Results are currently still pending at the time of this writing.

IL-7, one of the IL-2-related cytokines, also influences T cell proliferation and survival. It has been shown to selectively expand CTLs over Treg populations. Early phase clinical trials have shown IL-7 to be well tolerated. IL-15 promotes T cell proliferation and activation and supports the persistence of memory CD8+ T cells. IL-21 promotes T cell proliferation and enhancement of CTL and NK cell cytotoxicity. Both of these have shown modest preliminary results in early phase clinical trials in adults with non-bony tumors (Lee and Margolin 2011).

15.4.1.3 IL-6

IL-6 is known to mediate inflammation and causes stem cell differentiation. It has been shown to play a role in cancer pathogenesis, with its overexpression correlating with poorer prognosis. With the recent use of CAR T cells in clinical trials, it was found that the cytokine storm elicited was highly attributable to IL-6 secretion. Tocilizumab, a monoclonal antibody against the IL-6 receptor, has been demonstrated to reverse this phenomenon clinically (Teachey et al. 2013). Recent data suggest that IL-6 and IL-8 signaling may play a role in osteosarcoma metastasis (Bid et al. 2014), raising the possibility that agents disrupting these cytokines or their downstream signaling pathways may be worthy of testing in future clinical trials.

15.4.1.4 IL-12

IL-12 is produced in response to antigenic stimulation, with subsequent IFNγ production. It serves as a T cell and NK cell growth factor and promotes the Th1 phenotype differentiation of CD4+ T cells while enhancing cytotoxicity of CTLs. It reportedly provokes antiangiogenic effects as well. IL-12 has been evaluated in metastatic melanoma patients with poor overall results as a monotherapy but slightly improved results when combined with other cytokine therapy. Its effects seem to be dose and schedule-dependent, with notable induction of IL-10 as one of its therapeutic downfalls.

15.4.1.5 IL-18

IL-18 is known to stimulate NK cells and CTLs to secrete IFNγ, enhancing their cytotoxicity. It also serves to activate macrophages. Its safety profile has been documented in phase I clinical trials, but clinical responses have been modest thus far.

15.4.1.6 GM-CSF

GM-CSF is known to mediate hematopoiesis and monocyte/macrophage differentiation. It stimulates myelopoiesis and promotes dendritic cell maturation and activation. Its ability to stimulate immune responses has been demonstrated in several tumor models and shows promising results both when used alone and in combination with other immunotherapeutic agents. A recombinant version of this molecule is FDA approved for use to decrease time of neutropenia and thereby reduce infection risk following chemotherapy and to mobilize progenitor cells to peripheral blood for leukapheresis. As a single agent, it has shown to have antitumor effects when injected directly into metastatic melanoma lesions (Lee and Margolin 2011).

15.4.2 Adoptive Transfer of Immunologically Active Cells

The infusion of autologous immune cells has been studied in several cancer types. Whether it be NK cells or T cells, all have been shown to have some efficacy against solid tumors. The procedure can be quite lengthy, costly, and complex and involves the harvesting of a patient's cells, usually through apheresis. This is followed by priming of the cells with tumor antigens, expansion of the population in vitro, and reintroduction into the patient. The result is an HLA-matched infusion of tumor-specific activated immune cells and the possibility of the production of memory cells as well. Cytokine storm has been seen with infusion in these patients, and the infused cells have been shown to reach exhaustion and die off quickly in vivo.

Preclinically, activity of patient-derived cytokine-induced killer cells has been shown to be effective against autologous bone sarcomas (Sangiolo et al. 2014). Among pediatric bone tumors, Ewing sarcoma has been demonstrated to be susceptible to expanded NK cells (Cho et al. 2010). Osteosarcoma cells have also been shown to be sensitive to both allogeneic and autologous IL-15-induced NK cells (Buddingh et al. 2011). T cells primed against tumor antigens such as HER-2 have been demonstrated to target osteosarcomas expressing that antigen (Rainusso et al. 2012). $\gamma\delta$ T cell-based immunotherapy for osteosarcoma has also been shown to improve efficacy for treatment of osteosarcoma (Li 2013). Currently open clinical trials include NCT02100891, a phase II STIR trial of haploidentical transplant and donor natural killer cells for patients with high-risk solid tumors including Ewing sarcoma, opened in March of 2014.

15.4.3 Vaccines

Several versions of cancer vaccines have been developed, all of which expose the patient to tumor antigens with intent of inducing an antitumoral cellular immune response in situ and the generation of memory cells (Orentas et al. 2012a). Several ex vivo and in vivo versions of vaccines have been studied in which antigen-presenting cells are exposed either to peptides known to be expressed on the patient's tumor or whole autologous tumor lysates. These vaccines are often combined with immunologic adjuvants to further boost the immune response. Vaccine types encompass whole tumor cell vaccines, known antigen vaccines, DNA-based vaccines, and vector-based vaccines.

Whole tumor vaccines use irradiated autologous whole tumor cells. An advantage to this approach is that several antigenic epitopes may be present and stimulate a multimodal T cell repertoire. In addition, there is no need to identify tumor-specific antigens using whole tumor cells, making this an attractive approach for tumor types for which an antigen is unknown. Antigen vaccines use one or a few antigens rather than whole tumor cells, often combining several antigens in hopes of getting a stronger response. This vaccine type requires known tumor antigens. DNA vaccines use vectors given protein antigen-encoding DNA. Vector-based vaccines may be used to deliver more than one cancer antigen at a time. These are easier and less expensive to make than their counterparts. Dendritic cell vaccines can be either autologous or allogeneic. Dendritic cell-based immunotherapy has been reported to be a feasible, well-tolerated, and promising approach in the treatment of children with refractory malignant tumors (Suminoe et al. 2009). However, an early phase study of autologous dendritic cell vaccination was recently evaluated in patients with relapsed osteosarcoma and was found to be safe and feasible, but without evidence of much clinical benefit (Himoudi et al. 2012). Fusion of tumor cells with dendritic cells is also an effective method for introducing tumor antigens to dendritic cells, and this vaccine type has been shown to be a successful way to stimulate autologous T cells. Antitumor effects have been demonstrated using this vaccine type against osteosarcoma cells (Yu et al. 2005).

As of this writing, only one dendritic cell vaccine is FDA approved, a vaccine for hormone-resistant advanced stage prostate cancer (sipuleucel-T or Provenge) (Palucka and Banchereau 2013). This vaccine uses dendritic cells exposed to prostatic acid phosphatase (PAP) and has been shown to extend patient's lives by an average of 4 months. Side effects include fever, chills, fatigue, back and joint pain, nausea, and headache. Currently open vaccine trials include NCT01522820, targeting patients with NY-ESO-1 expressing solid tumors.

15.4.4 Checkpoint Inhibitors

Despite progress in immune-based therapies, there are several unresolved limitations to T cell-mediated therapies for solid tumors. Interference of T cell-facilitated elimination of cancer cells may occur due to several factors, such as decrease in access to tumor cells and T cell suppression. T cells may be physically excluded from tumors by abnormal tumor vascularization, and several clinical trials are currently in progress which target tumor pro-angiogenic factors. In addition, T cells are subject to intrinsic regulation (such as granule content) and extrinsic factors (such as the presence of suppressor cells or suppressive chemokines and cytokines) (Palucka and Banchereau 2013). Multiple studies have considered the tumor microenvironment as an entity in itself, operating as its own individual milieu independently of the surrounding host environment. Even more interesting is the commonly accepted notion that this microenvironment influences the efficacy of the host system to clear cancer cells, either through the stimulation of pro-tumoral cytokines or through the signaling of host immunosuppressive mechanisms, such as in the recruitment of myeloid-derived suppressor cells. Immunoediting, a tumor's ability to manipulate its microenvironment through tumor-derived cytokines, allows tumors to evolve and thus continued evasion of the immune response.

15.4.4.1 CTLA-4 Blockade

There are currently several studies looking at inhibitors of critical T cell "checkpoints" such as PD-1 and CTLA-4. In adult cancers such as melanoma, antibodies which block these receptors have shown encouraging results (Ott et al. 2013). The first approved antibody that blocks such immunoregulatory mechanisms, ipilimumab, is directed against CTLA-4, the T cell downregulatory molecule that normally prevents autoimmunity and allows self-tolerance. Ipilimumab prolongs T cell activation and promotes T cell proliferation, thus in effect "cutting the breaks" on the antitumoral adaptive immune response. Several phase III clinical trials demonstrated significant increases in survival rates for advanced stage melanoma patients (Kirkwood et al. 2012). Another anti-CTLA-4 antibody, tremelimumab, has also shown promising clinical activity in advanced melanoma patients. Currently, clinical trials using these agents are expanding to include other immunomodulatory agents such as IFNα (Kirkwood et al. 2012).

15.4.4.2 PD-1 and PD-L1 Blockade

PD-1, an inhibitory receptor in the same family as CTLA-4, is expressed on B cells, monocytes, activated T cells, and Treg cells (Kirkwood et al. 2012). Its presence has been implicated in T cell anergy and thus tumor immune escape (Kirkwood et al. 2012). Its ligands, PD-L1 and PD-L2, are expressed on peripheral tissues to suppress self-reactive lymphocytes and are variably expressed on APCs and induce T cell anergy or apoptosis. PD-Ls expressed on tumors can function to regulate Tregs, resulting in tumor-induced immune suppression. The presence of PD-L1 on tumor cells has been found to be inversely correlated with tumor-infiltrating lymphocytes and prognostic outcome in several cancer subtypes (Kirkwood et al. 2012). In earlier development, anti-PD-1-targeting monoclonal antibodies appear to be a promising immunoregulatory checkpoint blockade strategy, with PD-1 blockade enhancing tumor-specific CTL function and proliferation in melanomas (Kirkwood et al. 2012). MDX-1106 (ONO-4538) has been tested in a phase I and II studies for patients with relapsed or refractory solid tumors. No significant toxicities were observed and some objective responses were observed (Kirkwood et al. 2012). MDX-1105 (BMS-936559), a monoclonal antibody targeting PD-L1, is currently being tested in a phase I study for patients with solid tumors (Kirkwood et al. 2012).

15.4.4.3 Other Immunoregulatory Regulators

Other immunomodulatory regulator targets include those against CD40, a costimulatory molecule involved in the licensing of APCs and widely expressed by immune cells and multiple cancer subtypes alike, OX40 and OX40L, which function to enhance T cell expansion, survival, and cytokine production, and CD137 (4-1BB) and its ligand (Kirkwood et al. 2012).

15.4.5 Antibodies and CAR T Cells

Monoclonal antibody-based immunotherapy against tumor antigens has been shown to be an effective treatment method for both hematologic malignancies and solid tumors (Kirkwood et al. 2012). Antibodies function in part by binding their target antigen with the hypervariable region and engaging effector cells with their constant region, killing the target cell by stimulating antibody-dependent cellular cytotoxicity. Alternatively, more recently engineered bispecific T cell engager (BiTE) antibodies link the target cell and the immune cell with two separate but linked hypervariable regions. Similarly, CAR T cells are another strategy to direct effector cells to tumor cells. Early studies suggest both of these approaches have activity in certain leukemias, but their efficacy for solid tumors is less clear. Barriers to therapeutic efficacy include trafficking of the cells to the tumor and the immunosuppressive microenvironment. Nevertheless, preclinical studies show some efficacy and several clinical trials are already underway. Side effects observed thus far with monoclonal antibody therapies have been mild, with most representing allergic or hypersensitivity reactions (Kirkwood et al. 2012).

15.4.5.1 Anti-GD2

Targeting the ganglioside GD2 using a monoclonal antibody improved survival for patients with neuroblastoma (Yu et al. 2010). GD2 is expressed on Ewing sarcomas (Kailayangiri et al. 2012; Lipinski et al. 1986) and osteosarcoma (Roth et al. 2014). Several clinical trials of anti-GD2 antibodies, bispecific antibodies that recognize GD2 and CD3, and anti-GD2 CAR T cells in GD2+ sarcomas that include osteosarcoma and Ewing sarcoma are currently ongoing, and newer generations such as antibodies altered to elicit fewer side effects or conjugated to molecules such as IL-2 for improved efficacy are in development.

15.4.5.2 Anti-RANKL

The receptor activator of nuclear factor-kappaB (RANK) is a member of the tumor necrosis factor receptor family, and its activation by RANK ligand (RANKL) drives osteoclast development. The RANK/RANKL axis was shown to be active in mouse and human osteosarcoma cells (Gollamudi et al. 2010; Wittrant et al. 2006), and RANK expression is associated with a worse prognosis in patients (Bago-Horvath et al. 2014). Interruption of the pathway with an RANKL-Fc suggested it is important in cell migration and metastasis and tumor growth (Akiyama et al. 2010). Denosumab is an anti-RANKL antibody developed for treatment of osteoporosis. Its utility alone or in combination therapy for osteosarcoma has not been tested.

15.4.5.3 Anti-IGF-R1

As described above, various renditions of monoclonal antibodies directed against the human insulin-like growth factor-1 receptor (IGF-1R) have been developed and tested in solid tumors. Preclinically, cetuximab was shown to potentiate the cytotoxicity of resting NK cells against osteosarcoma (Pahl et al. 2012). In the pediatric realm, cixutumumab was found to be well tolerated but showed limited activity as a single agent in children with refractory solid tumors. Combinatorial studies with other IGF pathway inhibitors are currently ongoing (Weigel et al. 2014).

15.4.5.4 Anti-HER2

Human epidermal growth factor receptor 2 (HER2) is overexpressed in osteosarcoma and has been reported as a biomarker to predict poor therapeutic response and decreased survival (Ebb et al. 2012). A phase II trial conducted by Children's Oncology Group using the already established monoclonal antibody against HER2, trastuzumab, combined with conventional chemotherapy in metastatic osteosarcoma patients was shown to provide no significant improvement in outcomes (Ebb et al. 2012). Trastuzumab's therapeutic significance in osteosarcomas currently remains uncertain.

15.4.5.5 CAR T Cells

Chimeric antigen receptors, or CARs, are engineered T cell receptors with engrafted monoclonal antibody specificity and represent a means to produce a large number of cancer-specific T cells available for adoptive transfer. Because CAR Ts express single-chain engineered T cell receptors, they are capable of bypassing the MHC class I restriction of other T cell therapies. Three generations of CARs have been developed to date, with each new generation improving on its transmembrane and intramembranous costimulatory molecular domains. No single configuration has yet been accepted as universally optimal, making clinical applications unique and difficult to compare (Marr et al. 2012). Phase I clinical studies of CAR Ts have shown efficacy in leukemia (Kochenderfer et al. 2012), with a fraction of the T cells in these patients displaying a memory phenotype as well (Louis et al. 2011; Xu et al. 2014). Utilizing CAR technology against solid tumors has proven to be more challenging, as the tumor microenvironment is thought to play a role in the prevention of significant responses to CAR therapy (Han et al. 2013; Kakarla et al. 2013). Several antigenic targets are being used to arm CAR T cells, including those relevant for pediatric bone tumors, HER2 and GD2. NCT02107963 is a phase I clinical trial conducted by the NCI using anti-GD2 CARs in pediatric patients with non-neuroblastoma GD2+ solid tumors, opened in February 2014.

15.4.5.6 BiTE Cells

Bispecific T cell engagers, or BiTEs, are fusion proteins of two single-chain variable fragments (scFv) of different antibodies linked by a single peptide chain. One scFv binds T cells via the CD3 receptor, while the other scFv binds tumor cells via a tumor-specific antigen. These are used as a means to direct host CTLs against cancer cells independent of MHC class I expression or the presence of costimulatory molecules. However, this MHC-independent approach requires a known antigenic target. For example, blinatumomab (MT103) is an anti-CD19 (B cell surface molecule) BiTE used in the treatment of non-Hodgkin's lymphoma and acute lymphoblastic lymphoma (NCT00274742) and has several studies recruiting for use in acute leukemias (NCT01466179, NCT02000427, NCT02013167, NCT01471782). Once again, the tumor microenvironment poses an obstacle for the treatment of solid tumors which is not experienced with liquid tumors using this technology. Nonetheless, currently open clinical trials for pediatric bone tumors using BiTE therapies include NCT02173093, opened in July 2014. This is a phase I/II trial for pediatric patients with neuroblastoma and GD2-positive tumors such as osteosarcoma using OKT3 X humanized 3 F8 bispecific antibodies (GD2Bi).

15.5 Virotherapy

The use of viruses to lytically infect and kill tumor cells has long been sought as a cancer treatment strategy (Kelly and Russell 2007). In general, such viruses fall into two broad categories: wild-type, nonpathogenic viruses and attenuated, pathogenic viruses. It is becoming increasingly clear that in addition to direct lytic infection, the so-called oncolytic viruses can induce antitumor T cell immunity directed against tumor-associated antigens (Kaufman et al. 2010), in some cases by inducing an "immunogenic cell death" (Workenhe and Mossman 2014). Recent evidence suggests a third mechanism of tumor destruction induced by virus infection, production of a diffusible cytokine storm involving such proteins as IFNβ, TNFα, and TRAIL, which is particularly important for killing nearby but uninfected tumor cells (Beug et al. 2014). Finally, viruses can be engineered as gene delivery vehicles for the purposes of enhancing the immune response, inducing antiangiogenesis, activating prodrugs, etc. Thus, oncolytic virotherapy provides a platform for the creation of cancer therapeutics with diverse mechanisms of action. While still in its relative infancy, some such viruses have been tested in preclinical models of pediatric bone tumors, and initial clinical testing in pediatric patients has begun (Hammill et al. 2010).

15.5.1 Reolysin

Reovirus is a nonpathogenic virus that causes a subclinical infection or at most very mild respiratory and gastrointestinal symptoms. Derived from the Dearing strain of reovirus, Reolysin is among the most widely tested oncolytic viruses to date, primarily in phase II studies in combination with chemotherapy (Galanis et al. 2012). Preclinical studies suggested efficacy of pediatric sarcomas, including Ewing sarcoma and osteosarcoma, particularly in combination with chemotherapy or radiation therapy (Hingorani et al. 2011). The initial phase I trial in pediatric patients confirmed its safety as a single agent and with the addition of immunosuppressive doses of cyclophosphamide, though no patients experienced tumor response including seven with either osteosarcoma or Ewing sarcoma (Kolb et al. 2015), suggesting any efficacy from its use will likely be realized only in combination with other therapies.

15.5.2 Seneca Valley Virus

Similar to Reolysin, Seneca Valley virus (SVV-001, also known as NTX-010) is a nonpathogenic virus originally isolated as a contamination in tissue culture. This virus was originally found to preferentially be lytic for cells derived from neuroendocrine cancers (Reddy et al. 2007), and testing through the PPTP confirmed activity in some of these tumor models (Morton et al. 2010). Although there was some effect in a few Ewing sarcoma models, the observed preclinical efficacy was insufficient to warrant inclusion of these patients in the initial phase I clinical trial. Nevertheless, it is possible there may be utility of

this virus in some cases of Ewing sarcoma. Similar to the experience with Reolysin, the first pediatric phase I study of Seneca Valley virus confirmed its safety alone and in combination with cyclophosphamide, but there were no notable tumor responses (Burke et al. 2015).

15.5.3 HSV1716

Although wild-type HSV-1 is known to be neurotropic as it causes encephalitis and becomes latent in peripheral nerves, the virus and its attenuated derivatives are capable of infecting a wide range of cell types including models of pediatric bone tumors (Bharatan et al. 2002; Friedman et al. 2009). In a xenograft model of Ewing sarcoma, a combination of an oncolytic HSV-1 mutant with anti-VEGFA antibody (bevacizumab) was far more effective than either agent alone (Currier et al. 2013). The only clinical trial of an HSV-1 mutant in pediatric patients to date including those with malignant bone tumors has been with HSV1716, engineered for safety by deletion of the RL1 gene encoding the neurovirulence protein ICP34.5. The virus is being administered directly into tumor nodules or intravenously and has shown safety so far at the lower dose levels including in patients with osteosarcoma and Ewing sarcoma (Cripe 2015).

15.5.4 JX-594

Vaccinia virus is a nonpathogenic (in humans) cowpox virus that has been safely administered to millions of people as the small pox vaccine. Several variations of vaccinia virus have been tested in cancer patients, both by intratumoral and intravenous routes, demonstrating safety in adults with notable case reports of efficacy (Guse et al. 2011). The version currently in its most advanced clinical development is *pexasti-mogene devacirepvec* (also called Pexa-Vec or JX-594), a derivative of vaccinia created by deletion of the thymidine kinase gene to restrict virus replication to rapidly dividing cells and insertion of the gene encoding GM-CSF as an immune stimulant. An initial phase I trial of intratumoral Pexa-Vec in pediatric patients showed safety at the doses tested (Cripe et al. 2015). The trial included a patient with Ewing sarcoma who showed evidence of a transient therapeutic effect. As with the other viruses, vaccinia-derived vectors require further testing alone and in combination with other therapeutics to determine their utility for patients with pediatric bone tumors.

15.5.5 Other Vectors

There are a variety of other types of oncolytic viruses being developed and tested in academic medical centers and biopharmaceutical companies, including vectors derived from adenovirus, vesicular stomatitis virus, poliovirus, Maraba virus, and measles virus among others. It is too early to know the best routes of administration, doses, and ideal disease targets for each, but it is likely that some of these will exhibit activity in pediatric bone tumors.

15.6 Summary

Traditional treatments for pediatric bony cancers such as chemotherapy and radiation have only slowly improved over the past decades, with little to no significant progress in patient outcomes despite intensification of therapy. Researchers and practitioners alike have therefore sought to discover novel therapeutic approaches aimed at targeting tumors specifically and thereby limiting toxicities. New advances that show promise for pediatric bone tumors appear to be arising from a variety of vantage points, including small-molecule inhibitors, immunotherapies, and virotherapy. Each of these areas in turn is comprised of numerous different candidates and approaches. Although most have yet to be proven useful, there is certainly an eager anticipation among investigators that these targeted therapies will finally provide an avenue for progress in the treatment of pediatric bone malignancies.

References

Akers SN, Odunsi K, Karpf AR (2010) Regulation of cancer germline antigen gene expression: implications for cancer immunotherapy. Future Oncol 6:717–732

Akiyama T, Dass CR, Shinoda Y, Kawano H, Tanaka S, Choong PF (2010) Systemic RANK-Fc protein therapy is efficacious against primary osteosarcoma growth in a murine model via activity against osteoclasts. J Pharm Pharmacol 62:470–476

Bachner D, Schroder D, Gross G (2002) mRNA expression of the murine glycoprotein (transmembrane) nmb (Gpnmb) gene is linked to the developing retinal pigment epithelium and iris. Brain Res Gene Expr Patterns 1:159–165

Bagatell R, Norris R, Ingle AM, Ahern C, Voss S, Fox E, Little AR, Weigel BJ, Adamson PC, Blaney S (2014) Phase 1 trial of temsirolimus in combination with irinotecan and temozolomide in children, adolescents and young adults with relapsed or refractory solid tumors: a Children's Oncology Group Study. Pediatr Blood Cancer 61:833–839

Bago-Horvath Z, Schmid K, Rossler F, Nagy-Bojarszky K, Funovics P, Sulzbacher I (2014) Impact of RANK signalling on survival and chemotherapy response in osteosarcoma. Pathology 46:411–415

Bai RL, Paull KD, Herald CL, Malspeis L, Pettit GR, Hamel E (1991) Halichondrin B and homohalichondrin B, marine natural products binding in the vinca domain of tubulin. Discovery of tubulin-based mechanism of action by analysis of differential cytotoxicity data. J Biol Chem 266:15882–15889

Barber-Rotenberg JS, Selvanathan SP, Kong Y, Erkizan HV, Snyder TM, Hong SP, Kobs CL, South NL, Summer S, Monroe PJ et al (2012) Single enantiomer of YK-4-279 demonstrates specificity in targeting the oncogene EWS-FLI1. Oncotarget 3:172–182

Becker MA, Hou X, Harrington SC, Weroha SJ, Gonzalez SE, Jacob KA, Carboni JM, Gottardis MM, Haluska P (2012) IGFBP ratio confers resistance to IGF targeting and correlates with increased invasion and poor outcome in breast tumors. Clin Cancer Res Off J Am Assoc Cancer Res 18:1808–1817

Beug ST, Tang VA, LaCasse EC, Cheung HH, Beauregard CE, Brun J, Nuyens JP, Earl N, St-Jean M, Holbrook J et al (2014) Smac mimetics and innate immune stimuli synergize to promote tumor death. Nat Biotechnol 32:182–190

Bharatan NS, Currier MA, Cripe TP (2002) Differential susceptibility of pediatric sarcoma cells to oncolysis by conditionally replication-competent herpes simplex viruses. J Pediatr Hematol Oncol 24:447–453

Bid HK, Zhan J, Phelps DA, Kurmasheva RT, Houghton PJ (2012) Potent inhibition of angiogenesis by the IGF-1 receptor-targeting antibody SCH717454 is reversed by IGF-2. Mol Cancer Ther 11:649–659

Bid HK, London CA, Gao J, Zhong H, Hollingsworth RE, Fernandez S, Mo X, Houghton PJ (2013) Dual targeting of the type 1 insulin-like growth factor receptor and its ligands as an effective antiangiogenic strategy. Clin Cancer Res Off J Am Assoc Cancer Res 19:2984–2994

Bid HK, Roberts RD, Cam M, Audino A, Kurmasheva RT, Lin J, Houghton PJ, Cam H (2014) DeltaNp63 promotes pediatric neuroblastoma and osteosarcoma by regulating tumor angiogenesis. Cancer Res 74:320–329

Bjornsti MA, Houghton PJ (2004) The TOR pathway: a target for cancer therapy. Nat Rev Cancer 4:335–348

Bostedt KT, Schmid C, Ghirlanda-Keller C, Olie R, Winterhalter KH, Zapf J (2001) Insulin-like growth factor (IGF) I down-regulates type 1 IGF receptor (IGF 1R) and reduces the IGF I response in A549 non-small-cell lung cancer and Saos-2/B-10 osteoblastic osteosarcoma cells. Exp Cell Res 271:368–377

Braczkowski R, Schally AV, Plonowski A, Varga JL, Groot K, Krupa M, Armatis P (2002) Inhibition of proliferation in human MNNG/HOS osteosarcoma and SK-ES-1 Ewing sarcoma cell lines in vitro and in vivo by antagonists of growth hormone-releasing hormone: effects on insulin-like growth factor II. Cancer 95:1735–1745

Brenner JC, Ateeq B, Li Y, Yocum AK, Cao Q, Asangani IA, Patel S, Wang X, Liang H, Yu J et al (2011) Mechanistic rationale for inhibition of poly(ADP-ribose) polymerase in ETS gene fusion-positive prostate cancer. Cancer Cell 19:664–678

Brenner JC, Feng FY, Han S, Patel S, Goyal SV, Bou-Maroun LM, Liu M, Lonigro R, Prensner JR, Tomlins SA, Chinnaiyan AM (2012) PARP-1 inhibition as a targeted strategy to treat Ewing's sarcoma. Cancer Res 72:1608–1613

Buddingh EP, Schilham MW, Ruslan SE, Berghuis D, Szuhai K, Suurmond J, Taminiau AH, Gelderblom H, Egeler RM, Serra M et al (2011) Chemotherapy-resistant osteosarcoma is highly susceptible to IL-15-activated allogeneic and autologous NK cells. Cancer Immunol Immunother 60:575–586

Burke JM, Ahern C, Weigel B, Poirier J, Rudin C, Chen Y, Cripe TP, Bernhardt M, Blaney SM (2015) Phase I trial of Seneca Valley Virus (NTX-010) in children with relapsed/refractory solid tumors: a report of the Children's Oncology Group. Pediatr Blood Cancer 62:743–750

Carter PJ, Senter PD (2008) Antibody-drug conjugates for cancer therapy. Cancer J 14:154–169

Casanova M, Ferrari A, Spreafico F, Terenziani M, Massimino M, Luksch R, Cefalo G, Polastri D, Marcon I, Bellani FF (2002) Vinorelbine in previously treated advanced childhood sarcomas: evidence of activity in rhabdomyosarcoma. Cancer 94:3263–3268

Chawla SP, Staddon AP, Baker LH, Schuetze SM, Tolcher AW, D'Amato GZ, Blay JY, Mita MM, Sankhala KK, Berk L et al (2012) Phase II study of the mammalian target of rapamycin inhibitor ridaforolimus in patients with advanced bone and soft tissue sarcomas. J Clin Oncol Off J Am Soc Clin Oncol 30:78–84

Cho D, Shook DR, Shimasaki N, Chang YH, Fujisaki H, Campana D (2010) Cytotoxicity of activated natural killer cells against pediatric solid tumors. Clin Cancer Res 16:3901–3909

Choy E, Butrynski JE, Harmon D et al (2013) Translation of preclinical predictive sensitivity of Ewing sarcoma to PARP inhibition: phase II study of olaparib in adult patients with recurrent/metastatic Ewing sarcoma following failure of prior chemotherapy. Proceedings of the 104th Annual Meeting of the American Association for Cancer Research Abstr #LB-174

Chung JS, Dougherty I, Cruz PD Jr, Ariizumi K (2007a) Syndecan-4 mediates the coinhibitory function of DC-HIL on T cell activation. J Immunol 179: 5778–5784

Chung JS, Sato K, Dougherty II, Cruz PD Jr, Ariizumi K (2007b) DC-HIL is a negative regulator of T lymphocyte activation. Blood 109:4320–4327

Cohen BD, Baker DA, Soderstrom C, Tkalcevic G, Rossi AM, Miller PE, Tengowski MW, Wang F, Gualberto A, Beebe JS, Moyer JD (2005) Combination therapy enhances the inhibition of tumor growth with the fully human anti-type 1 insulin-like growth factor receptor monoclonal antibody CP-751,871. Clin Cancer Res 11:2063–2073

Coley WB (1933) The treatment of sarcoma of the long bones. Ann Surg 97:434–460

Cripe TP, Ngo MC, Geller JI, Louis CU, Currier MA, Racadio JM, Towbin AJ, Rooney DM, Pelusio A, Moon A et al (2015) Phase I study of intratumoral Pexa-Vec (JX-594), an oncolytic and immunotherapeutic vaccinia virus, in pediatric cancer patients. Mol Ther 23:602–608

Currier MA, Eshun FK, Sholl A, Chernoguz A, Crawford K, Divanovic S, Boon L, Goins WF, Frischer JS, Collins MH et al (2013) VEGF blockade enables oncolytic cancer virotherapy in part by modulating intratumoral myeloid cells. Mol Ther 21:1014–1023

Darnell JE Jr (2002) Transcription factors as targets for cancer therapy. Nat Rev Cancer 2:740–749

de Alava E, Panizo A, Antonescu CR, Huvos AG, Pardo-Mindan FJ, Barr FG, Ladanyi M (2000) Association of EWS-FLI1 type 1 fusion with lower proliferative rate in Ewing's sarcoma. Am J Pathol 156:849–855

De Bono JS, Mina LA, Gonzalez M, Curtin NJ, Wang E, Henshaw JW, Chadha M, Sachdev JC, Matei D, Jameson GS et al (2013) First-in-human trial of novel oral PARP inhibitor BMN 673 in patients with solid tumors. J Clin Oncol 31 (Suppl):abstr 2580

Delattre O, Zucman J, Plougastel B, Desmaze C, Melot T, Peter M, Kovar H, Joubert I, de Jong P, Rouleau G et al (1992) Gene fusion with an ETS DNA-binding domain caused by chromosome translocation in human tumours. Nature 359:162–165

Desbois-Mouthon C, Baron A, Blivet-Van Eggelpoel MJ, Fartoux L, Venot C, Bladt F, Housset C, Rosmorduc O (2009) Insulin-like growth factor-1 receptor inhibition induces a resistance mechanism via the epidermal growth factor receptor/HER3/AKT signaling pathway: rational basis for cotargeting insulin-like growth factor-1 receptor and epidermal growth factor receptor in hepatocellular carcinoma. Clin Cancer Res 15:5445–5456

Dilling MB, Dias P, Shapiro DN, Germain GS, Johnson RK, Houghton PJ (1994) Rapamycin selectively inhibits the growth of childhood rhabdomyosarcoma cells through inhibition of signaling via the type I insulin-like growth factor receptor. Cancer Res 54:903–907

Dobrynin P, Matyunina E, Malov SV, Kozlov AP (2013) The novelty of human cancer/testis antigen encoding genes in evolution. Int J Genom 2013:105108

DuBois SG, Krailo MD, Lessnick SL, Smith R, Chen Z, Marina N, Grier HE, Stegmaier K, and Children's Oncology (2009) Phase II study of intermediate-dose cytarabine in patients with relapsed or refractory Ewing sarcoma: a report from the Children's Oncology Group. Pediatr Blood Cancer 52:324–327

Ebb D, Meyers P, Grier H, Bernstein M, Gorlick R, Lipshultz SE, Krailo M, Devidas M, Barkauskas DA, Siegal GP et al (2012) Phase II trial of trastuzumab in combination with cytotoxic chemotherapy for treatment of metastatic osteosarcoma with human epidermal growth factor receptor 2 overexpression: a report from the Children's Oncology Group. J Clin Oncol 30:2545–2551

Edmonson JH, Green SJ, Ivins JC, Gilchrist GS, Creagan ET, Pritchard DJ, Smithson WA, Dahlin DC, Taylor WF (1984) A controlled pilot study of high-dose methotrexate as postsurgical adjuvant treatment for primary osteosarcoma. J Clin Oncol 2:152–156

Eilber F, Giuliano A, Eckardt J, Patterson K, Moseley S, Goodnight J (1987) Adjuvant chemotherapy for osteosarcoma: a randomized prospective trial. J Clin Oncol 5:21–26

Erkizan HV, Kong Y, Merchant M, Schlottmann S, Barber-Rotenberg JS, Yuan L, Abaan OD, Chou TH, Dakshanamurthy S, Brown ML et al (2009) A small molecule blocking oncogenic protein EWS-FLI1 interaction with RNA helicase A inhibits growth of Ewing's sarcoma. Nat Med 15:750–756

Eshleman JS, Carlson BL, Mladek AC, Kastner BD, Shide KL, Sarkaria JN (2002) Inhibition of the mammalian target of rapamycin sensitizes U87 xenografts to fractionated radiation therapy. Cancer Res 62:7291–7297

Ferrari S, Palmerini E (2007) Adjuvant and neoadjuvant combination chemotherapy for osteogenic sarcoma. Curr Opin Oncol 19:341–346

Fong PC, Yap TA, Boss DS, Carden CP, Mergui-Roelvink M, Gourley C, De Greve J, Lubinski J, Shanley S, Messiou C et al (2010) Poly(ADP)-ribose polymerase inhibition: frequent durable responses in BRCA carrier ovarian cancer correlating with platinum-free interval. J Clin Oncol 28:2512–2519

Fouladi M, Laningham F, Wu J, O'Shaughnessy MA, Molina K, Broniscer A, Spunt SL, Luckett I, Stewart CF, Houghton PJ et al (2007) Phase I study of everolimus in pediatric patients with refractory solid tumors. J Clin Oncol Off J Am Soc Clin Oncol 25:4806–4812

Friedman GK, Pressey JG, Reddy AT, Markert JM, Gillespie GY (2009) Herpes simplex virus oncolytic therapy for pediatric malignancies. Mol Ther 17:1125–1135

Gable KL, Maddux BA, Penaranda C, Zavodovskaya M, Campbell MJ, Lobo M, Robinson L, Schow S, Kerner JA, Goldfine ID, Youngren JF (2006) Diarylureas are small-molecule inhibitors of insulin-like growth factor I receptor signaling and breast cancer cell growth. Mol Cancer Ther 5:1079–1086

Galanis E, Markovic SN, Suman VJ, Nuovo GJ, Vile RG, Kottke TJ, Nevala WK, Thompson MA, Lewis JE, Rumilla KM et al (2012) Phase II trial of intravenous administration of Reolysin((R)) (Reovirus Serotype-3-dearing Strain) in patients with metastatic melanoma. Mol Ther 20:1998–2003

Garnett MJ, Edelman EJ, Heidorn SJ, Greenman CD, Dastur A, Lau KW, Greninger P, Thompson IR, Luo X, Soares J et al (2012) Systematic identification of genomic markers of drug sensitivity in cancer cells. Nature 483:570–575

Goel S, Mita AC, Mita M, Rowinsky EK, Chu QS, Wong N, Desjardins C, Fang F, Jansen M, Shuster DE et al (2009) A phase I study of eribulin mesylate (E7389), a mechanistically novel inhibitor of microtubule dynamics, in patients with advanced solid malignancies. Clin Cancer Res Off J Am Assoc Cancer Res 15: 4207–4212

Goetsch L, Gonzalez A, Leger O, Beck A, Pauwels PJ, Haeuw JF, Corvaia N (2005) A recombinant humanized anti-insulin-like growth factor receptor type I antibody (h7C10) enhances the antitumor activity of vinorelbine and anti-epidermal growth factor receptor therapy against human cancer xenografts. Int J Cancer 113:316–328

Gollamudi R, Ghalib MH, Desai KK, Chaudhary I, Wong B, Einstein M, Coffey M, Gill GM, Mettinger K, Mariadason JM et al (2010) Intravenous administration of Reolysin, a live replication competent RNA virus is safe in patients with advanced solid tumors. Invest New Drugs 28:641–649

Gorlick R, Maris JM, Houghton PJ, Lock R, Carol H, Kurmasheva RT, Kolb EA, Keir ST, Reynolds CP, Kang MH et al (2012) Testing of the Akt/PKB inhibitor MK-2206 by the Pediatric Preclinical Testing Program. Pediatr Blood Cancer 59:518–524

Grohar PJ, Woldemichael GM, Griffin LB, Mendoza A, Chen QR, Yeung C, Currier DG, Davis S, Khanna C, Khan J et al (2011) Identification of an inhibitor of the EWS-FLI1 oncogenic transcription factor by high-throughput screening. J Natl Cancer Inst 103: 962–978

Guerreiro AS, Boller D, Doepfner KT, Arcaro A (2006) IGF-IR: potential role in antitumor agents. Drug News Perspect 19:261–272

Guertin DA, Sabatini DM (2009) The pharmacology of mTOR inhibition. Sci Signal 2:pe24

Guse K, Cerullo V, Hemminki A (2011) Oncolytic vaccinia virus for the treatment of cancer. Expert Opin Biol Ther 11:595–608

Haluska P, Carboni JM, Loegering DA, Lee FY, Wittman M, Saulnier MG, Frennesson DB, Kalli KR, Conover CA, Attar RM et al (2006) In vitro and in vivo antitumor effects of the dual insulin-like growth factor-I/insulin receptor inhibitor, BMS-554417. Cancer Res 66:362–371

Hammill AM, Conner J, Cripe TP (2010) Oncolytic virotherapy reaches adolescence. Pediatr Blood Cancer 55:1253–1263

Han EQ, Li XL, Wang CR, Li TF, Han SY (2013) Chimeric antigen receptor-engineered T cells for cancer immunotherapy: progress and challenges. J Hematol Oncol 6:47

Himoudi N, Wallace R, Parsley KL, Gilmour K, Barrie AU, Howe K, Dong R, Sebire NJ, Michalski A, Thrasher AJ, Anderson J (2012) Lack of T-cell responses following autologous tumour lysate pulsed dendritic cell vaccination, in patients with relapsed osteosarcoma. Clin Transl Oncol 14:271–279

Hingorani P, Zhang W, Lin J, Liu L, Guha C, Kolb EA (2011) Systemic administration of reovirus (Reolysin) inhibits growth of human sarcoma xenografts. Cancer 117:1764–1774

Hofmann O, Caballero OL, Stevenson BJ, Chen YT, Cohen T, Chua R, Maher CA, Panji S, Schaefer U, Kruger A et al (2008) Genome-wide analysis of cancer/testis gene expression. Proc Natl Acad Sci U S A 105:20422–20427

Hong SH, Youbi SE, Hong SP, Kallakury B, Monroe P, Erkizan HV, Barber-Rotenberg JS, Houghton P, Uren A, Toretsky JA (2014) Pharmacokinetic modeling optimizes inhibition of the 'undruggable' EWS-FLI1 transcription factor in Ewing Sarcoma. Oncotarget 5:338–350

Horton JK, Wilson SH (2013) Predicting enhanced cell killing through PARP inhibition. Mol Cancer Res 11:13–18

Houchens DP, Ovejera AA, Riblet SM, Slagel DE (1983) Human brain tumor xenografts in nude mice as a chemotherapy model. Eur J Cancer Clin Oncol 19:799–805

Houghton PJ, Morton CL, Kolb EA, Gorlick R, Lock R, Carol H, Reynolds CP, Maris JM, Keir ST, Billups CA, Smith MA (2008) Initial testing (stage 1) of the mTOR inhibitor rapamycin by the pediatric preclinical testing program. Pediatr Blood Cancer 50:799–805

Houghton PJ, Morton CL, Gorlick R, Lock RB, Carol H, Reynolds CP, Kang MH, Maris JM, Keir ST, Kolb EA et al (2010a) Stage 2 combination testing of rapamycin with cytotoxic agents by the Pediatric Preclinical Testing Program. Mol Cancer Ther 9:101–112

Houghton PJ, Morton CL, Kang M, Reynolds CP, Billups CA, Favours E, Payne-Turner D, Tucker C, Smith MA (2010b) Evaluation of cytarabine against Ewing sarcoma xenografts by the pediatric preclinical testing program. Pediatr Blood Cancer 55:1224–1226

Hromas R, Klemsz M (1994) The ETS oncogene family in development, proliferation and neoplasia. Int J Hematol 59:257–265

Huang F, Greer A, Hurlburt W, Han X, Hafezi R, Wittenberg GM, Reeves K, Chen J, Robinson D, Li A et al (2009) The mechanisms of differential sensitivity to an insulin-like growth factor-1 receptor inhibitor (BMS-536924) and rationale for combining with EGFR/HER2 inhibitors. Cancer Res 69:161–170

Huang F, Hurlburt W, Greer A, Reeves KA, Hillerman S, Chang H, Fargnoli J, Graf Finckenstein F, Gottardis MM, Carboni JM (2010) Differential mechanisms of acquired resistance to insulin-like growth factor-i receptor antibody therapy or to a small-molecule inhibitor, BMS-754807, in a human rhabdomyosarcoma model. Cancer Res 70:7221–7231

Hudes G, Carducci M, Tomczak P, Dutcher J, Figlin R, Kapoor A, Staroslawska E, Sosman J, McDermott D, Bodrogi I et al (2007) Temsirolimus, interferon alfa, or both for advanced renal-cell carcinoma. N Engl J Med 356:2271–2281

Jackson-Booth PG, Terry C, Lackey B, Lopaczynska M, Nissley P (2003) Inhibition of the biologic response to insulin-like growth factor I in MCF-7 breast cancer cells by a new monoclonal antibody to the insulin-like growth factor-I receptor. The importance of receptor down-regulation. Horm Metab Res 35:850–856

Jain S, Vahdat LT (2011) Eribulin mesylate. Clin Cancer Res Off J Am Assoc Cancer Res 17:6615–6622

Jordan MA, Wilson L (2004) Microtubules as a target for anticancer drugs. Nat Rev Cancer 4:253–265

Jordan MA, Kamath K, Manna T, Okouneva T, Miller HP, Davis C, Littlefield BA, Wilson L (2005) The primary antimitotic mechanism of action of the synthetic halichondrin E7389 is suppression of microtubule growth. Mol Cancer Ther 4:1086–1095

Kailayangiri S, Altvater B, Meltzer J, Pscherer S, Luecke A, Dierkes C, Titze U, Leuchte K, Landmeier S, Hotfilder M et al (2012) The ganglioside antigen G(D2) is surface-expressed in Ewing sarcoma and allows for MHC-independent immune targeting. Br J Cancer 106:1123–1133

Kakarla S, Chow K, Mata M, Shaffer DR, Song XT, Wu MF, Liu H, Wang LL, Rowley DR, Pfizenmaier K, Gottschalk S (2013) Antitumor effects of chimeric receptor engineered human T cells directed to tumor stroma. Mol Ther 21:1611–1620

Kalebic T, Tsokos M, Helman LJ (1994) In vivo treatment with antibody against IGF-1 receptor suppresses growth of human rhabdomyosarcoma and down-regulates p34cdc2. Cancer Res 54:5531–5534

Kang Z, Yu Y, Zhu YJ, Davis S, Walker R, Meltzer PS, Helman LJ, Cao L (2013) Downregulation of IGFBP2 is associated with resistance to IGF1R therapy in rhabdomyosarcoma. Oncogene 33:5697

Kang MH, Reynolds CP, Maris JM, Gorlick R, Kolb EA, Lock R, Carol H, Keir ST, Wu J, Lyalin D et al (2014) Initial testing (stage 1) of the investigational mTOR kinase inhibitor MLN0128 by the pediatric preclinical testing program. Pediatr Blood Cancer 61:1486–1489

Kaufman HL, Kim DW, DeRaffele G, Mitcham J, Coffin RS, Kim-Schulze S (2010) Local and distant immunity induced by intralesional vaccination with an oncolytic herpes virus encoding GM-CSF in patients with stage IIIc and IV melanoma. Ann Surg Oncol 17:718–730

Kaufman B, Shapira-Frommer R, Schmutzler RK, Audeh MW, Friedlander M, Balmana J, Mitchell G, Fried G, Bowen K, Fielding A, Domchek SM (2013) Olaparib monotherapy in patients with advanced cancer and a germ-line BRCA1/2 mutation: an open-label phase II study. J Clin Oncol 31 (Suppl):abstr 11024

Kedar PS, Stefanick DF, Horton JK, Wilson SH (2012) Increased PARP-1 association with DNA in alkylation damaged, PARP-inhibited mouse fibroblasts. Mol Cancer Res 10:360–368

Kelly E, Russell SJ (2007) History of oncolytic viruses: genesis to genetic engineering. Mol Ther 15:651–659

Kirkwood JM, Butterfield LH, Tarhini AA, Zarour H, Kalinski P, Ferrone S (2012) Immunotherapy of cancer in 2012. CA Cancer J Clin 62:309–335

Kochenderfer JN, Dudley ME, Feldman SA, Wilson WH, Spaner DE, Maric I, Stetler-Stevenson M, Phan GQ, Hughes MS, Sherry RM et al (2012) B-cell depletion and remissions of malignancy along with cytokine-associated toxicity in a clinical trial of anti-CD19 chimeric-antigen-receptor-transduced T cells. Blood 119:2709–2720

Kofman S, Perlia CP, Economou SG (1973) Mithramycin in the treatment of metastatic Ewing's sarcoma. Cancer 31:889–893

Kolb EA, Kamara D, Zhang W, Lin J, Hingorani P, Baker L, Houghton P, Gorlick R (2010) R1507, a fully human monoclonal antibody targeting IGF-1R, is effective alone and in combination with rapamycin in inhibiting growth of osteosarcoma xenografts. Pediatr Blood Cancer 55:67–75

Kolb EA, Gorlick R, Lock R, Carol H, Morton CL, Keir ST, Reynolds CP, Kang MH, Maris JM, Billups C et al (2011) Initial testing (stage 1) of the IGF-1 receptor inhibitor BMS-754807 by the pediatric preclinical testing program. Pediatr Blood Cancer 56:595–603

Kolb EA, Gorlick R, Maris JM, Keir ST, Morton CL, Wu J, Wozniak AW, Smith MA, Houghton PJ (2012) Combination testing (Stage 2) of the Anti-IGF-1 receptor antibody IMC-A12 with rapamycin by the pediatric preclinical testing program. Pediatr Blood Cancer 58:729–735

Kolb EA, Gorlick R, Reynolds CP, Kang MH, Carol H, Lock R, Keir ST, Maris JM, Billups CA, Desjardins C et al (2013) Initial testing (stage 1) of eribulin, a novel tubulin binding agent, by the pediatric preclinical testing program. Pediatr Blood Cancer 60:1325–1332

Kolb EA, Sampson V, Stabley D, Walter A, Sol-Church K, Cripe TP, Hingorani P, Ahem C, Weigel B, Zwiebel J, Blaney SM (2015) A phase I trial and viral clearance study of reovirus (Reolysin) in children with relapsed or refractory extra-cranial solid tumors: a Children's Oncology Group phase I consortium report. Pediatr Blood Cancer 62:751–758

Krailo M, Ertel I, Makley J, Fryer CJ, Baum E, Weetman R, Yunis E, Barnes L, Bleyer WA, Hammond GD (1987) A randomized study comparing high-dose methotrexate with moderate-dose methotrexate as components of adjuvant chemotherapy in childhood nonmetastatic osteosarcoma: a report from the Childrens Cancer Study Group. Med Pediatr Oncol 15:69–77

Kuan CT, Wakiya K, Dowell JM, Herndon JE 2nd, Reardon DA, Graner MW, Riggins GJ, Wikstrand CJ, Bigner DD (2006) Glycoprotein nonmetastatic melanoma protein B, a potential molecular therapeutic target in patients with glioblastoma multiforme. Clin Cancer Res 12:1970–1982

Kurmasheva RT, Houghton PJ (2006) IGF-I mediated survival pathways in normal and malignant cells. Biochim Biophys Acta 1766:1–22

Kurmasheva RT, Dudkin L, Billups C, Debelenko LV, Morton CL, Houghton PJ (2009) The insulin-like growth factor-1 receptor-targeting antibody, CP-751,871, suppresses tumor-derived VEGF and synergizes with rapamycin in models of childhood sarcoma. Cancer Res 69:7662–7671

Lechner MG, Russell SM, Bass RS, Epstein AL (2011) Chemokines, costimulatory molecules and fusion proteins for the immunotherapy of solid tumors. Immunotherapy 3:1317–1340

Lee S, Margolin K (2011) Cytokines in cancer immunotherapy. Cancers (Basel) 3:3856–3893

Lee HJ, Yoon C, Schmidt B, Park do J, Zhang AY, Erkizan HV, Toretsky JA, Kirsch DG, Yoon SS (2013) Combining PARP-1 inhibition and radiation in Ewing sarcoma results in lethal DNA damage. Mol Cancer Ther 12:2591–2600

Li Z (2013) Potential of human gammadelta T cells for immunotherapy of osteosarcoma. Mol Biol Rep 40:427–437

Lipinski M, Braham K, Philip I, Wiels J, Philip T, Dellagi K, Goridis C, Lenoir GM, Tursz T (1986) Phenotypic characterization of Ewing sarcoma cell lines with monoclonal antibodies. J Cell Biochem 31:289–296

Liu WN, Lin JH, Cheng YR, Zhang L, Huang J, Wu ZY, Wang FS, Xu SG, Lin WP, Lan WB, Yang GX (2013) FIM-A, a phosphorus-containing sirolimus, inhibits the angiogenesis and proliferation of osteosarcomas. Oncol Res 20:319–326

Lock RB, Carol H, Morton CL, Keir ST, Reynolds CP, Kang MH, Maris JM, Wozniak AW, Gorlick R, Kolb EA et al (2012) Initial testing of the CENP-E inhibitor GSK923295A by the pediatric preclinical testing program. Pediatr Blood Cancer 58:916–923

Louis CU, Savoldo B, Dotti G, Pule M, Yvon E, Myers GD, Rossig C, Russell HV, Diouf O, Liu E et al (2011) Antitumor activity and long-term fate of chimeric antigen receptor-positive T cells in patients with neuroblastoma. Blood 118:6050–6056

MacEwen EG, Pastor J, Kutzke J, Tsan R, Kurzman ID, Thamm DH, Wilson M, Radinsky R (2004) IGF-1 receptor contributes to the malignant phenotype in human and canine osteosarcoma. J Cell Biochem 92:77–91

Mackall CL, Rhee EH, Read EJ, Khuu HM, Leitman SF, Bernstein D, Tesso M, Long LM, Grindler D, Merino M et al (2008) A pilot study of consolidative immunotherapy in patients with high-risk pediatric sarcomas. Clin Cancer Res 14:4850–4858

Marr LA, Gilham DE, Campbell JD, Fraser AR (2012) Immunology in the clinic review series; focus on cancer: double trouble for tumours: bi-functional and redirected T cells as effective cancer immunotherapies. Clin Exp Immunol 167:216–225

Masutani M, Nozaki T, Nakamoto K, Nakagama H, Suzuki H, Kusuoka O, Tsutsumi M, Sugimura T (2000) The response of Parp knockout mice against DNA damaging agents. Mutat Res 462:159–166

Meyers PA, Chou AJ (2014) Muramyl tripeptide-phosphatidyl ethanolamine encapsulated in liposomes (L-MTP-PE) in the treatment of osteosarcoma. Adv Exp Med Biol 804:307–321

Meyers PA, Schwartz CL, Krailo M, Kleinerman ES, Betcher D, Bernstein ML, Conrad E, Ferguson W, Gebhardt M, Goorin AM et al (2005) Osteosarcoma: a randomized, prospective trial of the addition of ifosfamide and/or muramyl tripeptide to cisplatin, doxorubicin, and high-dose methotrexate. J Clin Oncol 23:2004–2011

Mitsiades CS, Mitsiades NS, McMullan CJ, Poulaki V, Shringarpure R, Akiyama M, Hideshima T, Chauhan D, Joseph M, Libermann TA et al (2004) Inhibition of the insulin-like growth factor receptor-1 tyrosine kinase activity as a therapeutic strategy for multiple myeloma, other hematologic malignancies, and solid tumors. Cancer Cell 5:221–230

Morgenstern DA, Marzouki M, Bartels U, Irwin MS, Sholler GL, Gammon J, Yankanah R, Wu B, Samson Y, Baruchel S (2014) Phase I study of vinblastine and sirolimus in pediatric patients with recurrent or refractory solid tumors. Pediatr Blood Cancer 61:128–133

Moriceau G, Ory B, Mitrofan L, Riganti C, Blanchard F, Brion R, Charrier C, Battaglia S, Pilet P, Denis MG et al (2010) Zoledronic acid potentiates mTOR inhibition and abolishes the resistance of osteosarcoma cells to RAD001 (Everolimus): pivotal role of the prenylation process. Cancer Res 70:10329–10339

Morton CL, Houghton PJ, Kolb EA, Gorlick R, Reynolds CP, Kang MH, Maris JM, Keir ST, Wu J, Smith MA (2010) Initial testing of the replication competent Seneca Valley virus (NTX-010) by the pediatric preclinical testing program. Pediatr Blood Cancer 55:295–303

Motzer RJ, Escudier B, Oudard S, Hutson TE, Porta C, Bracarda S, Grunwald V, Thompson JA, Figlin RA, Hollaender N et al (2008) Efficacy of everolimus in advanced renal cell carcinoma: a double-blind, randomised, placebo-controlled phase III trial. Lancet 372:449–456

Murai J, Huang SY, Das BB, Renaud A, Zhang Y, Doroshow JH, Ji J, Takeda S, Pommier Y (2012) Trapping of PARP1 and PARP2 by Clinical PARP Inhibitors. Cancer Res 72:5588–5599

Murai J, Huang SY, Renaud A, Zhang Y, Ji J, Takeda S, Morris J, Teicher B, Doroshow JH, Pommier Y (2014a) Stereospecific PARP trapping by BMN 673 and comparison with olaparib and rucaparib. Mol Cancer Ther 13:433–443

Murai J, Josse R, Doroshow JH, Pommier Y (2014b) Schlafen 11 (SLFN11) is a critical determinant of cellular sensitivity to PARP inhibitors. Proceedings of the 105th Annual Meeting of the American Association for Cancer Research; 2014 Apr 5–9; San Diego, CA Philadelphia (PA): AACR, Abstr #1718

Murai J, Zhang Y, Morris J, Ji J, Takeda S, Doroshow JH, Pommier YG (2014c) Rationale for PARP inhibitors in combination therapy with camptothecins or temozolomide based on PARP trapping versus catalytic inhibition. J Pharmacol Exp Ther 349:408–416

Naing A, LoRusso P, Fu S, Hong DS, Anderson P, Benjamin RS, Ludwig J, Chen HX, Doyle LA, Kurzrock R (2012) Insulin growth factor-receptor (IGF-1R) antibody cixutumumab combined with the mTOR inhibitor temsirolimus in patients with refractory Ewing's sarcoma family tumors. Clin Cancer Res 18:2625–2631

Nguyen D, Zajac-Kaye M, Rubinstein L, Voeller D, Tomaszewski JE, Kummar S, Chen AP, Pommier Y, Doroshow JH, Yang SX (2011) Poly(ADP-ribose) polymerase inhibition enhances p53-dependent and -independent DNA damage responses induced by DNA damaging agent. Cell Cycle 10:4074–4082

Norris RE, Adamson PC, Nguyen VT, Fox E (2014) Preclinical evaluation of the PARP inhibitor, olaparib, in combination with cytotoxic chemotherapy in pediatric solid tumors. Pediatr Blood Cancer 61:145–150

Olmos D, Postel-Vinay S, Molife LR, Okuno SH, Schuetze SM, Paccagnella ML, Batzel GN, Yin D, Pritchard-Jones K, Judson I et al (2010) Safety, pharmacokinetics, and preliminary activity of the anti-IGF-1R antibody figitumumab (CP-751,871) in patients with sarcoma and Ewing's sarcoma: a phase 1 expansion cohort study. Lancet Oncol 11:129–135

Onaga M, Ido A, Hasuike S, Uto H, Moriuchi A, Nagata K, Hori T, Hayash K, Tsubouchi H (2003) Osteoactivin expressed during cirrhosis development in rats fed a choline-deficient, L-amino acid-defined diet, accelerates motility of hepatoma cells. J Hepatol 39:779–785

Orentas RJ, Lee DW, Mackall C (2012a) Immunotherapy targets in pediatric cancer. Front Oncol 2:3

Orentas RJ, Yang JJ, Wen X, Wei JS, Mackall CL, Khan J (2012b) Identification of cell surface proteins as potential immunotherapy targets in 12 pediatric cancers. Front Oncol 2:194

Ott PA, Hodi FS, Robert C (2013) CTLA-4 and PD-1/PD-L1 blockade: new immunotherapeutic modalities with durable clinical benefit in melanoma patients. Clin Cancer Res 19:5300–5309

Pahl JH, Ruslan SE, Buddingh EP, Santos SJ, Szuhai K, Serra M, Gelderblom H, Hogendoorn PC, Egeler RM, Schilham MW, Lankester AC (2012) Anti-EGFR antibody cetuximab enhances the cytolytic activity of natural killer cells toward osteosarcoma. Clin Cancer Res 18:432–441

Palucka K, Banchereau J (2013) Dendritic-cell-based therapeutic cancer vaccines. Immunity 39:38–48

Pappo AS, Patel SR, Crowley J, Reinke DK, Kuenkele KP, Chawla SP, Toner GC, Maki RG, Meyers PA, Chugh R et al (2011) R1507, a monoclonal antibody to the insulin-like growth factor 1 receptor, in patients with recurrent or refractory Ewing sarcoma family of tumors: results of a phase II Sarcoma Alliance for Research through Collaboration study. J Clin Oncol 29:4541–4547

Pappo AS, Vassal G, Crowley JJ, Bolejack V, Hogendoorn PC, Chugh R, Ladanyi M, Grippo JF, Dall G, Staddon AP et al (2014) A phase 2 trial of R1507, a monoclonal antibody to the insulin-like growth factor-1 receptor (IGF-1R), in patients with recurrent or refractory rhabdomyosarcoma, osteosarcoma, synovial sarcoma, and other soft tissue sarcomas: results of a Sarcoma Alliance for Research through Collaboration study. Cancer 120:2448–2456

Piha-Paul SA, Shin SJ, Vats T, Guha-Thakurta N, Aaron J, Rytting M, Kleinerman E, Kurzrock R (2014) Pediatric patients with refractory central nervous system tumors: experiences of a clinical trial combining bevacizumab and temsirolimus. Anticancer Res 34:1939–1945

Plummer R (2010) Perspective on the pipeline of drugs being developed with modulation of DNA damage as a target. Clin Cancer Res 16:4527–4531

Pollack VA, Alvarez E, Tse KF, Torgov MY, Xie S, Shenoy SG, MacDougall JR, Arrol S, Zhong H, Gerwien RW et al (2007) Treatment parameters modulating regression of human melanoma xenografts by an antibody-drug conjugate (CR011-vcMMAE) targeting GPNMB. Cancer Chemother Pharmacol 60:423–435

Pollak M, Richard M (1990) Suramin blockade of insulin-like growth factor I-stimulated proliferation of human osteosarcoma cells. J Natl Cancer Inst 82:1349–1352

Pratt CB, Champion JE, Fleming ID, Rao B, Kumar AP, Evans WE, Green AA, George S (1990) Adjuvant chemotherapy for osteosarcoma of the extremity. Long-term results of two consecutive prospective protocol studies. Cancer 65:439–445

Prieur A, Tirode F, Cohen P, Delattre O (2004) EWS/FLI-1 silencing and gene profiling of Ewing cells reveal downstream oncogenic pathways and a crucial role for repression of insulin-like growth factor binding protein 3. Mol Cell Biol 24:7275–7283

Rainusso N, Brawley VS, Ghazi A, Hicks MJ, Gottschalk S, Rosen JM, Ahmed N (2012) Immunotherapy targeting HER2 with genetically modified T cells eliminates tumor-initiating cells in osteosarcoma. Cancer Gene Ther 19:212–217

Reddy PS, Burroughs KD, Hales LM, Ganesh S, Jones BH, Idamakanti N, Hay C, Li SS, Skele KL, Vasko AJ et al (2007) Seneca Valley virus, a systemically deliverable oncolytic picornavirus, and the treatment of neuroendocrine cancers. J Natl Cancer Inst 99:1623–1633

Remsing LL, Bahadori HR, Carbone GM, McGuffie EM, Catapano CV, Rohr J (2003) Inhibition of c-src transcription by mithramycin: structure-activity relationships of biosynthetically produced mithramycin analogues using the c-src promoter as target. Biochemistry 42:8313–8324

Reynolds CP, Kang MH, Carol H, Lock R, Gorlick R, Kolb EA, Kurmasheva RT, Keir ST, Maris JM, Billups CA et al (2013) Initial testing (stage 1) of the phosphatidylinositol 3′ kinase inhibitor, SAR245408 (XL147) by the pediatric preclinical testing program. Pediatr Blood Cancer 60:791–798

Ripoll VM, Irvine KM, Ravasi T, Sweet MJ, Hume DA (2007) Gpnmb is induced in macrophages by IFN-gamma and lipopolysaccharide and acts as a feedback regulator of proinflammatory responses. J Immunol 178:6557–6566

Rose AA, Siegel PM (2007) Osteoactivin/HGFIN: is it a tumor suppressor or mediator of metastasis in breast cancer? Breast Cancer Res 9:403

Rose AA, Grosset AA, Dong Z, Russo C, Macdonald PA, Bertos NR, St-Pierre Y, Simantov R, Hallett M, Park M et al (2010) Glycoprotein nonmetastatic B is an independent prognostic indicator of recurrence and a novel therapeutic target in breast cancer. Clin Cancer Res 16:2147–2156

Rosen G, Nirenberg A, Caparros B, Juergens H, Kosloff C, Mehta BM, Marcove RC, Huvos AG (1981) Osteogenic sarcoma: eight-percent, three-year, disease-free survival with combination chemotherapy (T-7). Natl Cancer Inst Monogr 56:213–220

Roth M, Linkowski M, Tarim J, Piperdi S, Sowers R, Geller D, Gill J, Gorlick R (2014) Ganglioside GD2 as a therapeutic target for antibody-mediated therapy in patients with osteosarcoma. Cancer 120:548–554

Sachdev D, Yee D (2006) Inhibitors of insulin-like growth factor signaling: a therapeutic approach for breast cancer. J Mammary Gland Biol Neoplasia 11:27–39

Sachdev D, Yee D (2007) Disrupting insulin-like growth factor signaling as a potential cancer therapy. Mol Cancer Ther 6:1–12

Sachdev D, Li SL, Hartell JS, Fujita-Yamaguchi Y, Miller JS, Yee D (2003) A chimeric humanized single-chain antibody against the type I insulin-like growth factor (IGF) receptor renders breast cancer cells refractory to the mitogenic effects of IGF-I. Cancer Res 63:627–635

Sachdev D, Singh R, Fujita-Yamaguchi Y, Yee D (2006) Down-regulation of insulin receptor by antibodies against the type I insulin-like growth factor receptor: implications for anti-insulin-like growth factor therapy in breast cancer. Cancer Res 66:2391–2402

Sandhu SK, Schelman WR, Wilding G, Moreno V, Baird RD, Miranda S, Hylands L, Riisnaes R, Forster M, Omlin A et al (2013) The poly(ADP-ribose) polymerase inhibitor niraparib (MK4827) in BRCA mutation carriers and patients with sporadic cancer: a phase 1 dose-escalation trial. Lancet Oncol 14:882–892

Sangiolo D, Mesiano G, Gammaitoni L, Leuci V, Todorovic M, Giraudo L, Cammarata C, Dell'Aglio C, D'Ambrosio L, Pisacane A et al (2014) Cytokine-induced killer cells eradicate bone and soft-tissue sarcomas. Cancer Res 74:119–129

Schiewer MJ, Den R, Hoang DT, Augello MA, Lawrence YR, Dicker AP, Knudsen KE (2012) mTOR is a selective effector of the radiation therapy response in androgen receptor-positive prostate cancer. Endocr Relat Cancer 19:1–12

Schwartz GK, Tap WD, Qin LX, Livingston MB, Undevia SD, Chmielowski B, Agulnik M, Schuetze SM, Reed DR, Okuno SH et al (2013) Cixutumumab and temsirolimus for patients with bone and soft-tissue sarcoma: a multicentre, open-label, phase 2 trial. Lancet Oncol 14:371–382

Schwarzbich MA, Gutknecht M, Salih J, Salih HR, Brossart P, Rittig SM, Grunebach F (2012) The immune inhibitory receptor osteoactivin is upregulated in monocyte-derived dendritic cells by BCR-ABL tyrosine kinase inhibitors. Cancer Immunol Immunother 61:193–202

Scotlandi K, Benini S, Sarti M, Serra M, Lollini PL, Maurici D, Picci P, Manara MC, Baldini N (1996) Insulin-like growth factor I receptor-mediated circuit in Ewing's sarcoma/peripheral neuroectodermal tumor: a possible therapeutic target. Cancer Res 56:4570–4574

Scotlandi K, Benini S, Nanni P, Lollini PL, Nicoletti G, Landuzzi L, Serra M, Manara MC, Picci P, Baldini N (1998) Blockage of insulin-like growth factor-I receptor inhibits the growth of Ewing's sarcoma in athymic mice. Cancer Res 58:4127–4131

Scotlandi K, Manara MC, Nicoletti G, Lollini PL, Lukas S, Benini S, Croci S, Perdichizzi S, Zambelli D, Serra M et al (2005) Antitumor activity of the insulin-like growth factor-I receptor kinase inhibitor NVP-AEW541 in musculoskeletal tumors. Cancer Res 65:3868–3876

Shen C, Oswald D, Phelps D, Cam H, Pelloski CE, Pang Q, Houghton PJ (2013) Regulation of FANCD2 by the mTOR pathway contributes to the resistance of cancer cells to DNA double-strand breaks. Cancer Res 73:3393–3401

Smith JA, Wilson L, Azarenko O, Zhu X, Lewis BM, Littlefield BA, Jordan MA (2010a) Eribulin binds at microtubule ends to a single site on tubulin to suppress dynamic instability. Biochemistry 49:1331–1337

Smith MA, Seibel NL, Altekruse SF, Ries LA, Melbert DL, O'Leary M, Smith FO, Reaman GH (2010b) Outcomes for children and adolescents with cancer: challenges for the twenty-first century. J Clin Oncol 28:2625–2634

Smith MA, Hampton OA, Reynolds CP, Kang MH, Maris JM, Gorlick R, Kolb EA, Lock R, Carol H, Keir ST et al (2015) Initial testing (stage 1) of the PARP inhibitor BMN 673 by the pediatric preclinical testing program: PALB2 mutation predicts exceptional in vivo response to BMN 673. Pediatr Blood Cancer 62:91–98

Soldatenkov VA, Albor A, Patel BK, Dreszer R, Dritschilo A, Notario V (1999) Regulation of the human poly(ADP-ribose) polymerase promoter by the ETS transcription factor. Oncogene 18:3954–3962

Souhami RL, Craft AW, Van der Eijken JW, Nooij M, Spooner D, Bramwell VH, Wierzbicki R, Malcolm AJ, Kirkpatrick A, Uscinska BM et al (1997) Randomised trial of two regimens of chemotherapy in operable osteosarcoma: a study of the European Osteosarcoma Intergroup. Lancet 350:911–917

Spunt SL, Grupp SA, Vik TA, Santana VM, Greenblatt DJ, Clancy J, Berkenblit A, Krygowski M, Ananthakrishnan R, Boni JP, Gilbertson RJ (2011) Phase I study of temsirolimus in pediatric patients with recurrent/refractory solid tumors. J Clin Oncol Off J Am Soc Clin Oncol 29:2933–2940

Stehn JR, Haass NK, Bonello T, Desouza M, Kottyan G, Treutlein H, Zeng J, Nascimento PR, Sequeira VB, Butler TL et al (2013) A novel class of anticancer compounds targets the actin cytoskeleton in tumor cells. Cancer Res 73:5169–5182

Suminoe A, Matsuzaki A, Hattori H, Koga Y, Hara T (2009) Immunotherapy with autologous dendritic cells and tumor antigens for children with refractory malignant solid tumors. Pediatr Transplant 13:746–753

Sutow WW (1968) Vincristine (NSC-67574) therapy for malignant solid tumors in children (except Wilms' tumor). Cancer Chemother Rep Part 1 1(52):485–487

Sutow WW, Vietti TJ, Fernbach DJ, Lane DM, Donaldson MH, Lonsdale D (1971) Evaluation of chemotherapy in children with metastatic Ewing's sarcoma and osteogenic sarcoma. Cancer Chemother Rep Part 1 55:67–78

Taur JS, Desjardins CS, Schuck EL, Wong YN (2011) Interactions between the chemotherapeutic agent eribulin mesylate (E7389) and P-glycoprotein in CF-1 abcb1a-deficient mice and Caco-2 cells. Xenobiotica 41:320–326

Teachey DT, Rheingold SR, Maude SL, Zugmaier G, Barrett DM, Seif AE, Nichols KE, Suppa EK, Kalos M, Berg RA et al (2013) Cytokine release syndrome after blinatumomab treatment related to abnormal macrophage activation and ameliorated with cytokine-directed therapy. Blood 121:5154–5157

Thornton KA, Chen AR, Trucco MM, Shah P, Wilky BA, Gul N, Carrera-Haro MA, Ferreira MF, Shafique U, Powell JD et al (2013) A dose-finding study of temsirolimus and liposomal doxorubicin for patients with recurrent and refractory bone and soft tissue sarcoma. Int J Cancer J Int Cancer 133:997–1005

Tietze JK, Wilkins DE, Sckisel GD, Bouchlaka MN, Alderson KL, Weiss JM, Ames E, Bruhn KW, Craft N, Wiltrout RH et al (2012) Delineation of antigen-specific and antigen-nonspecific CD8(+) memory T-cell responses after cytokine-based cancer immunotherapy. Blood 119:3073–3083

Tolcher AW, Sarantopoulos J, Patnaik A, Papadopoulos K, Lin CC, Rodon J, Murphy B, Roth B, McCaffery I, Gorski KS et al (2009) Phase I, pharmacokinetic, and pharmacodynamic study of AMG 479, a fully human monoclonal antibody to insulin-like growth factor receptor 1. J Clin Oncol Off J Am Soc Clin Oncol 27:5800–5807

Tomihari M, Hwang SH, Chung JS, Cruz PD Jr, Ariizumi K (2009) Gpnmb is a melanosome-associated glycoprotein that contributes to melanocyte/keratinocyte adhesion in a RGD-dependent fashion. Exp Dermatol 18:586–595

Toretsky JA, Gorlick R (2010) IGF-1R targeted treatment of sarcoma. Lancet Oncol 11:105–106

Toretsky JA, Erkizan V, Levenson A, Abaan OD, Parvin JD, Cripe TP, Rice AM, Lee SB, Uren A (2006) Oncoprotein EWS-FLI1 activity is enhanced by RNA helicase A. Cancer Res 66:5574–5581

Towle MJ, Salvato KA, Budrow J, Wels BF, Kuznetsov G, Aalfs KK, Welsh S, Zheng W, Seletsky BM, Palme MH et al (2001) In vitro and in vivo anticancer activities of synthetic macrocyclic ketone analogues of halichondrin B. Cancer Res 61:1013–1021

Towle MJ, Salvato KA, Wels BF, Aalfs KK, Zheng W, Seletsky BM, Zhu X, Lewis BM, Kishi Y, Yu MJ, Littlefield BA (2011) Eribulin induces irreversible mitotic blockade: implications of cell-based pharmacodynamics for in vivo efficacy under intermittent dosing conditions. Cancer Res 71:496–505

Tse KF, Jeffers M, Pollack VA, McCabe DA, Shadish ML, Khramtsov NV, Hackett CS, Shenoy SG, Kuang B, Boldog FL et al (2006) CR011, a fully human monoclonal antibody-auristatin E conjugate, for the treatment of melanoma. Clin Cancer Res 12:1373–1382

Tutt A, Robson M, Garber JE, Domchek SM, Audeh MW, Weitzel JN, Friedlander M, Arun B, Loman N, Schmutzler RK et al (2010) Oral poly(ADP-ribose) polymerase inhibitor olaparib in patients with BRCA1 or BRCA2 mutations and advanced breast cancer: a proof-of-concept trial. Lancet 376:235–244

Wan X, Mendoza A, Khanna C, Helman LJ (2005) Rapamycin inhibits ezrin-mediated metastatic behavior in a murine model of osteosarcoma. Cancer Res 65:2406–2411

Wan X, Harkavy B, Shen N, Grohar P, Helman LJ (2007) Rapamycin induces feedback activation of Akt signaling through an IGF-1R-dependent mechanism. Oncogene 26:1932–1940

Wang Y, Hailey J, Williams D, Wang Y, Lipari P, Malkowski M, Wang X, Xie L, Li G, Saha D et al (2005) Inhibition of insulin-like growth factor-I receptor (IGF-IR) signaling and tumor cell growth by a fully human neutralizing anti-IGF-IR antibody. Mol Cancer Ther 4:1214–1221

Weigel B, Malempati S, Reid JM, Voss SD, Cho SY, Chen HX, Krailo M, Villaluna D, Adamson PC, Blaney SM (2014) Phase 2 trial of cixutumumab in children, adolescents, and young adults with refractory solid tumors: a report from the Children's Oncology Group. Pediatr Blood Cancer 61:452–456

Wittman MD, Balasubramanian B, Stoffan K, Velaparthi U, Liu P, Krishnanathan S, Carboni J, Li A, Greer A, Attar R et al (2007) Novel 1H-(benzimidazol-2-yl)-1H-pyridin-2-one inhibitors of insulin-like growth factor I (IGF-1R) kinase. Bioorg Med Chem Lett 17:974–977

Wittrant Y, Lamoureux F, Mori K, Riet A, Kamijo A, Heymann D, Redini F (2006) RANKL directly induces bone morphogenetic protein-2 expression in RANK-expressing POS-1 osteosarcoma cells. Int J Oncol 28:261–269

Witzig TE, Geyer SM, Ghobrial I, Inwards DJ, Fonseca R, Kurtin P, Ansell SM, Luyun R, Flynn PJ, Morton RF et al (2005) Phase II trial of single-agent temsirolimus (CCI-779) for relapsed mantle cell lymphoma. J Clin Oncol 23:5347–5356

Workenhe ST, Mossman KL (2014) Oncolytic virotherapy and immunogenic cancer cell death: sharpening the sword for improved cancer treatment strategies. Mol Ther 22:251–256

Wullschleger S, Loewith R, Hall MN (2006) TOR signaling in growth and metabolism. Cell 124:471–484

Xu Y, Zhang M, Ramos CA, Durett A, Liu E, Dakhova O, Liu H, Creighton CJ, Gee AP, Heslop HE et al (2014) Closely related T-memory stem cells correlate with in vivo expansion of CAR.CD19-T cells and are preserved by IL-7 and IL-15. Blood 123:3750–3759

Yee D (2012) Insulin-like growth factor receptor inhibitors: baby or the bathwater? J Natl Cancer Inst 104:975–981

Yi H, Fujimura Y, Ouchida M, Prasad DD, Rao VN, Reddy ES (1997) Inhibition of apoptosis by normal and aberrant Fli-1 and erg proteins involved in human solid tumors and leukemias. Oncogene 14:1259–1268

Yu Z, Ma B, Zhou Y, Zhang M, Qiu X, Fan Q (2005) Activation of antitumor cytotoxic T lymphocytes by fusion of patient-derived dendritic cells with autologous osteosarcoma. Exp Oncol 27:273–278

Yu AL, Gilman AL, Ozkaynak MF, London WB, Kreissman SG, Chen HX, Smith M, Anderson B, Villablanca JG, Matthay KK et al (2010) Anti-GD2 antibody with GM-CSF, interleukin-2, and isotretinoin for neuroblastoma. N Engl J Med 363:1324–1334

Zucman J, Delattre O, Desmaze C, Plougastel B, Joubert I, Melot T, Peter M, De Jong P, Rouleau G, Aurias A et al (1992) Cloning and characterization of the Ewing's sarcoma and peripheral neuroepithelioma t(11;22) translocation breakpoints. Genes Chromosomes Cancer 5:271–277

Survivorship

16

Stacy L. Whiteside and Anthony N. Audino

Contents

16.1 **Introduction** 294

16.2 **Survivorship Guideline Overview**....... 294
16.2.1 Children's Oncology Group Long-Term
Follow-Up Guidelines 295
16.2.2 National Comprehensive Cancer Network
Survivorship Guidelines................ 295
16.2.3 American Society of Clinical Oncology ... 295

16.3 **Treatment-Related Late Effects** 297
16.3.1 Cardiac Toxicity...................... 297
16.3.2 Renal Toxicity 298
16.3.3 Ototoxicity.......................... 300
16.3.4 Sexual Function and Infertility........... 301
16.3.5 Second Malignant Neoplasms (SMNs) 302

16.4 **Surgical Late Effects** 303

Conclusion 304

References................................ 305

S.L. Whiteside, CPNP-AC (✉) • A.N. Audino, MD
Division of Hematology/Oncology/BMT,
Nationwide Children's Hospital,
700 Children's Drive, Columbus, OH 43205, USA
e-mail: Stacy.whiteside@nationwidechildrens.org;
Anthony.audino@nationwidechildrens.org

Abstract

Advances in the treatment of childhood cancers and supportive care have resulted in marked improvements in survival rates. As of 2009, there were an estimated 363,000 survivors of childhood cancer in the United States; of these approximately 24 % have survived more than 30 years since their diagnosis, contributing to the growing number of long-term survivors of childhood and adult cancer in the United States (Mariotto et al. 2009). However, the use of chemotherapy, radiation, and/or surgery at an early age can contribute to complications that may not become apparent until years after the completion of therapy (Armenian and Robison 2013). A recent article from the Childhood Cancer Survivor Study (CCSS) cohort reported that two out of three survivors will develop a chronic health condition, and more than one-third will develop a condition that is severe or life-threatening (Oeffinger et al. 2006). To address the needs of this growing population, in 2005, the Institute of Medicine (IOM) published From Cancer Patient to Cancer Survivor: Lost in Transition, a report outlining the gaps in survivorship care. The report introduced the concept of survivorship care plans to summarize information critical to the individual's long-term care, such as the cancer diagnosis, treatment, and potential consequences; the timing and content of follow-up visits; tips on maintaining a healthy lifestyle and preventing recurrent or new cancers; legal rights

© Springer International Publishing Switzerland 2015
T.P. Cripe, N.D. Yeager (eds.), *Malignant Pediatric Bone Tumors - Treatment & Management*,
Pediatric Oncology, DOI 10.1007/978-3-319-18099-1_16

affecting employment and insurance; and the availability of psychological and support services (Hewitt et al. 2006). This report provided the basis for professional organizations including the Children's Oncology Group, National Comprehensive Cancer Network and the American Society of Clinical Oncology to publish evidenced-based guidelines for survivorship care for cancer survivors. It is crucial for healthcare professionals who care for cancer survivors at all stages of their survivorship to be familiar with actual and potential late effects survivors may experience throughout their lifetime.

16.1 Introduction

Advances in the treatment of childhood cancers and supportive care have resulted in marked improvements in survival rates. However, the use of chemotherapy, radiation, and/or surgery at an early age can contribute to complications that may not become apparent until years after the completion of therapy (Armenian and Robison 2013). A recent article from the Childhood Cancer Survivor Study (CCSS) cohort reported that two out of three survivors will develop a chronic health condition, and more than one-third will develop a condition that is severe or lifethreatening (Oeffinger et al. 2006). Several groups have published reports outlining gaps in survivorship care. In addition, these reports have introduced guidelines for survivorship care. These guidelines include testing to assess possible long-term affects of chemotherapy, radiation and/or surgery, including heart and renal function, as well as evaluation of hearing, sexual function, and work-up for secondary malignancies.

16.2 Survivorship Guideline Overview

The 2005 IOM report established five essential components of survivorship care that have been adapted and implemented by leading oncology professional organizations into their own individual

survivorship guidelines. These include the following:

1. Prevention of new and recurrent cancers and other late effects
2. Surveillance of cancer spread, recurrence, or second cancers
3. Assessment of late psychosocial and physical effects
4. Intervention for consequences of cancer and treatment (e.g., medical problems, symptoms, psychological distress, financial and social concerns)
5. Coordination of care between primary care providers and specialists to ensure that all of the survivor's health needs are met (NCCN 2014)

In 2011, the LIVESTRONG foundation convened a meeting of experts and stakeholders in the survivorship field to define essential components of survivorship care. After 2 days of consensus building, the group agreed on the following elements that all medical settings must provide for cancer survivors, either directly or through referral:

1. Survivorship care plan, psychosocial care plan, and treatment summary
2. Screening for new cancers and surveillance for recurrence
3. Care coordination strategy that addresses care coordination with PCPs and primary oncologists
4. Health promotion education
5. Symptom management and palliative care (https://assets-livestrong-org.s3.amazonaws.com/media/site_proxy/data/7e26de7ddcd2b7ace899e75f842e50c0075c4330.pdf)

In 2012, the Commission on Cancer (CoC) and the American College of Surgeons (ACS) updated their accreditation standards for hospital cancer programs (http://www.facs.org/cancer/coc/programstandards2012.html). Their patient-centered focus now includes the development and dissemination of a survivorship plan for all patients. This requirement is to be phased in by 2015.

16.2.1 Children's Oncology Group Long-Term Follow-Up Guidelines

The Children's Oncology Group (COG) is a 238-member National Cancer Institute-supported cooperative clinical trials group whose goals include minimizing the risk of long-term effects that may impact duration and/or quality of life in pediatric cancer survivors (Landier et al. 2006). The first version of the risk-based, exposure-related guidelines (*Long-Term Follow-up Guidelines for Survivors of Childhood, Adolescent, and Young Adult Cancer*) for use in directing follow-up care for survivors of pediatric malignancies was published in March of 2003. The COG guidelines represent a hybrid of evidence-based and consensus-driven approaches to guideline development and consist of clinically relevant screening recommendations that take into account the specialized health-care needs of pediatric cancer survivors (Landier et al. 2006). The guidelines are designed to standardize and direct follow-up care that facilitates early identification of and intervention for treatment-related complications (Landier et al. 2006). They also provide a platform for research into the efficacy and cost-effectiveness of health screening of this population. Recommendations for follow-up of individuals can be customized from the treatment exposure history including chemotherapy agents, radiation therapy and surgical history. The guideline supplies a patient treatment summary and an extensive list of "health links" offering detailed information on guideline-specific topics for survivors. The guidelines are updated at least every 5 years by a multidisciplinary task force who monitor the literature and report to the COG Long-Term Follow-up Guidelines Core Committee (Landier et al. 2004). Clinicians are advised to check the Children's Oncology Group website periodically for the latest updates and revisions to the guidelines which are posted at www.survivorshipguidelines.org (Table 16.1).

16.2.2 National Comprehensive Cancer Network Survivorship Guidelines

On January 31, 1995, this national alliance was created to develop and institute standards of care for the treatment of cancer and perform outcomes research. With 13 original NCCN Member Institutions, the goal was to ensure delivery of high-quality, cost-effective services to people with cancer across the country. NCCN became a developer and promoter of national programs to facilitate the fulfillment of NCCN Member Institution missions in education, research, and patient care. Now an alliance of 25 of the world's leading cancer centers, NCCN develops and communicates scientific, evaluative information to better inform the decision-making process between patients and physicians, ultimately improving patient outcomes. The NCCN Survivorship guidelines were originally released in 2013 and included eight distinct areas: anxiety and depression, cognitive function, exercise, fatigue, immunizations and infections, pain, sexual function, and sleep disorders. A new updated version was published in 2014. These guidelines, however, are not specifically intended to provide guidance for the care of survivors of childhood cancers and refer providers to the Children's Oncology group survivorship guidelines, as well as the NCCN guidelines for Adolescent and Young Adults available at www.NCCN.org.

16.2.3 American Society of Clinical Oncology

The American Society of Clinical Oncology published their guide to survivorship care in 2014 entitled *Providing High Quality Survivorship Care in Practice: An ASCO guide*. It further detailed high-quality survivorship care to include the following:

DEMOGRAPHICS		
Name:	**Sex:**	**Date of Birth:**

CANCER DIAGNOSIS		
Diagnosis: Ewing sarcoma	**Date of Diagnosis:**	**Date Therapy Completed:**

CHEMOTHERAPY: [x] Yes [ ] No *If yes, complete chart below*

Drug Name	Additional Information[†]
Vincristine	
Doxorubicin	375mg/m2
Cytoxan	10.8g/m2
Etoposide	3500mg/m2
Ifosfamide	72g/m2

[†]Anthracyclines: Include cumulative dose in mg/m^2 and age at first dose (see section 33 or 34 of Guidelines for isotoxic dose conversion);

Carboplatin: Indicate if dose was myeloablative and if patient was diagnosed at less than 1 year of age;

Methotrexate and Cytarabine: Indicate route of administration (i.e., IV, IM, SQ, PO, IT, IO);

IV Methotrexate and Cytarabine: Indicate if "high dose" (any single dose $\geq$1000 mg/m^2) or "standard dose" (all single doses <1000 mg/m^2)

Note: Cumulative doses, if known, should be recorded for all agents, particularly for alkylators and bleomycin.

RADIATION   [ ] Yes   [x] No   *If yes, complete chart below*

Site/Field*	Total Dose** (Gy)***

* For chest, thoracic spine, and upper abdominal radiation, include age at first dose   ** Total dose to each field should include boost dose, if given

*** Note: To convert cGy or rads to Gy, divide dose by 100 (example: 2400 cGy = 2400 rads = 24 Gy)

HEMATOPOIETIC CELL TRANSPLANT   [ ] Yes   [x] No   *If yes, answer question below*

Was this patient ever diagnosed with **chronic** graft-versus-host disease (cGVHD)?   [ ] Yes   [ ] No

SURGERY   [x] Yes   [ ] No   *If yes, complete chart below*

Procedure	Site (if applicable)	Laterality (if applicable)
Limb salvage 6/17/05	Proximal tibia	Right

OTHER THERAPEUTIC MODALITIES   [ ] Yes   [x] No   *If yes, answer questions below*

Did this patient receive radioiodine therapy (I-131 thyroid ablation)?	[ ] Yes [x] No
Did this patient receive systemic MIBG (in therapeutic doses)?	[ ] Yes [x] No
Did this patient receive bioimmunotherapy?	[ ] Yes [x] No

Summary prepared by:	**Date prepared:**

Table 16.1 Example of a summary of cancer treatment (abbreviated)

1. Surveillance for recurrence
2. Monitoring for and managing psychosocial and medical late effects
3. Providing screening recommendations for second cancers
4. Providing health education to survivors regarding their diagnoses, treatment exposures, and potential late and long-term effects
5. Providing referrals to specialists and resources as indicated
6. Familial genetic risk assessment (as appropriate)
7. Guidance about diet, exercise, and health promotion activities

8. Providing resources to assist with financial and insurance issues
9. Empowering survivors to advocate for their own health-care needs (Oeffinger et al. 2014).

This guide discusses how to build a survivorship care program for clinicians including models of care, implementation of a survivorship program, providing care, and measuring the quality of survivorship care. It also includes resources for transitioning care of survivors and working with primary care providers to continue high-quality health care addressing the unique needs of cancer survivors.

16.3 Treatment-Related Late Effects

16.3.1 Cardiac Toxicity

Cardiac toxicity during or following treatment for pediatric bone tumors is largely due to the inclusion of the anthracycline, doxorubicin, given at relatively high doses. Most treatment regimens for bone sarcomas require a minimum cumulative doxorubicin dose of 375 mg/m^2, with some as high as 600 mg/m^2. The pathophysiology of doxorubicin-induced cardiac damage is incompletely understood, but one important mechanism is thought to be cardiomyocyte death due to the production of free radicals and oxidative stress (Janeway and Grier 2010). Clinically apparent doxorubicin-associated cardiotoxicity presenting as congestive heart failure has been classified as acute, chronic, and late based on the timing of onset related to the doxorubicin administration (Janeway and Grier 2010). Acute cardiotoxicity, occurring after a single dose or course of doxorubicin is rare, particularly with modern chemotherapy regimens. Chronic doxorubicin-associated cardiotoxicity occurs within weeks to months of completing therapy. There are rare reports of late cardiotoxicity in which clinically apparent doxorubicin-induced heart failure occurs more than 1 year after the completion of therapy, particularly in association with periods of increased cardiac growth and demand such as puberty and pregnancy (Janeway and Grier 2010).

Data from the Childhood Cancer Survivor Study (CCSS) demonstrate that survivors of osteosarcoma have been reported to have a cumulative incidence of 10 % at 20 years for acute congestive heart failure for those patients who received >300 mg/m^2 (Nagarajan et al. 2011). The Rizzoli Institute has reported the study with the longest follow-up and most complete reporting of adverse events in patients with osteosarcoma. This study reported a 4 % incidence of severe doxorubicin-induced cardiotoxicity (Oeffinger et al. 2006). Cardiotoxicity was noted 1–12 weeks after the completion of therapy, with the exception of one patient who developed cardiac toxicity during the last trimester of pregnancy 8 years after completing treatment (Oeffinger et al. 2006). The Italian Sarcoma Group also reported their experience in patients treated for osteosarcoma from 1983 to 2006 with a reported incidence of cardiomyopathy of 2 % (Longhi et al. 2012). The median interval from the cessation of chemotherapy to the onset of cardiomyopathy was 2 months with a median total dose of doxorubicin of 480 mg/m^2 (Longhi et al. 2012).

Survivors of Ewing sarcoma reported in the CCSS were more likely than siblings to have arrhythmias (7.4 % vs. 2.9 %) and other serious cardiac conditions (4.5 % vs. 0.5 %) (Ginsberg et al. 2010). After adjusting for age, sex, and race/ethnicity, the relative risk of a survivor having an arrhythmia or serious cardiac event 5 or more years after diagnosis is 2.3 (95 % CI = 1.4–3.9) and 7.5 (95 % CI = 3.1–18.7), respectively (Ginsberg et al. 2010). The Scandinavian Sarcoma Study Group also demonstrated an increased incidence in heart disease and hypertension in Ewing sarcoma survivors compared to age- and gender-matched individuals from the general population, reporting an odds ratio for heart disease of 7.9 (95 % CI = 2.5–25.3; $p = 0.001$) (Aksnes et al. 2009). They described two patients treated before the age of 4 who developed cardiotoxicity, and concluded that age of exposure along with cumulative dose were independent risk factors (Aksnes et al. 2009). In the Italian Sarcoma Group report, the cardiotoxicity incidence was 1.3 %, with a median interval from the cessation of chemotherapy to the onset of cardiomyopathy of 3 months (Longhi et al. 2012). The median doxorubicin dose was 400 mg/m^2.

Cumulative dose is the most important factor affecting the risk of doxorubicin-associated cardiotoxicity, with a significant increase in the incidence of heart failure occurring after the administration of 550 mg/m^2 (Janeway and Grier 2010). Additional risk factors for doxorubicin-induced cardiotoxicity include older (greater than 40) and very young (less than 4 years) age, and female sex (Chrischilles et al. 2014). The number of patients who have doxorubicin-associated heart failure is much lower than the number of patients who develop echocardiographic abnormalities after treatment with doxorubicin.

Dexrazoxane is a topoisomerase 2 inhibitor that scavenges free radicals and chelates heavy metals. It is thought to protect the heart from doxorubicin-induced cardiotoxicity by forming complexes with iron, preventing both tissue damage and the formation of free radicals (Janeway and Grier 2010). Two randomized controlled studies in children show that dexrazoxane decreases the risk of short-term, subclinical cardiac toxicity without increasing infectious complications (Wexler et al. 1996; Moghrabi et al. 2007). Additional studies are required to determine whether dexrazoxane decreases the risk of late cardiotoxicity. A recent study reported an increased incidence of secondary malignancies in patients with Hodgkin's disease who were randomized to receive dexrazoxane, but concerns have been raised about the methodology of the study (Hellmann 2007; Lipshultz et al. 2007; Tebbi et al. 2007). A trial in which children with leukemia were randomized to receive dexrazoxane did not show an increase in secondary leukemias in patients who received dexrazoxane (Barry et al. 2008). Dexrazoxane has not been systematically assessed in any bone sarcoma studies, so it is not possible at this time to make an evidence-based guideline for or against its use.

The Children's Oncology Group long-term follow-up guidelines recommend detailed history of shortness of breath, orthopnea, chest pain, palpitations, or if under 25 years abdominal symptoms including nausea or vomiting. Physical exam should include assessment of cardiac murmur, S3, S4, increased P2 sound, pericardial rub, rales, wheezes, jugular venous distension, and peripheral edema. Echocardiogram at entry into long-term follow-up is recommended, and then periodically based on age at treatment, radiation dose, and cumulative anthracycline dose. EKG is recommended at entry into long-term follow-up, repeat as clinically indicated (COG 2013) (Table 16.2).

16.3.2 Renal Toxicity

The treatment-related nephrotoxicity for bone tumor patients is primarily due to the chemotherapeutic agents, namely, cisplatin, methotrexate, and ifosfamide. Cisplatin and methotrexate have been a standard of care in the treatment of osteosarcoma since the 1970s, and remaining two of the three drug combination routinely utilized for localized osteosarcoma. Ifosfamide was introduced in first-line therapy of childhood soft tissue sarcomas and bone sarcomas since the 1980s and continues to be used for bone sarcomas today.

The nephrotoxicity of cisplatin is considered dose-related and includes a variable reduction of glomerular filtration rate (GFR) along with tubular dysfunction. Cisplatin directly damages the tubular epithelial cells, resulting in a pathology resembling acute tubular necrosis that leads to increased magnesium loss in the urine expressed as increased renal magnesium (Mg) excretion and hypomagnesaemia (Janeway and Grier 2010). Cisplatin-induced hypokalemia and hypocalcemia are the result of both altered renal processing in the presence of hypomagnesaemia and increased kidney losses. In 12–20 % of patients, cisplatin-associated hypomagnesaemia persists after the completion of chemotherapy (Stohr et al. 2007). About 60 % of children receiving median cisplatin doses of 500–600 mg/m^2 have decreased glomerular function at the completion of therapy (Skinner et al. 1998). However, these deficits in glomerular filtration seem to be mild, and improvement is common. In two long-term follow-up studies of osteosarcoma survivors receiving ifosfamide in addition to standard therapy with methotrexate/adriamycin/cisplatin therapy, the incidence of glomerular impairment was low and the extent of dysfunction was minimal (Koch Nogueira et al. 1998; Arndt et al. 1999). The risk of cisplatin-associated nephrotoxicity is associated with higher dose rates and greater dose intensity. Consequently, prolonged infusions and fractionated doses administered

Table 16.2a Recommended frequency of echocardiogram (or comparable cardiac imaging) following anthracyclines

Age at treatment	Radiation with potential impact to the heart	Anthracycline dose	Recommended frequency
<1 year old	Yes	Any	Every year
	No	<200 mg/m^2	Every 2 years
		≥200 mg/m^2	Every year
1–4 years old	Yes	Any	Every year
	No	<100 mg/m^2	Every 5 years
		≥100 mg/m^2 to <300 mg/m^2	Every 2 years
		≥300 mg/m^2	Every year
≥5 years old	Yes	<300 mg/m^2	Every 2 years
		≥300 mg/m^2	Every year
	No	<200 mg/m^2	Every 5 years
		≥200 mg/m^2 to <300 mg/m^2	Every 2 years
		≥300 mg/m^2	Every year
Any age with decrease in serial function			Every year

Table 16.2b Recommended frequency of echocardiogram (or comparable cardiac imaging) following radiation

Age at treatment	Radiation dose	Anthracycline dose	Recommended frequency
<5 years old	Any	None	Every 2 years
		Any	Every year
≥5 years old	<30 Gy	None	Every 5 years
	≥30 Gy	None	Every 2 years
	Any	<300 mg/m^2	Every 2 years
		≥300 mg/m^2	Every year
Any age with decrease in serial function			Every year

over several days have been recommended (Launay-Vacher et al. 2008).

Methotrexate and its metabolites can precipitate in the renal tubules causing acute renal insufficiency and failure (Janeway and Grier 2010). Early studies of high-dose methotrexate done in the 1970 demonstrated that nephrotoxicity was common, and the mortality rate following high-dose methotrexate was as high as 6 % (Von Hoff et al. 1977). The use of aggressive hydration and alkalization of urine as well as the use of leucovorin rescue along with routine monitoring of methotrexate levels has decreased the incidence of nephrotoxicity following high-dose methotrexate to 1–8 % (Janeway and Grier 2010). Unfortunately, severe and fatal cases of high-dose methotrexate-associated nephrotoxcity still occur in patients with osteosarcoma (Widemann et al. 2004). Methotrexate-induced nephrotoxicity is typically an acute treatment side effect and rarely causes long-term renal damage as a single agent. However, it may contribute to the cumulative effects of other nephrotoxic agents.

Many studies have demonstrated that tubular toxicity develops as a result of treatment with ifosfamide. Both glomerular and tubular function may be affected by ifosfamide, and a variety of tubular disorders, such as Fanconi syndrome and hypophosphatemic rickets, have been described. The combination of cisplatin and ifosfamide is particularly hazardous, since evidence suggests that ifosfamide nephrotoxicity is possibly potentiated by cisplatin. Ifosfamide-related proximal tubular damage is typically observed with a reduction in glomerular filtration rate, hypophosphatemia, and glycosuria (Oberlin et al. 2009). In one study by the Children's Oncology Group, in which the cumulative dose of ifosfamide was 71 g/m^2, Fanconi syndrome was described in approximately 7 % of patients (Goorin et al. 2002). Fanconi syndrome is a global proximal tubule defect in which resorption of glucose, amino acids, phosphate, and bicarbonate in the proximal tubule is impaired. Excessive urinary losses result in metabolic acidosis, hypophosphatemia, and hypokalemia. Although less prevalent, glomerular dysfunction can also develop, usually in patients who have evidence of tubular toxicity (Janeway and Grier 2010). When measured 6 months after the completion of therapy, 9 % of patients who received a median ifosfamide dose of 62 g/m^2 had a glomerular filtration rate below 60 ml/min/1.73 m^2. Although glomerular dysfunction is usually mild, acute renal failure can also occur, particularly at high cumulative doses. In most patients, ifosfamide-associated nephrotoxicity remains stable over time. A small proportion of patients will have significant improvements or worsening of both tubular and glomerular function (Heney et al. 1991). The risk of ifosfamide-associated nephrotoxicity is associated with higher cumulative doses, younger age at the time of administration, preexisting renal dysfunction, exposure to other nephrotoxic drugs, and treatment with cisplatin (Loebstein et al. 1999). Other than aggressive hydration, there are no specific therapies or modifications that are known to protect against the development of ifosfamide-related nephrotoxicity.

The COG long-term follow-up guidelines recommend annual blood pressure monitoring, annual urinalysis, and serum chemistries including BUN, creatinine at baseline and as clinically indicated for patients who received cisplatin and/or ifosfamide to monitor for renal toxicity (COG 2013).

16.3.3 Ototoxicity

Hearing loss as a late effect of therapy can occur after exposure to cancer-therapeutic agents such as platinum compounds and cranial radiation. Platinum agents cisplatin and carboplatin have improved cure rates in many childhood cancers including bone sarcomas, but their use may result in irreversible high-frequency sensorineural hearing loss. The deficit is progressive with increasing cumulative dosing (Grewal et al. 2010). In general, approximately 50 % of children treated with cisplatin-based regimens reportedly develop some degree of permanent hearing loss (Knight et al. 2005). With cumulative doses in excess of 400 mg/m^2, typical for osteosarcoma treatment, up to 90 % of young children may suffer moderate-to-severe deficits, with severe hearing loss seen in up to 25 % (Knight et al. 2005).

The mechanism of platinum cochlear toxicity is through interference with signal transduction from the Organ of Corti in the cochlea (Grewal et al. 2010). Three sites of damage occur: the outer hair cells (effector cells), the spiral ganglion (main nerve supply to the cochlea), and the stria vascularis (primary blood supply) (Rybak et al. 2007). Chemotherapy-related damage begins in the first row of outer hair cells at the base of the cochlea, where high-frequency sounds are processed. Therefore, the use of platinum compounds can result in bilateral sensorineural hearing loss, which initially involves the higher frequencies (4,000–8,000 Hz) (Schell et al. 1989). With increasing doses of chemotherapy, or when compounded by other ototoxic factors such as radiation or aminoglycoside use, loss of hair cells can progress apically in the cochlea to involve the speech frequencies. High-frequency hearing sensitivity is critical for the understanding of speech. The speech frequencies are considered to be 500–2,000 Hz.

Major risk factors for hearing loss are younger age, higher cumulative dose of chemotherapy, central nervous system tumors, and concomitant CNS radiation. Individual susceptibility to cisplatin is variable. Dolan et al. demonstrated that 38–47 % of human variation in susceptibility to cisplatin-induced ototoxicity is due to genetic variables (Dolan et al. 2004). Children are more susceptible to ototoxicity from platinum agents than adults. For cisplatin, the risk of significant hearing loss involving the speech frequencies (500–2,000 Hz) usually occurs with cumulative doses that exceed 400 mg/m^2 in pediatric patients, whereas adults may tolerate doses up to 600 mg/m^2 before significant hearing loss involving the speech frequencies occurs (Schell et al. 1989). For carboplatin, ototoxicity has been reported to occur at similar cumulative doses in excess of 400 mg/m^2. Other factors that may contribute to hearing loss include medications such as aminoglycoside antibiotics and loop diuretics, impaired renal function, and coexisting ear pathology such as chronic otitis or middle ear effusions (Grewal et al. 2010).

Clinically detectable hearing loss may require more than one cycle of a platinum agent to occur. Knight et al. reported a series of children who were receiving platinum compounds for a variety of oncologic diagnoses found a median time to observation of ototoxicity to be 135 days (Knight et al. 2005). No patient in that series showed improvement in hearing, suggesting that hearing loss is permanent. Progressive hearing loss as long as 136 months from the end of therapy with platinum compounds has been reported in a cohort of survivors of pediatric solid tumors (Bertolini et al. 2004).

Several otoprotectants are in clinical and preclinical trials, although their efficacy is unclear at present. Because cisplatin ototoxicity alters the antioxidant system of the outer hair cells, several agents that reduce oxidative stress in the cochlea have been tested (Rybak and Ramkumar 2007). Sodium thiosulfate is currently being tested by the Children's Oncology Group in an intervention trial of pediatric patients treated with cisplatin (Hyppolito et al. 2006). Preclinical data indicated that this antioxidant confers otoprotection without affecting cytotoxicity (Neuwelt et al. 2006). After encouraging results in adult patients with ovarian cancer, amifostine as an otoprotectant was studied in children with high-risk germ cell tumors and osteosarcoma who received platinum-based regimens. Amifostine unfortunately did not lessen the risk of unacceptable hearing loss in either group and was limited by emesis in the patients with osteosarcoma (Gallegos-Castorena et al. 2007). In a retrospective review of patients with osteosarcoma, the incidence of ototoxicity was lower in patients who received cisplatin in two divided doses of 60 mg/m^2/dose given 24 h apart than those who received a single dose of 120 mg/m^2 (Lewis et al. 2009). The current standard treatment for osteosarcoma uses divided dosing of 60 mg/m^2/dose daily over 2 days.

The Children's Oncology Group long-term follow-up guidelines recommend a complete audiological evaluation consisting of air conduction, bone conduction, speech audiometry, and tympanometry for all survivors at risk for hearing loss on entry into long-term follow-up and more frequently if any change is noted (COG 2013). The general principles of management of hearing loss include awareness on the part of parents and providers, appropriate referrals to audiologists and otolaryngologists, and implementation of amplification and other adaptive strategies where indicated (Grewal et al. 2010).

16.3.4 Sexual Function and Infertility

When considering late effects in cancer survivors, sexual functioning in adolescent and young adult survivors of childhood cancer has been particularly neglected in the literature, despite increasing reports of the importance of sexual functioning on quality of life. The psychosocial difficulties that cancer survivors experience including significant changes in peer relationships, disturbed body image, worry about the future, difficulties with intimate relationships, diminished quality of life, can influence psychosexual functioning (Ford et al. 2014). Additionally, treatment-related factors that may influence sexual functioning include disruptions in normal pubertal development, premature ovarian failure, and the burden of medical comorbidities (Ford et al. 2014). Zebrack et al. surveyed nearly 600 survivors aged 18–39 regarding their sexual functioning, health-related quality of life, psychological distress, and life satisfaction (Zebrack et al. 2010). Fifty-two percent of female survivors and 32 % of male survivors reported at least "a little problem" in one or more areas of sexual functioning (Zebrack et al. 2010). These findings are consistent with other studies of sexual functioning in childhood cancer survivors which report that females survivors are twice as likely than their male counterparts to report marked sexual impairment (Bober et al. 2013). It has been postulated that young women may perceive changes such as the impact of treatment on body image and psychosexual development as being more traumatic than male peers, and this is one reason why female survivors may be more vulnerable to cancer-related sexual dysfunction (Oeffinger et al. 2006). Moreover, long-term effects of treatment on menopausal status and vaginal health (e.g., vaginal dryness or vaginal atrophy) may additionally be related to the loss of sexual function in this group of young women (Oeffinger et al. 2006).

Although examination of sexual functioning in a mixed group of cancer survivors allows for greater power for analysis, it fails to consider the unique difficulties tumor site specific groups may face. This most certainly is true for survivors of bone tumors, who face a unique gamut of issues related to body image and sexual functioning. Few studies have examined the unique issues of patients who have undergone treatment for bone tumors. Most studies have examined this population related to their local control measures including limb salvage, amputation, and Van Nes rotationplasty. In one recent study, almost half of the young adult survivors of bone cancer in childhood who had undergone a Van Nes rotationplasty expressed some limitation in initiating intimate relationships as a result of the rotationplasty (Veenstra et al. 2000). In another study, adolescent and young adult bone cancer survivors who had undergone amputation reported a significantly more active sex life (88 %) than those who had limb-sparing surgeries (75 %) which has been re-demonstrated in other studies of limb salvage survivors (Refaat et al. 2002). Additionally, fear of infertility, disclosure of cancer history, and concern for health of future offspring also may impact sexual functioning and intimate relationships. Refer to Chap. 5 for a more detailed discussion of fertility issues.

The Children's Oncology Group long-term follow-up guidelines recommend a detailed reproductive history for patients receiving alkylating agents with annual visits including pubertal onset, sexual functioning, and medication use, as medications can have a substantial impact on sexual functioning (COG 2013). Sexual history includes vaginal dryness and libido for females; and erections, nocturnal emissions, and libido for males. It also recommends annual tanner staging until sexual maturity for all patients, with semen analysis at the request of a sexually mature patient, or serum FSH if unable to obtain semen analysis for males (COG 2013). For females, obtain a baseline of serum FSH, LH, estradiol at age 13 and as clinically indicated in patients with delayed or arrested puberty, irregular menses, primary or secondary amenorrhea, and/or clinical signs of estrogen deficiency (COG 2013). A sexual health assessment should be a part of comprehensive survivorship clinics including attention to functioning and the psychological component of health and wellbeing, including self-image, subjective attitude

toward one's own sexuality and relationships with intimate partners (Zebrack et al. 2010). Clinicians must be skillful in their approach and informed of the developmental and psychosocial needs unique to young adults with cancer and geared toward making young people feel comfortable discussing personal issues and providing appropriate referrals to reproductive providers and counselors.

16.3.5 Second Malignant Neoplasms (SMNs)

The improved survival of children and young adults with cancer has resulted in one of the most ominous and significant long-term problems associated with therapy, the development of second malignant neoplasms. Childhood cancer survivors are at significant risk for development of malignant neoplasms. This risk is approximately tenfold greater than the general population, and an important health-related concern for the aging childhood cancer survivor population (Armenian and Robison 2013). SMNs are the leading cause of treatment-related mortality in long-term cancer survivors (Armenian and Robison 2013). Commonly reported solid SMNs include breast, thyroid, soft tissue and bone sarcomas, skin and brain cancer, and there is a strong and well-defined association with radiation exposure that is characterized by a latency that exceeds 10 years (Armenian and Robison 2013). Other SMNs such as therapy-associated leukemia (t-MDS/AML) are notable for their shorter latency, typically less than 10 years from primary cancer diagnosis, and association with alkylating agents and topoisomerase II inhibitor chemotherapy (Bhatia and Sklar 2002). Survivors who develop a first SMN are at an especially high risk of multiple occurrences of subsequent neoplasms, such that within 20 years from their original diagnosis the estimated cumulative incidence of another neoplasm is 47 % (Armenian and Robison 2013). Data collection regarding genetic predisposition syndromes and molecular epidemiologic studies are ongoing to address the role of genetics in the development of SMNs.

The Childhood Cancer Survivor Study (CCSS) has collected data on perhaps the largest cohort of relatively long-term survivors and began to analyze the relations between anticancer treatment and SMN development (Meadows et al. 2009). Overall female survivors were at greater risk than male survivors for the occurrence of any SMN (RR=1.64) (Meadows et al. 2009). Age at the time of original diagnosis was also an important risk factor; children younger at diagnosis are at an increased overall risk of SMNs and specific risk of thyroid and CNS SMNs (Meadows et al. 2009). Exposure to increased doses of alkylating agents, anthracyclines, and epidodophyllotoxins, all components of bone tumor treatment, was also associated with an increased risk of any SMN (Meadows et al. 2009). The cumulative incidence of SMNs in Ewing sarcoma survivors in the study at 25 years from their original diagnosis was 9 %, with a median time from first diagnosis to first SMN of 14.5 years (range 4–32 years) (Ginsberg et al. 2010). SMNS included breast cancer, osteosarcoma, papillary thyroid cancer, acute myelogenous leukemia, and five sarcomas (Ginsberg et al. 2010). In contrast, the cumulative incidence for osteosarcoma survivors at 25 years was 5.4 % with breast cancer as the leading SMN, followed by skin cancer, gastrointestinal cancer, thyroid, and soft-tissue or bone sarcomas (Nagarajan et al. 2011).

The Children's Oncology Group long-term follow-up guidelines recommend annual detailed history of fatigue, bleeding, or easy bruising as well as dermatologic exam assessing for pallor, petechiae, or purpura. Complete blood count and bone marrow exam should be performed as clinically indicated. Clinicians should counsel patients to report any fatigue, pallor, petechiae, or bone pain. Survivors should be aware of their risk of secondary cancers and maintain a healthy lifestyle including avoiding smoking or excessive alcohol intake, eating healthy well-balanced diet, maintaining regular exercise, and regular use of sunscreen.

It is well recognized that radiation exposure is a considerable risk for solid secondary malignant neoplasms. Excluding 11 nonmelanoma skin cancers, there were 36 SMNs reported among 34 participants in the CCSS analysis of Ewing sarcoma patients (Ginsberg et al. 2010). Of these patients, 86.7 % had received radiation therapy (Ginsberg et al. 2010). Of the 403 Ewing sarcoma survivor participants, the

survivors who received radiation had a SMN incidence ratio was 6.6 % (95 % CI=4.5–9.6), and for those survivors who did not receive radiation the standardized incidence ratio was 3.3 (CI=1.1–10.2, P=.28) (Ginsberg et al. 2010). As expected, thyroid cancer and secondary sarcomas were found most frequently in or near the radiation field. The standardized incidence ratio for breast cancer among women treated with whole-lung radiation was 36.0 (95 % CI=15.5–83.5) with an excess absolute risk of 5.6 (Ginsberg et al. 2010). Among women not treated with chest radiation, the standard incidence ratio was 17.0 (95 % CI-7.8–37.2) with an excess absolute risk of 3.2 (Ginsberg et al. 2010).

The Children's Oncology Group long-term follow-up guidelines recommend annual breast exam beginning at puberty until the age of 25, then every 6 months for all females who have had radiation fields involving the breast. For radiation doses greater than or equal to 20 Gy yearly mammography is recommended beginning 8 years after radiation or at age 25, whichever comes first. Breast MRI is recommended yearly as an adjunct to mammography beginning 8 years after radiation or at age 25, whichever occurs last. In radiation fields that include bone, detailed history should include bone pain and physical exam with palpation of any bones in irradiated field. X-ray or other diagnostic imaging should be considered in patients with clinical symptoms (COG 2013).

16.4 Surgical Late Effects

Amputation and limb-sparing surgery prevent local recurrence of bone tumors by removal of all gross and microscopic disease. If optimally executed, both procedures accomplish an en bloc excision of tumor with a margin of normal uninvolved tissue. The type of surgical procedure, the primary tumor site, and the age of the patient affect the risk of postsurgical complications (Oeffinger et al. 2009). Complications in survivors treated with amputation include prosthetic fit problems, chronic pain in the residual limb, phantom limb pain, and bone overgrowth (Nagarajan et al. 2002; Aulivola et al. 2004). While limb-sparing surgeries may offer a more aesthetically pleasing outcome, complica-

Table 16.3 Bone and joint late effects

Predisposing therapy	Musculoskeletal effects	Health screening
Radiation impacting musculoskeletal system	Hypoplasia; fibrosis; reduced/uneven growth (scoliosis, kyphosis); limb length discrepancy	Exam: bones and soft tissues in radiation fields History: psychosocial assessment, with attention to: educational and/or vocational progress, depression, anxiety, posttraumatic stress, social withdrawal
Radiation impacting musculoskeletal system	Radiation-induced fracture	Exam of affected bone
Methotrexate; corticosteroids (dexamethasone, prednisone); radiation impacting skeletal structures; HSCT	Reduced bone mineral density	Bone mineral density test (DXA or quantitative CT)
Amputation	Amputation-related complications (impaired cosmesis, functional/activity limitations, residual limb integrity, chronic pain, increased energy expenditure)	History: pain, functional/activity limitations. Exam: residual limb integrity. Prosthetic evaluation
Limb-sparing surgery	Limb-sparing surgical complications (functional/activity limitations, fibrosis, contractures, chronic infection, chronic pain, limb length discrepancy, increased energy expenditure, prosthetic malfunction [loosening, nonunion, fracture])	History: pain, functional/activity limitations Exam: residual limb integrity. Radiograph of affected limb. Orthopedic evaluation

CT computed tomography, *DXA* dual-energy X-ray absorptiometry, *GVHD* graft-versus-host disease, *HSCT* hematopoietic stem cell transplantation

tions have been reported more frequently in survivors who underwent these procedures than in those treated with amputation. Complications after limb-sparing surgery include nonunion, pathologic fracture, aseptic loosening, limb-length discrepancy, endoprosthetic fracture, and limited joint range of motion (Nagarajan et al. 2002; Kaste et al. 2001). Occasionally, refractory complications develop after limb-sparing surgery and require amputation (Eiser et al. 2001; Renard et al. 2000).

A number of studies have compared functional outcomes after amputation and limb-sparing surgery, but results have been limited by inconsistent methods of functional assessment and small cohort sizes. Overall, data suggest that limb-sparing surgery results in better function than amputation, but differences are relatively modest (Nagarajan et al. 2002; Renard et al. 2000). Similarly, long-term quality of life outcomes among survivors undergoing amputation and limb-sparing procedures have not differed substantially (Eiser et al. 2001). A longitudinal analysis of health status among extremity sarcoma survivors in the CCSS indicates an association between lower extremity amputation and increasing activity limitations with age, and an association between upper extremity amputation and lower educational attainment (Marina et al. 2013) (Table 16.3).

Conclusion

Survivors of pediatric bone tumors face lifelong challenges related to their treatment. Health-care providers, both adult oncologists and primary care physicians, rate childhood sarcoma survivors as a population of patients that they feel the least comfortable treating (Landier et al. 2006). In comparison to adult oncologists, primary care physicians reported a lower level of knowledge regarding both common childhood cancers and associations of late effects with treatment exposures (Landier et al. 2006). While their reported level of knowledge of these factors was higher than primary care providers, adult oncologists still were substantially less knowledgeable than pediatric oncologists scoring a mean of 2.66, compared to 1.88 for primary care providers, while pediatric oncologists scored a mean of 4.41 (score range 1–5 with 5 representing self-reported highest level of knowledge, comfort, or interest) (Landier et al. 2006). Survivors of pediatric bone tumors experience multiple and sometimes significant health issues related to their treatment that may increase their risk of early mortality and diminish quality of life. Knowledge about risk factors for late effects is essential to provide timely preventative or corrective interventions, since many treatment effects have delayed manifestations related to growth, development, and aging (Landier et al. 2006). Published evidence-based guidelines can provide the optimal surveillance plan and screening evaluations based on a personalized plan that integrates risks related to the previous cancer, cancer therapy, genetic predispositions, lifestyle behaviors, and comorbid health conditions. The full benefits of risk-based health care cannot be realized unless survivors and health-care providers have accurate information about cancer diagnosis, treatment modalities, and potential cancer-related health risks to guide recommendations for screening and risk-reducing interventions, regardless of treatment setting or provider (Landier et al. 2006).

References

Aksnes LH, Bauer HC, Dahl AA, Fossa SD, Hjorth L, Jebsen N, Lernedal H, Hall KS (2009) Health status at long-term follow-up in patients treated for extremity localized Ewing Sarcoma or osteosarcoma: a Scandinavian sarcoma group study. Pediatr Blood Cancer 53:84–89

Armenian SH, Robison LL (2013) Childhood cancer survivorship: an update on evolving paradigms for understanding pathogenesis and screening for therapy-related late effects. Curr Opin Pediatr 25:16–22

Arndt C, Morgenstern B, Hawkins D, Wilson D, Liedtke R, Miser J (1999) Renal function following combination chemotherapy with ifosfamide and cisplatin in patients with osteogenic sarcoma. Med Pediatr Oncol 32:93–96

Aulivola B, Hile CN, Hamdan AD, Sheahan MG, Veraldi JR, Skillman JJ, Campbell DR, Scovell SD, Logerfo FW, Pomposelli FB Jr (2004) Major lower extremity amputation: outcome of a modern series. Arch Surg 139:395–399, discussion 399

Barry EV, Vrooman LM, Dahlberg SE, Neuberg DS, Asselin BL, Athale UH, Clavell LA, Larsen EC, Moghrabi A, Samson Y, Schorin MA, Cohen HJ, Lipshultz SE, Sallan SE, Silverman LB (2008) Absence of secondary malignant neoplasms in children with high-risk acute lymphoblastic leukemia treated with dexrazoxane. J Clin Oncol 26:1106–1111

Bertolini P, Lassalle M, Mercier G, Raquin MA, Izzi G, Corradini N, Hartmann O (2004) Platinum compound-related ototoxicity in children: long-term follow-up reveals continuous worsening of hearing loss. J Pediatr Hematol Oncol 26:649–655

Bhatia S, Sklar C (2002) Second cancers in survivors of childhood cancer. Nat Rev Cancer 2:124–132

Bober SL, Zhou ES, Chen B, Manley PE, Kenney LB, Recklitis CJ (2013) Sexual function in childhood cancer survivors: a report from Project REACH. J Sex Med 10:2084–2093

Chrischilles, EA, Mcdowell BD, Rubenstein L, Charlton M, Pendergast J, Juarez GY and Arora NK (2014) Survivorship care planning and its influence on long-term patient-reported outcomes among colorectal and lung cancer survivors: the CanCORS disease-free survivor follow-up study. J Cancer Surviv

COG (2013) Long-term follow-up guidelines for survivors of childhood, adolescent and young adult cancers, version 4.0 [online]. Children's Oncology Group, Monrovia, Available: www.survivorshipguidelines.org

Dolan ME, Newbold KG, Nagasubramanian R, Wu X, Ratain MJ, Cook EH Jr, Badner JA (2004) Heritability and linkage analysis of sensitivity to cisplatin-induced cytotoxicity. Cancer Res 64:4353–4356

Eiser C, Darlington AS, Stride CB, Grimer R (2001) Quality of life implications as a consequence of surgery: limb salvage, primary and secondary amputation. Sarcoma 5:189–195

Ford JS, Kawashima T, Whitton J, Leisenring W, Laverdiere C, Stovall M, Zeltzer L, Robison LL, Sklar CA (2014) Psychosexual functioning among adult female survivors of childhood cancer: a report from the childhood cancer survivor study. J Clin Oncol 32:3126–3136

Gallegos-Castorena S, Martinez-Avalos A, Mohar-Betancourt A, Guerrero-Avendano G, Zapata-Tarres M, Medina-Sanson A (2007) Toxicity prevention with amifostine in pediatric osteosarcoma patients treated with cisplatin and doxorubicin. Pediatr Hematol Oncol 24:403–408

Ginsberg JP, Goodman P, Leisenring W, Ness KK, Meyers PA, Wolden SL, Smith SM, Stovall M, Hammond S, Robison LL, Oeffinger KC (2010) Long-term survivors of childhood Ewing sarcoma: report from the childhood cancer survivor study. J Natl Cancer Inst 102:1272–1283

Goorin AM, Harris MB, Bernstein M, Ferguson W, Devidas M, Siegal GP, Gebhardt MC, Schwartz CL, Link M, Grier HE (2002) Phase II/III trial of etoposide and high-dose ifosfamide in newly diagnosed metastatic osteosarcoma: a pediatric oncology group trial. J Clin Oncol 20:426–433

Grewal S, Merchant T, Reymond R, Mcinerney M, Hodge C, Shearer P (2010) Auditory late effects of childhood cancer therapy: a report from the Children's Oncology Group. Pediatrics 125:e938–e950

Hellmann K (2007) Dexrazoxane-associated risk for secondary malignancies in pediatric Hodgkin's disease: a claim without evidence. J Clin Oncol 25:4689–4690, author reply 4690–1

Heney D, Wheeldon J, Rushworth P, Chapman C, Lewis IJ, Bailey CC (1991) Progressive renal toxicity due to ifosfamide. Arch Dis Child 66:966–970

Hewitt ME, Ganz PA, Institute of Medicine (U.S.), American Society of Clinical Oncology (U.S.) (2006) From cancer patient to cancer survivor: lost in transition : an American Society of Clinical Oncology and Institute of Medicine Symposium. National Academies Press, Washington, D.C

Hyppolito MA, De Oliveira JA, Rossato M (2006) Cisplatin ototoxicity and otoprotection with sodium salicylate. Eur Arch Otorhinolaryngol 263:798–803

Janeway KA, Grier HE (2010) Sequelae of osteosarcoma medical therapy: a review of rare acute toxicities and late effects. Lancet Oncol 11:670–678

Kaste SC, Neel MN, Rao BN, Thompson VF, Pratt CB (2001) Complications of limb-sparing procedures using endoprosthetic replacements about the knee for pediatric skeletal sarcomas. Pediatr Radiol 31:62–71

Knight KR, Kraemer DF, Neuwelt EA (2005) Ototoxicity in children receiving platinum chemotherapy: underestimating a commonly occurring toxicity that may influence academic and social development. J Clin Oncol 23:8588–8596

Koch Nogueira PC, Hadj-Aissa A, Schell M, Dubourg L, Brunat-Mentigny M, Cochat P (1998) Long-term nephrotoxicity of cisplatin, ifosfamide, and methotrexate in osteosarcoma. Pediatr Nephrol 12: 572–575

Landier W, Bhatia S, Eshelman DA, Forte KJ, Sweeney T, Hester AL, Darling J, Armstrong FD, Blatt J, Constine LS, Freeman CR, Friedman DL, Green DM, Marina N, Meadows AT, Neglia JP, Oeffinger KC, Robison LL, Ruccione KS, Sklar CA, Hudson MM (2004) Development of risk-based guidelines for pediatric cancer survivors: the Children's Oncology Group Long-Term Follow-Up Guidelines from the Children's Oncology Group Late Effects Committee and Nursing Discipline. J Clin Oncol 22:4979–4990

Landier W, Wallace WH, Hudson MM (2006) Long-term follow-up of pediatric cancer survivors: education, surveillance, and screening. Pediatr Blood Cancer 46:149–158

Launay-Vacher V, Rey JB, Isnard-Bagnis C, Deray G, Daoughars M (2008) Prevention of cisplatin nephrotoxicity: state of the art and recommendations from the European Society of Clinical Pharmacy Special Interest Group on Cancer Care. Cancer Chemother Pharmacol 61:903–909

Lewis MJ, Dubois SG, Fligor B, Li X, Goorin A, Grier HE (2009) Ototoxicity in children treated for osteosarcoma. Pediatr Blood Cancer 52:387–391

Lipshultz SE, Lipsitz SR, Orav EJ (2007) Dexrazoxane-associated risk for secondary malignancies in pediatric Hodgkin's disease: a claim without compelling evidence. J Clin Oncol 25:3179, author reply 3180

Loebstein R, Atanackovic G, Bishai R, Wolpin J, Khattak S, Hashemi G, Gobrial M, Baruchel S, Ito S, Koren G (1999) Risk factors for long-term outcome of ifosfamide-induced nephrotoxicity in children. J Clin Pharmacol 39:454–461

Longhi A, Ferrari S, Tamburini A, Luksch R, Fagioli F, Bacci G, Ferrari C (2012) Late effects of chemotherapy and radiotherapy in osteosarcoma and Ewing sarcoma patients: the Italian Sarcoma Group Experience (1983–2006). Cancer 118:5050–5059

Marina N, Hudson MM, Jones KE, Mulrooney DA, Avedian R, Donaldson SS, Popat R, West DW, Fisher P, Leisenring W, Stovall M, Robison LL, Ness KK (2013) Changes in health status among aging survivors of pediatric upper and lower extremity sarcoma: a report from the childhood cancer survivor study. Arch Phys Med Rehabil 94:1062–1073

Mariotto AB, Rowland JH, Yabroff KR, Scoppa S, Hachey M, Ries L, Feuer EJ (2009) Long-term survivors of childhood cancers in the United States. Cancer Epidemiol Biomarkers Prev 18:1033–1040

Meadows AT, Friedman DL, Neglia JP, Mertens AC, Donaldson SS, Stovall M, Hammond S, Yasui Y, Inskip PD (2009) Second neoplasms in survivors of childhood cancer: findings from the Childhood Cancer Survivor Study cohort. J Clin Oncol 27:2356–2362

Moghrabi A, Levy DE, Asselin B, Barr R, Clavell L, Hurwitz C, Samson Y, Schorin M, Dalton VK, Lipshultz SE, Neuberg DS, Gelber RD, Cohen HJ, Sallan SE, Silverman LB (2007) Results of the Dana-Farber Cancer Institute ALL Consortium Protocol 95-01 for children with acute lymphoblastic leukemia. Blood 109:896–904

Nagarajan R, Neglia JP, Clohisy DR, Robison LL (2002) Limb salvage and amputation in survivors of pediatric lower-extremity bone tumors: what are the long-term implications? J Clin Oncol 20:4493–4501

Nagarajan R, Kamruzzaman A, Ness KK, Marchese VG, Sklar C, Mertens A, Yasui Y, Robison LL, Marina N (2011) Twenty years of follow-up of survivors of childhood osteosarcoma. Cancer 117:625–634

NCCN. 07/22/2014. NCCN clinical practice guidelines in oncology: survivorship; version 2.2014 [Online]. Available: www.nccn.org

Neuwelt EA, Gilmer-Knight K, Lacy C, Nicholson HS, Kraemer DF, Doolittle ND, Hornig GW, Muldoon LL (2006) Toxicity profile of delayed high dose sodium thiosulfate in children treated with carboplatin in conjunction with blood-brain-barrier disruption. Pediatr Blood Cancer 47:174–182

Oberlin O, Fawaz O, Rey A, Niaudet P, Ridola V, Orbach D, Bergeron C, Defachelles AS, Gentet JC, Schmitt C, Rubie H, Munzer M, Plantaz D, Deville A, Minard V,

Corradini N, Leverger G, De Vathaire F (2009) Long-term evaluation of Ifosfamide-related nephrotoxicity in children. J Clin Oncol 27:5350–5355

Oeffinger KC, Mertens AC, Sklar CA, Kawashima T, Hudson MM, Meadows AT, Friedman DL, Marina N, Hobbie W, Kadan-Lottick NS, Schwartz CL, Leisenring W, Robison LL (2006) Chronic health conditions in adult survivors of childhood cancer. N Engl J Med 355:1572–1582

Oeffinger KC, Hudson MM, Landier W (2009) Survivorship: childhood cancer survivors. Prim Care 36:743–780

Oeffinger KC, Argenbright K, McCabe M, Ng A, Rodriguez MA, Surbone A, Waisman J (2014) Providing high quality survivorship care in practice: an ASCO guide

Refaat Y, Gunnoe J, Hornicek FJ, Mankin HJ (2002) Comparison of quality of life after amputation or limb salvage. Clin Orthop Relat Res 397:298–305

Renard AJ, Veth RP, Schreuder HW, van Loon CJ, Koops HS, van Horn JR (2000) Function and complications after ablative and limb-salvage therapy in lower extremity sarcoma of bone. J Surg Oncol 73:198–205

Rybak LP, Ramkumar V (2007) Ototoxicity. Kidney Int 72:931–935

Rybak LP, Whitworth CA, Mukherjea D, Ramkumar V (2007) Mechanisms of cisplatin-induced ototoxicity and prevention. Hear Res 226:157–167

Schell MJ, McHaney VA, Green AA, Kun LE, Hayes FA, Horowitz M, Meyer WH (1989) Hearing loss in children and young adults receiving cisplatin with or without prior cranial irradiation. J Clin Oncol 7:754–760

Skinner R, Pearson AD, English MW, Price L, Wyllie RA, Coulthard MG, Craft AW (1998) Cisplatin dose rate as a risk factor for nephrotoxicity in children. Br J Cancer 77:1677–1682

Stohr W, Paulides M, Bielack S, Jurgens H, Koscielniak E, Rossi R, Langer T, Beck JD (2007) Nephrotoxicity of cisplatin and carboplatin in sarcoma patients: a report from the late effects surveillance system. Pediatr Blood Cancer 48:140–147

Tebbi CK, London WB, Friedman D, Villaluna D, De Alarcon PA, Constine LS, Mendenhall NP, Sposto R, Chauvenet A, Schwartz CL (2007) Dexrazoxane-associated risk for acute myeloid leukemia/myelodysplastic syndrome and other secondary malignancies in pediatric Hodgkin's disease. J Clin Oncol 25: 493–500

Veenstra KM, Sprangers MA, van der Eyken JW, Taminiau AH (2000) Quality of life in survivors with a Van Ness-Borggreve rotationplasty after bone tumour resection. J Surg Oncol 73:192–197

von Hoff DD, Penta JS, Helman LJ, Slavik M (1977) Incidence of drug-related deaths secondary to high-dose methotrexate and citrovorum factor administration. Cancer Treat Rep 61:745–748

Wexler LH, Andrich MP, Venzon D, Berg SL, Weaver-Mcclure L, Chen CC, Dilsizian V, Avila N, Jarosinski P, Balis FM, Poplack DG, Horowitz ME (1996) Randomized trial of the cardioprotective agent ICRF-187 in pediatric sarcoma patients treated with doxorubicin. J Clin Oncol 14:362–372

Widemann BC, Balis FM, Kempf-Bielack B, Bielack S, Pratt CB, Ferrari S, Bacci G, Craft AW, Adamson PC (2004) High-dose methotrexate-induced nephrotoxicity in patients with osteosarcoma. Cancer 100:2222–2232

Zebrack BJ, Foley S, Wittmann D, Leonard M (2010) Sexual functioning in young adult survivors of childhood cancer. Psychooncology 19:814–822